EAT WELL STAY WELL

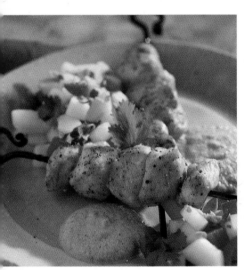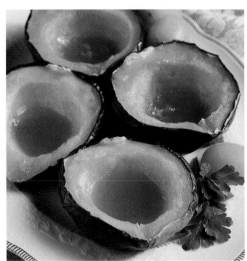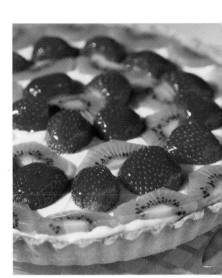

Reader's Digest

EAT WELL

500 Delicious Recipes Made with Healing Foods

STAY WELL

Reader's Digest Association, Inc.
Pleasantville, New York • Montreal

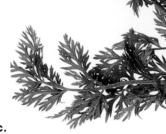

Reader's Digest Cooking, Home, Consumer Books

GROUP EDITORIAL DIRECTOR
Carol A. Guasti

GROUP DESIGN DIRECTOR
Joan Mazzeo

RESEARCH EDITOR
Linda Ingroia

Project Development Staff

DESIGN DIRECTOR
Perri DeFino

SENIOR EDITOR
Lee Fowler

EDITOR
Judith Cressy

Reader's Digest General Books

EDITOR-IN-CHIEF
David Palmer

EXECUTIVE EDITOR
Gayla Visalli

MANAGING EDITOR
Christopher Cavanaugh

Copyright © 1998 The Reader's Digest Association, Inc.

Copyright © 1998 The Reader's Digest Association (Canada) Ltd.

Copyright © 1998 Reader's Digest Association Far East Ltd.

Philippine Copyright © 1998 The Reader's Digest Association Far East Ltd.

All rights reserved. Unauthorized reproduction, in any manner, is prohibited.

Reader's Digest and the Pegasus logo are registered trademarks of The Reader's Digest Association, Inc.

Printed in the United States of America

Address any comments about EAT WELL, STAY WELL to Editor, U.S. General Books, Customer Service, Reader's Digest, Pleasantville, NY 10570

To order additional copies of EAT WELL, STAY WELL, call 1-800-846-2100

You can also visit us on the World Wide Web at www.readersdigest.com

Library of Congress Cataloging-in-Publication Data

Eat well, stay well : 500 delicious recipes made with healing foods.
    p. cm.
    Includes index.
    ISBN 0-7621-0124-5 (hbk.)
    1. Nutrition. 2. Diet therapy. 3. Health. I. Reader's Digest Association.
II. Title: Reader's Digest eat well, stay well
RA784.E162 1998
641.5'63--dc21   98-28078
                      CIP

Produced by Rebus, Inc.

PUBLISHER
Rodney M. Friedman

DIRECTOR, RECIPE DEVELOPMENT & PHOTOGRAPHY
Grace Young

EDITORIAL DIRECTOR, FOOD GROUP
Kate Slate

WRITER
Bonnie J. Slotnick

ASSISTANT EDITOR
James W. Brown, Jr.

ART DIRECTOR
Timothy Jeffs

DESIGN ASSISTANT
Yoheved Gertz

SENIOR RECIPE DEVELOPER
Sandra Rose Gluck

RECIPE DEVELOPER
Paul Piccuito

RECIPE TESTERS
Iris Carulli, Michelle Steffens

PHOTOGRAPHERS
Beatriz daCosta, Mark Ferri, Lisa Koenig, Steven Mark Needham

PHOTOGRAPHERS' ASSISTANTS
Alix Berenberg, Todd Chalfant, Phill Chevalier, Katie Bleacher Everard, Christopher Lilly, Inbal Nahari, Robert Piazza, Robert Presciutti, Lisa Silvestri, Tanya Stroedel

FOOD STYLISTS
A.J. Battifarano, Roscoe Betsill, Delores Custer, Paul S. Grimes, Helen Jones, Karen Pickus, Diane Simone Vezza

ASSISTANT FOOD STYLISTS
Margarette Adams, Charles Davis, Tracy Donovan, Danielle Gorman, Julie Grimes, Amy Lord, Cara Morris, Eric Robledo, Megan Schlow

PROP STYLIST
Debrah Donahue

DECORATIVE BACKGROUNDS
Sue Israel

NUTRITION CONSULTANT
Jeanine Barone

NUTRITIONISTS
Hill Nutrition Associates

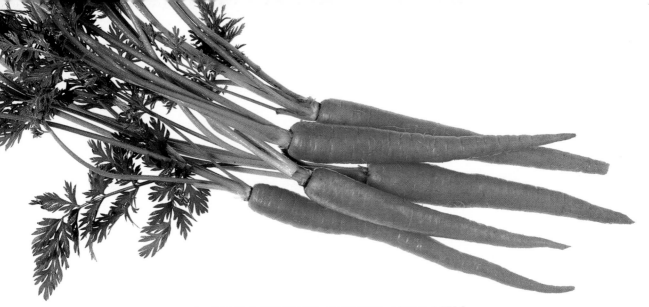

EATING WELL IS THE KEY TO GOOD HEALTH

Nearly every day, researchers announce another exciting discovery regarding the foods we eat and how they affect our health. We now know, for instance, that vitamins and minerals add up to more than we thought: Some help fight heart disease, cancer, and cataracts. And some vitamin- and mineral-rich foods—fruits, vegetables, legumes, grains, and seeds— also contain newly-discovered compounds, called phytochemicals, that have surprisingly powerful health-preserving properties. But you don't need to turn vegetarian to maximize your chances of a long, healthy life:

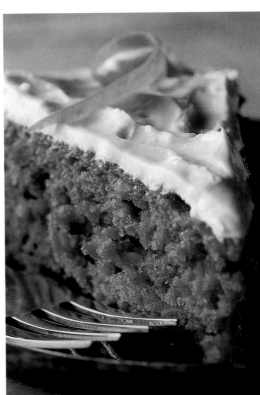

Meat, poultry, fish, eggs, and dairy products also supply health-giving, and possibly life-extending, nutrients. *Eat Well, Stay Well* clues you in to the foods that can help you avoid illness and achieve optimal health. Our recipes offer tempting, delicious ways to serve these foods—from party-perfect appetizers to scrumptious desserts; each food and every recipe is accompanied by a nutritional analysis. And in the front of the book you'll find a comprehensive nutrition glossary, as well as a chapter of photo-illustrated cooking techniques.

Contents

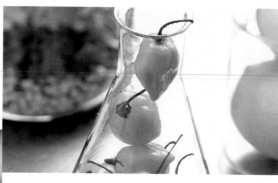
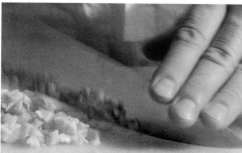
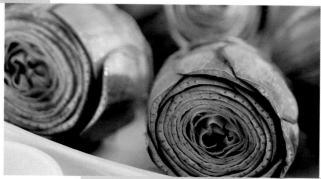
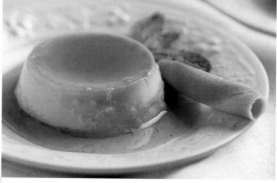

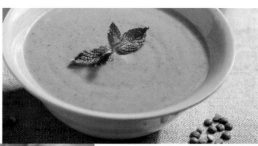
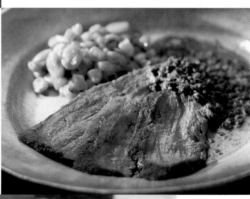
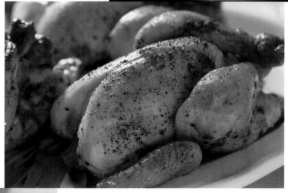
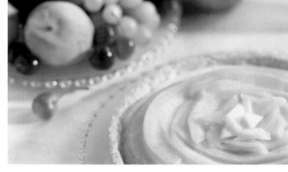

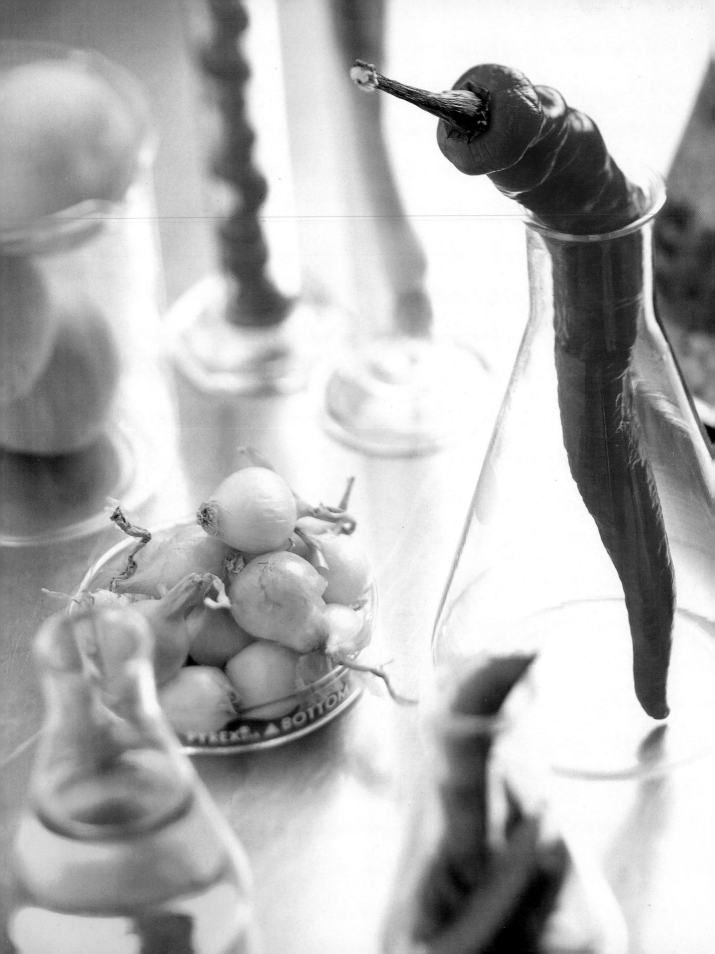

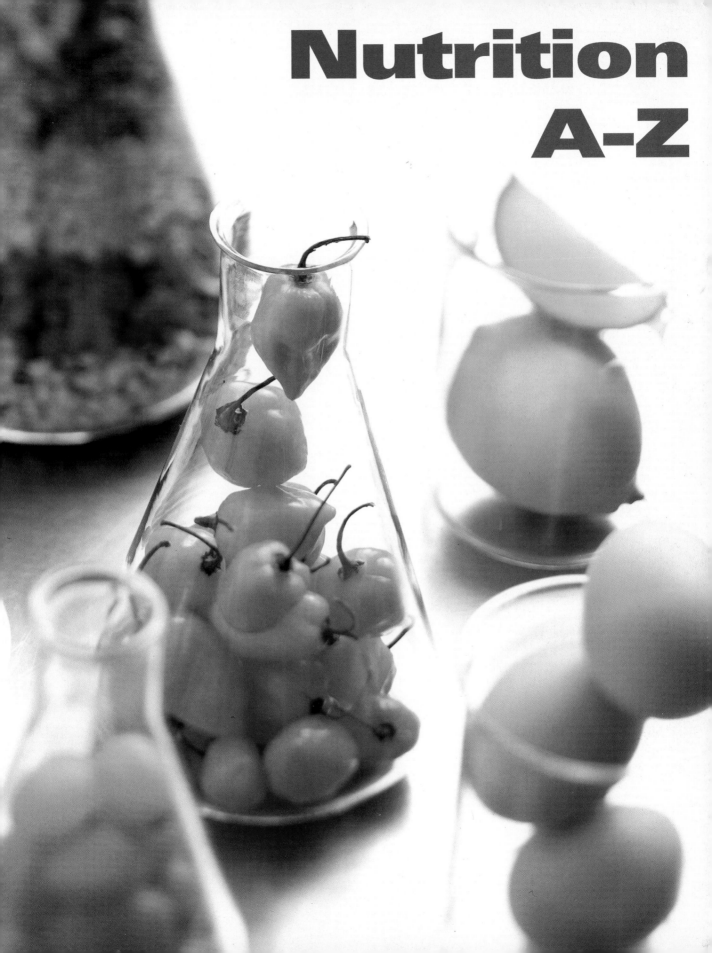

Nutrition
A-Z

ALLYL SULFIDES: These PHYTOCHEMICALS are found in onion-family plants —onions, leeks, scallions, chives, shallots, and garlic. Allyl sulfides are sulfur compounds that seem to suppress cholesterol production and lower blood pressure; they may also have cancer-fighting properties in that they may deactivate certain hormones that promote tumor growth.

AMINO ACIDS: The building blocks of PROTEIN. Of the 21 amino acids, nine are *essential,* meaning that your body cannot produce enough to meet its needs: You must get additional supplies of these amino acids from food. The essential amino acids are histidine, isoleucine, leucine, lysine, methionine, phenylalanine, threonine, tryptophan, and valine. Some amino acids—cysteine, tyrosine, arginine, proline, and glycine—are considered "conditionally essential" because the body can produce them only under certain circumstances.

ANTICARCINOGENS: Substances that fight cancer. Research has shown that many substances in food may be anticarcinogenic. They include VITAMIN C, VITAMIN E, BETA CAROTENE, and a host of PHYTOCHEMICALS, such as ELLAGIC ACID, ISOFLAVONES, and SULFORAPHANE.

ANTIOXIDANTS: Compounds that deactivate and repair the damage caused by FREE RADICALS, thus preventing the onset of certain diseases. A number of antioxidants are found in food. For instance, vitamins C and E and BETA CAROTENE are known to be antioxidants; scientists are currently researching the antioxidant capabilities of the many different plant compounds called PHYTOCHEMICALS.

ASCORBIC ACID: *see* VITAMIN C

BETA CAROTENE: The most common of the 600 or more CAROTENOIDS, beta carotene gives color to carrots, cantaloupe, and other orange and yellow fruits and vegetables; it's found in dark-green vegetables, too, but its orange color is obscured by the green color of chlorophyll. Beta carotene is a vitamin A precursor; that is, the body converts available beta carotene into as much vitamin A as it requires. Beta carotene is a cancer fighter and may also help prevent cataracts, in both cases partly through its ANTIOXIDANT function. Beta carotene also seems to enhance immune function.

BETA GLUCANS: The type of soluble DIETARY FIBER found in barley and oats. Beta glucans have been shown to lower blood cholesterol levels.

BIOTIN: One of the B vitamins, biotin is made by the human body, so deficiencies of it are virtually unknown. Biotin plays a role in the metabolism of proteins and carbohydrates. Good food sources include eggs, dairy products, legumes, whole grains, and CRUCIFEROUS VEGETABLES.

BORON: A trace MINERAL that works in conjunction with CALCIUM and MAGNESIUM to build strong bones. Boron is found in most fruits; grapes are a good source, as are dried fruits, such as raisins.

BRASSICA: The cabbage family of vegetables, which includes cabbage, broccoli, Brussels sprouts, cauliflower, and mustard greens. These plants are also called CRUCIFEROUS VEGETABLES.

CAFFEINE: A natural stimulant found in coffee, tea, colas, and, to a lesser extent, chocolate. Caffeine increases the heart rate and enhances mental alertness. Taken in moderation, caffeine can help wake you up or keep you alert; if you're not accustomed to it, however, it can make you irritable and anxious. Caffeine promotes calcium loss and may increase the risk of osteoporosis. And there is some evidence that caffeine may increase the risk of miscarriage. Although not all experts agree, it's probably a good idea to cut down on caffeine if you are pregnant.

CALCIUM: A major dietary MINERAL that builds and restores bones and teeth and is essential in the prevention of osteoporosis, the "brittle bone disease"

GOOD SOURCES OF CALCIUM

Food	Amount	Calcium (mg)
BROCCOLI, FRESH, COOKED	1 cup chopped	72
BUTTERMILK, LOW-FAT	1 cup	285
CHEESE, CHEDDAR	1 ounce	205
CHEESE, MOZZARELLA, PART SKIM	1 ounce	183
CHEESE, PARMESAN	1 ounce	390
CHEESE, RICOTTA, PART-SKIM	½ cup	337
CHEESE, SWISS	1 ounce	272
COLLARD GREENS, FRESH, COOKED	1 cup chopped	226
KALE, FRESH, COOKED	1 cup chopped	94
MILK, SKIM	1 cup	302
SALMON, CANNED SOCKEYE, DRAINED, EATEN WITH BONES	3 ounces	203
SARDINES, CANNED, EATEN WITH BONES	2 sardines	92
SESAME SEEDS, UNHULLED	2 tablespoons	175
SOY MILK, CALCIUM-FORTIFIED	1 cup	80
TOFU, PROCESSED WITH CALCIUM SULFATE (NIGARI)	¼ block	129
YOGURT, LOW-FAT PLAIN	8 ounces	415
YOGURT, NONFAT PLAIN	8 ounces	452

that can cause bone fractures in older people, especially women. Adequate calcium intake is especially important before age 35—when your body is still building bone—but also after age 35, to maintain strong bones for a lifetime. Another function of calcium is that it helps regulate muscle contractions, including heartbeat. Some research indicates that an adequate supply of calcium may help counteract high blood pressure. Many dairy foods, especially milk and yogurt, are excellent sources of calcium; some dark-green leafy vegetables, such as kale, are also good sources, as are the types of canned fish (sardines and salmon) that are eaten bones and all.

CALORIE: A unit used to measure the energy potential in food and the amount of energy used by the body. (Technically, a calorie is the amount of heat required to raise the temperature of 1 gram of water 1°C.) We get calories from the carbohydrates, proteins, and fat in the foods we eat. Carbohydrates and protein have 4 calories per gram, while fat has 9 calories per gram.

The basic rule for weight maintenance in terms of calories is that "calories out" should equal "calories in": If you consume just the amount of calories that your body needs to maintain itself and to power your daily activities, your weight will remain fairly constant. However, if you consistently consume more calories than you need, they will be stored as fat and you will gain weight.

CAPSAICIN: A PHYTOCHEMICAL found in hot peppers (chilies) and concentrated in the seeds and ribs. Aside from the "heat" it adds to foods, capsaicin may act as an anticoagulant, preventing blood from clotting and sticking to blood-vessel walls. Researchers believe that capsaicin may protect DNA from CARCINOGENS, and may help kill *Helicobacter pylori*—the bacteria now known to cause most stomach ulcers. The hotness of capsaicin can also help clear up nasal congestion (think of how a spoonful of super-spicy salsa seems to go right through your head) and can be useful when you have a cold. Capsaicin is potent enough to burn skin, so when you are cooking with chili peppers, wear rubber gloves, or else be sure to wash your hands with soap and water afterward. Never touch your eyes after handling chilies.

CARBOHYDRATES (SIMPLE OR COMPLEX): Along with PROTEIN and FAT, one of the three MACRO-NUTRIENTS—the major components of foods.

Carbohydrates—which are either sugars (simple carbohydrates) or starches (complex carbohydrates)—are carbon compounds that the body turns into GLU-COSE, its basic fuel. Carbohydrates are found in all foods from plant sources—fruits, vegetables, legumes, and grains. Foods rich in complex carbohydrates should make up a large part of your diet: They supply energy and usually also contain other valuable nutrients, such as vitamins, minerals, and fiber. Foods that contain large amounts of simple carbohydrates may supply little else of redeeming nutritional value.

Naturally sweet fruits are a notable exception: They contain valuable nutrients in addition to sugar in the form of fructose or sucrose.

CARCINOGEN: A substance that causes the growth of cancer.

CAROTENOIDS: These PHYTOCHEM-ICALS are the yellow, orange, and red pigments found in fruits and vegetables. There are 600 or more carotenoids. The body converts some carotenoids, including BETA CAROTENE, into vitamin A. Other carotenoids include LUTEIN, LYCOPENE, and ZEAXAN-THIN. Scientists are researching the antioxidant and other cancer-fighting properties of foods containing carotenoids.

CHLORINE: An element that in its compound forms (chlorides) is a mineral essential to maintaining the acid balance in the body's cells. Most of our dietary needs for this mineral are met by table salt (sodium chloride).

CHOLESTEROL: A waxy, fatlike substance present in every cell in animals, including humans. Cholesterol is essential to several of the body's functions, including the manufacture of vitamin D, hormones, and skin oils, so we need a certain amount of cholesterol. But when excess cholesterol circulates in the blood, it adheres to the artery walls, forming a substance

GOOD SOURCES OF BETA CAROTENE

Food	Amount	Beta Carotene (mg)
APRICOTS, DRIED	½ cup	11.2
APRICOTS, FRESH	3 medium	3.7
BROCCOLI, RAW	1 cup florets	1.3
CANTALOUPE	1 cup diced	4.7
CARROTS, RAW	1 medium	4.8
COLLARD GREENS, RAW	2 cups chopped	1.8
KALE, RAW	2 cups chopped	6.4
MANGO	1 cup sliced	2.2
PUMPKIN, FRESH, RAW	1 cup	3.6
SPINACH, RAW	1 cup	1.2
SWEET POTATO, RAW	1 medium	11.6
SWISS CHARD, RAW	2 cups chopped	2.6
WATERCRESS, RAW	2 cups chopped	2.8
WINTER SQUASH, RAW	1 cup cubes	2.8

called plaque that can limit blood flow and contribute to stiffening of the arteries—a condition called atherosclerosis. This can eventually lead to a heart attack or stroke.

The body produces all the cholesterol it requires, but there is also cholesterol in some foods; this dietary cholesterol does not go directly into your bloodstream. If you do consume a lot of dietary cholesterol, however, it will have the *indirect* effect of elevating your blood cholesterol level; but consumption of saturated fat actually does much more to raise blood cholesterol—especially LDL cholesterol (*see below*)—than does consumption of cholesterol.

Only foods from animal sources (meat, poultry, seafood, eggs, and dairy products) contain cholesterol. There is no cholesterol in foods from plant sources—and that includes fatty foods like nuts, avocados, and coconuts, as well as vegetable, seed, and nut oils.

Cholesterol circulates in the bloodstream in units, called lipoproteins, that also contain fat and protein. There are two types of lipoproteins:

• *Low-density lipoprotein,* or LDL, carries cholesterol from the liver to other parts of the body. This is the cholesterol that leaves deposits on blood vessel walls. Sometimes referred to as "bad" cholesterol.

• *High-density lipoprotein,* or HDL, performs the reverse task, carrying cholesterol from the body's tissues back to the liver—which includes removing some of the cholesterol deposits from the blood vessels. Hence, HDL is sometimes called "good" cholesterol.

Your goal should be a low *total* blood cholesterol level (under 200 milligrams per deciliter), but the *balance* of lipoproteins is equally important: A high level of HDL (above 35mg/dl and preferably around 60mg/dl) and a low level of LDL (below 130mg/dl) is desirable. A diet low in total fat, and, more important, low in saturated fat, will help you toward this goal: Eating plenty of fiber, especially soluble fiber, is also a good idea. An exercise program can also help lower your blood cholesterol.

CHROMIUM: A trace MINERAL that helps the body turn GLUCOSE into energy, chromium also helps reg-

ulate the action of the hormone insulin. Some experts believe that chromium deficiency is fairly common, but it's easy to get an adequate amount of this mineral: Chromium is found in meat, seafood, eggs, nuts, whole grains, dairy products, fruit, and potatoes (be sure to eat the skin).

COBALAMIN: *see* VITAMIN B12

COPPER: A trace MINERAL that aids in the formation of genetic matter, red blood cells, bones, and connective tissue. Copper also supports the functioning of the immune system. Copper deficiencies are rare. Among the best sources are shellfish (especially oysters), sunflower seeds, nuts, lentils, and whole grains.

CRUCIFEROUS VEGETABLES: The word "cruciferous," which means "cross-shaped," describes a family of vegetables with cross-shaped flowers. Cruciferous vegetables are also called brassicas, or cabbage family vegetables. They include cabbage, broccoli, Brussels sprouts, cauliflower, and kale, as well as mustard greens, turnips, and rutabaga. These vegetables contain PHYTO-CHEMICALS called INDOLES, which seem to offer protection against some forms of cancer. Cruciferous vegetables are also rich in vitamin C, and most are good sources of DIETARY FIBER. Those that are dark green or yellow, such as broccoli and rutabaga, also contain BETA CAROTENE.

D **DAILY REFERENCE VALUES (DRVs):** These standards, created by the Food and Drug Administration, set a suggested intake of nutrients for which there were no RECOMMENDED DIETARY ALLOWANCES. These include fat, saturated fat, carbohydrate, cholesterol, fiber, sodium, and potassium. The DRVs are one component of the DAILY VALUES shown on food labels (*see sample label on page 23*).

DAILY VALUES (DVs): These guidelines, created by the Food and Drug Administration, are the basis for the

GOOD SOURCES OF DIETARY FIBER

Food	Amount	Dietary Fiber (g)
APPLE, WITH SKIN	1 large	6
ARTICHOKE	1 medium	7
BARLEY, PEARLED, COOKED	1 cup	6
BLACKBERRIES, FRESH	1 cup	7
BROWN RICE, COOKED	1 cup	4
FIGS, DRIED	½ cup	12
KIDNEY BEANS, COOKED	1 cup	11
LENTILS, COOKED	1 cup	16
OATMEAL, COOKED	1 cup	4
PEAR, WITH SKIN	1 medium	4
POTATO, BAKED, WITH SKIN	1 medium	7
PRUNES	½ cup	6
SPLIT PEAS, COOKED	½ cup	6
WHEAT BRAN	¼ cup	6
WHEAT GERM	¼ cup	4
WINTER SQUASH, BAKED	1 cup cubes	6

nutrition information on the new food labels that first appeared in 1994. The Daily Values, which comprise the DAILY REFERENCE VALUES (DRVs) and REFERENCE DAILY INTAKES (RDIs), are suggested amounts of nutrients for a healthy person consuming 2,000 calories a day. The food labels show nutrient content in terms of "% Daily Values." The DVs also serve as standards by which companies may be permitted to label foods with claims such as "high-fiber" or "low-fat."

DIETARY FIBER: The parts of foods from plant sources (fruits, vegetables, legumes, grains, nuts, and seeds) that we eat, but, for the most part, cannot digest. Though indigestible, fiber performs some vital functions in the body. There are two basic types of fiber: Insoluble (insoluble in water) and soluble.

Insoluble fiber, which used to be known as roughage, is bulky material that helps move waste through the digestive tract. This promotes regular bowel function and may also reduce the risk of colon cancer. Some good sources of insoluble fiber are wheat bran and whole grains, the skins of apples and pears, and vegetables such as potatoes, carrots, and broccoli.

Soluble fiber is found in oats, barley, beans, and many fruits and vegetables. Some types of soluble fiber have been found to help lower blood cholesterol. Soluble fiber also helps control blood-sugar levels.

Many health experts agree that Americans should at least double their fiber consumption, for a total of 20 to 30 grams per day. In addition to the known benefits of fiber itself, foods that are naturally high in fiber (i.e., foods from plant sources) are rich in other important nutrients.

E **ELLAGIC ACID:** Found in strawberries, raspberries, cranberries, and some other fruits, nuts, and vegetables, this PHYTOCHEMICAL shows promise as a cancer preventive through its ability to inactivate CARCINOGENS and inhibit the formation of FREE RADICALS.

ENDOSPERM: The inner kernel of a whole grain, which contains most of the starch and protein.

ENRICHED:
Foods labeled
"enriched" must contain at least
10 percent more of the DAILY VALUE for a certain nutrient than was in the original food. Typically, enriched foods are flours, breads, pastas, and cereals made from refined grain products, such as white flour or refined cornmeal. Enrichment is intended to compensate for vitamins and minerals lost in milling. The added nutrients in these products are usually iron, riboflavin, thiamin, niacin, and folate. *See also* FORTIFIED.

F **FAT:** One of the three MACRONUTRIENTS found in the foods we eat. Dietary fats are vital to many of the body's functions; for instance, vitamins A, D, E, and K are fat-soluble, and will not be absorbed by the body in the absence of sufficient dietary fat. And fats are important in cooking: They carry flavor, lock in moisture, and help keep baked goods tender.

Although some dietary fat is necessary, excessive fat intake can lead to obesity and also increase the risk of heart disease, diabetes, and cancer.

Fats are composed of chains of fatty acids, of which there are a number of different types. These fatty acids are classified as either saturated or unsaturated, according to the number of hydrogen atoms they contain.

• *Saturated fatty acids* carry a full complement of hydrogen atoms.
• *Monounsaturated fatty acids* are missing one pair of hydrogen atoms.
• *Polyunsaturated fatty acids* lack two or more pairs of hydrogen atoms.

Fats are classified according to the proportions of fatty acids they contain: e.g., highly saturated, highly polyunsaturated, etc. Highly saturated fats are mostly animal fats, such as those found in butter, lard, meat, and poultry; palm, palm kernel, and coconut oil are also highly saturated. Saturated fats are usually solid at room temperature. Highly polyunsaturated fats include corn, safflower, and sesame oils, while olive and canola oils are highly monounsaturated fats.

Hydrogenated fats form another category. These are vegetable oils that have been specially treated with hydrogen to make them solid at room temperature and resistant to rancidity. Hydrogenation creates what are called "trans fatty acids" by saturating unsaturated fatty acids and changing their structure.

The different types of dietary fat have different effects on the body. Mono- and polyunsaturated fats have been shown to lower total cholesterol levels. Highly saturated fats raise total blood cholesterol and, in particular, LDL, or "bad" cholesterol. Trans fats have a similar, and possibly worse, effect: They raise

COMPARING COOKING OILS

Type of Oil	% Poly-unsaturated	% Mono-unsaturated	% Saturated
AVOCADO	14	74	12
CANOLA	32	62	6
CORN	59	24	13
OLIVE	9	72	14
PEANUT	32	46	17
SAFFLOWER	75	12	9
SESAME	40	40	18
SOYBEAN	59	23	14
SUNFLOWER	66	20	10
BUTTER (FOR COMPARISON)	4	29	62

Note: Some percentages do not add up to 100% because water and other substances make up the total composition of the oil.

overall cholesterol and LDL, and perhaps also lower HDL. So from a health standpoint, liquid fats (cooking oils) are a better choice than solid fats (butter, lard, shortening, or margarine).

Of course, overall fat intake is important, too. Health authorities recommend that adults get no more than 30 percent of their daily calories from fat; some researchers call for an even lower fat intake. (Note that this recommendation applies to food intake over the course of a day or a week, and not to a single dish or meal.) But most Americans need to to cut down on saturated fat as well: It should account for no more than one-third of your total fat intake. The most effective way to do this is to eat less red meat. The first step in cutting down on trans fats is to read labels: Hydrogenated fats are often used in margarines, cookies, crackers, and potato chips. Solid vegetable shortening sold for cooking and baking is also a hydrogenated fat, and this type of fat is widely used to cook fast-food french fries (ask before you order).

FIBER: *see* DIETARY FIBER

FLAVONOIDS: These PHYTOCHEMICALS are found mostly in fruits and vegetables, including citrus fruits, cranberries, onions, soybeans, carrots, and broccoli, and also in tea and wine. They act as ANTIOXIDANTS. High flavonoid intake has been linked to reduced risk of coronary heart disease; one of the known effects of these phytochemicals is that they keep platelets from clumping together and blocking blood vessels. Flavonoids may also inhibit enzymes responsible for the spread of malignant cells.

FLUORIDE: This mineral contributes to the formation of bones and teeth. Many Americans get fluoride from their water supply; canned salmon and sardines, eaten with their bones, are also good sources of this mineral, as are black and green tea.

FOLATE: This B vitamin—also called folacin or folic acid—is vital to tissue growth and thus plays a role in the prevention of certain birth defects, so it is particularly important that women of childbearing age get enough of this nutrient. Folate may also help

GOOD SOURCES OF FOLATE

Food	Amount	Folate (mcg)
ARTICHOKE, COOKED	1 medium	61
ASPARAGUS, COOKED	1 cup pieces	131
AVOCADO	½ medium	57
BLACKBERRIES, FRESH	1 cup	49
BROCCOLI, COOKED	1 cup chopped	78
BRUSSELS SPROUTS, COOKED	1 cup	94
CHICK-PEAS, COOKED	1 cup	282
GREEN PEAS, FRESH, COOKED	1 cup	101
LENTILS, COOKED	1 cup	358
ORANGE JUICE, FRESH	1 cup	75
PEANUTS, RAW	1 ounce	68
PINTO BEANS, COOKED	1 cup	294
ROMAINE LETTUCE	2 cups shredded	152
SPINACH, RAW	2 cups	117
WHEAT GERM	¼ cup	81
WILD RICE, COOKED	1 cup	43

prevent cancer of the cervix. And folate is one of three B vitamins that help fight heart disease by lowering levels of HOMOCYS-TEINE, an AMINO ACID that may contribute to arterial blockage. Folate is found in leafy vegetables (the word "folate" is related to "foliage"), but also in legumes, whole grains, nuts, pork, and shellfish. Because of this vitamin's importance, cereals and many other refined grain products are also enriched with folate.

FORTIFIED: Food labeled "fortified" must contain at least 10 percent more of the DAILY VALUE for a certain nutrient than was in the original food. In the case of "fortified" (as compared to "enriched") foods, the added nutrients were either not originally present or present in insignificant amounts. One of the most common fortified foods is milk, which has vitamins A and D added to it.

FREE RADICALS: These are unstable compounds (oxygen compounds, among others) formed in the body during normal metabolic processes. These unstable, highly reactive molecules attempt to bind with other elements, creating even more unstable molecules and setting up a chain reaction that can damage basic genetic material (DNA) as well as other cell structures and tissues. This cellular damage, if uncorrected, can eventually result in cancer and other diseases (free radicals are suspected of playing a role in heart disease, cataracts, arthritis, and neurological diseases). External factors can promote the formation of free radicals: These include exposure to heat, radiation, environmental pollutants, including cigarette smoke, and drinking alcohol. The body has its own mechanisms for self-repair, but certain nutrients, which function as ANTIOXIDANTS, can also aid in repairing the damage caused by free radicals. These antioxidant nutrients include VITAMIN C, VITAMIN E, and BETA CAROTENE. Other CAROTENOIDS, such as LYCOPENE, LUTEIN, and ZEAXANTHIN, are currently being researched for possible antioxidant effects.

G GENISTEIN: This compound belongs to the category of PHYTOCHEMICALS called ISOFLAVONES. Genistein, found in soybeans and soy products (tofu, soy milk, etc.), may block the formation of new blood vessels; this in turn slows the growth of tumors.

GLUCOSE: Your body turns most of the CARBOHYDRATES you eat into its basic energy source, glucose. Glucose is carried in the bloodstream for distribution to the cells when energy is required, or stored as GLYCOGEN.

GLYCOGEN: Excess GLUCOSE not utilized by the body is converted into glycogen, a form in which it can be stored in the muscles or liver.

H HDL: *see* CHOLESTEROL

HEME IRON: *see* IRON

HOMOCYSTEINE: An AMINO ACID that circulates in the blood; people with elevated homocysteine levels are at increased risk of arterial blockage, resulting in a heart attack or stroke. Normally, three of the B vitamins (FOLATE, VITAMIN B6, and VITAMIN B12) assist in the conversion of homocysteine into other non-damaging amino acids; however, if these vitamins are in short supply (due to dietary deficiency, or a genetic problem) the homocysteine in the bloodstream will continue to pose a risk.

I INDOLES: Nitrogen compounds found in CRUCIFEROUS VEGETABLES. Indoles seem to have the ability to convert the active form of estrogen (which can promote the growth of breast tumors) into an inactive form. Indoles may be protective against other cancers as well.

IODINE: Required for normal cell metabolism, this mineral is essential to the functioning of the thyroid gland. Most of our dietary iodine comes from iodized salt, but the mineral is also found in seafood and dairy products, among other foods.

IRON: This mineral plays a key role in the blood's distribution of oxygen to the body. A serious shortage of iron—iron-deficiency anemia—produces fatigue and impaired immunity. Iron is found in red meat, poultry, fish, egg yolks, legumes, nuts, dried fruits, leafy greens, and enriched foods such as breakfast cereals, bread, and pasta. There are two types of iron in food: Heme and nonheme iron.

• *Heme iron,* found in meat and other foods from animal sources, is easily absorbed by the body.

• *Nonheme iron,* found in foods from plant sources, is less readily absorbed, but you can enhance absorption by consuming some vitamin C-rich foods along with the vegetarian iron sources. Some examples are beans (nonheme iron) with cabbage (vitamin C); prunes or raisins (nonheme iron) with orange juice (vitamin C); and kale (nonheme iron) with tomatoes (vitamin C). You can also add iron to your diet by cooking in iron pots; if the food you cook is acidic (tomatoes, for example), the food will pick up even more iron from the pot.

ISOFLAVONES: PHYTOCHEMI-CALS found in legumes, including soybeans. Isofla-vones are phytoestrogens—plant substances that mimic estrogen's action in the body. Some researchers believe that a diet rich in isoflavones may protect against "hormone sensitive" cancers, such as those of the breast and prostate. Isoflavones also lower total cholesterol while raising HDL.

ISOTHIOCYANATES: The class of PHYTOCHEMICALS, found in CRUCIFEROUS VEGETABLES, that includes SULFORAPHANE. Isothiocyanates stimulate anticancer enzymes.

LDL: *see* CHOLESTEROL

LACTOSE: The type of sugar found in milk. Some people, called lactose-intolerant, have difficulty digesting lactose, but such people can more easily digest cheese (most of the lactose is removed in processing) and cultured dairy products, such as yogurt and buttermilk. Specially treated milk, in which the lactose is predigested through the addition of lac-

tase (an enzyme), is widely available.

LEGUMES: A family of plants characterized by the seed-bearing pods that grow on them. All beans and peas, as well as lentils and peanuts, are members of this group of plants. Legumes are very healthful foods, being good sources of protein, iron, B vitamins, and fiber.

LIMONENES: Compounds found in the peels of citrus fruits that may deactivate certain CARCINOGENS.

LIPOPROTEINS: *see* CHOLESTEROL

LUTEIN: A CAROTENOID found in kale, spinach, parsley, red bell peppers, avocados, and other fruits and vegetables. This PHYTOCHEMICAL may protect against age-related macular degeneration, the leading cause of blindness in the elderly.

LYCOPENE: One of the CAROTENOIDS, this PHYTOCHEMI-CAL is found in tomatoes and tomato products, red bell peppers, watermelon, pink grapefruit, apricots, and some other fruits and vegetables. Studies have shown that a diet that includes plenty of tomato products can be protective against prostate cancer. The lycopene is best absorbed by the body if the tomatoes are cooked, as they are in tomato sauce, paste, or purée. Lycopene also seems to have protective effects against other types of cancer, including tumors of the colon, cervix, and bladder.

LYSINE: *see* AMINO ACIDS

MACRONUTRIENTS: The food components—PROTEIN, CARBOHY-DRATES, and FAT—from which we get energy.

MAGNESIUM: This mineral works with its allies, CALCIUM, MOLYBDENUM, POTASSIUM, and PHOSPHO-RUS, to build and maintain bones and teeth; magnesium also contributes to the functioning of the

IMPORTANT MINERALS AT A GLANCE

Mineral	The roles it plays	Where to find it
CALCIUM	Builds and maintains bone strength and density; helps regulate heartbeat and muscle contraction	Dairy products, sardines and salmon eaten with bones, dark leafy greens
CHLORINE	Helps maintain fluid and acid balance	Table salt
CHROMIUM	Metabolism of carbohydrates and fats	Seafood, whole grains, potato skins
COPPER	Formation of red blood cells; for healthy bones, nerves, immune system	Shellfish, nuts, beans, sunflower seeds, whole grains
FLUORIDE	Keeps teeth and bones strong	Fluoridated water; sardines and salmon (with bones); black or green tea
IODINE	Necessary for function of the thyroid gland, cell metabolism	Iodized salt; fish; produce grown in iodine-rich soil
IRON	Essential to formation of hemoglobin; component of enzymes and proteins	Red meat, eggs, legumes, nuts, fortified cereals; foods cooked in iron pots
MAGNESIUM	Aids in bone growth, nerve and muscle function	Whole grains, leafy greens, nuts, soybeans, bananas, apricots, spices
MANGANESE	Aids in reproduction and energy production; helps build bones	Nuts, whole grains, beans, coffee, green and black tea
MOLYBDENUM	Helps build strong bones and teeth	Grains, dark leafy greens, beans
PHOSPHORUS	Helps build bones and teeth and form cell membranes and genetic material	Meat, poultry, fish, dairy products, legumes, nuts
POTASSIUM	Helps regulate muscle contraction, nerve impulses, function of heart and kidneys, fluid balance	Bananas, potatoes, avocados, dried fruits, dairy products, beans
SELENIUM	Component of an enzyme that acts as an antioxidant; detoxifies toxic metals	Brazil nuts, fish, shellfish, red meat, grains, chicken, garlic
SODIUM	Helps regulate fluid balance and blood pressure	Table salt, salt and sodium compounds added to prepared foods
ZINC	Involved in activity of enzymes for cell division, growth, and repair as well as proper functioning of immune system; maintains taste and smell acuity	Oysters, crabmeat, meat, eggs, milk

nerves and muscles. Magnesium is found in whole grains, leafy greens, meat, fish, dairy products, nuts, seeds, legumes, avocados, and bananas.

MANGANESE: A trace mineral, manganese plays a role in reproduction and in the production of energy. It is also a component of ANTIOXIDANT enzymes. Good sources include whole grains, nuts, beans, and egg yolks.

MINERALS: Inorganic elements that originate in the soil; some minerals act as nutrients. Of the 16 nutrient minerals, seven—CALCIUM, COPPER, IODINE, IRON, MAGNESIUM, SELENIUM, and ZINC—have been assigned RDAs, and five other minerals—COPPER, MANGANESE, FLUORIDE, CHROMIUM, and MOLYBDENUM—have been assigned "estimated safe and adequate dietary intakes." The *macro-minerals,* of which we need to consume relatively large amounts, are calcium, chloride, magnesium, phosphorus, potassium, sodium, and sulfur. The other minerals, which our bodies require in minute amounts, are called *trace minerals.*

Minerals are required for formation of bones, teeth, and nails, as well as other parts of the body. They are components of enzymes and play roles in the regulation of the nervous and digestive systems and in heart function.

Unlike vitamins, minerals cannot be destroyed by overcooking food. But if you boil mineral-rich foods (such as vegetables) for a long time and then discard the cooking liquid, you will be pouring some of the minerals down the drain. To conserve the mineral content when cooking vegetables, steam, braise, or microwave them whenever possible; if blanching in a large quantity of water, do it quickly—in a matter of seconds or minutes. *See also* BORON, CHLORINE, CHROMIUM, FLUORIDE, MAGNESIUM, MANGANESE, MOLYBDENUM, PHOSPHORUS, POTASSIUM, and SODIUM.

MOLYBDENUM: This trace MINERAL is a component of various enzymes; it also helps strengthen bones and teeth. Molybdenum deficiency is almost unknown. Milk, legumes, and grains are all good sources.

MONOTERPENES: PHYTOCHEMICALS that function as ANTIOXIDANTS and seem to protect against heart disease and cancer. Monoterpenes are found in citrus fruits, berries, parsley, broccoli, and cabbage.

MONOUNSATURATED FAT: *see* FAT

NIACIN: One of the B vitamins (vitamin B3), niacin is important in the body's production of energy from food. It is also required for normal growth and the synthesis of DNA (genetic material). In addition, niacin helps keep the skin, nerves, and digestive system healthy. Lean meat, poultry, and seafood are excellent sources of niacin; milk, legumes, and fortified cereals also supply good amounts of this vitamin.

OMEGA-3: This term describes two types of polyunsaturated fatty acids (*see* FAT). The preeminent source of omega-3 fatty acids is seafood. Omega-3s are unique in their ability to lower levels of TRIGLYCERIDES in the blood. In addition, omega-3s function as blood thinners, lessening the likelihood of a heart attack or stroke. (Some researchers believe that omega-3s help lower total cholesterol and/or LDL, or "bad" cholesterol, but the studies are inconclusive.) In addition, omega-3s also seem to protect against certain forms of cancer and, because they have anti-inflammatory powers, may be effective against rheumatoid arthritis. The best sources of omega-3 fatty acids are fatty fish, such as salmon, mackerel, anchovies, sardines, and herring; many leaner fish and shellfish are also good sources.

GOOD SOURCES OF OMEGA-3 FATTY ACIDS

Type of seafood	Fat (g)*	Omega-3 (mg)*
BASS, STRIPED	2.3	754
BLUEFISH	4.2	771
GROUPER	0.1	247
HALIBUT	2.3	363
HERRING, PACIFIC	3.9	1,658
MACKEREL, SPANISH	6.3	1,341
POLLOCK, ATLANTIC	0.1	421
POMPANO	9.5	568
SALMON, ATLANTIC	6.3	1,436
SALMON, CHINOOK (KING)	10.4	1,355
SEA BASS	2.0	595
SNAPPER	1.3	311
SWORDFISH	4.0	639
TROUT, RAINBOW	3.4	568
TUNA, BLUEFIN	4.9	1,173
CLAMS	1.0	142
CRAB, BLUE	1.1	320
MUSSELS, BLUE	2.2	441
OYSTERS, EASTERN	2.5	439
SCALLOPS	0.8	198
SHRIMP	1.7	480

*PER 3½ OUNCES RAW

OXALIC ACID (OXALATES): A natural compound found in some vegetables, including spinach, Swiss chard, beet greens, and rhubarb. Oxalic acid binds with calcium and iron, thus limiting the body's absorption of these minerals. Vegetarians should not depend on these vegetables for iron and calcium.

PANTOTHENIC ACID: This B vitamin (B5) helps the body convert food into energy; it also plays a role in synthesizing hormones and other body chemicals. Deficiencies of pantothenic acid are virtually unknown.

PECTIN: A type of soluble DIETARY FIBER, pectin is found in apples, citrus fruits, berries, bananas, and grapes, as well as other fruits, vegetables, legumes, and nuts. (Pectin is also sold in powdered form for use in making jams and jellies.) This type of soluble fiber helps reduce cholesterol, and thus may help prevent heart disease. Pectin also helps regulate intestinal function.

PHOSPHORUS: This bone-building MINERAL is also important for energy production and the formation of cells. Phosphorus is found in a great variety of foods, notably fish, meat, poultry, dairy products, eggs, peas, beans, and nuts. Phosphorus deficiencies are rare.

PHYTOCHEMICALS: Chemical compounds found in plants; some are produced to protect the plants against natural enemies. Ongoing research, however, demonstrates that some phytochemicals also boost immunity and help fight diseases, including cancer and heart disease. Phytochemicals include ALLYL SULFIDES, BETA CAROTENE and other CAROTENOIDS, CAPSAICIN, ELLAGIC ACID, FLAVONOIDS, GENISTEIN, INDOLES, ISOTHIOCYANATES, LIMONENES, LUTEIN, LYCOPENE, RESVERATROL, SAPONINS, SINIGRIN, TRITERPENOIDS, and ZEAXANTHIN.

PHYTOESTROGENS: These compounds, found in plants, mimic the action of the estrogen produced by the human body. Phytoestrogens may protect against both cancer and heart disease. Soybeans and foods made from them are rich sources of phytoestrogens.

REFERENCE DAILY INTAKES (RDIs)

Nutrient	Amount
VITAMIN A	5,000 IU•
VITAMIN C	60 mg★
CALCIUM	1,000 mg
IRON	18 mg
VITAMIN D	400 IU
VITAMIN E	30 IU
VITAMIN K	80 mcg♦
THIAMIN	1.5 mg
RIBOFLAVIN	1.7 mg
NIACIN	20 mg
VITAMIN B6	2.0 mg
FOLATE	400 mcg
VITAMIN B12	6 mcg
BIOTIN	300 mcg
PANTOTHENIC ACID	10 mg
PHOSPHORUS	1,000 mg
IODINE	150 mcg
MAGNESIUM	400 mg
ZINC	15 mg
SELENIUM	70 mcg
COPPER	2.0 mg
MANGANESE	2.0 mg
CHROMIUM	120 mcg
MOLYBDENUM	75 mg
CHLORIDE	3,400 mg

•international units   ★ milligrams   ♦ micrograms

POLYPHENOLS: PHYTOCHEMICALS that show promise as disease-fighters in several different arenas. They act as antioxidants and, in the laboratory, have been shown to have antiviral and anticarcinogenic properties. FLAVONOIDS, ISOFLAVONES, and ELLAGIC ACID are all polyphenols.

POLYUNSATURATED FAT: *see* FAT

POTASSIUM: This MINERAL is crucial to the regulation of muscle contraction and nerve impulses and thus helps regulate heart contractions. It also helps control fluid balance in the cells as well as blood pressure. Some studies have indicated that a diet rich in potassium may reduce the risk of high blood pressure and stroke. The REFERENCE DAILY INTAKES do not include potassium, but the DAILY REFERENCE VALUES recommend an intake of 3,500 mg. Potassium is found in most foods; white and sweet potatoes, bananas, avocados, dried apricots, prunes, beef, plain yogurt, and milk are some particularly good sources. Dried beans also supply good amounts of potassium.

PROTEIN: The basic building material of our bodies, protein consists of chains of AMINO ACIDS. Some foods provide complete protein; that is, they have a full complement of essential amino acids. Foods from animal sources—meat, poultry, seafood, eggs, and dairy products—fall into this category. Among plant-derived foods, only soybeans contain complete protein; all other plant foods are deficient in one or more essential amino acids. Still, even if you are a vegetarian (or eat little meat), you needn't worry about getting complete protein as long as you eat a wide range of foods over the course of each day. For instance, the amino acids that are in short supply in grains are found in legumes, so a combination such as peanut butter on bread, or bean chili with rice, will help restore the balance. If you consume sufficient protein, you needn't monitor your amino acid intake; it will take care of itself. For vegetarians, eating whole grains and legumes will increase protein intake, as will eating dairy products.

PYRIDOXINE: *see* VITAMIN B6

RECOMMENDED DIETARY ALLOWANCES (RDAs): Established by the National Academy of Sciences, the RDAs are standards that specify the amount of nutrients required daily for the maintenance of good health. That is, they set the minimum intakes of vitamins, minerals, and protein needed for the average person to stay healthy. There are different RDAs for infants, children, men, and women of different ages, as well as special standards for pregnant and lactating women.

REFERENCE DAILY INTAKES (RDIs): These dietary standards, based on the RDAs, make up one part of the DAILY VALUES used on food labels (*see sample label, at right*) to give the nutritional values for vitamins and minerals. The remaining information on labels comes from the DAILY REFERENCE VALUES. In contrast to the RDAs, the RDIs (*see chart, opposite page*) are single values, and do not vary according to age or gender.

RESVERATROL: A PHYTOCHEMICAL found in grapes, grape juice, and wine—and also in peanuts. It may lower cholesterol and seems to protect against coronary artery disease.

RIBOFLAVIN: This B vitamin (B2), found in dairy products, lean meats, eggs, nuts, legumes, leafy greens, and enriched breads and cereals, plays essential roles in the production of red blood cells, energy production, and growth. Studies show that older women seem to need more riboflavin than other people, and researchers believe that many elderly people do not consume enough riboflavin.

SALT: *see* SODIUM

SAPONINS: PHYTOCHEMICALS found in potatoes, onions, leeks, garlic, and other vegetables, as well as legumes. Saponins are ANTIOXIDANTS that may reduce blood cholesterol and fight cancer.

SATURATED FAT: *see* FAT

SELENIUM: This trace MINERAL may have cancer-fighting properties: It forms a part of an enzyme, glutathione peroxidase, that is an ANTIOXIDANT.

Selenium also helps detoxify poisonous metals, such as mercury. Selenium is found in Brazil nuts, fish, shrimp, oysters, chicken, whole grains, dried beans, and garlic.

SINIGRIN: A PHYTOCHEMICAL found in CRUCIFEROUS VEGETABLES that gives them their slightly bitter flavor; Brussels sprouts are especially rich in sinigrin. In the laboratory, sinigrin has been shown to suppress the development of precancerous cells.

Nutrition Facts

Serving Size 1 cup (248g)
Servings Per Container 4

Amount Per Serving

CALORIES 150	Calories from Fat 36

	% Daily Value*
TOTAL FAT 4g	**6%**
Saturated Fat 2.5g	**12%**
CHOLESTEROL 20mg	**7%**
SODIUM 170mg	**7%**
TOTAL CARBOHYDRATE 17g	**6%**
Dietary Fiber 0g	**0%**
Sugars 17g	
PROTEIN 13g	

Vitamin A	4%	•	Vitamin C	6%
Calcium	40%	•	Iron	2%

* Percent Daily Values are based on a 2,000 calorie diet. Your daily values may be higher or lower depending on your calorie needs:

	Calories	2,000	2,500
Total Fat	Less than	65g	80g
Sat Fat	Less than	20g	25g
Cholesterol	Less than	300mg	300mg
Sodium	Less than	2,400mg	2,400mg
Total Carbohydrate		300g	375g
Dietary Fiber		25g	30g

Calories per gram:
Fat 9   •   Carbohydrate 4   •   Protein 4

◆ % DAILY VALUES BASED ON DAILY REFERENCE VALUES (DRVs)
★ % DAILY VALUES BASED ON REFERENCE DAILY INTAKES (RDIs)

SODIUM: A MINERAL that is vital for maintaining proper fluid balance in the body. The problem for most people, however, is getting *too much* sodium. This mineral is found not only in table salt, but also (as a part of various chemical compounds) in most processed foods, particularly canned goods, fast foods, cheese, and smoked meats. Sodium occurs naturally in fresh foods as well, although usually at moderate levels. Excess sodium elevates blood pressure in many people (however, not everyone with high blood pressure is sodium-sensitive), and it can also contribute to such problems as osteoporosis.

SOLANINE: A bitter natural compound in potatoes that can rise to mildly toxic levels if the potatoes have been improperly stored (in too warm a place, or exposed to light). Potatoes that have sprouted or taken on a greenish tinge have high levels of solanine; either peel the greenish skin off (solanine only goes about 1/16 inch deep) or discard the potatoes.

STARCH: *see* CARBOHYDRATES

STEROLS: PHYTOCHEMICALS found in monounsatured and polyunsaturated vegetable oils, some vegetables (including cucumbers), and some shellfish. Sterols have a cholesterol-lowering effect.

SUGAR: *see* CARBOHYDRATES

SULFORAPHANE: A PHYTOCHEMICAL found in CRUCIFEROUS VEGETABLES such as broccoli, cabbage, and Brussels sprouts. Sulforaphane stimulates the production of enzymes that rid the body of CARCINOGENS.

THIAMIN: One of the B vitamins (B1), thiamin helps the body transform food into energy. Pork is a leading source of thiamin; fish, sunflower seeds, rice, and pasta also supply good amounts of this vitamin. Many breads and cereals are enriched with thiamin.

TOCOPHEROL: *see* VITAMIN E

TRACE MINERALS: *see* MINERALS

TRANS FAT: *see* FAT

TRIGLYCERIDES: Triglycerides are fats that circulate in the bloodstream. Some come from food we eat, but the body also assembles its own triglycerides. High blood triglyceride levels usually accompany low levels of "good" CHOLESTEROL (HDL) and are often present in people who are overweight. Blood triglycerides can often be lowered through weight loss, decreased consumption of saturated fat, and exercise. The omega-3 fatty acids found in seafood have also been shown to help lower triglycerides.

TRITERPENOIDS: Found in citrus fruits, grains, and cruciferous vegetables, these PHYTOCHEMICALS help deactivate certain hormones that promote tumor growth; they also slow down the rapid cell division that is characteristic of malignant tumors.

VITAMINS: These nutrients, required by the body in minute amounts, are organic compounds that regulate reactions taking place in the body. They enable the body to convert food to energy and help the body to protect itself from disease and to heal itself when injured. We get most of the vitamins we need from foods (or from supplements); the body produces a few vitamins, but not in the quantities it actually requires.

The B-complex vitamins and vitamin C are water soluble; any excess of these vitamins is excreted in urine, rather than stored. So it's important to replenish your body's supply of these vitamins regularly.

Water-soluble vitamins, especially vitamin C, can be lost if foods that contain them, such as vegetables and fruits, are cooked too long, over too high heat, or in too much liquid (if the liquid is then discarded). Try steaming or microwaving, and always cook these foods as quickly as possible (or eat them raw).

The fat-soluble vitamins—A, D, E, and K—are stored in the liver and in body fat, so you don't need to renew your supply as often. These vitamins are less likely to be lost in cooking, although high heat (as used in frying) can destroy the vitamin E in vegetable oils.

IMPORTANT VITAMINS AT A GLANCE

Vitamin	The roles it plays	Where to find it
BIOTIN	Important in the metabolism of protein, carbohydrates, and fats	Eggs, dairy products, mushrooms, whole grains
FOLATE (FOLACIN, FOLIC ACID)	Fights heart disease; adequate intake reduces risk of birth defects and some cancers	Leafy greens, asparagus, broccoli, beans, orange juice, enriched cereals
VITAMIN A	Important for healthy eyes; also maintains health of skin, teeth, bones	As beta carotene (which the body converts to vitamin A) in yellow, orange, and dark-green produce; as preformed vitamin A in eggs, fortified milk, fish
VITAMIN B1 (THIAMIN)	Conversion of carbohydrates into energy; brain, nerve cell, and heart function	Pork, fish, sunflower seeds, rice, enriched breads and cereals
VITAMIN B2 (RIBOFLAVIN)	Conversion of food to energy; growth; red blood cell production	Dairy products, meat, poultry, fish, leafy greens, nuts
VITAMIN B3 (NIACIN)	Conversion of food to energy; health of skin, nerves, digestive system	Nuts, meat, fish, poultry, dairy products
VITAMIN B5 (PANTOTHENIC ACID)	Conversion of food to energy; production of essential body chemicals	Found in nearly all foods
VITAMIN B6 (PYRIDOXINE)	Important in chemical reactions of proteins and amino acids in the body; production of red blood cells	Poultry, beef, fish, bananas, beans, nuts, fortified cereals
VITAMIN B12 (COBALAMIN)	Essential for development of red blood cells, nervous system function	Meat, poultry, seafood, eggs, dairy products, fortified soy milk
VITAMIN C	Antioxidant; helps reduce risk of cancer, cataracts; also essential for healthy gums and teeth, wound healing; enhances iron absorption	Citrus fruit, red peppers and chilies, strawberries, kiwifruit, cantaloupe, broccoli, potatoes
VITAMIN D	For strong bones and teeth; also seems to reduce risk of colon cancer	Milk, dairy products, fatty fish
VITAMIN E	Antioxidant; helps prevent heart disease	Nuts, vegetable oil, avocados, leafy greens, almonds, pumpkin and sunflower seeds
VITAMIN K	Essential for normal blood clotting; may aid in calcium absorption	Broccoli, Brussels sprouts, cabbage, leafy greens, milk, soybeans, eggs

VITAMIN A: Known as a vision enhancer, vitamin A is also important for healthy skin, teeth, and bones. This vitamin may have some anticarcinogenic powers, but many of the disease-fighting properties formerly attributed to it actually belong to BETA CAROTENE and the other CAROTENOIDS that are precursors of vitamin A (that is, the body converts them into vitamin A). The best sources of vitamin A, in the form of beta carotene, are dark green, orange, or yellow fruits and vegetables, such as apricots, mangos, spinach, kale, carrots, pumpkin, and sweet potatoes. Preformed vitamin A is found in egg yolks, dairy products, fish, and organ meats.

VITAMIN B COMPLEX: BIOTIN, FOLATE, NIACIN, PANTOTHENIC ACID, RIBOFLAVIN, THIAMIN, and VITAMINS B6 and B12 make up this group of vitamins.

VITAMIN B1: *see* THIAMIN

VITAMIN B2: *see* RIBOFLAVIN

VITAMIN B3: *see* NIACIN

VITAMIN B5: *see* PANTOTHENIC ACID

VITAMIN B6 (PYRIDOXINE): This vitamin aids in the body's utilization of protein and in the production of red blood cells. Pyridoxine works with other B vitamins to help keep levels of HOMOCYSTEINE low. Vitamin B6 plays a role in antibody production, so an adequate supply of this nutrient strengthens immunity. Many elderly people do not get as much of this vitamin as they should for optimal health. Some good sources of B6 are chicken, beef, fish, beans, bananas, and enriched cereals.

VITAMIN B12 (COBALAMIN): Vitamin B12 plays a role in the formation of red blood cells and in the functioning of the nervous system. A very important role of vitamin B12 is that it enables the body to utilize FOLATE, thus helping to keep HOMOCYSTEINE levels down. This vitamin is plentiful in meat,

GOOD SOURCES OF VITAMIN C

Food	Amount	Vitamin C (mg)
ASPARAGUS, FRESH, COOKED	1 cup pieces	20
BROCCOLI, FRESH, COOKED	1 cup chopped	116
BRUSSELS SPROUTS, FRESH, COOKED	1 cup	97
CABBAGE, FRESH, COOKED	1 cup shredded	30
CANTALOUPE	1 cup cubes	68
CHILI PEPPER, RED, RAW	1 medium	109
GRAPEFRUIT JUICE, FRESH SQUEEZED	1 cup	94
HONEYDEW MELON	large wedge	40
KALE, FRESH, COOKED	1 cup chopped	53
KIWIFRUIT	1 large	68
MANGO	1 cup sliced	46
ORANGE JUICE, FRESH SQUEEZED	1 cup	124
ORANGE	1 navel	80
PAPAYA	1 cup cubes	87
POTATO, WHITE, BAKED, WITH SKIN	1 medium	26
RED BELL PEPPER, RAW	½ cup chopped	142
STRAWBERRIES, FRESH	1 cup sliced	94
TOMATO, FRESH, FULLY RIPE	1 medium	24

poultry, fish, eggs, and dairy products—that is, foods from animal sources. Strict vegetarians can get B12 from soy products, such as soy milk, that are fortified with this vitamin.

VITAMIN C (ASCORBIC ACID): This water-soluble vitamin is an important ANTIOXIDANT. It helps the body build new cells and repair damaged ones, and promotes the absorption of dietary iron. Researchers are investigating vitamin C as a line of defense against many diseases, including several types of cancer, heart disease, cataracts, and the common cold. The body does not produce vitamin C and does not retain stores of the vitamin for very long, so you should eat C-rich foods often. Most fruits and vegetables have some C, and the following are particularly rich in this important nutrient: citrus fruits and juices, strawberries, kiwifruit, cabbage, peppers, melon, broccoli, and potatoes.

VITAMIN D: A fat-soluble vitamin, D works in concert with calcium and phosphorus to build and maintain strong bones and teeth. This makes it a crucial nutrient in the prevention of osteoporosis. Vitamin D may also reduce the risk of colon cancer. When your skin is exposed to sunshine, it causes your body to produce vitamin D; however, in the winter in northern latitudes, you may not be exposed to enough sun to synthesize sufficient amounts of the vitamin. You can also get vitamin D from foods, notably milk, which has vitamin D added to it. This vitamin is also found in fatty fish, such as salmon, mackerel, and herring, and in some enriched cereals.

VITAMIN E (TOCOPHEROL): A potent ANTIOXIDANT, vitamin E is a fat-soluble vitamin. Research indicates that vitamin E helps prevent heart disease, in part by reducing the harmful effects of LDL CHOLESTEROL, and by preventing blood clots. Vitamin E is also under investigation as a treatment for osteoarthritis. Vitamin E is found in some fatty foods, including vegetable oils, avocados, nuts, and seeds, but also in brown rice and dark leafy greens. However, it is almost impossible to get sufficient vitamin E from food to have an antioxidant effect; many health authorities recommend supplements.

VITAMIN K: This fat-soluble vitamin facilitates blood clotting; it may also play a role in calcium absorption, thus helping to prevent osteoporosis. The body makes most of the vitamin K it needs, but K is also found in dark leafy greens, broccoli, Brussels sprouts, and many other fruits and vegetables.

W **WATER:** Although not a nutrient, water plays a vital role in many body processes, making possible the functions of every cell and organ. Water lubricates the joints, rids the body of waste, and regulates body temperature. You need two to three quarts (eight to twelve 8-ounce glasses) of water just to replace what's lost through normal body functions. Of course, you don't need to take in all this liquid by drinking water: You also replenish fluids with other beverages, such as milk or juice, and by eating foods (such as soups and most fruits and vegetables), that have a high water content. Because fiber absorbs water, anyone who eats lots of fiber (and almost everyone should) also needs to drink plenty of fluids.

Z **ZEAXANTHIN:** One of the CAROTENOIDS, zeaxanthin, like LUTEIN, may help prevent age-related macular degeneration, the leading cause of blindness in the elderly. Kale and broccoli are two good sources of zeaxanthin.

ZINC: An important MINERAL with many functions, zinc is involved in cell division, repair, and growth, as well as immune function, and keeps your senses of taste and smell working properly. A Dutch study suggests that high zinc levels are associated with a reduced risk of cancer. Zinc deficiency is rare, although it is sometimes seen in vegans (vegetarians who eat no animal products at all, including dairy products or eggs). Slight zinc deficiencies have also been noted in elderly people. Good sources of zinc include seafood, meat, eggs, and dairy products.

Since ancient times, food has been used to prevent and cure disease. Recently, this concept has been seen in a whole new light, thanks to research that has shown that many substances in foods—from vitamins and minerals to fiber and phytochemicals—play roles in disease prevention. The recommendations in this chart are for foods that have proven or possible disease-fighting qualities. It is not meant as a prescription and definitely not as a list of cures for diseases. Consult your physician or a nutritionist for personal advice before making dramatic changes in your diet.

Disorder	Consume plenty of
ACNE	Carrots, cantaloupe, and dark leafy greens for vitamin A. Poultry and fish for zinc. Yogurt for its active cultures.
ANEMIA (IRON DEFICIENCY)	Meat, poultry, fish, legumes, dried fruit, dark leafy greens, enriched cereals for iron. Citrus fruits, cabbage, broccoli, red bell peppers, kale, strawberries, kiwifruit for vitamin C, which enhances iron absorption. Onions, which have a similar effect.
ARTHRITIS	Seafood for omega-3 fatty acids (for rheumatoid arthritis only). Citrus fruits for vitamin C and flavonoids. Dark leafy greens, orange and yellow fruits and vegetables for beta carotene.
CANCER	Orange and yellow vegetables, tomatoes, red bell peppers, chilies; dark leafy greens, cabbage family vegetables (broccoli, Brussels sprouts, cauliflower), garlic, onions, orange fruits (apricots and nectarines), citrus (including red grapefruit), berries, grapes, watermelon, whole grains, legumes (especially soy), nuts, seafood, lean poultry, low-fat dairy products. These foods supply beta-carotene, lycopene, indoles, ellagic acid, and other phytochemicals; folate, vitamins C and E, calcium and selenium; and omega-3 fatty acids.
CATARACTS AND OTHER EYE DISORDERS	Kale, spinach, parsley, green peas, celery, carrots, sweet potatoes, potatoes, citrus fruits, kiwifruit, bananas; wheat germ and whole grains; lean meat, poultry, and fish. These supply the antioxidants lutein and beta carotene, as well as vitamins C and E, the B vitamins, zinc, and selenium.
COLDS	Citrus fruits, strawberries, kiwifruit, red bell peppers, broccoli, and cabbage for vitamin C. Chilies for capsaicin. Onions and garlic as decongestants. Whole grains, legumes, seafood, and meat for zinc.
CONSTIPATION AND OTHER INTESTINAL ILLS	Whole-grain breads and cereals, fruits (including prunes, figs, and other dried fruits), and vegetables (especially root vegetables) for insoluble fiber.
DIABETES	Plenty of whole grains, fruits, and vegetables; moderate portions of lean meat, poultry and fish—these add up to a low-fat, high-fiber diet, and weight control is a prime factor in diabetes prevention.

Disorder	Consume plenty of
HEART DISEASE	Fruits (including citrus, berries, apples), vegetables (including dark leafy greens), legumes, wheat germ, whole grains (including oats), nuts, unsaturated oils, low-fat dairy products, tofu, seafood. These supply the antioxidant vitamins C and E, as well as soluble and insoluble fiber, calcium, and omega-3 fatty acids. Garlic, ginger, onions, chilies, grapes, and wine supply heart-healthy phytochemicals.
HIGH BLOOD PRESSURE	Low-fat dairy products (including vitamin D-fortified products), dark leafy greens, and tofu for calcium. Fruits and vegetables (including bananas, avocados, dried apricots, potatoes, and tomato sauce) for potassium. Citrus fruits, strawberries, kiwifruit, and red bell peppers for vitamin C. Garlic, onions, and celery for their phytochemicals. Fish and shellfish for omega-3 fatty acids. And follow an overall low-fat diet for weight control.
HIGH CHOLESTEROL	Fruit (including citrus fruits—especially grapefruit—apples, blackberries, raspberries, bananas, dried apricots, and figs), oat bran, barley, carrots, and legumes (especially soybeans) for soluble fiber. A wide variety of other fruits and vegetables for their antioxidant powers. Low-fat dairy products for calcium; milk for vitamin D. Unsaturated vegetable oils (in place of—not in addition to—saturated fats). Garlic, onions, and their relatives also seem to lower cholesterol. Alcohol—in moderate amounts—raises HDL, or "good" cholesterol.
HIGH TRIGLYCERIDES	Fish and seafood for omega-3 fatty acids. Chilies for capsaicin.
OSTEOPOROSIS	Dairy products, canned fish with bones, and dark leafy greens for calcium. Grapes, apples, and pears for boron. Whole grains and nuts for magnesium and manganese. Fortified milk, fish, and enriched cereals for vitamin D and phosphorus. Poultry, lean meat, and beans for phosphorus.
STROKE	Fruits and vegetables for vitamin C and other antioxidants. Fish for omega-3s. Nuts and seeds for vitamin E. Fruit for potassium and soluble fiber. Garlic for its phytochemicals, which lower blood pressure.
TOOTH DECAY AND GUM DISEASE	Dairy products, leafy greens, and canned salmon and sardines (with their bones) for calcium. Citrus fruits and buckwheat for bioflavonoids (phytochemicals). Cheddar cheese, cherries, apples, tea, and grape juice help fight decay after you eat sugary foods. Crisp fruits and vegetables act as natural "toothbrushes" and supply vitamin C.
URINARY TRACT INFECTION	Cranberries and blueberries contain substances that fight UTIs. Eat other fruits and vegetables for vitamin C. Drink plenty of water.
WEIGHT CONTROL	Complex carbohydrates and fresh fruits and vegetables for energy, vitamins, minerals, and a feeling of fullness without fat. Low-fat dairy products, lean poultry, and fish for protein. Drink plenty of water.

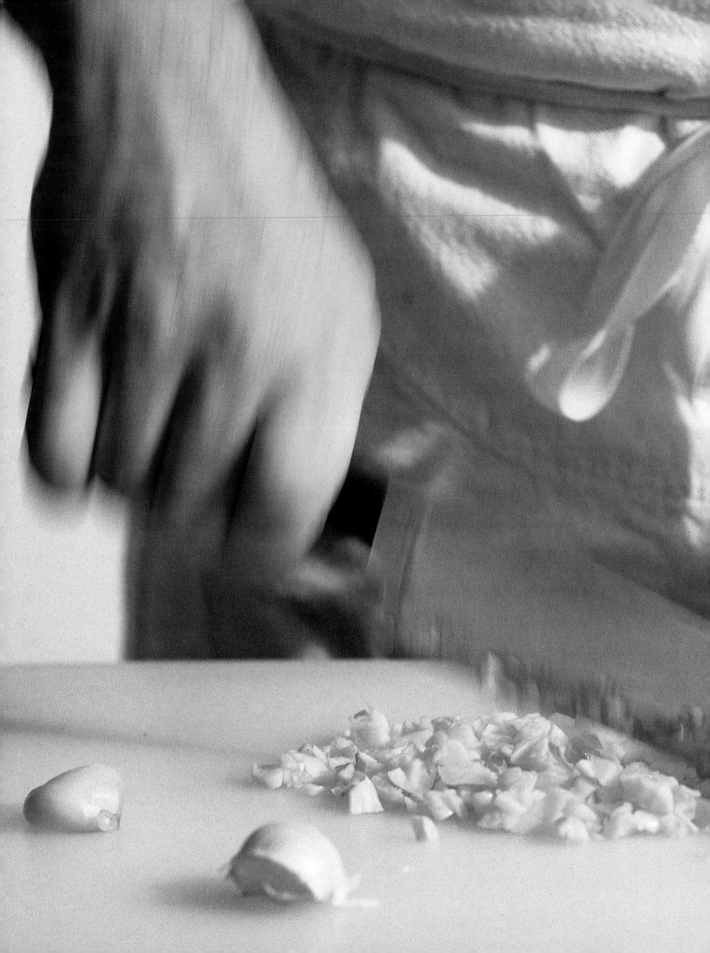

Techniques

ROASTING BELL PEPPERS

1 ▶

It's easy to roast and peel peppers if you cut them into flat sections. Start by cutting off the top and bottom.

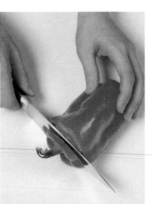

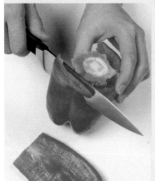

◀ 2

Cut the pepper into flat panels; remove the seeds and ribs from the inside of each piece. Place the pieces, skin-side up, on a broiler pan and broil until the skin is well charred.

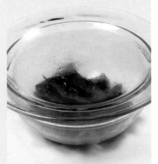

3 ▶

Place the charred peppers in a bowl and cover with a plate; let the peppers steam for a few minutes to loosen the skins.

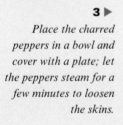

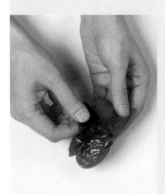

◀ 4

After steaming, the charred skin will pull off easily. If not, scrape the pepper with a knife.

PEELING TOMATOES

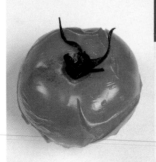

◀ 1

To peel tomatoes, drop them into a big pot of boiling water; blanch for about 20 seconds, or until the skin splits.

2 ▶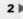

Lift the tomatoes out of the boiling water and let stand for a minute or so to cool; then peel off the loosened skin with your fingers.

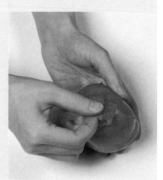

SOFTENING SUN-DRIED TOMATOES

◀ 1

Reconstitute sun-dried tomatoes by soaking them in boiling water. Let stand for 5 to 10 minutes, or until softened.

2 ▶

Drain the tomatoes; save the liquid for use in the recipe, or in a soup or sauce. Use scissors to snip the tomatoes into strips or dice.

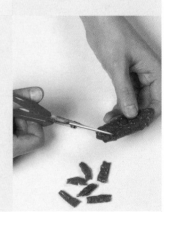

CUTTING CARROTS INTO JULIENNE

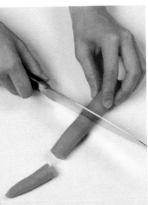

1 ▶

First cut the carrot (or zucchini, summer squash, celery, etc.) into 2-inch lengths.

◀ 2

Then cut the 2-inch pieces lengthwise into ¼-inch-thick slices.

3 ▶

Finally, cut the slices into julienne strips that are about ¼ inch wide.

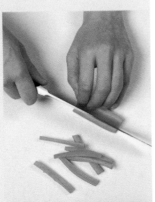

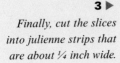

CUTTING ZUCCHINI INTO RIBBONS

◀ 1

Slice zucchini or summer squash into ribbons with a vegetable peeler. To serve, steam or blanch the ribbons, then sauté briefly.

STEAMING VEGETABLES

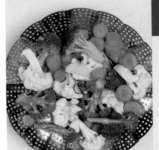

◀ 1

Steaming is one of the most healthful ways to cook vegetables. This inexpensive collapsible steamer is widely available.

2 ▶

This is an Asian bamboo steamer. It comes with its own lid and is used over a wok. Place a shallow layer of vegetables in the bottom of the steamer; don't fill it.

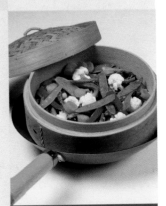

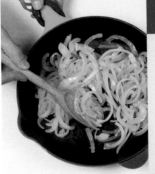

CARAMELIZING ONIONS

◀ 1

Cook thinly sliced onions, covered, over medium heat, stirring often, for 10 minutes, or until very soft.

2 ▶

Uncover the pan and cook, stirring occasionally, for 10 minutes longer, or until the onions are nicely browned but still soft. Adding a pinch of sugar to the onions will speed the process.

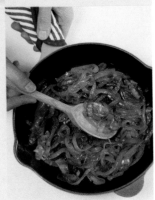

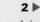

PREPARING ASPARAGUS

1 ▶

To remove the tough end from an asparagus stalk, bend the stalk not far from the bottom. The tough part will snap off.

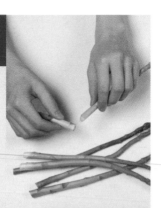

SHREDDING CABBAGE

◀ 1

Start by halving the head lengthwise, through the core. Then cut each half in half again, lengthwise.

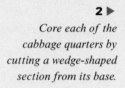

2 ▶

Core each of the cabbage quarters by cutting a wedge-shaped section from its base.

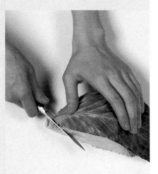

◀ 3

Cut crosswise slices from each quarter to produce strips or shreds.

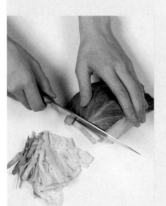

SNIPPING HERBS

◀ 1

It's easier to snip herbs, such as dill or parsley, with scissors than to chop them with a knife.

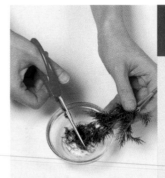

PEELING RUTABAGA

1 ▶

Rutabagas have a thick skin and a thick coat of wax. Peel off both wax and skin with a sturdy paring knife.

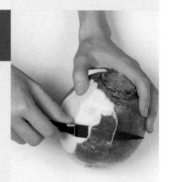

PEELING GARLIC CLOVES

◀ 1

To crack the skin, place a clove under the flat side of a knife blade (sharp edge away from you); smack blade with the heel of your hand.

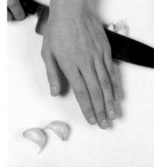

STRINGING SNOW PEAS

1 ▶

String snow peas and sugar snap peas by pinching the tips of the pods, then pulling the strings off both front and back.

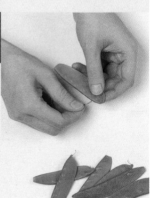

PARING CITRUS FRUIT

1 ▶

When peeling citrus fruits for use in recipes, use a paring knife to remove all of the white pith, which is bitter.

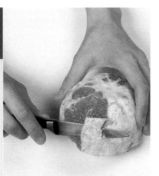

GRATING CITRUS ZEST

◀ 1

Cover the face of the grater with a sheet of plastic wrap before grating the zest; clean-up will be much easier.

JUICING CITRUS

1 ▶

You don't need an electrical appliance to squeeze citrus juice. This cheap, practical wooden reamer does the job quickly.

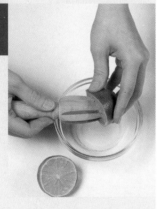

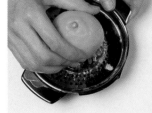

◀ 2

There are also juicers with a strainer top set into a bowl or cup to catch the juice. The container at the bottom is sometimes conveniently marked as a measuring cup.

CORING AND SLICING APPLES

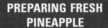

◀ 1

A timesaver when you need apple wedges, a corer-slicer does two jobs at once. Use it on a peeled or unpeeled apple.

PREPARING FRESH PINEAPPLE

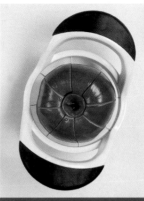

1 ▶

Delicious fresh pineapple is worth the trouble of preparing it. To start, twist off the leafy "crown."

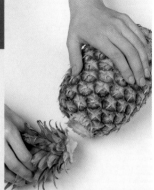

◀ 2

Stand the pineapple on the work surface and use a chef's knife to slice downward through the rind; don't cut too deeply or you'll lose a lot of the fruit.

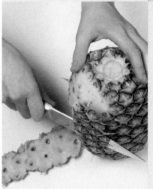

3 ▶

The "eyes" run in a fairly even diagonal pattern around the fruit. Cut long diagonal notches about ¼ inch deep around the pineapple to remove the eyes.

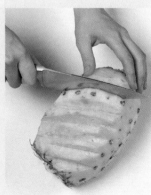

PREPARING MANGO

1 ▶

A mango has a large, flat seed in the center. To avoid it, cut away each "cheek" of the fruit, leaving the center piece intact.

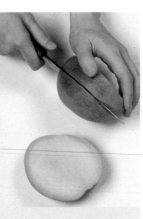

◀ 2

It's hard to peel mango flesh; try this method instead. Score the fruit into cubes, cutting to, but not through, the skin.

3 ▶

Push the skin side of the mango slice upward to turn the whole thing "inside out."

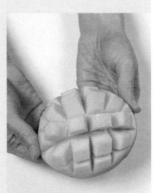

◀ 4

Then simply slice the mango cubes off the skin. (Finally, slice the remaining strip of flesh off the pit and cube it as well.)

FREEZING BERRIES

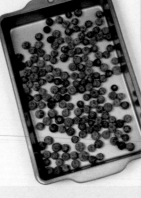

◀ 1

Freeze berries this way to keep them from crushing: Spread the berries in a shallow pan and freeze them rock-hard.

2 ▶

Then pour the frozen berries into freezer bags. For many recipes, you can use them without thawing. This method works for freezing any kind of berries.

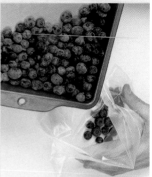

ADDING CORNSTARCH TO FRUIT SAUCE

◀ 1

For a glossy sauce, stir a mixture of cornstarch and cold water into cooked fruit. Simmer, stirring gently.

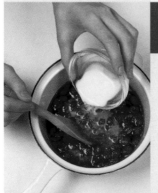

2 ▶

In a few minutes the juices will be glossy and thick. Remove the sauce from the heat as soon as it thickens since overcooking can "break" the sauce.

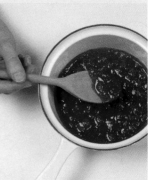

BAKING BREAD

1 ▶

Dissolve yeast in warm water to which a little sugar has been added. If the yeast is properly "live," the mixture will foam.

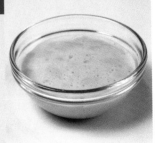

◀ 2

To knead dough, push into it with the heel of your hand to stretch it away from you. Fold back the stretched portion, then give the dough a quarter turn. Repeat until the dough is smooth and elastic.

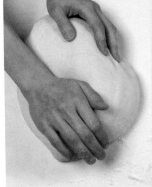

3 ▶

Let the dough rise, covered, in a warm, draft-free spot. When the dough is doubled in size and does not spring back when poked with your fingers, punch it down with your fist.

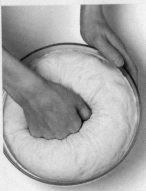

◀ 4

If making a conventional loaf, shape the dough into a rectangle whose width matches the pan's length, then fold in the sides and place the loaf in the pan seam-side down. Set aside to rise.

TRANSFERRING DOUGH TO PIE PLATE

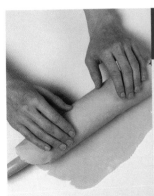

◀ 1

When the pie dough is rolled out to the proper size, roll the dough partway onto the pin, using a light touch.

2 ▶

Carefully place the rolling pin over the pie plate so that the edge of the dough hangs over about 1 inch. Unroll the dough, then press it gently into the plate.

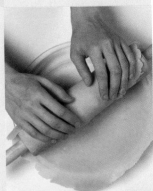

TOASTING NUTS

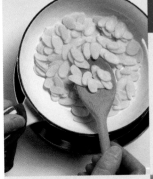

◀ 1

Toast nuts in a dry skillet over moderate heat, stirring and shaking the pan frequently, for 5 to 7 minutes.

2 ▶

When the nuts are a light golden color and fragrant, immediately turn them out of the pan, or they will overcook from the skillet's retained heat.

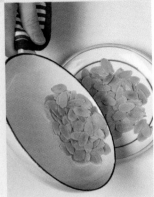

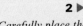

MAKING LOW-FAT WHIPPED "CREAM"

1 ▶

Soften gelatin in water in a heatproof cup. Place the cup in simmering water for about 2 minutes to dissolve the gelatin; cool.

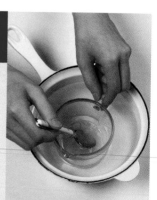

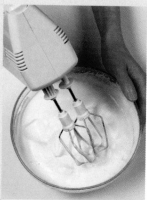

◀ 2

For maximum volume, pre-chill evaporated milk in a large mixing bowl for 30 minutes in the freezer. Then begin beating at medium speed. Beat until the milk is foamy.

3 ▶

Increase the mixer speed to high and beat until the milk holds soft peaks when the beaters are lifted (with mixer turned off). If the recipe requires it, continue beating until stiff peaks form.

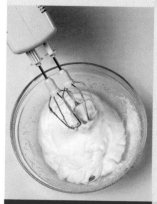

◀ 4

Fold the cooled gelatin mixture into the milk. Then chill the whipped milk in the refrigerator for 15 minutes, or until you can mound it with a spoon.

BEATING EGG WHITES

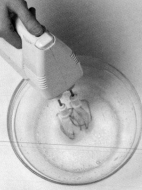

◀ 1

Have egg whites at room temperature. Use a clean, dry bowl and beaters. Starting at medium-low speed, beat until frothy.

2 ▶

Increase the mixer speed to medium and continue beating until the whites have become foamy and increased in volume.

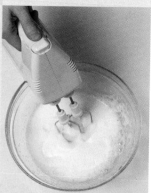

◀ 3

Continue beating, occasionally tilting the bowl and moving the beaters around to incorporate as much air as possible. Beat until egg whites are stiff but still look moist and glossy.

MAKING YOGURT CHEESE IN A COFFEE FILTER

1 ▶

You can drain the whey from yogurt in a coffee filter. In 2 hours the yogurt will be slightly thickened; in 12 hours it will be quite firm.

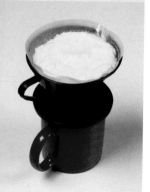

BONING SALMON FILLETS

1 ▶
Salmon fillets sometimes contain pin-bones. Pull them out with large tweezers or needle-nose pliers.

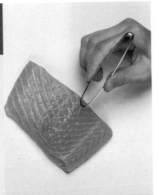

QUARTERING SCALLOPS

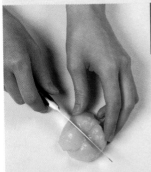

◀ 1
To use sea scallops in a recipe that calls for bay scallops, cut the sea scallops in quarters, to about bay-scallop size.

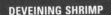

DEVEINING SHRIMP

1 ▶
You can devein shrimp with a paring knife or scissors, but these shelling and deveining tools make it even easier.

◀ 2
To shell and devein the shrimp in one stroke, slip the tool into the back of the shell and slide it toward the tail. The shell should come off in one piece.

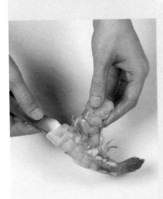

BAKING FOOD IN PACKETS

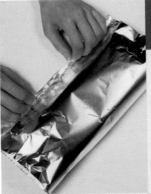

◀ 1
Place the food on one side of a sheet of foil. Fold the foil over and crimp the long edges together, leaving a little breathing room.

2 ▶
When the long side is sealed, fold over the short ends and crimp them, again leaving a little room. This seals in the moisture so that the food will steam in the oven.

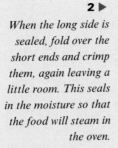

CHECKING LIVE CLAMS

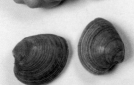

◀ 1
Before cooking clams, check to see if they're still alive by rapping them on the counter. Discard any that don't snap shut.

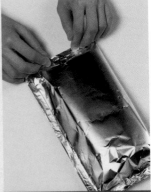

DEBEARDING MUSSELS

1 ▶
Before cooking mus-sels, scrub the shells under running water with a stiff brush and pull out the hairlike "beards."

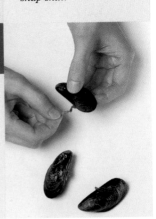

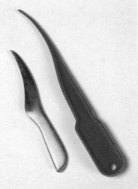

BREADING CHICKEN BREASTS

1 ▶

Rinse the chicken breasts and pat dry. Lightly beat egg whites in a shallow bowl, then dip the chicken in the egg.

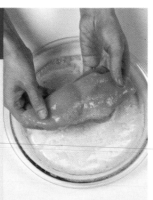

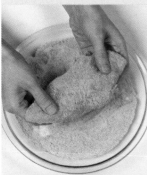

◀ 2

Shake off excess egg, then dip both sides of each chicken breast in the bread crumbs. Gently shake off any excess crumbs.

ROASTING CHICKEN

1 ▶

Rinse and dry chicken. Remove and discard the pockets of fat from the cavity. Set aside the bag of giblets for use in stocks, if desired.

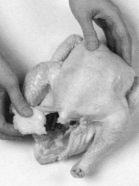

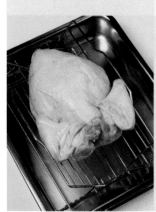

◀ 2

Place the chicken breast-side down on a rack. The rack lets the fat drain off; starting the chicken breast-side down keeps the white meat moist (turn the chicken halfway through cooking time).

DEGLAZING A ROASTING PAN

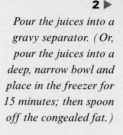

◀ 1

After roasting meat or poultry, add liquid (broth, wine, etc.) to the pan and stir to scrape the brown bits from the bottom.

2 ▶

Pour the juices into a gravy separator. (Or, pour the juices into a deep, narrow bowl and place in the freezer for 15 minutes; then spoon off the congealed fat.)

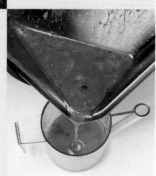

◀ 3

The gravy separator lets you pour off the juices while leaving the fat behind. To make gravy, pour the pan juices into a saucepan.

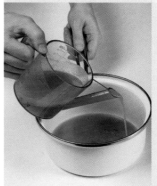

4 ▶

Add a mixture of flour and water to the pan juices, then cook, stirring, over medium heat until the gravy is thickened.

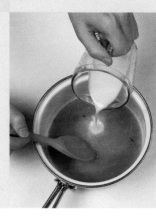

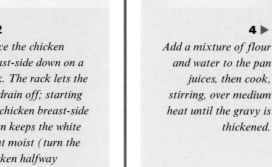

CUTTING FLANK STEAK FOR STIR-FRYING

1 ▶

A stir-fry requires meat that's cut into uniform strips. With flank steak, start by cutting the steak in half lengthwise.

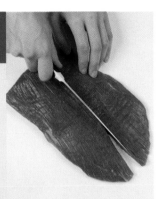

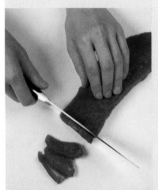

◀ 2

Then cut each half crosswise into strips about ¼ inch thick.

BROILING AND CARVING FLANK STEAK

1 ▶

Lean cuts like flank steak are best broiled on a nonstick broiler pan. (Other nonstick pans should not go under the broiler.)

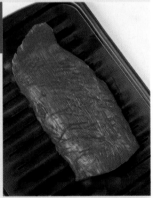

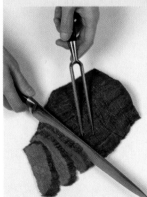

◀ 2

For truly tender flank steak, cook it only to medium-rare. Carve it across the grain, on a sharp angle to the surface.

MAKING MEDALLIONS FROM BONE-IN CHOPS

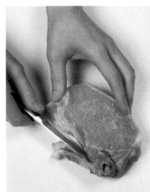

◀ 1

You can make boneless pork medallions from loin pork chops ½ to ¾ inch thick. First, cut away the bone.

2 ▶

Then trim all the fat from the edges of the chop with a paring knife.

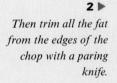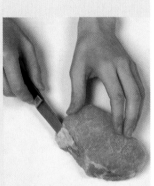

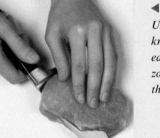

◀ 3

Using a large, sharp knife, carefully halve each pork chop horizontally to make two thin slices.

4 ▶

If the recipe calls for pork scallops, place the medallions between sheets of plastic wrap and pound with a meat mallet or small, heavy skillet to a ¼-inch thickness.

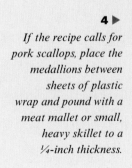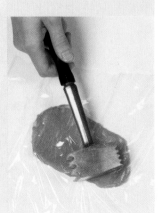

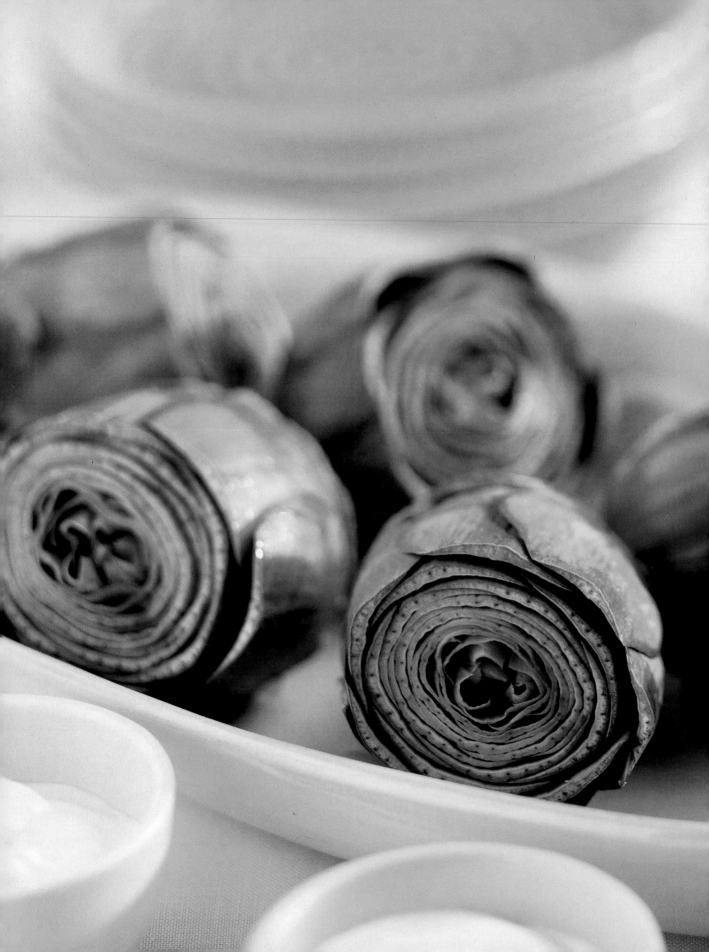

Vegetables

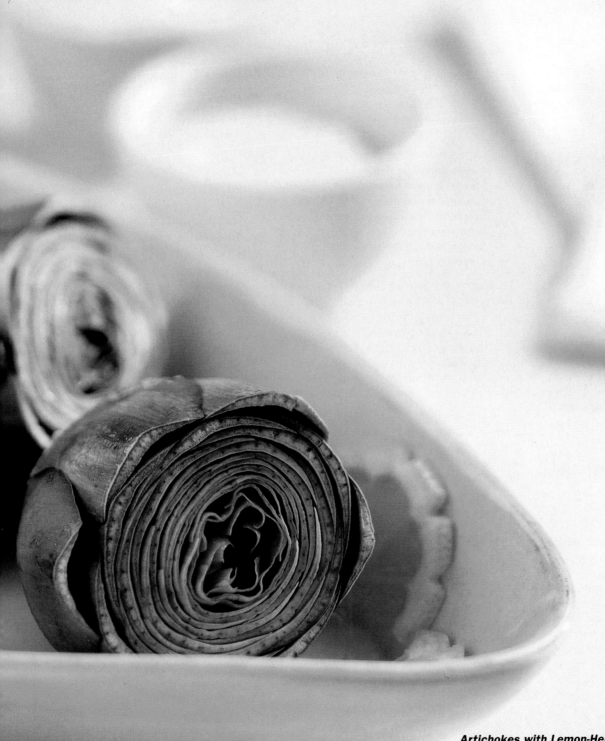

Artichokes with Lemon-Herb Mayonnaise

Artichokes

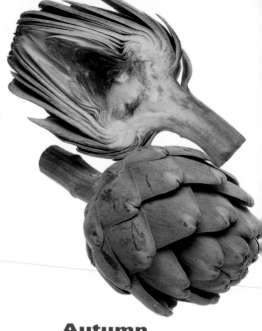

Nutritional power

Actually the bud from a thistle-like plant, artichokes are high in fiber, folate, and potassium, and supply a surprising amount of vitamin C as well.

Healthy Highlights

PER 1 LARGE	
Calories	76
Fiber	8.7g
Protein	5g
Total Fat	0.2g
Saturated Fat	0.1g
Cholesterol	0mg
Sodium	152mg

NUTRIENTS	
	% Daily Value
Vitamin C	32%
Folate	28%
Magnesium	24%
Potassium	20%
Copper	19%
Iron	11%
Vitamin B6	10%

Did you know? . . .

When artichokes are first picked, much of their carbohydrate is in the form of inulin, which is an indigestible starch. With time, though, the inulin is converted to sugar. So it's hard to be very specific about calorie counts when it comes to artichokes, but they're always quite low.

Artichokes with Lemon-Herb Mayonnaise

PREP: 30 MINUTES / COOK: 25 MINUTES

A whole artichoke is a pleasurably "slow" food to eat, making it a most convivial appetizer.

- 6 large whole artichokes
- 6 cloves garlic, peeled
- ½ teaspoon dried rosemary, crumbled
- ½ cup light mayonnaise
- 2 teaspoons grated lemon zest
- ¼ cup lemon juice
- 1 teaspoon dried tarragon
- ½ teaspoon salt

1. With a stainless-steel knife, trim the artichoke stems to about 1 inch. With your fingers, snap off any discolored leaves from the bottoms. Cut off 1 inch from the tops of the artichokes. (For a nicer presentation, cut off about ½ inch from the tops of all the remaining outer leaves.) Peel the stems.

2. Choose a pot large enough to hold a steamer basket and 6 artichokes comfortably. Fill the pot with 1 inch of water. Add the garlic and rosemary, and bring to a boil. Add the steamer basket with the artichokes, cover, and steam for 30 minutes (adding water as necessary) or until a heart is tender when pierced with a knife. Set the artichokes upside down to drain. Discard the garlic and rosemary.

3. Meanwhile, in a small bowl, combine the mayonnaise, lemon zest, lemon juice, tarragon, and salt. Serve the hot steamed artichokes with the dipping sauce. Serves 6.

Per serving: Calories 153; Fiber 9g; Protein 6g; Total Fat 7g; Saturated Fat 1g; Cholesterol 7mg; Sodium 582mg

Autumn Artichoke Stew

PREP: 15 MINUTES / COOK: 30 MINUTES

Frozen artichoke hearts are a great timesaver and, unlike marinated artichokes, they have no added oil or salt.

- 2 teaspoons olive oil
- 1 onion, finely chopped
- 2 cloves garlic, minced
- 2 large carrots, halved lengthwise and thinly sliced
- 2 ounces ham, finely chopped
- 2 packages (9 ounces each) frozen artichoke hearts
- ½ cup dry red wine or chicken broth
- ⅔ cup chicken broth
- ½ teaspoon dried thyme
- ¼ teaspoon salt
- ¼ cup chopped parsley
- 2 teaspoons unsalted butter

1. In a large nonstick skillet, heat the oil over moderate heat. Add the onion and garlic, and sauté for 7 minutes or until the onion is soft. Add the carrots and ham, and cook for 4 minutes or until the carrots are crisp-tender.

2. Stir in the artichoke hearts and cook for 3 minutes. Add the wine, bring to a boil, and cook for 3 minutes or until the liquid is reduced by half.

3. Add the broth, ⅔ cup of water, the thyme, and salt, and return to a boil. Reduce to a simmer and cook, uncovered, for 12 minutes, or until the arti-

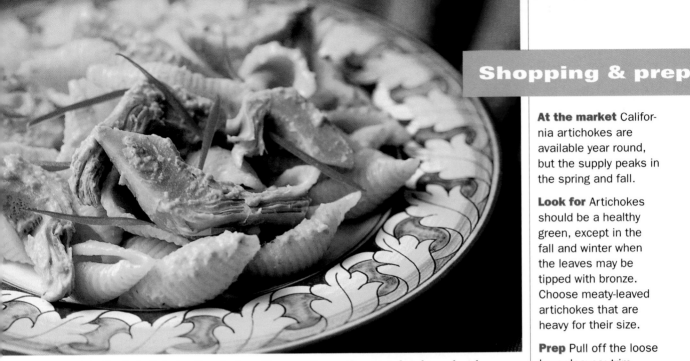

Pasta Shells & Artichoke Hearts in a Creamy Green Sauce is brightened with thin slivers of crisp red bell pepper.

At the market California artichokes are available year round, but the supply peaks in the spring and fall.

Look for Artichokes should be a healthy green, except in the fall and winter when the leaves may be tipped with bronze. Choose meaty-leaved artichokes that are heavy for their size.

Prep Pull off the loose lower leaves; trim stem to about 1 inch. Slice about 1 inch off the top of the artichoke.

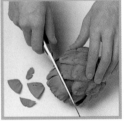

Trimming the top of the artichoke eliminates some of the sharp, inedible leaf tips.

Basic cooking Steam whole artichokes in a steamer basket over boiling water for 20 to 40 minutes, or until an inner petal can easily be pulled out. To microwave, rinse but do not dry the artichokes, then wrap individually in plastic wrap and cook at high, allowing 9 to 15 minutes for 4 artichokes. Let stand for 3 minutes, then check for doneness as above.

---

choke hearts are tender. Add the chopped parsley and butter, stirring to melt the butter. Serves 4.

Per serving: Calories 154; Fiber 10g; Protein 7g; Total Fat 7g; Saturated Fat 2g; Cholesterol 13mg; Sodium 580mg

---

Pasta Shells & Artichoke Hearts in a Creamy Green Sauce

PREP: 10 MINUTES / COOK: 20 MINUTES

This fiber-rich dinner dish features a light, clean-tasting sauce made from peas. The sauce is enriched with a touch of reduced-fat sour cream.

- 1 **tablespoon olive oil**
- 4 **cloves garlic, minced**
- 2 **packages (9 ounces each) frozen artichoke hearts, thawed**
- ¾ **cup chicken broth**
- 8 **ounces medium pasta shells**
- 1 **cup frozen peas, thawed**
- 1 **tablespoon lemon juice**
- ½ **teaspoon dried tarragon**
- ½ **teaspoon each salt and black pepper**
- ¼ **cup reduced-fat sour cream**
- 2 **teaspoons flour**
- ¼ **cup finely slivered red bell pepper**

1. In a large skillet, heat the oil over moderate heat. Add the garlic and sauté for 1 minute. Add the artichoke hearts and cook, stirring, for 1 minute or until well coated. Add the broth and ¾ cup of water, and bring to a boil. Reduce to a simmer, cover, and cook for 15 minutes or until the artichokes are tender.

2. Meanwhile, in a large pot of boiling water, cook the pasta according to package directions until firm-tender. Drain, reserving ¼ cup of the pasta cooking liquid.

3. In a food processor, combine the reserved pasta cooking liquid, the peas, lemon juice, tarragon, salt, and black pepper, and process until smooth. Pour the sauce into the skillet with the artichokes and bring to a boil.

4. In a small bowl, whisk together the sour cream and flour. Stir the sour cream mixture into the skillet and cook for 1 minute or until the sauce is lightly thickened. Pour over the hot pasta, tossing to combine. Sprinkle with the slivered red bell pepper. Serves 2 to 3.

Per serving: Calories 359; Fiber 11g; Protein 14g; Total Fat 7g; Saturated Fat 2g; Cholesterol 5mg; Sodium 584mg

Asparagus

Nutritional power
Asparagus is an impressive source of folate. It also provides vitamin C, beta carotene, and alpha carotene.

Healthy Highlights

PER 1 CUP COOKED	
Calories	43
Fiber	2.9g
Protein	5g
Total Fat	0.6g
Saturated Fat	0.1g
Cholesterol	0mg
Sodium	20mg

NUTRIENTS	
	% Daily Value
Folate	66%
Vitamin C	32%
Vitamin A	19%
Thiamin	15%
Manganese	14%
Riboflavin	14%

Did you know? . . . Throw out the water after cooking asparagus and you discard nutrients, too. So try to include the cooking liquid in the dish (as in the Bisque recipe at right).

If stored at room temperature, fresh asparagus will lose as much as half of its vitamin C within two days. The vegetable's delicate taste and texture will suffer as well.

Creamy Asparagus & Sweet Potato Bisque

PREP: 15 MINUTES / COOK: 35 MINUTES

- 1½ pounds asparagus, trimmed and cut into 1-inch lengths (trimmings reserved)
- 1 large sweet potato (8 ounces), peeled and cut into ½-inch cubes
- 2 teaspoons olive oil
- 1 onion, halved and thinly sliced
- 2 tablespoons flour
- 1 cup chicken broth
- ½ teaspoon dried marjoram
- ⅛ to ¼ teaspoon cayenne pepper
- ½ teaspoon salt
- ¾ cup low-fat (1%) milk
- 3 ounces baked ham, finely diced

1. In a medium pot, bring 2½ cups of water to a boil. Add 8 of the asparagus tips and cook 2 minutes to blanch. Remove with a slotted spoon and set aside for garnish.

2. Add the sweet potato to the boiling water and cook for 10 minutes or until tender. Remove with a strainer or slotted spoon. Add the asparagus trimmings, reduce to a simmer, cover, and cook for 10 minutes. Reserving the liquid, strain and discard the trimmings. You should have 2 cups of liquid.

3. Meanwhile, in a medium saucepan, heat the oil over moderately low heat. Add the onion and sauté for 7 minutes

or until light golden. Stir in the flour until well coated. Add the reserved cooking liquid, the broth, the remaining asparagus, the marjoram, cayenne, and salt, and bring to a boil. Reduce to a simmer, cover, and cook for 7 minutes or until the asparagus are tender.

4. Transfer the mixture to a food processor and process to a smooth purée. Return the purée to the pan and stir in the milk, ham, and sweet potato. Cook for 2 minutes or until heated through. Serve the soup garnished with the reserved asparagus tips. Serves 4.

Per serving: Calories 194; Fiber 4g; Protein 13g; Total Fat 6g; Saturated Fat 2g; Cholesterol 14mg; Sodium 889mg

Linguine with Roasted Asparagus & Pecans

PREP: 10 MINUTES / COOK: 20 MINUTES

Toasted pecans add a crunchy accent to pasta tossed with tender asparagus and a creamy lemon sauce. Roasting the asparagus intensifies its flavor.

- 2 pounds asparagus, trimmed and cut into 1-inch lengths
- 1 tablespoon olive oil
- ¼ cup pecan halves
- 8 ounces linguine
- 2 cloves garlic, minced
- 3 tablespoons reduced-fat sour cream
- ⅓ cup chicken broth
- ½ teaspoon grated lemon zest
- ½ teaspoon salt
- ¼ teaspoon pepper

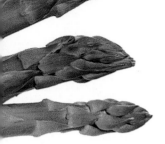

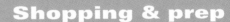
1. Preheat the oven to 450°F. Bring a large pot of water to a boil.

2. In a large glass baking dish, toss the asparagus and oil together. Bake for 15 minutes or until the asparagus are lightly browned. In a separate pan, bake the pecan halves for 5 minutes or until fragrant and lightly toasted. When cool enough to handle, chop the pecans.

3. Meanwhile, add the pasta to the boiling water and cook according to package directions until firm-tender, adding the garlic during the final 3 minutes of cooking. Drain the pasta and transfer to a large bowl.

4. In a small bowl, combine the sour cream, broth, lemon zest, salt, and pepper. Add the sour cream mixture to the pasta, tossing to coat. Add the asparagus (and any juices from the baking dish) and the pecans, tossing gently to combine. Serves 4.

Per serving: Calories 359; Fiber 4g; Protein 16g; Total Fat 11g; Saturated Fat 2g; Cholesterol 4mg; Sodium 375mg

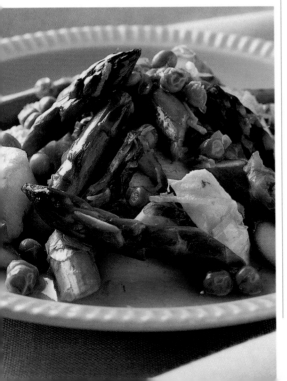

Asparagus & Chicken Stir-Fry

PREP: 15 MINUTES / COOK: 10 MINUTES

Stir-fries can feature all sorts of flavors; soy sauce is not a requirement. Here, the taste of the vegetables themselves predominates, subtly underscored by the lemon zest.

- 1 tablespoon olive oil
- 3 scallions, thinly sliced
- ¾ pound skinless, boneless chicken breasts, cut across the grain into ½-inch-wide pieces
- 1½ pounds asparagus, trimmed and cut into 2-inch lengths
- 1 cup frozen peas
- ½ cup chicken broth
- ½ teaspoon grated lemon zest
- ¼ teaspoon salt
- 3 radishes, cut into thin matchsticks
- 1 teaspoon cornstarch blended with 1 tablespoon water

1. In a large skillet, heat 2 teaspoons of the oil over moderate heat. Add the scallions and sauté for 1 minute or until they are wilted. Add the chicken and sauté for 3 minutes or until it is no longer pink.

2. Add the remaining 1 teaspoon oil and the asparagus, and sauté for 2 minutes to coat the asparagus.

3. Add the peas, broth, ½ cup of water, the lemon zest, and salt, and bring to a boil. Reduce to a simmer and cook, uncovered, for 2 minutes or until the chicken and asparagus are just cooked through.

4. Stir in the radishes and the cornstarch mixture, and cook, stirring, for 1 minute or until the sauce is lightly thickened. Serves 4.

Per serving: Calories 199; Fiber 3g; Protein 27g; Total Fat 5g; Saturated Fat 1g; Cholesterol 49mg; Sodium 368mg

***Asparagus & Chicken Stir-Fry** teams plump asparagus with tender chicken breast, green peas, and radishes.*

At the market
Although imported asparagus may be available in the autumn and winter, local crops, sold from spring through midsummer, will be fresher and tastier.

Look for Asparagus should be a bright spring green. Whether fat or skinny, stalks should be full and round, trimmed ends moist, and buds tight and unwilted.

Prep Hold each stalk with both hands, close to the base, then bend the stalk until it snaps. The stalk should break where the tough part begins.

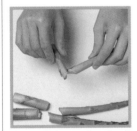

Snap off the tough ends of asparagus stalks; discard or use to flavor broth.

Basic cooking Steam whole stalks for 3 to 5 minutes, or until the thickest part is tender. To microwave 1 pound of asparagus, arrange stalks in shallow dish with tips toward center. Add ¼ cup water, cover, and cook at high for 5 to 7 minutes. Let stand, covered, for 5 minutes.

Beets

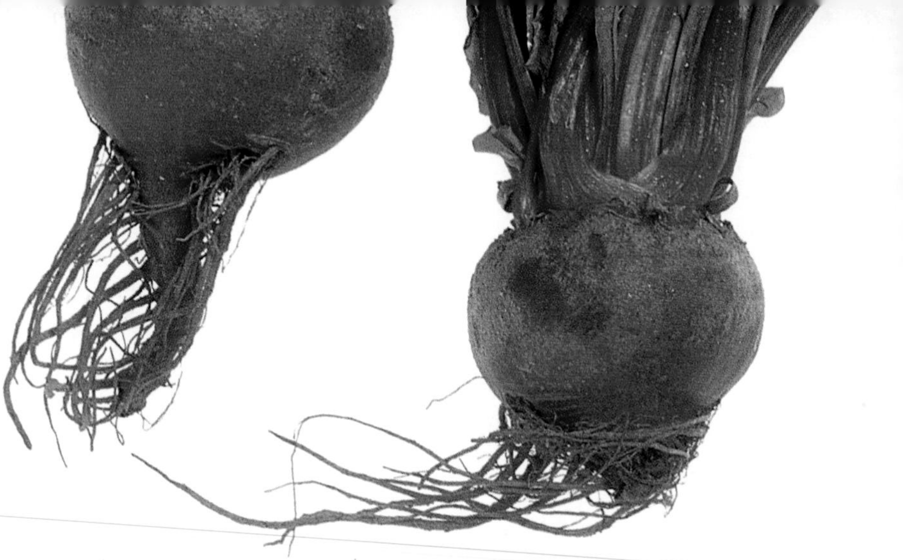

Nutritional power
Deliciously sweet (yet low in calories), beets provide significant amounts of folate, vitamin C, potassium, and other minerals.

Healthy Highlights

PER 1 CUP COOKED

Calories	75
Fiber	3.4g
Protein	3g
Total Fat	0.3g
Saturated Fat	0g
Cholesterol	0mg
Sodium	131mg

NUTRIENTS

	% Daily Value
Folate	34%
Manganese	28%
Potassium	17%
Vitamin C	10%

Did you know? . . .
If you buy beets with nice fresh tops, cook those greens as you would spinach or kale. They're rich in vitamin C, calcium, and iron.

Beets, like Brussels sprouts, contain a substance that hinders thiamin absorption—but this won't be a problem for anyone with a balanced diet.

Beet & Watercress Salad with Walnuts

PREP: 15 MINUTES
COOK: 1 HOUR 15 MINUTES

To save time, microwave the beets (see "Basic cooking") rather than roasting them.

2½	pounds fresh beets
½	teaspoon grated orange zest
½	cup orange juice
1	tablespoon no-salt-added tomato paste
1	tablespoon olive oil
½	teaspoon Dijon mustard
½	teaspoon salt
4	cups packed watercress, large stems trimmed
¼	cup coarsely chopped walnuts

1. Preheat the oven to 450°F. Wrap each beet separately in foil. Place on a baking sheet and bake for 1 hour and 15 minutes or until the beets are tender.

2. Unwrap the beets and when cool enough to handle, using a paper towel to keep your hands from getting stained, slip the beets out of their skins. Cut each beet into 8 wedges.

3. In a medium bowl, whisk together the orange zest, orange juice, tomato paste, oil, mustard, and salt. Add the beets, watercress, and walnuts, tossing well to combine. Serve at room temperature or chilled. Serves 4.

Per serving: Calories 184; Fiber 3g; Protein 5g; Total Fat 8g; Saturated Fat 1g; Cholesterol 0mg; Sodium 443mg

Chunky Beet, Potato & Beef Soup

PREP: 30 MINUTES / COOK: 35 MINUTES

Here's a healthy, hearty version of borscht, the famous eastern European beet soup. You can make it ahead of time and reheat it.

2	teaspoons olive oil
6	scallions, thinly sliced
4	cloves garlic, minced
2½	pounds fresh beets, peeled and cut into ½-inch cubes
¾	pound all-purpose potatoes, peeled and cut into ½-inch cubes
2	carrots, thinly sliced
¼	cup red wine vinegar
4	teaspoons sugar
1	teaspoon salt
¼	teaspoon pepper
¾	pound well-trimmed beef sirloin, cut into ¼-inch chunks
¼	cup reduced-fat sour cream

1. In a large saucepan, heat the oil over moderate heat. Add the scallions and garlic, and sauté for 2 minutes or until the scallions are tender.

2. Add the beets, potatoes, carrots, vinegar, sugar, salt, pepper, and 4½ cups of water. Bring to a boil, reduce to a simmer, cover, and cook for 30 minutes or until the beets and potatoes are tender. Add the beef and cook for 3 minutes or until just cooked through. Serve topped with a dollop of sour cream. Serves 4.

Per serving: Calories 335; Fiber 5g; Protein 24g; Total Fat 8g; Saturated Fat 3g; Cholesterol 57mg; Sodium 765mg

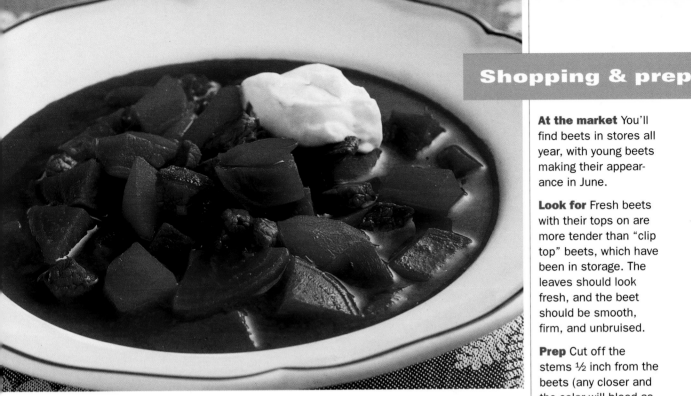

Chunky Beet, Potato & Beef Soup is a welcoming dish on a chilly winter day.

Chocolate-Spice Brownies

PREP: 10 MINUTES / COOK: 30 MINUTES

- 1½ cups flour
- 1½ teaspoons baking powder
- ¼ teaspoon baking soda
- 1 teaspoon cinnamon
- ¼ teaspoon grated nutmeg
- ¼ teaspoon salt
- ½ cup plus 1 tablespoon unsweetened cocoa powder
- 1 teaspoon vanilla extract
- 1 can (14½ ounces) sliced beets, drained
- ½ cup low-fat (1.5%) buttermilk
- ½ cup granulated sugar
- ½ cup packed dark brown sugar
- 3 tablespoons vegetable oil
- 3 egg whites
- ¼ cup chopped walnuts or pecans
- ½ cup marshmallow creme

1. Preheat the oven to 350°F. Spray an 8-inch square baking pan with nonstick cooking spray; set aside.

2. On a sheet of wax paper, combine the flour, baking powder, baking soda, cinnamon, nutmeg, and salt. In a small bowl, whisk together ½ cup of the cocoa powder, ⅓ cup of warm water, and the vanilla. In a food processor, process the beets and buttermilk to a smooth purée.

3. In a large bowl, with an electric mixer, beat the granulated sugar, brown sugar, and oil until combined. Add the egg whites one at a time, beating well after each addition. Beat in the cocoa mixture and the beet purée. Fold the flour mixture into the batter. Fold in the chopped nuts.

4. Spoon the batter into the prepared pan, smoothing the top. Bake for 30 minutes or until a cake tester inserted in the center comes out just clean. Cool for 30 minutes in the pan on a rack, then invert onto the rack to cool completely.

5. Meanwhile, in a small bowl, combine the marshmallow creme, 2 teaspoons of water, and the remaining 1 tablespoon cocoa. Spread the frosting over the cooled cake, then cut into 12 brownies. Makes 12 brownies.

Per brownie: Calories 208; Fiber 2g; Protein 4g; Total Fat 6g; Saturated Fat 1g; Cholesterol 0mg; Sodium 216mg

Shopping & prep

At the market You'll find beets in stores all year, with young beets making their appearance in June.

Look for Fresh beets with their tops on are more tender than "clip top" beets, which have been in storage. The leaves should look fresh, and the beet should be smooth, firm, and unbruised.

Prep Cut off the stems ½ inch from the beets (any closer and the color will bleed as the beets cook). Scrub the beets gently but thoroughly, being careful not to nick the skin.

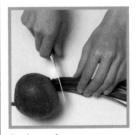

Don't cut the stems too close to the beet, or the color will bleed.

Basic cooking Bake whole beets wrapped in foil at 450° for 1 to 2 hours (time will depend on the age and size of beets). Simmer whole beets, covered, in boiling water for 40 minutes to 2 hours. Steam sliced or diced beets for 5 to 10 minutes. Microwave 1 pound whole beets with ¼ cup water, covered, for 10 minutes.

Bell peppers

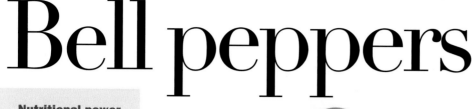

Nutritional power

Peppers—especially red ones—are a super source of vitamin C. They also contain flavonoids, which seem to fight cancer in several different ways.

Healthy Highlights

Green Bell Pepper
PER 1 CUP RAW

Calories	40
Fiber	2.7g
Protein	1g
Total Fat	0.3g
Saturated Fat	0g
Cholesterol	0mg
Sodium	3mg

NUTRIENTS

	% Daily Value
Vitamin C	222%
Vitamin A	19%
Vitamin B6	19%

Did you know? . . .
The longer a pepper ripens, the sweeter and more healthful it becomes. A red bell pepper supplies nearly 11 times the beta carotene of a green pepper—and half again as much vitamin C.

Ounce for ounce, a red bell pepper contains four times as much vitamin C as an orange.

Bread Salad with Roasted Peppers

PREP: 15 MINUTES / COOK: 20 MINUTES

If you use a regular (waxed) cucumber for this salad, be sure to peel it.

> Roasted Red Peppers (at right)
> 3   cups Italian or French bread cubes (1 inch)
> 1   large tomato, diced
> 1½ cups diced (½ inch) European cucumber
> 3   ounces feta cheese, crumbled
> ¼   cup coarsely chopped Gaeta, Calamata, or other brine-cured olives

1. Prepare the Roasted Red Peppers as directed, but omit the salt and garlic.

2. Preheat the oven to 375°F. Spread the bread cubes on a baking sheet and bake, tossing occasionally, for 7 minutes or until lightly crisped, but not browned.

3. In a large salad bowl, combine the peppers and their marinade with the toasted bread, the tomato, cucumber, feta, and olives, tossing well. Serve at room temperature or chilled. Serves 4.

Per serving: Calories 227; Fiber 4g; Protein 7g; Total Fat 12g; Saturated Fat 4g; Cholesterol 19mg; Sodium 551mg

Roasted Red Peppers

PREP: 10 MINUTES / COOK: 10 MINUTES

Roasting peppers transforms them, rendering them savory and slightly smoky-tasting. The traditional method of roasting peppers calls for holding a whole pepper directly over a flame and turning it as it chars. Here the process is considerably streamlined.

> 4   large red bell peppers, cut lengthwise into flat panels (see how-to photo)
> 2   tablespoons balsamic vinegar
> 1   tablespoon olive oil
> ¼   teaspoon salt
> 1   clove garlic, crushed and peeled

1. Preheat the broiler. Place the pepper pieces, skin-side up, on the broiler rack and broil 4 inches from the heat for 12 minutes or until the skin is blackened. When the peppers are cool enough to handle, peel them and cut into 2-inch-wide strips.

2. In a medium bowl, combine the vinegar, oil, and salt. Add the garlic and the peppers, tossing well. Cover and refrigerate for at least 1 hour or up to 3 days. Remove and discard the garlic before serving. Makes 3 cups.

Per ½ cup: Calories 39; Fiber 1g; Protein 1g; Total Fat 2g; Saturated Fat 0g; Cholesterol 0mg; Sodium 92mg

Tex-Mex Stuffed Peppers

PREP: 15 MINUTES / COOK: 25 MINUTES

- 2   red bell peppers
- 2   green bell peppers
- 4   teaspoons olive oil
- 3   scallions, thinly sliced
- 3   cloves garlic, minced
- 1   cup rice
- ½   teaspoon salt
- ½   teaspoon ground cumin
- ⅛   teaspoon cayenne pepper (optional)
- 1½ cups canned black beans, rinsed and drained
- 4   ounces Monterey jack cheese, shredded
- 2   plum tomatoes, coarsely chopped

1. Slice off the top ½ inch of each pepper at the stem end and reserve. Remove and discard the ribs and seeds. Discard the stems and finely chop the reserved pepper tops; set aside.

2. In a medium saucepan, heat the oil over moderate heat. Add the scallions and garlic, and sauté for 2 minutes or until softened. Add the chopped pepper pieces and cook, stirring occasionally, for 4 minutes or until crisp-tender.

3. Add the rice, salt, cumin, cayenne, and 2¼ cups of water. Bring to a boil, reduce to a simmer, cover, and cook for 17 minutes or until the rice is tender. Stir in the beans and cheese, and cook just until the cheese has melted and the beans are piping hot.

4. Meanwhile, in a large pot of boiling water, cook the peppers for 4 minutes or until softened. Spoon the rice mixture into the pepper halves, top with the chopped tomato, and serve. Serves 4.

Per serving: Calories 413; Fiber 6g; Protein 16g; Total Fat 14g; Saturated Fat 6g; Cholesterol 30mg; Sodium 629mg

At the market Green peppers are always available; imported red and yellow peppers, which can be quite expensive, are sold year-round, too. (Look for orange, brown, and purple peppers, as well). In the summer, seek out locally grown peppers and stock up while prices are low (seed and chop or roast the peppers, then freeze them).

Look for Peppers should be smooth, unblemished, and bright in color. Choose peppers that are heavy for their size: Hefty peppers have thick, meaty walls.

Prep If you're slicing or chopping peppers, halve them lengthwise and pull off the stem and cap; pull out the ribs and seeds with your fingers. For roasting, slice the pepper lengthwise into flat panels.

Bread Salad with Roasted Peppers *is a satisfying variation on an Italian classic.*

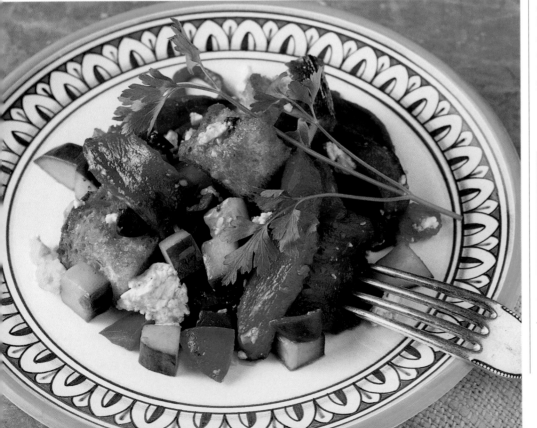

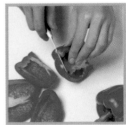

It's easier to peel roasted peppers if you stem them and cut them into relatively flat pieces instead of roasting them whole.

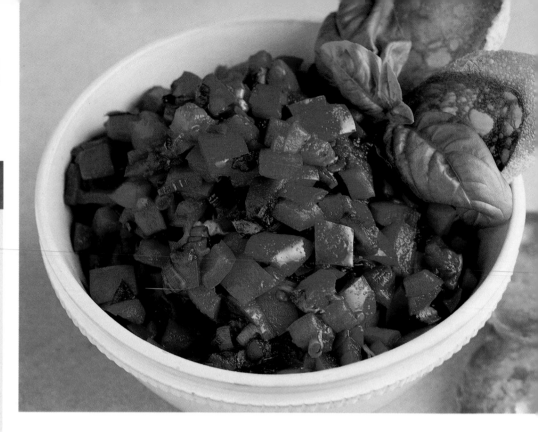

Red Pepper Relish is sweet, sour, hot, herby, and vividly colorful.

Healthy Highlights

Red Bell Pepper
PER 1 CUP RAW

Calories	40
Fiber	3.0g
Protein	1g
Total Fat	0.3g
Saturated Fat	0g
Cholesterol	0mg
Sodium	3mg

NUTRIENTS

	% Daily Value
Vitamin C	472%
Vitamin A	170%
Vitamin B6	19%

Did you know? . . .

Because of their high vitamin C content, bell peppers are a good choice to serve with iron-rich foods such as beef. The vitamin C enhances iron absorption.

You can add a lot of nutritional value to a salad (such as tuna, chicken, or pasta) by serving it in a "bowl" made from a seeded bell pepper.

Bell peppers belong to the same species as chili peppers, but sweet peppers lack the tongue-tingling heat of chilies because they do not contain capsaicin.

Pipérade

PREP: 20 MINUTES / COOK: 10 MINUTES

Here's a lightened version of a traditional bell pepper and scrambled egg dish from the Basque region of France. Extra egg whites stand in for some of the yolks, and cottage cheese adds a satisfying richness.

- 1   tablespoon olive oil
- 3   red bell peppers, cut into ¼-inch-wide strips
- 2   green bell peppers, cut into ¼-inch-wide strips
- 1   onion, halved and thinly sliced
- 4   cloves garlic, minced
- ¾   teaspoon salt
- 1   large tomato, finely chopped
- 2   eggs
- 4   egg whites
- ¼   cup low-fat (1%) cottage cheese
- 1   tablespoon flour
- ½   teaspoon black pepper

1. In a large nonstick skillet, heat the oil over moderate heat. Add the bell peppers, onion, garlic, and ¼ teaspoon of the salt, and sauté for 5 minutes or until the peppers are crisp-tender. Add the tomato and cook, stirring, for 7 minutes or until the liquid has evaporated.

2. Meanwhile, in a food processor, combine the whole eggs, egg whites, cottage cheese, flour, black pepper, and the remaining ½ teaspoon salt, and process until smooth.

3. Pour the egg mixture into the skillet, reduce the heat to low, and cook, stirring, for 3 minutes or until set. Serves 4.

Per serving: Calories 159; Fiber 3g; Protein 11g; Total Fat 6g; Saturated Fat 1g; Cholesterol 107mg; Sodium 564mg

Pepper Steak

PREP: 15 MINUTES / COOK: 10 MINUTES

- 1   tablespoon olive oil
- 4   green bell peppers, cut into ½-inch-wide strips
- 1   onion, halved and thinly sliced
- 4   cloves garlic, minced
- 1   pound well-trimmed beef sirloin, cut into ½-inch-wide strips
- ½   cup chicken broth
- 2   tablespoons sherry
- 1   tablespoon lower-sodium soy sauce
- 2   teaspoons cornstarch
- ½   teaspoon crushed red pepper flakes

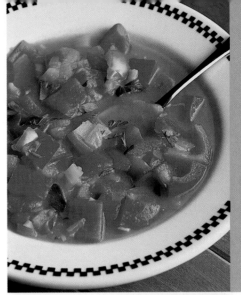

1. In a large nonstick skillet, heat 2 teaspoons of the oil over moderate heat. Add the bell peppers, onion, and garlic, and sauté for 5 minutes.

2. Add the remaining 1 teaspoon oil and the beef, and sauté for 2 minutes or until no longer pink. In a small bowl, whisk the broth, sherry, and soy sauce into the cornstarch. Stir in the red pepper flakes and ½ cup of water. Pour into the skillet, bring to a boil, and cook, stirring, for 1 minute or until lightly thickened. Serves 4.

Per serving: Calories 242; Fiber 2g; Protein 26g; Total Fat 9g; Saturated Fat 2g; Cholesterol 76mg; Sodium 352mg

Red Pepper Relish

PREP: 15 MINUTES / COOK: 20 MINUTES
CHILL: 1 HOUR

Serve this lively condiment with broiled chicken or fish and reap the benefits: A half-cup serving supplies more than three times the Daily Value for vitamin C.

- ½ **cup balsamic or red wine vinegar**
- ¼ **cup firmly packed light brown sugar**
- 4 **large red bell peppers, cut into ½-inch squares**
- 1 **large tomato, diced**
- 3 **scallions, thinly sliced**
- ½ **teaspoon salt**
- ⅛ **teaspoon cayenne pepper**
- ⅓ **cup chopped fresh basil**

1. In a medium saucepan, combine the vinegar and sugar. Bring to a boil over moderate heat, stirring to dissolve the sugar. Add the bell peppers, tomato, scallions, salt, and cayenne. Reduce to a simmer, cover, and cook for 5 minutes or until the peppers are tender.

2. Reserving the cooking liquid, drain the relish and transfer to a bowl. Return the liquid to the saucepan, bring to a boil, and cook for 5 to 10 minutes or until reduced by half. Stir in the basil. Pour the liquid over the relish and cool to room temperature. Refrigerate for at least 1 hour. Makes 3 cups.

Per ½ cup: Calories 67; Fiber 2g; Protein 1g; Total Fat 0g; Saturated Fat 0g; Cholesterol 0mg; Sodium 193mg

Pepper Soup In a covered saucepan, simmer 3 diced red bell peppers, 1 diced green bell pepper, 1 small diced onion, 2 cloves minced garlic, 1 cup chopped tomatoes, 1 cup chicken broth, 1 tsp. ground coriander, and ½ tsp. salt until flavorful. Stir in some chopped parsley. Serves 4. *[Cal 48; Fat 1g; Sod 543mg]*

Pasta with Red Pepper Sauce
In small pan of boiling water, blanch 3 cloves garlic for 2 minutes. In food processor, purée the garlic, 2 cups bottled roasted red peppers, ½ cup chicken broth, 2 tbsp. tomato paste, 1 tbsp. olive oil, and ¼ tsp. pepper. Cook 12 ounces fusilli pasta. Toss with pepper purée and sprinkle with 2 tbsp. Parmesan. Serves 4. *[Cal 394; Fat 6g; Sod 393mg]*

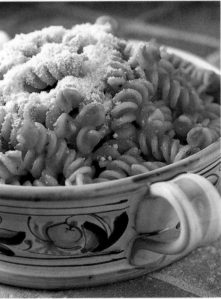

Multi-Pepper Stir-Fry
In a large nonstick skillet, sauté 2 each sliced red and yellow bell peppers, 1 sliced green bell pepper, and 2 cloves minced garlic in 1 tbsp. olive oil until crisp-tender. Add ¼ cup chopped basil, 2 tbsp. red wine vinegar, 1 tsp. sugar, and ½ tsp. salt, and cook for 2 minutes. Serves 4. *[Cal 64; Fat 4g; Sod 276mg]*

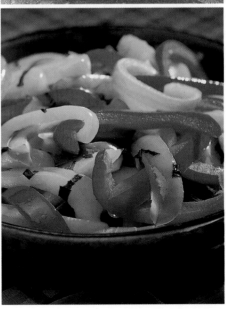

Broccoli

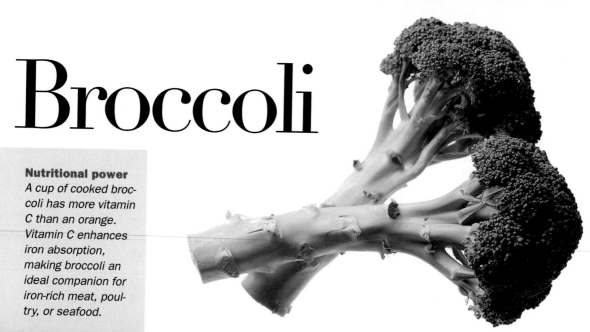

Nutritional power
A cup of cooked broccoli has more vitamin C than an orange. Vitamin C enhances iron absorption, making broccoli an ideal companion for iron-rich meat, poultry, or seafood.

Healthy Highlights

PER 1 CUP COOKED	
Calories	44
Fiber	4.5g
Protein	5g
Total Fat	0.5g
Saturated Fat	0.1g
Cholesterol	0mg
Sodium	41mg

NUTRIENTS	
	% Daily Value
Vitamin C	193%
Vitamin A	43%
Folate	20%
Manganese	17%
Potassium	15%
Riboflavin	11%
Vitamin B6	11%

Did you know? . . .
Broccoli is not only rich in disease-fighting vitamin C, it also contains phytochemicals—including beta carotene, sulforaphane, and indoles—which protect against or slow the growth of some types of cancer.

Broccoli & Barley Soup

PREP: 10 MINUTES / COOK: 35 MINUTES

- 1 tablespoon olive oil
- 1 onion, finely chopped
- 3 cloves garlic, minced
- 2 carrots, thinly sliced
- ⅔ cup quick-cooking barley
- ½ cup chicken broth
- 1 can (14½ ounces) no-salt-added stewed tomatoes
- ¾ teaspoon salt
- ½ teaspoon pepper
- ½ teaspoon dried tarragon
- 4 cups small broccoli florets

1. In a large saucepan or Dutch oven, heat the oil over moderate heat. Add the onion and garlic, and sauté for 5 minutes or until softened. Add the carrots and sauté for 4 minutes.

2. Add the barley, stirring to coat. Stir in 3½ cups of water, the broth, tomatoes, salt, pepper, and tarragon. Bring to a boil, breaking up the tomatoes with a spoon. Reduce to a simmer, cover, and cook for 20 minutes or until the barley is tender.

3. Add the broccoli and cook for 5 minutes or until just tender. Serves 4.

Per serving: Calories 222; Fiber 11g; Protein 9g; Total Fat 5g; Saturated Fat 1g; Cholesterol 0mg; Sodium 631mg

Shrimp with Broccoli, Tomatoes & Basil

PREP: 20 MINUTES / COOK: 20 MINUTES

The variety of vegetables here gives you a hearty helping of vitamin C; the broccoli, shrimp, and rice supply plenty of iron.

- 1 cup rice
- ¾ teaspoon salt
- 4 teaspoons olive oil
- 3 scallions, thinly sliced
- 3 cloves garlic, minced
- 6 cups small broccoli florets
- 2 cups cherry tomatoes, halved
- ½ cup chopped fresh basil
- ⅓ cup chicken broth
- 1 pound medium shrimp, peeled and deveined
- ¾ teaspoon cornstarch blended with 1 tablespoon water

1. In a medium saucepan, bring 2¼ cups of water to a boil. Add the rice and ¼ teaspoon of the salt, reduce to a simmer, cover, and cook for 17 minutes or until the rice is tender.

2. Meanwhile, in a large nonstick skillet, heat 1 teaspoon of the oil over moderate heat. Add the scallions and garlic, and sauté for 2 minutes or until the scallions are tender.

3. Add the remaining 1 tablespoon oil to the skillet along with the broccoli, stirring to coat. Add the tomatoes,

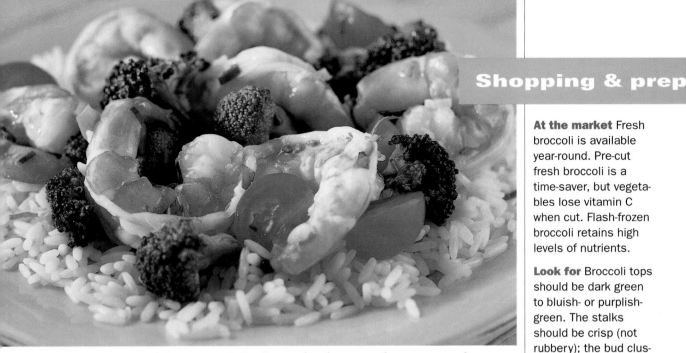

Shrimp with Broccoli, Tomatoes & Basil is perfect for a casual company meal.

basil, broth, and the remaining ½ teaspoon salt, and cook, stirring frequently, for 3 minutes or until the tomatoes begin to soften. Add the shrimp and ⅓ cup of water, and cook for 3 minutes or until the shrimp are just cooked through and the broccoli is crisp-tender.

4. Bring to a boil, add the cornstarch mixture, and cook, stirring, for 1 minute or until the sauce is lightly thickened. Spoon over the rice and serve hot. Serves 4.

Per serving: Calories 390; Fiber 8g; Protein 30g; Total Fat 8g; Saturated Fat 1g; Cholesterol 140mg; Sodium 727mg

Chicken, Broccoli & Pasta Casserole

PREP: 10 MINUTES / COOK: 40 MINUTES

Here's comfort food without the fat. We've used lean chicken breast, low-fat milk, and just one ounce of Cheddar per serving.

- **8** ounces medium pasta shells
- **3½** cups low-fat (1%) milk
- **⅓** cup flour
- **¾** teaspoon salt
- **¼** teaspoon cayenne pepper
- **2** packages (10 ounces each) frozen chopped broccoli, thawed
- **1** cup shredded Cheddar cheese (4 ounces)
- **4** skinless, boneless chicken breast halves (about 5 ounces each)
- **½** teaspoon dried rosemary, crumbled

1. Preheat the oven to 375°F. In a large pot of boiling water, cook the pasta according to package directions until firm-tender. Drain the pasta well and then transfer to a 13 x 9 x 2-inch baking dish.

2. In a medium saucepan, whisk the milk into the flour. Stir in ½ teaspoon of the salt and the cayenne. Bring to a boil over moderate heat and cook, stirring constantly, for 5 minutes or until lightly thickened. Add the broccoli and Cheddar, and cook, stirring, for 1 minute or until the cheese is melted.

3. Pour the broccoli-cheese mixture over the pasta in the baking dish. Place the chicken on top and sprinkle with the rosemary and the remaining ¼ teaspoon salt. Cover with foil and bake for 25 minutes or until the chicken is cooked through. Serves 4.

Per serving: Calories 645; Fiber 4g; Protein 59g; Total Fat 15g; Saturated Fat 8g; Cholesterol 121mg; Sodium 825mg

At the market Fresh broccoli is available year-round. Pre-cut fresh broccoli is a time-saver, but vegetables lose vitamin C when cut. Flash-frozen broccoli retains high levels of nutrients.

Look for Broccoli tops should be dark green to bluish- or purplish-green. The stalks should be crisp (not rubbery); the bud clusters should be compact, not opened or yellowed.

Prep Cut off broccoli florets of desired size and set aside. If stalks are tough, peel off outer skin before cutting up the stalks for cooking.

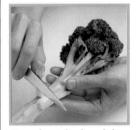

To peel, catch edge of skin between thumb and knife blade, and pull upward.

Basic cooking Steam broccoli florets for 5 to 8 minutes (stalks a bit longer). To microwave 1 pound broccoli stalks, arrange spoke-fashion, add ¼ cup water, cover, and cook at high for 6 to 10 minutes. Let stand for 3 minutes.

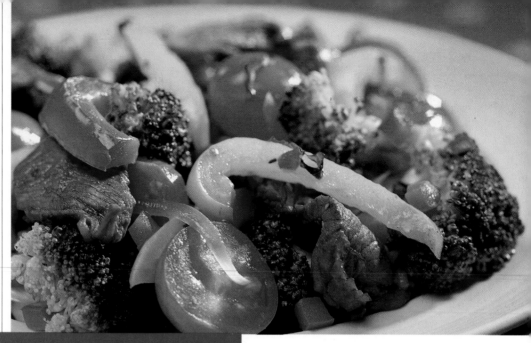

**Italic Beef &
Broccoli Sauté**

*A wealth of vege-
tables—tomatoes,
peppers, onion, and
garlic—rounds out
this family-pleasing
main dish.*

Did you know? . . .
Cooked broccoli offers
even more benefits
than raw. Cooking the
vegetable ups the
indole content by free-
ing a crucial enzyme.

The carotenoids in broccoli help fight one of the major causes of blindness in the elderly.

Broccoli contains dithi-
olthiones, which trigger
the formation of en-
zymes that may stop
carcinogens from dam-
aging DNA.

Broccoli is a rich
source of lutein and
zeaxanthin, two carot-
enoids. According to a
Harvard University
study, these sub-
stances may protect
against macular degen-
eration, the leading
cause of irreversible
blindness in adults
over 65. Lutein also
seems to offer lung
cancer protection.

There may be broccoli
sprouts in your future:
Scientists have bred
sprouts (like alfalfa
sprouts) with 30 to 50
times the concentra-
tion of cancer-fighting
phytochemicals found
in regular broccoli.

Italian Beef & Broccoli Sauté

PREP: 25 MINUTES / COOK: 20 MINUTES

3	pickled red cherry peppers
¾	pound well-trimmed beef sirloin, thinly sliced
2	tablespoons balsamic vinegar
2	cloves garlic, minced
2	teaspoons olive oil
1	red onion, thinly sliced
1	yellow or red bell pepper, slivered
6	cups small broccoli florets
¾	teaspoon dried oregano
2	cups cherry tomatoes, halved
⅓	cup chopped fresh basil
½	teaspoon salt

1. Mince one of the cherry peppers. In
a medium bowl, combine the minced
pepper, the beef, vinegar, and garlic.
Let stand for 15 minutes. Meanwhile,
dice the remaining cherry peppers.

2. In a large skillet, heat the oil over
moderate heat. Add the onion and bell
pepper, and cook for 5 minutes. Add
the broccoli and oregano, reduce the
heat to moderately low, cover, and
cook, stirring occasionally, for 10 minutes or until the broccoli is crisp-tender.

3. Push the vegetables to one side,
increase the heat to moderately high,
and add the reserved cherry peppers
and the beef and its marinade. Sauté
for 2 minutes. Add the cherry tomatoes,
basil, and salt, and sauté for 2 minutes
or until heated through. Serves 4.

*Per serving: Calories 231; Fiber 8g;
Protein 26g; Total Fat 7g; Saturated Fat 2g;
Cholesterol 52mg; Sodium 416mg*

Hearty Broccoli, Potato & Smoked Turkey Stew

PREP: 20 MINUTES / COOK: 35 MINUTES

1	tablespoon olive oil
1	large onion, finely chopped
3	cloves garlic, minced
2	carrots, cut into 1-inch lengths
¾	pound all-purpose potatoes, peeled and cut into ½-inch chunks
¾	cup chicken broth
½	teaspoon dried tarragon
¼	teaspoon pepper
1	bunch of broccoli
½	pound smoked turkey, unsliced, cut into ½-inch chunks
1	cup frozen corn kernels

1. In a large saucepan, heat the oil
over moderate heat. Add the onion and
garlic, and sauté for 7 minutes. Add the
carrots and potatoes, stirring to coat.

2. Add the broth, tarragon, pepper, and ¾ cup of water. Bring to a boil, reduce to a simmer, cover, and cook for 17 minutes or until the potatoes and carrots are almost tender.

3. Meanwhile, trim the tough stem ends of the broccoli. Cut the broccoli tops into small florets. Peel the stalks and thinly slice. Add the broccoli to the skillet, cover, and cook for 5 minutes.

4. Add the turkey and corn, and cook for 3 minutes or just until heated through. Serves 4.

Per serving: Calories 274; Fiber 9g; Protein 20g; Total Fat 7g; Saturated Fat 1g; Cholesterol 30mg; Sodium 837mg

Broccoli-Stuffed Potatoes

PREP: 10 MINUTES / COOK: 55 MINUTES

To save time, microwave the potatoes instead of baking them.

- 4 **large (8-ounce) baking potatoes**
- 1 **cup low-fat (1%) cottage cheese**
- ¼ **cup reduced-fat sour cream**
- ¼ **teaspoon salt**
- ½ **teaspoon dried tarragon**
- ¼ **teaspoon cayenne pepper**
- 1 **package (10 ounces) chopped frozen broccoli, thawed**

1. Preheat the oven to 400°F. Pierce the potatoes with a fork and bake for 45 minutes. Leave the oven on.

2. Meanwhile, in a food processor, process the cottage cheese until creamy. Transfer to a medium bowl and stir in the sour cream, salt, tarragon, and cayenne. Stir in the broccoli.

3. Split each potato open and scrape out most of the flesh with a fork, leaving a ⅓-inch shell. Stir the potato flesh into the broccoli-cottage cheese mixture. Spoon the mixture back into the potato shells, place on a baking sheet, and return to the oven for 10 minutes or until heated through. Serves 4.

Per serving: Calories 251; Fiber 5g; Protein 14g; Total Fat 3g; Saturated Fat 1g; Cholesterol 7mg; Sodium 402mg

Creamy Broccoli Soup Sauté 1 small onion in 2 tsp. olive oil until tender. Add 10-oz. package frozen broccoli, 1½ cups chicken broth, ¼ tsp. marjoram or oregano, and pinch of cayenne. Simmer until broccoli is tender. Purée with 1 cup reduced-fat (2%) milk. Heat through to serve. Serves 4. *[Cal 89; Fat 4g; Sod 443mg]*

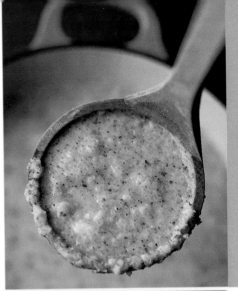

Broccoli Pizza In a nonstick skillet, sauté 6 cups broccoli florets and 2 cloves minced garlic in 2 tsp. olive oil until crisp-tender. In a 450°F oven, bake a large prebaked pizza shell until lightly crisped. Top with 1 cup part-skim ricotta, 2 tbsp. Parmesan, and the broccoli. Sprinkle with ½ cup coarsely chopped roasted red pepper and bake until heated through. Serves 6. *[Cal 326; Fat 10g; Sod 548mg]*

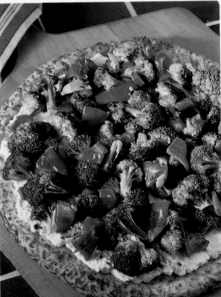

Broccoli, Roasted Pepper & Olive Salad In a bowl, combine 3 tbsp. balsamic vinegar, 1 tbsp. olive oil, and 2 tsp. Dijon mustard. Steam 6 cups broccoli florets until crisp-tender. Add to bowl along with 1 cup sliced roasted red peppers and ⅓ cup chopped green olives. Toss. Serves 4. *[Cal 119; Fat 6g; Sod 485mg]*

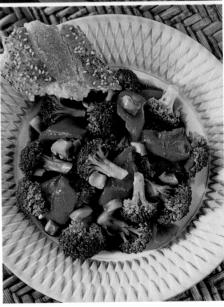

Brussels sprouts

Nutritional power
When the USDA tested some common fruits and vegetables for their overall antioxidant power, Brussels sprouts ranked number five.

Healthy Highlights

PER 1 CUP COOKED	
Calories	61
Fiber	4.1g
Protein	4g
Total Fat	0.8g
Saturated Fat	0.2g
Cholesterol	0mg
Sodium	33mg

NUTRIENTS	
	% Daily Value
Vitamin C	162%
Folate	23%
Vitamin A	22%
Manganese	18%
Potassium	17%
Vitamin B6	14%

Did you know? . . .
The slightly bitter undertone you can sometimes taste in Brussels sprouts comes from sinigrin, a natural compound in the plant that helps keep away insects. Of course, the substance is not toxic to humans—in fact, it shows promise in combating the early stages of colon cancer.

Warm Winter Salad

PREP: 20 MINUTES / COOK: 15 MINUTES

This substantial first course (or side dish) is a tempting change from light, leafy salads.

- ½ pound small red potatoes, quartered
- 1 container (10 ounces) Brussels sprouts, quartered
- 1 red apple, cut into ½-inch chunks
- 2 stalks celery, thinly sliced
- 3 scallions, thinly sliced
- ½ cup apple juice
- ⅓ cup distilled white vinegar
- 2 tablespoons flour
- 1 tablespoon spicy brown mustard
- 1 tablespoon drained white horseradish
- 1 teaspoon olive oil
- ½ teaspoon caraway seeds
- ½ teaspoon salt

1. In a large pot of boiling water, cook the potatoes for 5 minutes. Add the Brussels sprouts and cook for 5 to 8 minutes or until firm-tender. Drain and place in a salad bowl along with the apple, celery, and scallions.

2. In a small saucepan, whisk together the apple juice, vinegar, flour, mustard, horseradish, oil, caraway seeds, and salt. Bring to a simmer, whisking, over moderate heat. Cook for 2 minutes to develop the flavors. Pour the hot dressing over the vegetables, tossing to combine. Serve warm or at room temperature. Serves 4.

Per serving: Calories 151; Fiber 7g; Protein 4g; Total Fat 2g; Saturated Fat 0g; Cholesterol 0mg; Sodium 365mg

Brussels Sprouts & Mushrooms à la Grecque

PREP: 20 MINUTES / COOK: 20 MINUTES

- 1 tablespoon olive oil
- 2 onions, diced
- 2 pounds small mushrooms, quartered
- 2 containers (10 ounces each) Brussels sprouts, halved
- 1 cup chicken broth
- ½ teaspoon dried oregano
- 4 teaspoons Dijon mustard
- 2 teaspoons honey
- ½ teaspoon salt
- ¼ teaspoon pepper
- 2 teaspoons cornstarch blended with 2 tablespoons water
- 2 tablespoons lemon juice

1. In a large nonstick skillet, heat the oil over moderate heat. Add the onions and sauté for 6 minutes or until softened. Add the mushrooms and sauté for 4 minutes or until beginning to brown.

2. Add the Brussels sprouts, broth, 1 cup of water, and the oregano, and bring to a boil. Reduce to a simmer, cover, and cook for 8 minutes or until the Brussels sprouts are just tender. Stir in the mustard, honey, salt, and pepper.

3. Bring to a simmer, stir in the cornstarch mixture, and cook, stirring, for 2 minutes or until lightly thickened. Off the heat, stir in the lemon juice. Serve warm or at room temperature. Serves 6.

Per serving: Calories 140; Fiber 8g; Protein 7g; Total Fat 4g; Saturated Fat 1g; Cholesterol 0mg; Sodium 470mg

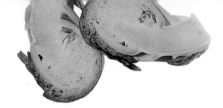

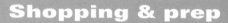
Sautéed Sprouts with Chicken & Chestnuts

PREP: 25 MINUTES / COOK: 20 MINUTES

Reminiscent of Thanksgiving dinner, this one-pan meal has a tangy apple-wine sauce. Each serving supplies 167 mg of calcium—most of it from the chestnuts.

- 2 **containers (10 ounces each) Brussels sprouts, halved**
- 4 **teaspoons olive oil**
- ¾ **pound skinless, boneless chicken breasts, cut into ¾-inch chunks**
- ¾ **teaspoon each dried thyme and tarragon**
- ½ **cup dry white wine**
- 2 **tablespoons flour**
- 1 **cup apple juice**
- ⅔ **cup water-packed canned chestnuts**
- 1 **teaspoon salt**
- ½ **teaspoon pepper**
- 2 **tablespoons reduced-fat sour cream**

1. In a large nonstick skillet, bring 1 inch of water to a boil. Add the Brussels sprouts, cover, and cook for 10 minutes or until they are tender at the stem end. Drain.

2. In the same skillet, heat the oil over moderate heat. Add the chicken and sauté for 3 minutes or until the chicken is browned. Add the thyme and tarragon, and cook for 1 minute or until the herbs are fragrant.

3. Add the wine to the skillet and bring to a simmer, scraping up any browned bits clinging to the bottom of the pan. Boil for 2 minutes or until the liquid is reduced by half.

4. In a small bowl, whisk together the flour and apple juice. Stir the apple juice mixture into the skillet along with the Brussels sprouts, chestnuts, salt, and pepper. Cook for 2 minutes or until heated through and thickened. Off the heat, stir in the sour cream. Serves 4.

Per serving: Calories 306; Fiber 10g; Protein 26g; Total Fat 7g; Saturated Fat 2g; Cholesterol 52mg; Sodium 655mg

At the market Brussels sprouts are a fall and winter vegetable, but you can find them in spring and summer, too. They're sold in small and large tubs, loose, or on the stalk.

Look for Rich green color indicates freshness; avoid sprouts that are yellowed or wilted. Pick small, compact sprouts with undamaged leaves.

Prep Trim stems, but not too close to the base of the sprout or the leaves may fall off during cooking. (If you buy sprouts on the stalk, you'll need to cut them off before cooking.)

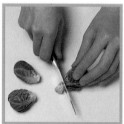

Slice most of the stem off each sprout, but leave on a bit as a base.

Basic cooking Steam whole Brussels sprouts for 6 to 12 minutes, depending on size. To microwave 1 pound sprouts, place in a dish with ¼ cup water, cover, and cook 4 to 8 minutes, depending on size. Let stand for 3 minutes.

Warm Winter Salad *Mustard and horseradish lend a bold bite to the creamy dressing.*

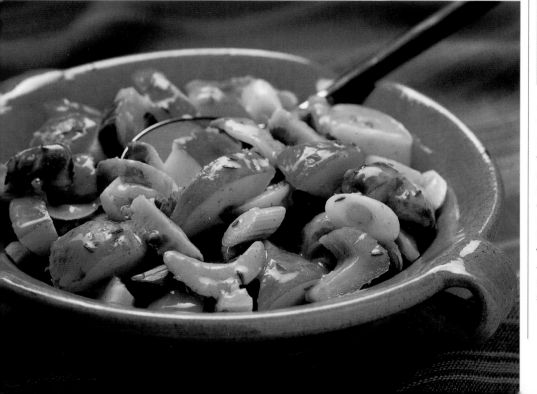

Cabbage

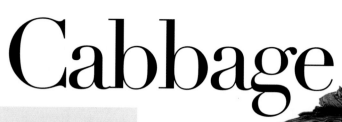

Nutritional power

*This versatile veg-
etable, a good
source of vitamin C,
is also rich in
indoles. Preliminary
studies suggest that
these phytochemi-
cals may help pre-
vent breast cancer.*

Healthy Highlights

Green Cabbage
PER 1 CUP RAW

Calories	22
Fiber	2.0g
Protein	1g
Total Fat	0.2g
Saturated Fat	0g
Cholesterol	0mg
Sodium	16mg

NUTRIENTS

	% Daily Value
Vitamin C	48%

Red Cabbage
PER 1 CUP RAW

Calories	19
Fiber	1.4g
Protein	1g
Total Fat	0.2g
Saturated Fat	0g
Cholesterol	0mg
Sodium	8mg

NUTRIENTS

	% Daily Value
Vitamin C	67%

Old-Fashioned Stuffed Cabbage Rolls

PREP: 40 MINUTES / COOK: 1 HOUR

*A meatless filling makes this homestyle
favorite low in fat and high in fiber.*

- ½   ounce dried mushrooms
- 1   cup boiling water
- 1   small head of green cabbage (1¼ pounds)
- 1½ teaspoons olive oil
- ½   cup finely chopped red bell pepper
- 2   carrots, shredded
- 3   scallions, chopped
- ¾   teaspoon dried thyme
- 1   can (14½ ounces) no-salt-added stewed tomatoes, chopped with their juice
- ½   cup quick-cooking brown rice
- ½   teaspoon salt
- 2   tablespoons snipped fresh dill
- ⅓   cup shredded Swiss cheese
- ½   cup chicken broth
- 1   teaspoon cornstarch blended with 1 tablespoon water

1. In a small heatproof bowl, combine the dried mushrooms and the boiling water and let stand for 15 minutes or until softened. Reserving the soaking liquid, scoop out the dried mushrooms and chop them. Strain the soaking liq- uid through a coffee filter or a paper towel-lined sieve. Measure out ¾ cup and discard any remainder.

2. Meanwhile, bring a large pot of water to a boil. Add the whole head of cabbage and cook for 3 minutes to soft- en the leaves. Peel back and cut off 4 leaves, being careful not to tear them. Repeat twice more (returning the water to a boil each time) to remove a total of 12 leaves. Chop enough of the remain- ing cabbage to measure 1½ cups.

3. In a large nonstick skillet, heat the oil over moderate heat. Add the bell pepper and chopped cabbage, and sauté for 8 minutes. Add the car- rots, scallions, and thyme, and sauté for 2 minutes.

4. Add the chopped mushrooms, the reserved soaking liquid, 1 cup of the tomatoes, the brown rice, and salt. Bring to a simmer and cook for 20 min- utes or until the rice is almost tender. Transfer the mixture to a bowl and stir in 1 tablespoon of the dill and the cheese; set aside to cool slightly.

5. Spoon ¼ cup of the filling into the center of each leaf. Fold the bottom up and the sides in, then roll up. Place the rolls in a large skillet, seam-side down, and add the broth, ½ cup of water, the

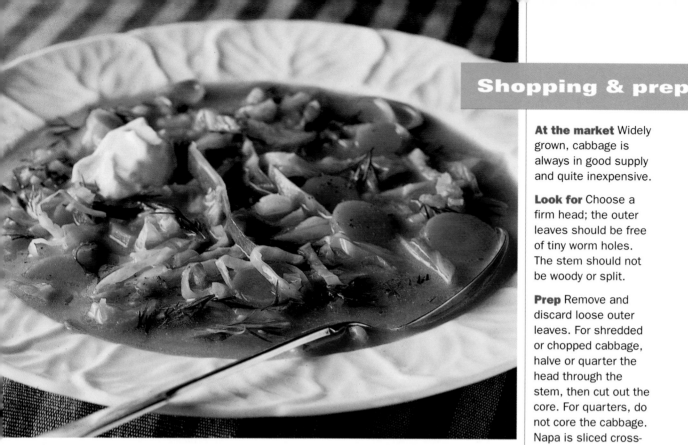

Creamy Cabbage & Carrot Soup has a warming touch of ground ginger in the broth.

At the market Widely grown, cabbage is always in good supply and quite inexpensive.

Look for Choose a firm head; the outer leaves should be free of tiny worm holes. The stem should not be woody or split.

Prep Remove and discard loose outer leaves. For shredded or chopped cabbage, halve or quarter the head through the stem, then cut out the core. For quarters, do not core the cabbage. Napa is sliced cross-wise to shred it; the leaves and stalk of bok choy may be cooked together, or the stalks cut off and cooked separately.

Basic cooking Steam shredded cabbage 5 to 8 minutes, wedges 12 to 20. Microwave 1 pound cabbage wedges in a dish with ¼ cup liquid; cook, covered, 6 to 8 minutes. Cook shredded cabbage the same way for 4 to 6 minutes.

remaining tomatoes, and the remaining 1 tablespoon dill. Bring to a simmer, cover, and cook for 20 minutes or until the cabbage is tender.

6. Transfer the rolls to a serving dish. Bring the cooking liquid in the skillet to a boil. Stir in the cornstarch mixture and cook, stirring, for 1 minute or until lightly thickened. Pour the sauce over the rolls and serve. Serves 4.

Per serving: Calories 196; Fiber 9g; Protein 8g; Total Fat 6g; Saturated Fat 2g; Cholesterol 9mg; Sodium 495mg

Creamy Cabbage & Carrot Soup

PREP: 15 MINUTES / COOK: 40 MINUTES
You can make this soup with crinkly Savoy cabbage, which is rich in beta carotene.

- 1 tablespoon olive oil
- 1 large onion, finely chopped
- 4 cloves garlic, minced
- 2 carrots, thinly sliced
- 8 cups shredded green cabbage
- 2½ cups chicken broth
- ¾ cup snipped fresh dill
- ⅓ cup no-salt-added tomato paste
- ¾ teaspoon ground ginger
- ¼ teaspoon each salt and pepper
- ⅓ cup reduced-fat sour cream

1. In a large Dutch oven or flame-proof casserole, heat the oil over moderate heat. Add the onion and garlic, and sauté for 7 minutes or until the onion is soft. Add the carrots and sauté for 5 minutes or until the carrots are crisp-tender.

2. Stir in the cabbage, cover, and cook, stirring occasionally, for 10 minutes or until the cabbage is wilted.

3. Add the broth, 2½ cups of water, the dill, tomato paste, ginger, salt, and pepper. Bring to a boil, reduce to a simmer, cover, and cook for 15 minutes or until the cabbage is very tender. Stir the sour cream into the soup. Serves 4.

Per serving: Calories 179; Fiber 6g; Protein 6g; Total Fat 8g; Saturated Fat 2g; Cholesterol 7mg; Sodium 862mg

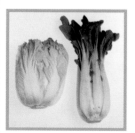

Napa (left) and bok choy, two Chinese cabbages.

Healthy Highlights

Napa Cabbage

PER 1 CUP RAW

Calories	12
Fiber	2.4g
Protein	1g
Total Fat	0.2g
Saturated Fat	0g
Cholesterol	0mg
Sodium	7mg

NUTRIENTS

	% Daily Value
Vitamin C	35%
Vitamin A	18%
Folate	15%

Bok Choy

PER 1 CUP COOKED

Calories	20
Fiber	2.7g
Protein	3g
Total Fat	0.3g
Saturated Fat	0g
Cholesterol	0mg
Sodium	58mg

NUTRIENTS

	% Daily Value
Vitamin A	87%
Vitamin C	73%
Potassium	21%
Folate	17%
Calcium	16%
Vitamin B6	14%
Manganese	12%

Did you know? . . .
Because of its dark green leaves, bok choy is richer in beta carotene than regular green cabbage. Both bok choy and Napa supply more calcium than green cabbage.

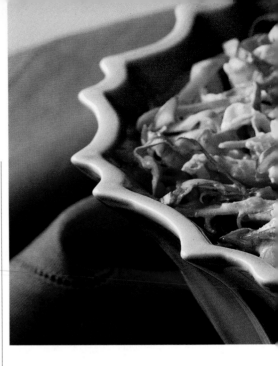

Colcannon

PREP: 25 MINUTES / COOK: 35 MINUTES

A traditional Irish recipe (also enjoyed in Scotland), colcannon is a simple combination of mashed potatoes and cabbage.

- 1½ pounds small all-purpose potatoes
- ⅓ cup low-fat (1%) milk
- ¾ teaspoon salt
- 3 slices (1¾ ounces) smoky bacon, coarsely chopped
- 2 cups finely chopped onions
- 3 cloves garlic, minced
- 8 cups green cabbage chunks (1 inch)
- ¼ teaspoon pepper

1. In a medium pot of boiling water, cook the potatoes for 25 minutes or until tender. When cool enough to handle, peel the potatoes and transfer to a medium bowl. With a potato masher or electric mixer, beat in the milk and ¼ teaspoon of the salt; set aside.

2. Meanwhile, in a large skillet, cook the bacon in ¼ cup of water over moderate heat for 7 minutes or until the bacon is crisp and has rendered its fat. With a slotted spoon, transfer the bacon to a plate.

3. Add the onions and garlic to the skillet and cook, stirring frequently, for 10 minutes or until the onion is golden brown and very tender. Add the cabbage, pepper, the remaining ½ teaspoon salt, and the bacon, and cook, stirring frequently, for 15 minutes or until the cabbage is tender but not mushy.

4. Stir in the mashed potatoes and cook, stirring frequently, for 5 minutes or until the potatoes are piping hot. Serves 6.

Per serving: Calories 186; Fiber 5g; Protein 5g; Total Fat 5g; Saturated Fat 2g; Cholesterol 6mg; Sodium 497mg

Stir-Fried Bok Choy with Garlic Sauce

PREP: 15 MINUTES / COOK: 15 MINUTES

The garlic in this sauce is simmered in broth to soften its pungency. Sesame oil gives the sauce a nutlike flavor.

- 2 teaspoons peanut or olive oil
- 10 cloves garlic, minced
- 1 tablespoon chopped fresh ginger
- ¼ cup chicken broth
- 1 red bell pepper, cut into ½-inch squares
- 2 carrots, halved lengthwise and thinly sliced
- 4 cups 1-inch strips of bok choy, Napa cabbage, or green cabbage
- 1 teaspoon sugar
- ½ teaspoon salt
- 2 teaspoons sesame oil

1. In a large nonstick skillet, heat the peanut oil over moderately low heat. Add the garlic and ginger, and sauté for 1 minute or until slightly softened. Add the broth and ¼ cup of water, cover, and cook for 7 minutes or until the garlic and ginger are very soft.

2. Add the bell pepper and carrots, and cook for 1 minute. Add the bok choy and toss with the other ingredients until well coated. Sprinkle with the sugar and salt and cook for 4 minutes (6 minutes if using green cabbage) or

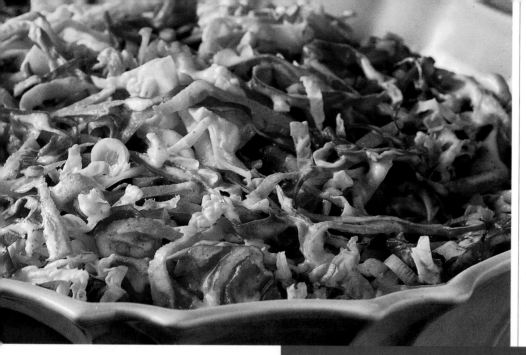

Three-Cabbage Slaw with Creamy Honey-Mustard Dressing
To boost flavor and nutrition, there are carrots and scallions in the mix, as well.

Did you know? . . .
Cabbage contains isothiocyanates, which appear to stimulate the production of cancer-fighting enzymes.

until the cabbage is tender. Drizzle with the sesame oil and serve hot. Serves 4.

Per serving: Calories 87; Fiber 2g; Protein 2g; Total Fat 5g; Saturated Fat 1g; Cholesterol 0mg; Sodium 399mg

Warm Red Cabbage with Pears

PREP: 15 MINUTES / COOK: 10 MINUTES

- 2 teaspoons olive oil
- 1 small red onion, finely chopped
- 1 tablespoon minced fresh ginger
- 2 cloves garlic, minced
- 6 cups shredded red cabbage
- 2 pears, peeled and cut into ½-inch slices
- ½ teaspoon salt
- ¼ cup balsamic vinegar

1. In a large nonstick skillet, heat the oil over moderate heat. Add the onion, ginger, and garlic, and sauté for 5 minutes or until the onion is tender.

2. Add the cabbage, pears, and salt, and sauté for 5 minutes or until the cabbage is crisp-tender. Sprinkle with the vinegar, cook for 1 minute, and serve hot or at room temperature. Serves 4.

Per serving: Calories 114; Fiber 5g; Protein 2g; Total Fat 3g; Saturated Fat 0g; Cholesterol 0mg; Sodium 289mg

Both bok choy and Napa supply more calcium than regular green cabbage.

Three-Cabbage Slaw with Creamy Honey-Mustard Dressing

PREP: 20 MINUTES / CHILL: 1 HOUR

You can also make this slaw with one type of cabbage—an all-Napa slaw, for example, is particularly crisp and delicate.

- ¼ cup cider vinegar
- ⅓ cup reduced-fat sour cream
- 2 tablespoons honey
- 2 tablespoons spicy brown mustard
- 1 teaspoon olive oil
- ¾ teaspoon salt
- 6 cups shredded red and green cabbage
- 2 cups shredded Napa cabbage
- 4 carrots, shredded
- 2 scallions, thinly sliced

1. In a large bowl, whisk together the vinegar, sour cream, honey, mustard, oil, and salt.

2. Add the cabbages, carrots, and scallions, tossing to combine. Refrigerate for 1 hour or until chilled. Serves 6.

Per serving: Calories 101; Fiber 3g; Protein 3g; Total Fat 3g; Saturated Fat 1g; Cholesterol 4mg; Sodium 372mg

Red cabbage provides more vitamin C than green; crinkly Savoy, which has medium-green leaves, has a significant amount of beta carotene.

Buy a whole cabbage, rather than a head that has been halved: When cabbage is cut, it loses vitamin C.

You can avoid the lingering, sulfurous odor of boiled cabbage by cooking it quickly in lots of water, in an uncovered pot.

Although plain cabbage is (like most vegetables) virtually fat-free, a one-cup serving of mayonnaise-dressed deli coleslaw may contain as much as 16 grams of fat.

Carrots

Nutritional power
Carrots are the lead-ing source of beta carotene in the American diet. They also contain flavo-noids, phytochemi-cals that function as antioxidants.

Healthy Highlights

PER 1 CUP RAW	
Calories	52
Fiber	3.7g
Protein	1g
Total Fat	0.2g
Saturated Fat	0g
Cholesterol	0mg
Sodium	43mg

NUTRIENTS	
	% Daily Value
Vitamin A	686%
Vitamin C	18%
Potassium	13%

Did you know? . . .
As part of a National Cancer Institute study, scientists devised a vegetable "cocktail" packed with disease-fighting ingredients: Carrot juice was a main component.

Flavonoids, found in carrots, may inhibit enzymes responsible for the spread of malignant cells. Research indicates that they may also fight heart disease.

Chicken & Carrot Stew

PREP: 20 MINUTES / COOK: 20 MINUTES

- 1 tablespoon olive oil
- 4 skinless, boneless chicken breast halves (1 pound total), cut crosswise into quarters
- 2 tablespoons flour
- 1 large onion, cut into 1-inch chunks
- 3 cloves garlic, minced
- 1 pound peeled "baby" carrots
- ⅔ cup chicken broth
- ½ teaspoon dried marjoram
- ½ teaspoon salt
- ¼ teaspoon ground ginger
- ¼ teaspoon pepper

1. In a large nonstick skillet, heat the oil over moderate heat. Dredge the chicken in the flour, shaking off the excess. Sauté for 2 minutes per side or until lightly browned. With a slotted spoon, transfer the chicken to a plate.

2. Add the onion and garlic to the pan and sauté for 7 minutes or until the onion is tender. Add the carrots, tossing to coat. Add the broth, ⅔ cup of water, the marjoram, salt, ginger, and pepper, and bring to a boil. Reduce to a simmer and cook for 7 minutes or until the carrots are crisp-tender.

3. Add the chicken, cover, and cook for 4 minutes or until the chicken and carrots are tender. Serves 4.

Per serving: Calories 248; Fiber 5g; Protein 29g; Total Fat 5g; Saturated Fat 1g; Cholesterol 66mg; Sodium 565mg

Carrot Cake with Cream Cheese Frosting

PREP: 15 MINUTES / COOK: 45 MINUTES

One of the few vegetables suitable for use in a dessert, carrots bring sweetness, moisture, and pleasing texture to this popular cake. This recipe is lower in fat than most.

- 1 cup flour
- 1 teaspoon baking soda
- 1 teaspoon cinnamon
- ½ teaspoon ground ginger
- ¼ teaspoon ground cardamom
- ¼ teaspoon salt
- 3 tablespoons peanut or other vegetable oil
- ½ cup granulated sugar
- ½ cup packed light brown sugar
- 1 egg
- 2 egg whites
- 2¼ cups shredded carrots
- ¼ cup golden raisins
- 2 tablespoons sunflower seeds
- 3 ounces reduced-fat cream cheese (Neufchâtel)
- ¾ cup marshmallow creme

1. Preheat the oven to 350°F. Spray an 8-inch round cake pan with nonstick cooking spray. Line the bottom of the pan with a round of wax paper and spray it with nonstick cooking spray.

2. On a sheet of wax paper, sift together the flour, baking soda, cinna-mon, ginger, cardamom, and salt. In a large bowl, with an electric mixer, beat the oil, granulated sugar, and brown sugar until light and fluffy. Beat in the

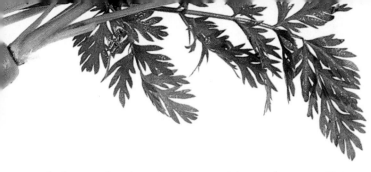

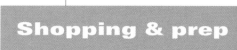

whole egg, then beat in the egg whites. Fold in the carrots, raisins, and sunflower seeds. Fold in the flour mixture until just combined.

3. Spoon the batter into the prepared pan. Bake for 30 minutes or until a cake tester inserted in the center comes out clean. Cool in the pan on a rack for 20 minutes, then invert onto the rack to cool completely.

4. In a medium bowl, with an electric mixer, beat the cream cheese until smooth. Beat in the marshmallow creme until well combined. Spread over the cooled cake. Serves 8.

Per serving: Calories 306; Fiber 2g; Protein 5g; Total Fat 9g; Saturated Fat 2g; Cholesterol 32mg; Sodium 318mg

Carrot Cake with Cream Cheese Frosting *Sunflower seeds and raisins power up the nutrition in this luscious cake.*

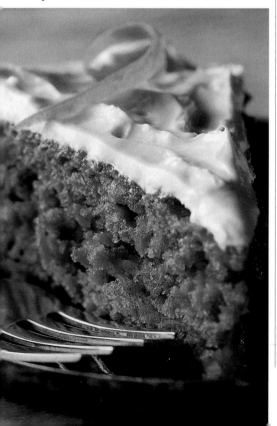

Carrot-Apricot Muffins with Pecans

PREP: 22 MINUTES / COOK: 30 MINUTES

Dried apricots, brimming with beta carotene, potassium, iron, and fiber, are a healthful addition to these pecan-flecked muffins.

- ¼ **cup pecans**
- 2 **cups flour**
- 1¾ **teaspoons baking powder**
- ¾ **teaspoon cinnamon**
- ¼ **teaspoon salt**
- ½ **cup unsweetened applesauce**
- ¼ **cup granulated sugar**
- ¼ **cup packed light brown sugar**
- 3 **tablespoons vegetable oil**
- 1 **egg**
- 1 **egg white**
- 2 **cups packed shredded carrots**
- ⅓ **cup coarsely chopped dried apricots**

1. Preheat the oven to 375° F. Line a 2½-inch muffin pan with paper liners or spray with nonstick cooking spray; set the pan aside.

2. In a small baking pan, toast the pecans for 5 minutes or until lightly fragrant. When cool enough to handle, coarsely chop.

3. In a medium bowl, combine the flour, baking powder, cinnamon, and salt. In a separate bowl, combine the applesauce, granulated sugar, brown sugar, oil, whole egg, and egg white. Stir in the pecans, carrots, and apricots.

4. Make a well in the center of the dry ingredients and stir in the applesauce mixture until just moistened. Spoon into the prepared muffin cups and bake for 30 minutes or until a cake tester inserted in the center of a muffin comes out just clean. Makes 12 muffins.

Per serving: Calories 187; Fiber 2g; Protein 4g; Total Fat 6g; Saturated Fat 1g; Cholesterol 18mg; Sodium 139mg

At the market Carrots are always in good supply. They're sold "topped" (minus their leaves) in plastic bags, and in bunches with leaves attached. "Baby" carrots (trimmed to thumb size) are sold washed and peeled.

Look for Carrot bags often have orange lines printed on them, making the carrots look brighter. Don't be fooled: Turn the bag over and check through the clear side. The leaves on bunched carrots should be springy and a fresh green.

Prep Peel carrots with a vegetable peeler, then slice, dice, or chop as needed.

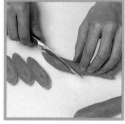

Carrot slices cut on a long diagonal are pretty, and they cook quickly.

Basic cooking Steam cut-up carrots (or cook them in a small amount of orange or apple juice) for 3 to 4 minutes. To microwave 1 pound of cut-up carrots, place in a dish, add 2 tablespoons water, cover, and cook at high for 4 to 6 minutes.

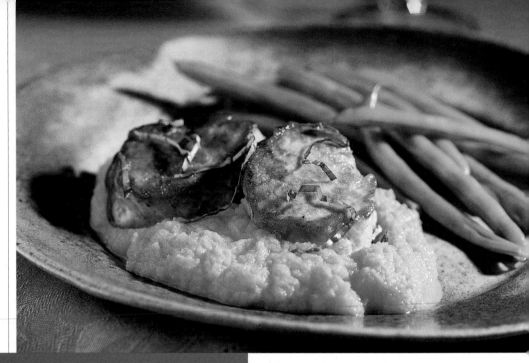

Pork Medallions with Roasted Carrot Purée *The carrots are roasted to concentrate their sweetness, then puréed and seasoned.*

Did you know? . . .
A USDA study suggests that calcium pectate, a type of soluble fiber found in carrots, has a cholesterol-lowering effect.

Cooking breaks down carrots' tough cell walls, releasing more beta carotene.

Raw carrots are a nutritious snack, but you should eat cooked carrots, too: Cooking breaks down the vegetable's tough cell walls, releasing more beta carotene. Cooking also brings out carrots' natural sweetness.

Carrots really can be good for your eyes: Beta carotene, in its antioxidant capacity, may help prevent cataracts.

If you eat lots of carrots, the palms of your hands (and the soles of your feet) may turn yellow-orange. This is harmless—just an accumulation of carotenoids—and the color will fade with time . . . and it's no reason to cut down on your carrot intake.

Pork Medallions with Roasted Carrot Purée
PREP: 15 MINUTES / COOK: 35 MINUTES

    1   pound carrots, thinly sliced
    3   cloves garlic, peeled
    5   teaspoons olive oil
    ½   cup chicken broth
    1   tablespoon no-salt-added tomato paste
    ½   teaspoon salt
    ⅛   teaspoon cayenne pepper
    1   pound well-trimmed pork tenderloin, cut into 8 slices
    2   tablespoons flour
    2   tablespoons slivered fresh basil

1. Preheat the oven to 450°F. In a metal baking pan, toss together the carrots, garlic, and 2 teaspoons of the olive oil. Bake, tossing the carrots occasionally, for 25 minutes or until the carrots are tender.

2. Transfer the carrots to a food processor and purée along with the broth, ½ cup of water, the tomato paste, salt, and cayenne. Set aside.

3. In a large nonstick skillet, heat the remaining 3 teaspoons oil over moderately high heat. Dredge the pork in the flour, shaking off the excess. Sauté for 2 minutes per side or until browned and cooked through. Transfer to a plate.

4. Wipe out the skillet, add the carrot purée, and bring to a boil. Spoon onto 4 plates, top with the pork, and sprinkle with the basil. Serves 4.

Per serving: Calories 278; Fiber 4g; Protein 25g; Total Fat 12g; Saturated Fat 3g; Cholesterol 75mg; Sodium 503mg

Moroccan-Style Carrot Salad
PREP: 25 MINUTES / COOK: 5 MINUTES
MARINATE: 1 HOUR

    1   pound carrots, diagonally sliced
    1   red bell pepper, diced
    ½   cup orange juice
    3   tablespoons lemon juice
    1   tablespoon honey
    2   teaspoons vegetable oil
    1   teaspoon ground cumin
    1   teaspoon ground coriander
    ½   teaspoon salt
    ¼   teaspoon ground ginger
    ⅓   cup chopped cilantro
    ⅓   cup chopped dates
    ¼   cup chopped black olives

1. In a steamer or colander set over a pot of boiling water, steam the carrots for 5 minutes. Add the bell pepper and steam for 1 minute or until the carrots and pepper are crisp-tender.

2. In a serving bowl, whisk together the orange juice, lemon juice, honey, oil, cumin, coriander, salt, and ginger. Stir in the cilantro, dates, and olives.

3. Add the carrots and pepper to the dressing, tossing to coat. Let sit at room temperature for at least 1 hour before serving. Serves 4.

Per serving: Calories 159; Fiber 5g; Protein 2g; Total Fat 4g; Saturated Fat 0g; Cholesterol 0mg; Sodium 392mg

Vegetable Antipasto

PREP: 20 MINUTES / COOK: 15 MINUTES
MARINATE: 4 HOURS

- 1 **cup vegetable or chicken broth**
- ½ **cup dry white wine**
- ½ **teaspoon dried oregano**
- ⅛ **teaspoon crushed red pepper flakes**
- 1 **pound carrots, diagonally sliced**
- 2 **cups cauliflower florets**
- ¼ **pound green beans, halved crosswise**
- ½ **cup pickled pepperoncini peppers**
- ¼ **cup white wine vinegar**
- 1 **teaspoon olive oil**
- ½ **teaspoon salt**
- ½ **cup cubed (¾ inch) part-skim mozzarella cheese**
- ½ **cup chopped fresh basil**

1. In a large skillet, bring the broth, wine, oregano, and red pepper flakes to a simmer. Add the carrots, cover, and cook for 6 minutes. Add the cauliflower and beans, return to a simmer, and cook for 8 minutes.

2. Transfer the vegetables and liquid to a medium bowl, stir in the pepperoncini, vinegar, oil, and salt. Cover and refrigerate for at least 4 hours or overnight. Just before serving, stir in the mozzarella and basil. Serves 4.

Per serving: Calories 149; Fiber 6g; Protein 6g; Total Fat 4g; Saturated Fat 2g; Cholesterol 8mg; Sodium 910mg

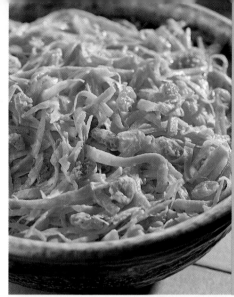

Carrot Slaw In a bowl, combine ¼ cup light mayonnaise, 2 tbsp. white vinegar, 1 tsp. Dijon mustard, and ¼ tsp. pepper. Add ⅓ cup golden raisins and 1 lb. carrots, shredded; toss to combine. Serves 4. *[Cal 137; Fat 5g; Sod 186mg]*

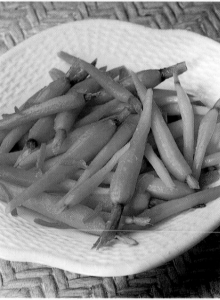

Orange-Glazed Carrots Steam 1 lb. very small, peeled carrots (or pre-peeled "baby" carrots), until crisp-tender. In a large skillet, heat ¼ cup orange juice, 2 tbsp. orange marmalade (or apricot jam), 2 tsp. unsalted butter, and ½ tsp. salt. Add the carrots and cook over moderate heat until nicely glazed. Serves 4. *[Cal 97; Fat 2g; Sod 319mg]*

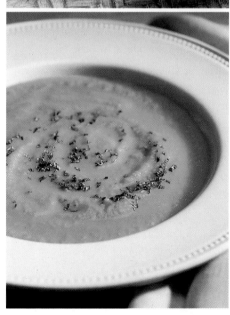

Creamy Carrot & Mint Soup In a saucepan, combine 3 cups thinly sliced carrots, 1 tbsp. rice, 1 cup chicken broth, 1 cup water, 1 tsp. sugar, ½ tsp. salt, and ¼ tsp. cayenne. Simmer, covered, for 17 minutes or until the rice is tender. Purée in a food processor along with 1 cup reduced-fat (2%) milk. Reheat and stir in ⅓ cup chopped fresh mint. Serves 4. *[Cal 88; Fat 2g; Sod 596mg]*

Cauliflower

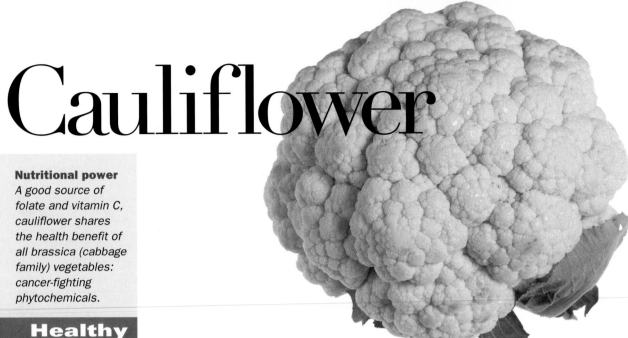

Nutritional power
A good source of folate and vitamin C, cauliflower shares the health benefit of all brassica (cabbage family) vegetables: cancer-fighting phytochemicals.

Healthy Highlights

PER 1 CUP COOKED	
Calories	29
Fiber	3.3g
Protein	2g
Total Fat	0.6g
Saturated Fat	0.1g
Cholesterol	0mg
Sodium	19mg

NUTRIENTS	
	% Daily Value
Vitamin C	92%
Folate	14%
Vitamin B6	11%

Did you know? . . .
Broccoflower, a new cross between cauliflower and broccoli, is more nutritious than cauliflower: Broccoflower, which has green curd rather than white, has more vitamin C and also some beta carotene.

Cauliflower quickly loses its folacin to the cooking water when boiled. When possible, steam, braise, or roast it.

Cauliflower-Onion Relish with Carrots & Peppers

PREP: 15 MINUTES / COOK: 15 MINUTES

A zesty side dish for a cookout, this colorful relish is great with grilled chicken breasts and turkey burgers.

- 1 cup distilled white vinegar
- ½ cup sugar
- 2 tablespoons mustard seeds
- 1½ teaspoons turmeric
- ½ teaspoon salt
- 1 head of cauliflower, cut into florets
- 2 carrots, thinly sliced
- 1 red onion, cut into ½-inch chunks
- 1 red bell pepper, diced
- 2 tablespoons yellow mustard

1. In a large saucepan, bring the vinegar, sugar, mustard seeds, turmeric, and salt to a boil over moderate heat.

2. Add the cauliflower, carrots, onion, and bell pepper, and return to a boil. Reduce to a simmer, cover, and cook for 12 minutes or until the cauliflower is tender. Cool to room temperature, stir in the yellow mustard. Serve warm, at room temperature, or chilled. Serves 4.

Per serving: Calories 213; Fiber 7g; Protein 6g; Total Fat 2g; Saturated Fat 0g; Cholesterol 0mg; Sodium 413mg

Roasted Cauliflower with Tomatoes & Garlic

PREP: 10 MINUTES / COOK: 45 MINUTES

Roasting the vegetables intensifies their flavor and helps preserve B vitamins. Squeeze the garlic out of its skin and spread on toasted bread as an accompaniment.

- 2 tablespoons olive oil
- 8 cloves garlic, unpeeled
- ½ teaspoon dried rosemary, crumbled
- 1 head of cauliflower, cut into florets
- 1½ cups chopped plum tomatoes (about 4)
- ½ teaspoon salt

1. Preheat the oven to 425°F. In a 13 x 9-inch glass baking dish, combine the oil, garlic, and rosemary. Place in the oven and when the oil is hot but not smoking, add the cauliflower. Roast, turning the cauliflower occasionally, for 20 minutes or until lightly browned.

2. Add the tomatoes and salt, tossing well. Roast for 20 minutes or until the tomatoes are piping hot and the cauliflower is tender. Serves 4.

Per serving: Calories 119; Fiber 5g; Protein 4g; Total Fat 7g; Saturated Fat 1g; Cholesterol 0mg; Sodium 303mg

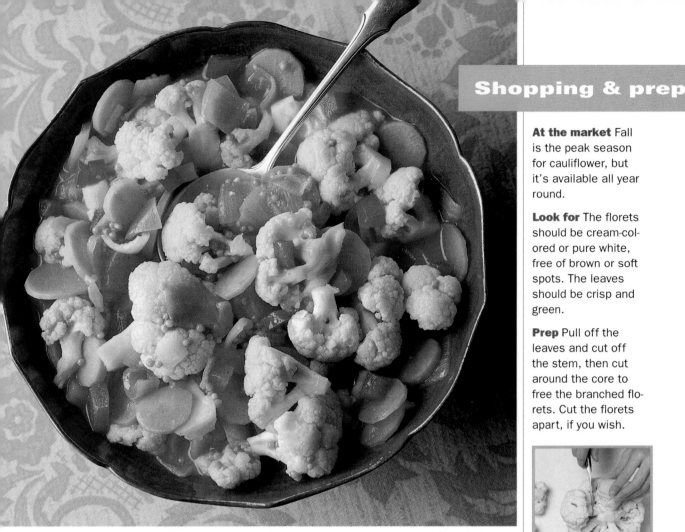

Cauliflower-Onion Relish with Carrots & Peppers dresses up simple meals.

At the market Fall is the peak season for cauliflower, but it's available all year round.

Look for The florets should be cream-colored or pure white, free of brown or soft spots. The leaves should be crisp and green.

Prep Pull off the leaves and cut off the stem, then cut around the core to free the branched florets. Cut the florets apart, if you wish.

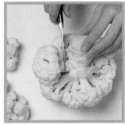

Use a small, sharp knife to cut the cauliflower florets from the stem.

Basic cooking Steam cauliflower florets for 3 to 5 minutes; a whole head, cored, for 15 to 20 minutes. Microwave 1 pound cauliflower florets with ¼ cup water; cover and cook at high for 4 to 7 minutes; let stand for 3 minutes.

Cauliflower with Deviled Cheese Sauce

PREP: 10 MINUTES / COOK: 10 MINUTES

As homey and rich as old-fashioned macaroni and cheese, this comforting dish has the added benefits of the fiber and phytochemicals from the cauliflower.

1½ cups low-fat (1%) milk
3 tablespoons flour
1 cup shredded medium to sharp Cheddar cheese (4 ounces)
2 tablespoons grated Parmesan cheese
½ teaspoon spicy brown mustard
¼ teaspoon cayenne pepper
¼ teaspoon salt
1 head of cauliflower, cut into florets
¼ cup snipped fresh chives or scallion greens

1. In a medium saucepan, whisk the milk into the flour. Bring to a boil over moderate heat, reduce to a simmer, and cook, stirring constantly, for 5 minutes or until the sauce is lightly thickened. Remove from the heat. Whisk in the Cheddar cheese, Parmesan cheese, mustard, cayenne, and salt, whisking the sauce until smooth.

2. Meanwhile, in a steamer or colander set over a pot of boiling water, steam the cauliflower for 5 minutes or until crisp-tender. Transfer the hot cauliflower to the pan of sauce, stirring to coat. Serve the cauliflower sprinkled with the chives. Serves 4.

Per serving: Calories 223; Fiber 4g; Protein 15g; Total Fat 11g; Saturated Fat 7g; Cholesterol 35mg; Sodium 433mg

Chili peppers

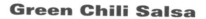

Nutritional power

Capsaicin, which makes chilies hot, is an antioxidant; it may protect DNA from carcinogens. It may also help kill the bacteria that cause most stomach ulcers.

Healthy Highlights

PER ¼ CUP RAW	
Calories	15
Fiber	0.6g
Protein	1g
Total Fat	0.1g
Saturated Fat	0g
Cholesterol	0mg
Sodium	3mg

NUTRIENTS	
	% Daily Value
Vitamin C	152%

Did you know? . . .
Red chilies contain more than ten times the beta carotene of green chilies.

Chilies are a leading source of vitamin C. They're not usually downed in large quantities—but the more, the healthier.

Capsaicin is concentrated in the seeds and ribs; to cool the heat, remove them.

Capsaicin acts as an anticoagulant, thus may help prevent heart attacks.

Thai Chicken Curry

PREP: 20 MINUTES / COOK: 10 MINUTES

Unlike Indian curries, which are primarily seasoned with dried ground spices, Thai curries are flavored with fresh herbs, fresh chilies, and coconut milk. Serve this fragrant curry over white or brown rice.

- ⅓ cup flaked coconut
- 4 scallions, thinly sliced
- 3 cloves garlic, crushed and peeled
- 3 tablespoons lime juice
- 2 tablespoons lower-sodium soy sauce
- 2 fresh jalapeño peppers, stemmed
- 1 tablespoon chopped fresh ginger
- ½ teaspoon each ground coriander and cumin
- 2 teaspoons olive oil
- ¾ pound skinless, boneless chicken breasts, cut across the grain into ¼-inch-wide strips
- ½ pound green beans, cut into 1-inch lengths
- 3 plum tomatoes, coarsely chopped

1. In a food processor or blender, combine the coconut, scallions, garlic, lime juice, soy sauce, jalapeños, ginger, coriander, cumin, and 1 cup of water, and process until smooth; set aside.

2. In a large skillet, heat the oil over moderate heat. Add the chicken and green beans, and sauté for 3 minutes or until the chicken is lightly browned.

3. Add the tomatoes and scallion purée to the skillet and bring to a boil. Reduce to a simmer, cover, and cook for 4 minutes or until the beans are crisp-tender and the chicken is cooked through. Serves 4.

Per serving: Calories 187; Fiber 2g; Protein 22g; Total Fat 6g; Saturated Fat 2g; Cholesterol 49mg; Sodium 383mg

Green Chili Salsa

PREP: 15 MINUTES / COOK: 10 MINUTES

Spoon this snappy sauce over vegetables, use it to top chicken or fish, or serve with chips.

- 1 green bell pepper, cut lengthwise into flat panels
- 6 fresh jalapeño peppers, seeded and finely chopped
- 1 can (4½ ounces) chopped mild green chilies, drained
- ½ cup chopped cilantro
- 2 tablespoons lime juice
- 1 tablespoon olive oil
- ½ teaspoon each dried oregano and ground cumin
- ¼ teaspoon salt

1. Preheat the broiler. Place the bell pepper pieces, skin-side up, on the broiler rack and broil 4 inches from the heat for 12 minutes, or until the skin is blackened. When the peppers are cool enough to handle, peel and dice them.

2. Transfer the bell peppers to a medium bowl. Add the jalapeños, mild green chilies, cilantro, lime juice, and oil. Stir in the oregano, cumin, and salt. Makes 2 cups.

Per ½ cup: Calories 55; Fiber 1g; Protein 1g; Total Fat 4g; Saturated Fat 1g; Cholesterol 0mg; Sodium 334mg

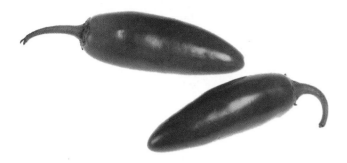

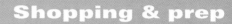

Chunky Corn & Chili Soup

PREP: 20 MINUTES / COOK: 30 MINUTES

The rainbow assortment of vegetables in this recipe signals a healthy variety of nutrients.

- 1   tablespoon olive oil
- 6   scallions, thinly sliced
- 2   cloves garlic, minced
- 1   red bell pepper, cut into ½-inch squares
- 1½ cups chicken broth
- ¾   pound sweet potatoes, peeled and cut into ½-inch cubes
- 1½ cups chopped plum tomatoes (about 4)
- 1   can (4½ ounces) chopped mild green chilies, drained
- 2   fresh jalapeño peppers, seeded and finely chopped
- ½   teaspoon dried oregano
- 1   cup frozen corn kernels
- 1   tablespoon lime juice

1. In large saucepan, heat the oil over moderate heat. Add the scallions and garlic, and sauté for 2 minutes or until tender. Add the bell pepper and sauté for 4 minutes or until crisp-tender.

2. Stir in the broth, 1½ cups of water, the sweet potatoes, tomatoes, mild green chilies, jalapeños, and oregano, and bring to a boil. Reduce to a simmer, cover, and cook for 20 minutes or until the sweet potatoes are tender. Uncover, stir in the corn and lime juice, and cook for 3 minutes or until the corn is heated through. Serves 4.

Per serving: Calories 181; Fiber 5g; Protein 4g; Total Fat 5g; Saturated Fat 1g; Cholesterol 0mg; Sodium 610mg

At the market Most supermarkets sell fresh jalapeños; some stock a wider variety. Latin and Asian stores are good sources for chilies. You can substitute canned mild green chilies or pickled jalapeños, but note that these contain virtually no vitamin C.

Look for Fresh chilies should be glossy, colorful, plump, and unwrinkled.

Prep The capsaicin in chilies can burn your skin and eyes; wear rubber gloves when handling chilies, or wash your hands well with soap and water afterward. Halve chilies lengthwise and scrape out seeds and ribs with a paring knife; leave some ribs for more heat. A jalapeño can be mild as a bell pepper or fiery hot, so before you cook, taste a sliver of the chili: Add a pinch of red pepper flakes to the dish if the chili is too mild.

Chunky Corn & Chili Soup looks like a bowl of confetti and tastes like a Mexican fiesta.

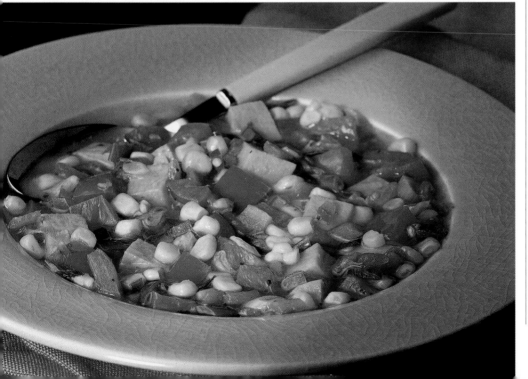

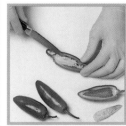

Rubber gloves protect you from the burning capsaicin as you scrape out the seeds.

Cooking greens

Nutritional power
These dark, leafy greens have a lot to offer: disease-fighting carotenoids, indoles, and isothiocyanates, as well as vitamin C, calcium, and iron.

Healthy Highlights

Kale
PER 1 CUP COOKED

Calories	42
Fiber	2.6g
Protein	3g
Total Fat	0.5g
Saturated Fat	0.1g
Cholesterol	0mg
Sodium	30mg

NUTRIENTS

	% Daily Value
Vitamin A	192%
Vitamin C	88%
Manganese	27%

Swiss Chard
PER 1 CUP COOKED

Calories	35
Fiber	3.7g
Protein	3g
Total Fat	0.1g
Saturated Fat	0g
Cholesterol	0mg
Sodium	313mg

NUTRIENTS

	% Daily Value
Vitamin A	110%
Vitamin C	53%
Magnesium	38%
Potassium	32%
Iron	22%
Vitamin E	17%
Calcium	10%

Swiss Chard Quiche
PREP: 30 MINUTES / CHILL: 1 HOUR
COOK: 1 HOUR

CRUST
- 1 cup flour
- 2 teaspoons sugar
- ¼ teaspoon salt
- ¼ cup (½ stick) unsalted butter, cut into pieces
- 3 tablespoons reduced-fat sour cream

FILLING
- 8 cups packed Swiss chard or spinach leaves, coarsely chopped
- ¼ teaspoon sugar
- 2 eggs
- 3 egg whites
- ¾ cup reduced-fat (2%) milk
- ¼ cup low-fat (1%) cottage cheese
- 1 tablespoon flour
- 1 cup shredded Monterey jack cheese

1. For the crust: In a medium bowl, combine the flour, sugar, and salt. With a pastry blender or 2 knives, cut in the butter until the mixture resembles coarse meal. Add the sour cream and stir just until combined. Flatten into a disk, wrap in plastic wrap, and refrigerate for at least 1 hour or overnight.

2. Preheat the oven to 375°F. On a lightly floured surface, roll the dough out to a 13-inch round. Fit the dough into a 10-inch tart pan with a removable bottom. With a fork, prick the bottom of the shell in several places. Line with foil and weight down with pie weights or dried beans. Bake for 15 minutes or until the edges begin to brown and the bottom is set. Remove the weights and cool on a wire rack.

3. For the filling: Rinse the chard and place it, with the water still clinging to it, in a large skillet over moderate heat. Sprinkle with the sugar, cover, and cook for 5 minutes or until wilted. Uncover and cook for 5 minutes or until the liquid has evaporated. Set aside.

4. In a food processor, combine the whole eggs, egg whites, milk, cottage cheese, and flour, and process until smooth. Transfer to a medium bowl and stir in the Monterey jack.

5. Place the tart shell on a baking sheet with sides. Spread the chard over the bottom of the tart shell. Pour the egg mixture over and bake for 30 minutes or until the custard is set. Serve warm or at room temperature. Serves 6.

Per serving: Calories 302; Fiber 1g; Protein 14g; Total Fat 17g; Saturated Fat 10g; Cholesterol 117mg; Sodium 401mg

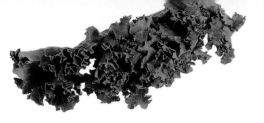

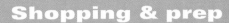

Mixed Greens Frittata

PREP: 15 MINUTES / COOK: 20 MINUTES

- 4 teaspoons olive oil
- 2 cloves garlic, minced
- 8 cups mixed greens, such as kale, Swiss chard, and spinach, torn into bite-size pieces
- 2 eggs
- 4 egg whites
- ¼ cup low-fat (1%) cottage cheese
- ¼ cup grated Parmesan cheese
- 1 tablespoon flour
- ½ teaspoon salt

1. In a large broilerproof nonstick skillet, heat 2 teaspoons of the oil over moderate heat. Add the garlic and cook for 2 minutes. Add the greens and cook, stirring often, for 7 minutes or until very tender. Transfer the greens to a plate and wipe out the skillet.

2. In a food processor, combine the whole eggs, egg whites, cottage cheese, Parmesan, flour, and salt. Add the

Swiss Chard Quiche is the perfect centerpiece for a company brunch or a Sunday-night supper.

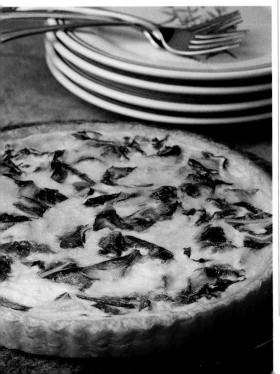

remaining 2 teaspoons oil to the skillet and heat over moderate heat. Add the greens, pour the egg mixture over, and cook without stirring for 10 minutes or until the eggs are set around the edges and slightly wobbly in the center.

3. Preheat the broiler. Broil the frittata 6 inches from the heat for 1 minute or just until the center is set. Serves 4.

Per serving: Calories 172; Fiber 4g; Protein 14g; Total Fat 9g; Saturated Fat 3g; Cholesterol 111mg; Sodium 611mg

Sautéed Greens with Bacon & Hot Pepper

PREP: 15 MINUTES / COOK: 20 MINUTES

You can also make this with spinach. Use two bunches and add them in Step 3; cook, covered, for 3 to 4 minutes—just until wilted.

- 1 bunch of kale (1 pound), tough stems removed
- 2 slices bacon, cut crosswise into ¼-inch-wide strips
- 1 large red onion, finely chopped
- 4 cloves garlic, minced
- ½ teaspoon crushed red pepper flakes
- ½ teaspoon salt

1. Bring a large pot of water to a boil. Add the kale in batches and cook for 3 minutes to wilt. Reserving 1¼ cups of the cooking liquid, drain the kale.

2. In a large nonstick skillet, cook the bacon in ¼ cup of the reserved cooking liquid over moderate heat for 4 minutes or until the bacon has rendered its fat. Remove the bacon with a slotted spoon. Add the onion and garlic, and cook for 7 minutes or until the onion is soft. Stir in the red pepper flakes.

3. Add the kale, bacon, salt, and the remaining 1 cup cooking liquid. Cook for 4 minutes or until the kale is tender. Serves 4.

Per serving: Calories 126; Fiber 6g; Protein 4g; Total Fat 7g; Saturated Fat 3g; Cholesterol 8mg; Sodium 388mg

At the market Kale is most abundant in the fall and winter, while Swiss chard is in best supply from spring through late fall. Other greens are sold all year: Try collards, broccoli rabe, and beet and mustard greens.

Look for Greens should have fresh, vivid color. Stalks should be plump and moist; leaves should be crisp and free of holes or spots. Small leaves are more tender than large ones.

Prep Wash greens well: They can be gritty. Trim Swiss chard stems with a knife (stems are edible, too, but require longer cooking than leaves).

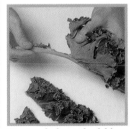

To stem kale easily, fold each leaf in half, then pull off the stem.

Basic cooking Steam washed leaves in their own moisture: tender young leaves for about 2 minutes, sturdier greens for up to 15 minutes. Microwave washed greens, covered, for 4 to 7 minutes. (Cooking times depend on type of greens.)

Broccoli Rabe

PER ¼ POUND RAW

Calories	20
Fiber	3.0
Protein	3g
Total Fat	0g
Saturated Fat	0g
Cholesterol	0mg
Sodium	20mg

NUTRIENTS

	% Daily Value
Vitamin C	121%
Vitamin A	51%

Collard Greens

PER 1 CUP COOKED

Calories	51
Fiber	5.3g
Protein	3g
Total Fat	0.4g
Saturated Fat	0g
Cholesterol	0mg
Sodium	30mg

NUTRIENTS

	% Daily Value
Vitamin A	104%
Vitamin C	38%
Manganese	21%

Did you know? . . .
Other cooking greens that are nutrition powerhouses include beet, turnip, mustard, and dandelion greens. Beet and turnip greens are considerably more nutritious than their roots when it comes to vitamin C, beta carotene, calcium, iron, and folate.

Southern-Style Braised Greens & Corn

PREP: 15 MINUTES / COOK: 35 MINUTES

Fresh greens are a mainstay of Southern cooking—not just collards but also turnip, beet, and mustard greens. Feel free to substitute other greens for the collards in this recipe.

- 2 teaspoons olive oil
- 3 ounces Virginia ham or smoked turkey, cut into ¼-inch dice
- 6 scallions, thinly sliced
- 2 cloves garlic, finely chopped
- 10 cups firmly packed collard greens, torn into bite-size pieces, or 2 packages (10 ounces each) frozen collard greens
- ½ cup chicken broth
- ½ teaspoon pepper
- ½ teaspoon dried marjoram
- ¼ teaspoon salt
- 1½ cups frozen corn kernels
- 4 teaspoons balsamic or red wine vinegar

1. In a large nonstick skillet, heat the oil over moderate heat. Add the ham, scallions, and garlic, and sauté for 3 minutes or until the scallions are soft.

2. Add the greens, stirring to coat. Add the broth, pepper, marjoram, and salt, and cook, partially covered, for 30 minutes or until the greens are wilted and very tender.

3. Stir in the corn and cook just until heated through. Stir in the vinegar and serve the greens with their cooking liquid. Pass additional vinegar at the table. Serves 4.

Per serving: Calories 210; Fiber 11g; Protein 12g; Total Fat 5g; Saturated Fat 1g; Cholesterol 13mg; Sodium 646mg

Portuguese Greens Soup with Sausages

PREP: 20 MINUTES / COOK: 45 MINUTES

This recipe calls for fresh chorizo, a spicy Mexican pork sausage. If you can't find chorizo, use a second Italian sausage link. You can also make this soup with spinach, but add it at the very end and cook until just wilted.

- 1 teaspoon olive oil
- 1 sweet Italian sausage link (2½ ounces), cut into ½-inch-thick slices
- 1 large onion, finely chopped
- 2 cloves garlic, minced
- 1 can (10 ounces) red kidney beans, rinsed and drained
- 1 fresh chorizo sausage link (3 ounces), cut into ½-inch-thick slices
- 1 cup chicken broth
- 2 tablespoons no-salt-added tomato paste
- ½ teaspoon pepper
- 10 cups firmly packed kale and Swiss chard leaves, torn into bite-size pieces
- 1 tablespoon red wine vinegar

1. In a nonstick Dutch oven, heat the oil over moderate heat. Add the Italian sausage and cook, turning occasionally, for 4 minutes or until the sausage is browned and the fat has been rendered.

2. Add the onion and garlic to the pan and sauté for 7 minutes or until soft. Add the beans, chorizo, broth, 3 cups of water, the tomato paste, and pepper. Bring to a boil, reduce to a simmer, and add the greens. Cook, uncovered, for 30 minutes or until the sausages are cooked through and the greens are as tender as you like them. Stir in the vinegar and serve. Serves 4.

Per serving: Calories 293; Fiber 9g; Protein 15g; Total Fat 16g; Saturated Fat 5g; Cholesterol 32mg; Sodium 978mg

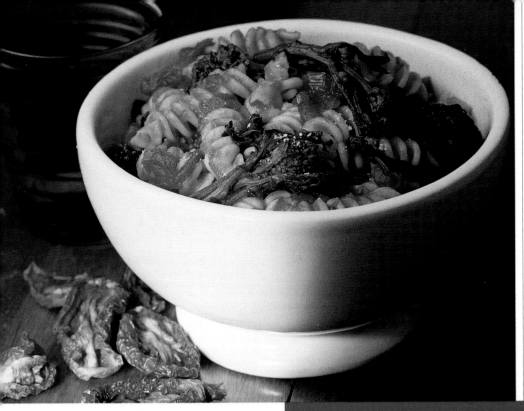

Pasta with Broccoli Rabe & Sun-Dried Tomatoes In Italy, garlic-sautéed greens are a classic partner for pasta.

Did you know? . . .
Most cooking greens are rich in calcium and iron, but some types of greens (such as beet greens, Swiss chard, and sorrel) contain compounds that interfere with mineral absorption. For the greatest benefits, eat a variety of greens.

Pasta with Broccoli Rabe & Sun-Dried Tomatoes

PREP: 15 MINUTES / COOK: 25 MINUTES

You can substitute broccoli for the rabe. Cut the broccoli tops into small florets; peel the stems and cut them into 1-inch pieces.

- ½ cup sun-dried tomatoes (not oil-packed)
- 1 large bunch of broccoli rabe (1¼ pounds), cut into 1-inch lengths
- 8 ounces fusilli pasta
- 1 tablespoon olive oil
- 4 cloves garlic, minced
- 1 to 1½ teaspoons crushed red pepper flakes
- 2 tablespoons no-salt-added tomato paste
- ¾ teaspoon salt
- ¼ teaspoon black pepper
- ⅓ cup golden raisins (optional)
- ⅓ cup grated Parmesan cheese

1. To a large pot of boiling water, add the sun-dried tomatoes and cook for 5 minutes or until softened. With a slotted spoon, remove the sun-dried tomatoes and when cool enough to handle, coarsely chop.

2. Add the broccoli rabe to the boiling water and cook for 4 minutes or until crisp-tender. With a slotted spoon, transfer the broccoli rabe to a colander. Add the pasta to the boiling water and cook according to package directions until firm-tender. Reserving 1½ cups of the cooking liquid, drain the pasta and transfer to a large serving bowl.

3. Meanwhile, in a large skillet, heat the oil over low heat. Add the garlic and red pepper flakes, and sauté for 3 minutes. Add the sun-dried tomatoes, broccoli rabe, tomato paste, salt, black pepper, and reserved cooking liquid. Cook, stirring, for 4 minutes or until the broccoli rabe is heated through and tender. Add to the hot pasta along with the raisins and Parmesan, tossing well to combine. Serves 4.

Per serving: Calories 339; Fiber 4g; Protein 16g; Total Fat 6g; Saturated Fat 2g; Cholesterol 5mg; Sodium 580mg

When fruits and vegetables were tested for antioxidant power, kale ranked second.

For a recent USDA study, common fruits and vegetables were analyzed for their antioxidant power. Among all the vegetables studied, kale ranked second. (Garlic was number one.)

For a change, try preparing some of your favorite cabbage recipes (such as stuffed cabbage) with cooking greens. Just be sure to adjust the cooking times so that the greens don't cook to mush.

Fennel

Nutritional power
Along with its unique flavor, this favorite Italian vegetable offers fiber, vitamin C, and potassium, as well as respectable amounts of iron and calcium.

Healthy Highlights

PER 1 CUP RAW	
Calories	27
Fiber	2.7g
Protein	1g
Total Fat	0.2g
Saturated Fat	0g
Cholesterol	0mg
Sodium	45mg

NUTRIENTS	
	% Daily Value
Vitamin C	17%
Potassium	12%

Did you know? . . .
Recipes that call for fennel sometimes suggest celery as an alternative, but the nutritional difference is significant. Although they're similar in texture, fennel has considerably more fiber. Fennel also provides more calcium, potassium, and vitamin C than celery. And of course, there's that wonderful licorice-like flavor.

Pork & Fennel Sauté

PREP: 15 MINUTES / COOK: 25 MINUTES

A dish where the produce outweighs the meat is likely to be a healthful one. With fennel, onion, garlic, and apple, this is a sure winner.

- 1 **bulb fennel (1¼ pounds)**
- 1 **pound well-trimmed pork tenderloin, cut into 8 slices**
- 2 **tablespoons flour**
- 4 **teaspoons olive oil**
- 1 **onion, finely chopped**
- 2 **cloves garlic, minced**
- 1 **McIntosh apple, cut into ¼-inch-thick wedges**
- ½ **cup chicken broth**
- ½ **teaspoon salt**
- ¼ **teaspoon pepper**
- 2 **tablespoons reduced-fat sour cream**

1. Cut off the fennel stalks and fronds. Finely chop 2 tablespoons of the fronds and reserve; discard the stalks. Cut the bulb in half lengthwise and thinly slice crosswise. Set aside.

2. With the heel of your hand, lightly flatten the pieces of pork. On a sheet of wax paper, dredge the pork in the flour, shaking off the excess. In a large non-stick skillet, heat 1 tablespoon of the oil over moderately high heat. Add the pork and cook for 3 minutes per side or until browned and just cooked through. With a slotted spoon, transfer the pork to a plate.

3. Add the remaining 1 teaspoon oil, the onion, and garlic to the skillet and sauté for 5 minutes or until softened.

Add the sliced fennel and sauté for 5 minutes or until crisp-tender. Add the apple and sauté for 5 minutes or until crisp-tender.

4. Stir in the broth, ½ cup of water, the salt, and pepper, and bring to a boil. Reduce to a simmer, return the pork to the pan, and cook for 1 minute or until cooked through. Spoon the pork and fennel mixture onto 4 plates. Whisk the sour cream and reserved fennel fronds into the sauce, spoon over the pork, and serve. Serves 4.

Per serving: Calories 282; Fiber 3g; Protein 26g; Total Fat 12g; Saturated Fat 3g; Cholesterol 77mg; Sodium 579mg

Fennel & Potato Hash with Caramelized Onions

PREP: 25 MINUTES / COOK: 40 MINUTES

Served with a salad, this meatless hash will make a small but satisfying meal. For a more substantial dish, add cubed cooked beef or chicken, and cook, stirring, until heated through. Or top the hash with a poached egg.

- 1 **pound all-purpose potatoes**
- 2 **bulbs fennel (2½ pounds total)**
- 1 **tablespoon olive oil**
- 2 **large onions, finely chopped**
- 2 **cloves garlic, minced**
- ¾ **teaspoon salt**
- ¼ **teaspoon pepper**

1. In a large pot of boiling water, cook

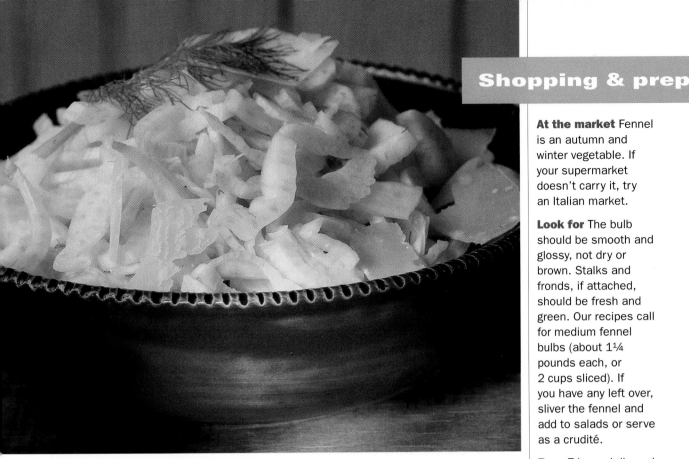

Fresh Fennel Salad with Lemon Serve this simple and refreshingly crunchy salad before or alongside a rich main course.

At the market Fennel is an autumn and winter vegetable. If your supermarket doesn't carry it, try an Italian market.

Look for The bulb should be smooth and glossy, not dry or brown. Stalks and fronds, if attached, should be fresh and green. Our recipes call for medium fennel bulbs (about 1¼ pounds each, or 2 cups sliced). If you have any left over, sliver the fennel and add to salads or serve as a crudité.

Prep Trim and discard stalks; save fronds for garnishing and flavoring. Halve the bulb lengthwise, then slice it crosswise.

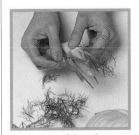

Don't discard fennel fronds—they're rich in flavor and vitamin C.

Basic cooking Steam sliced or chopped fennel for 10 to 15 minutes. Braise halved fennel bulbs (or sliced fennel) in a skillet with just enough boiling liquid to cover; cook for 25 to 40 minutes, or until tender.

---

the potatoes for 30 minutes or until tender. Drain and when cool enough to handle, peel and thinly slice.

2. Meanwhile, cut off the fennel stalks and fronds. Finely chop ¼ cup of the fronds and reserve; discard the stalks. Cut the bulb in half lengthwise and thinly slice crosswise. Set aside.

3. In a large nonstick skillet, heat the oil over moderate heat. Add the onions and garlic, and sauté for 12 minutes or until the onions are golden brown.

4. Add the sliced fennel to the skillet and cook, stirring, for 10 minutes or until crisp-tender. Add the potatoes, sprinkle with the salt and pepper, and cook, stirring frequently, for 10 minutes or until the potatoes and fennel are tender. Stir in the chopped fennel fronds and serve. Serves 4.

Per serving: Calories 204; Fiber 6g; Protein 6g; Total Fat 4g; Saturated Fat 1g; Cholesterol 0mg; Sodium 648mg

Fresh Fennel Salad with Lemon

PREP: 10 MINUTES

- ¼ cup lemon juice
- 4 teaspoons olive oil
- ½ teaspoon salt
- 2 bulbs fennel (2½ pounds total)
- ¼ cup shaved Parmesan cheese

1. In a medium bowl, whisk together the lemon juice, 2 tablespoons of water, the oil, and salt.

2. Cut off the fennel stalks and fronds. Finely chop ¼ cup of the fronds and add to the bowl of dressing; discard the stalks. Cut the bulb in half lengthwise and thinly slice crosswise. Add the fennel to the bowl and toss well to combine. Serve the salad sprinkled with the Parmesan. Serves 4.

Per serving: Calories 104; Fiber 2g; Protein 5g; Total Fat 6g; Saturated Fat 2g; Cholesterol 4mg; Sodium 598mg

Garlic

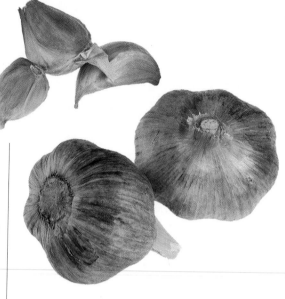

Nutritional power
Used medicinally since ancient times, garlic is now being studied by scientists. It may fight cancer and heart disease, and lower blood pressure.

Healthy Highlights

PER ½ OUNCE RAW	
Calories	22
Fiber	0.3g
Protein	1g
Total Fat	0.1g
Saturated Fat	0g
Cholesterol	0mg
Sodium	3mg

NUTRIENTS	
	% Daily Value
Manganese	13%

Did you know? . . .
Garlic contains sulfur compounds that may speed the breakdown of carcinogens (cancer-causing substances).

A study in China's Shandong province showed that the more garlic people ate, the less likely they were to develop stomach cancer.

Garlic has been shown to lower blood pressure and blood cholesterol, and to inhibit clotting.

Chicken Breasts with Roasted Garlic Sauce

PREP: 10 MINUTES / COOK: 1 HOUR

Yes, there are two full heads (not cloves) of garlic in this savory chicken dish, but roasting mellows and sweetens the garlic.

- 2 heads of garlic (5 ounces total)
- 4 skinless, boneless chicken breast halves (4 ounces each)
- 2 tablespoons flour
- 2 teaspoons olive oil
- ½ cup chicken broth
- ¼ teaspoon dried rosemary, crumbled
- ¼ teaspoon each salt and pepper
- ½ teaspoon grated lemon zest
- 1 tablespoon lemon juice
- 2 tablespoons chopped parsley

1. Preheat the oven to 450°F. Wrap each head of garlic in foil. Bake for 45 minutes or until very soft when squeezed. When cool enough to handle, cut off the stem end from each head of garlic, squeeze the garlic pulp into a small bowl, and mash with a fork.

2. Dredge the chicken in the flour, shaking off the excess. In a large nonstick skillet, heat the oil over moderate heat. Add the chicken and cook for 8 minutes or until lightly browned on both sides.

3. Add the mashed garlic, the broth, ½ cup of water, the rosemary, salt, pepper, and lemon zest, and bring to a boil. Reduce to a simmer, cover, and cook, stirring occasionally, for 4 minutes or until the sauce coats the chicken and the chicken is cooked through. Stir the lemon juice and parsley into the sauce. Serve the chicken topped with the sauce. Serves 4.

Per serving: Calories 210; Fiber 1g; Protein 29g; Total Fat 4g; Saturated Fat 1g; Cholesterol 66mg; Sodium 347mg

White Bean Garlic Dip

PREP: 10 MINUTES / COOK: 5 MINUTES

This velvety and aromatic bean purée is a smart alternative to a dip based on cream cheese or sour cream. Serve it with raw vegetables as dippers.

- 10 cloves garlic
- 1 can (19 ounces) cannellini beans, rinsed and drained
- 2 tablespoons reduced-fat sour cream
- 1 tablespoon lemon juice
- 2 teaspoons sesame oil
- ½ teaspoon ground coriander
- ¼ teaspoon salt
- ¼ cup chopped parsley
- 1 teaspoon paprika

1. In a small pot of boiling water, cook the garlic for 3 minutes to blanch. Drain, reserving 2 tablespoons of the cooking liquid. Peel the garlic.

2. In a food processor, combine the garlic, reserved cooking liquid, and beans, and process to a smooth purée. Add the sour cream, lemon juice, sesame oil, coriander, and salt, and process briefly to blend. Transfer the mixture to a small serving bowl. Serve sprinkled with the parsley and paprika. Makes 2 cups.

Per ¼ cup: Calories 71; Fiber 3g; Protein 4g; Total Fat 2g; Saturated Fat 0g; Cholesterol 1mg; Sodium 155mg

Creamy Garlic Soup with Herbed Croutons

PREP: 30 MINUTES / COOK: 45 MINUTES

To make the task of peeling three heads of garlic easier, blanch the unpeeled garlic cloves in boiling water for 1 to 2 minutes.

- 3 slices (1 ounce each) firm-textured white sandwich bread
- 1 tablespoon olive oil
- 1 tablespoon grated Parmesan cheese
- ½ teaspoon each dried thyme and sage
- 1½ cups chicken broth
- 3 heads of garlic (7 ounces total), peeled
- ¾ pound all-purpose potatoes, peeled and thinly sliced
- ¼ teaspoon salt
- 3 tablespoons light mayonnaise
- ¼ cup chopped parsley

1. Preheat the oven to 375°F. Brush the bread with the oil. Cut the bread into ½-inch squares, then toss with the Parmesan and ¼ teaspoon each of the thyme and sage. Spread the squares on a baking sheet and bake for 5 minutes or until lightly crisped.

2. In a medium saucepan, combine the broth, garlic, and the remaining ¼ teaspoon each thyme and sage. Bring to a simmer, cover, and cook for 25 minutes or until the garlic is very soft.

3. Meanwhile, in another medium saucepan, bring 2 cups of water to a boil. Add the potatoes and cook for 12 minutes or until very tender; drain.

4. Transfer the garlic mixture to a food processor and process to a smooth purée. Return the purée to the pan. Add the potatoes, their cooking liquid, and the salt, and bring to a boil. Reduce to a simmer, add the mayonnaise, and cook, whisking, for 2 minutes or until the soup is lightly thickened. Serve the soup topped with the croutons and sprinkled with the parsley. Serves 4.

Per serving: Calories 256; Fiber 3g; Protein 7g; Total Fat 9g; Saturated Fat 2g; Cholesterol 5mg; Sodium 766mg

At the market A kitchen staple, garlic is always in good supply.

Look for Choose a full, plump head of garlic with taut, unbroken outer skin. Pass up heads with shriveled cloves or green shoots sprouting from the top.

Prep Separate the cloves from the head; avoid piercing the skin on the remaining cloves. To peel, place each clove under the flat side of a broad knife blade; strike the blade with your fist. This will crack and loosen the peel, making it easy to remove.

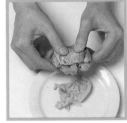

After roasting, garlic pulp can be squeezed out of the skin—no peeling required.

Basic cooking Blanching whole, unpeeled garlic cloves for just a few minutes tempers the pungent flavor a bit and makes the garlic easier to peel. Roasting a whole head of garlic, wrapped in foil, renders it sweet and spreadable. Roast at 450° for about 45 minutes.

Chicken Breasts with Roasted Garlic Sauce *Serve with potatoes to sop up the sauce.*

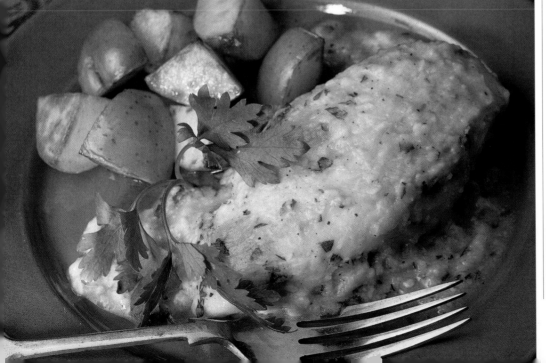

Ginger

Nutritional power
Revered in Asia for both stimulant and calmative powers, ginger shows promise as a remedy for seasickness, morning sickness, and other stomach ills.

Healthy Highlights

PER ½ OUNCE RAW	
Calories	10
Fiber	0.3g
Protein	0g
Total Fat	0.1g
Saturated Fat	0g
Cholesterol	0mg
Sodium	2mg

Did you know? . . .
For centuries, various forms of ginger have been used to quell nausea. Several studies have investigated this effect, and in Germany, ginger is approved as a medical treatment for motion sickness and also for heartburn.

One teaspoon of ground ginger contains .5mg of manganese—that's 25% of the Daily Value for this mineral, which is involved in energy production and helps build strong bones.

Scallop & Oriental Vegetable Sauté

PREP: 20 MINUTES / COOK: 10 MINUTES

- 3 tablespoons lower-sodium soy sauce
- 4 teaspoons lemon juice
- 1 tablespoon grated plus ⅓ cup slivered fresh ginger
- 1 pound sea scallops, halved
- 2½ teaspoons vegetable oil
- 1½ pounds Napa cabbage, sliced
- 1½ cups snow peas, halved lengthwise
- 6 scallions, sliced
- 4 cloves garlic, minced
- 1 tablespoon rice vinegar
- 1 teaspoon cornstarch blended with 1 tablespoon water
- ¾ teaspoon honey
- ¾ teaspoon sesame oil

1. In a medium bowl, combine the soy sauce and lemon juice with the grated ginger. Add the scallops, tossing to coat. Let marinate for 15 minutes.

2. Meanwhile, in a large nonstick skillet, heat the vegetable oil over moderately high heat. Add the cabbage and sauté for 4 minutes. Stir in the slivered ginger, the snow peas, scallions, and garlic, and sauté for 2 minutes. With a slotted spoon, transfer the vegetables to a serving dish.

3. Add the scallops and their marinade to the pan. Cook for 2 minutes or until the scallops are just opaque. With a slotted spoon, transfer the scallops to the serving dish. Add the vinegar, cornstarch mixture, and honey to the pan and cook, stirring, for 1 minute or until the sauce is lightly thickened. Stir in the sesame oil and pour the sauce over the scallops and vegetables. Serves 4.

Per serving: Calories 215; Fiber 4g; Protein 24g; Total Fat 5g; Saturated Fat 1g; Cholesterol 38mg; Sodium 657mg

Homemade Ginger Ale

PREP: 5 MINUTES / COOK: 30 MINUTES

Bottled ginger ale just can't compare to this potent, peppery syrup; there's far more real ginger in this homemade brew. If you let the ginger cool in the liquid in Step 1 instead of straining it right away, you will get a "hotter" ginger syrup.

- ¾ cup thinly sliced unpeeled fresh ginger
- 1 cup sugar
- 3 strips (2 x ½ inch) lemon zest
- ⅛ teaspoon whole black peppercorns
- ⅛ teaspoon allspice berries (optional) Seltzer

1. In a medium saucepan, bring 2 cups of water and the ginger to a boil over moderate heat. Reduce the heat to low, cover, and simmer for 25 minutes. Reserving the liquid, strain and discard the ginger.

2. In the same saucepan, combine the ginger liquid, the sugar, lemon zest, peppercorns, and allspice over low heat. Bring to a boil and boil for 2 minutes. Cover the syrup and let stand until cooled to room temperature. Strain the ginger syrup and refrigerate.

3. To serve, pour ¼ cup of the syrup into a tall glass. Add ¾ cup of cold seltzer; add ice if you wish. Serves 8.

Per serving: Calories 100; Fiber 0g; Protein 0g; Total Fat 0g; Saturated Fat 0g; Cholesterol 0mg; Sodium 1mg

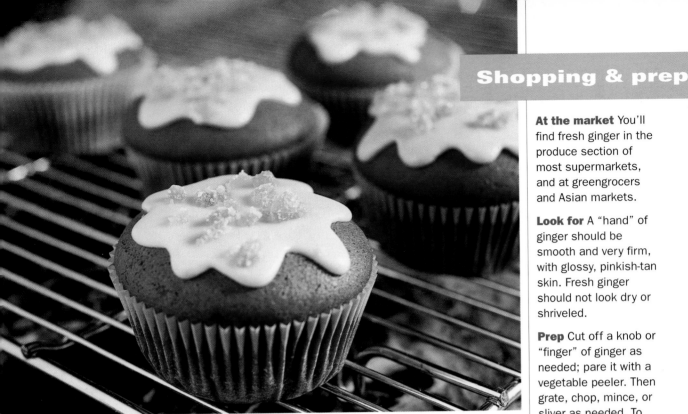

Gingerbread Cupcakes with Ginger Glaze are homey yet sophisticated party fare.

At the market You'll find fresh ginger in the produce section of most supermarkets, and at greengrocers and Asian markets.

Look for A "hand" of ginger should be smooth and very firm, with glossy, pinkish-tan skin. Fresh ginger should not look dry or shriveled.

Prep Cut off a knob or "finger" of ginger as needed; pare it with a vegetable peeler. Then grate, chop, mince, or sliver as needed. To make ginger juice, see below.

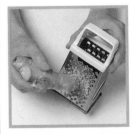

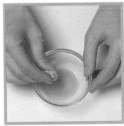

To make ginger juice, first grate the desired amount of ginger (a 2-inch piece of ginger will yield about 2 teaspoons juice). To extract the juice, squeeze the grated ginger with your fingers, press it in a tea strainer, or wring it in a square of cheesecloth.

Gingerbread Cupcakes with Ginger Glaze

PREP: 15 MINUTES / COOK: 25 MINUTES

"Triple-gingerbread" we might have said— these cupcakes are made with fresh ginger juice as well as ground ginger, and are decorated with crystallized ginger.

1⅓	**cups flour**
1	**tablespoon ground ginger**
1	**teaspoon dry mustard**
1	**teaspoon baking soda**
½	**teaspoon cinnamon**
¼	**teaspoon salt**
⅛	**teaspoon ground cloves**
½	**cup packed dark brown sugar**
¼	**cup molasses**
3	**tablespoons vegetable oil**
2	**egg whites**
½	**cup low-fat (1.5%) buttermilk**
1	**piece (2 inches) of fresh ginger**
½	**cup confectioners sugar**
2	**tablespoons chopped crystallized ginger (optional)**

1. Preheat the oven to 350°F. Line a 2½-inch muffin tin with paper liners; set aside. On a sheet of wax paper, combine the flour, ginger, mustard, baking soda, cinnamon, salt, and cloves.

2. In a bowl, with an electric mixer, beat the brown sugar, molasses, and oil until well combined. Beat in the egg whites, one at a time, until well incorporated and light in texture. Alternately fold the flour mixture and the buttermilk into the sugar mixture, beginning and ending with the flour mixture. Spoon into the prepared muffin cups and bake for 20 minutes or until a cake tester inserted in the center of a cupcake comes out clean. Cool in the pan on a wire rack.

3. Grate the ginger on the fine side of a box grater. Squeeze the ginger to extract the juice and measure out 2 teaspoons. In a small bowl, combine the confectioners sugar and ginger juice. Spread the tops of the cooled cupcakes with the ginger glaze. Sprinkle with the crystallized ginger. Makes 12 cupcakes.

Per serving: Calories 163; Fiber 0g; Protein 3g; Total Fat 4g; Saturated Fat 1g; Cholesterol 1mg; Sodium 171mg

Mushrooms

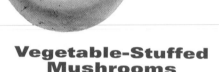

Nutritional power
Very low in calories, yet packed with meaty flavor, mushrooms also contain substances that may enhance immune function and slow tumor growth.

Healthy Highlights

PER 1 CUP RAW	
Calories	18
Fiber	0.8g
Protein	2g
Total Fat	0.3g
Saturated Fat	0g
Cholesterol	0mg
Sodium	3mg

NUTRIENTS	
	% Daily Value
Riboflavin	18%
Copper	17%
Niacin	15%

Did you know? . . .
Mushrooms contain compounds called triterpenoids, which seem to fight cancer by inhibiting certain steps in the formation of tumors.

Cooking mushrooms breaks down their fibrous cell walls, making some of their nutrients more available to the body.

Pasta with Creamy Mushroom Sauce

PREP: 25 MINUTES / COOK: 25 MINUTES

- 12 ounces fusilli pasta
- 2 teaspoons vegetable oil
- 5 scallions, thinly sliced
- 4 cloves garlic, minced
- ½ pound fresh shiitake mushrooms, trimmed, halved, and thinly sliced
- 1 pound button mushrooms, halved and thinly sliced
- ½ teaspoon salt
- 2 tablespoons flour
- 2 cups reduced-fat (2%) milk
- ½ teaspoon pepper
- 1 teaspoon unsalted butter
- ¼ cup grated Parmesan cheese

1. In a large pot of boiling water, cook the pasta according to package directions until firm-tender. Drain well and transfer to a large serving bowl.

2. Meanwhile, in a large nonstick skillet, heat the oil over moderate heat. Add the scallions and garlic, and sauté for 2 minutes. Add the shiitakes, cover, and cook, stirring occasionally, for 5 minutes or until tender.

3. Add the button mushrooms and sprinkle with the salt. Cover and cook, stirring occasionally, for 5 minutes. Increase the heat to high, uncover, and cook for 4 minutes or until the liquid has evaporated. Sprinkle with the flour, stirring until absorbed. Gradually add the milk and cook, stirring, for 5 minutes or until the sauce is lightly thickened. Stir in the pepper.

4. Add the sauce, butter, and Parmesan to the hot pasta, tossing well to coat. Serves 4.

Per serving: Calories 495; Fiber 5g; Protein 22g; Total Fat 9g; Saturated Fat 4g; Cholesterol 16mg; Sodium 442mg

Vegetable-Stuffed Mushrooms

PREP: 20 MINUTES / COOK: 20 MINUTES

- 24 large or 12 extra-large mushrooms, stems removed
- 2 teaspoons vegetable oil
- 1 onion, finely chopped
- 3 cloves garlic, minced
- 1 carrot, finely chopped
- 1 red bell pepper, finely chopped
- ½ cup chicken broth
- ½ teaspoon dried oregano
- 3 tablespoons grated Parmesan cheese
- 2 tablespoons chopped parsley

1. Preheat the oven to 400°F. In a medium pot of boiling water, cook the mushroom caps for 2 minutes to blanch. Drain on paper towels.

2. In a large skillet, heat the oil over moderate heat. Add the onion and garlic, and sauté for 5 minutes. Add the carrot and pepper, and cook for 4 minutes. Add the broth and oregano, and cook for 4 minutes or until the vegetables are very soft. Remove from the heat; stir in the Parmesan and parsley.

3. Spoon the mixture into the mushroom caps. Place on a baking sheet and bake for 10 minutes or until piping hot. Serves 4.

Per serving: Calories 107; Fiber 3g; Protein 6g; Total Fat 4g; Saturated Fat 1g; Cholesterol 3mg; Sodium 216mg

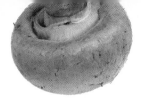

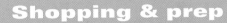

Fresh & Dried Mushroom Soup

PREP: 20 MINUTES / COOK: 30 MINUTES

Dried porcini have a special flavor, but they can be pricey. The inexpensive imported dried mushrooms sold in supermarkets make an acceptable substitute in this recipe.

- ½ **cup dried porcini or other imported dried mushrooms (¾ ounce)**
- 1 **cup boiling water**
- 2 **teaspoons vegetable oil**
- 1 **large onion, finely chopped**
- 4 **cloves garlic, minced**
- ½ **pound fresh shiitake mushrooms, trimmed, halved, and thinly sliced**
- 1 **pound button mushrooms, thinly sliced**
- ¼ **cup dry sherry or chicken broth**
- 1½ **cups chicken broth**
- 1 **large tomato, finely chopped**
- ½ **teaspoon dried tarragon**
- ½ **teaspoon pepper**

1. In a small bowl, combine the dried mushrooms and boiling water, and let stand for 10 minutes or until softened.

Reserving the liquid, scoop out the dried mushrooms and coarsely chop. Strain the soaking liquid through a coffee filter or a paper towel-lined sieve.

2. In a large saucepan, heat the oil over moderate heat. Add the onion and garlic, and sauté for 5 minutes or until the onion has softened. Stir in the dried mushrooms. Add the shiitakes and sauté for 5 minutes or until they are soft. Add the button mushrooms and cook, stirring frequently, for 5 minutes or until they begin to give up liquid.

3. Add the reserved soaking liquid and bring to a boil. Add the sherry and cook for 5 minutes or until reduced by half. Add the broth, 1½ cups of water, the tomato, tarragon, and pepper. Bring to a boil, reduce to a simmer, cover, and cook for 10 minutes or until the soup is richly flavored. Serves 4.

Per serving: Calories 133; Fiber 5g; Protein 7g; Total Fat 4g; Saturated Fat 1g; Cholesterol 0mg; Sodium 408mg

At the market White mushrooms are in the market all year round. If you can't find shiitake or other "exotic" mushrooms at the supermarket, try a gourmet shop.

Look for Fresh mushrooms should look clean, plump, and moist; pass up those that are dry or darkening. The gills (under the caps) should be tightly closed.

Prep Trim the stem bases of white mushrooms; trim the entire stem from shiitakes. Wipe mushrooms with a damp paper towel or a soft brush, if necessary. Soak dried mushrooms in boiling water to soften, then drain. If using the soaking liquid in the dish, strain it through a coffee filter or paper towel to remove any grit.

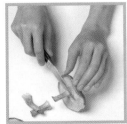

Shiitake stems are too tough to eat. Trim them close to the base of the cap.

Basic cooking Simmer mushrooms in a little broth to give them extra flavor with no added fat. Cook for 3 to 5 minutes.

Vegetable-Stuffed Mushrooms make a healthful start for a festive meal.

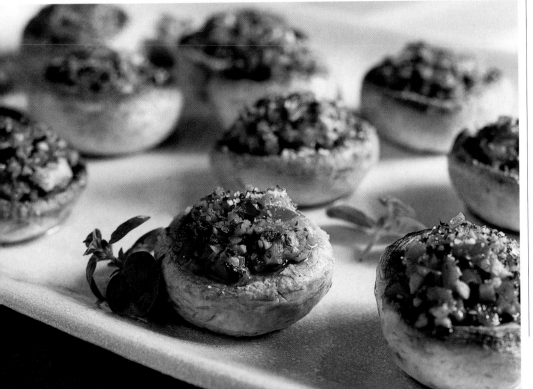

Onions

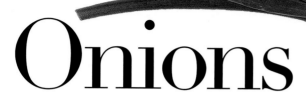

Nutritional power
Onion-family vegetables offer cancer-fighting compounds and antioxidant flavonoids; they also seem to help lower blood pressure and cholesterol.

Healthy Highlights

Onions
PER 1 CUP COOKED

Calories	92
Fiber	2.9g
Protein	3g
Total Fat	0.4g
Saturated Fat	0.1g
Cholesterol	0mg
Sodium	6mg

NUTRIENTS

	% Daily Value
Vitamin C	18%
Manganese	16%
Vitamin B6	14%
Potassium	12%

Scallions
PER ½ CUP RAW

Calories	16
Fiber	1.3g
Protein	1g
Total Fat	0.1g
Saturated Fat	0g
Cholesterol	0mg
Sodium	8mg

NUTRIENTS

	% Daily Value
Vitamin C	15%

Chicken with Smothered Onions
PREP: 10 MINUTES / COOK: 35 MINUTES

- **4 teaspoons vegetable oil**
- **4 skinless, boneless chicken breast halves (4 ounces each)**
- **2 tablespoons flour**
- **1 large Spanish onion (1¼ pounds), halved and thinly sliced**
- **½ teaspoon sugar**
- **½ teaspoon salt**
- **⅓ cup chicken broth**
- **¼ teaspoon dried rosemary, crumbled**
- **¼ teaspoon pepper**
- **2 tablespoons chopped parsley**

1. In a large nonstick skillet, heat 2 teaspoons of the oil over moderate heat. Dredge the chicken in the flour, shaking off the excess. Add the chicken to the pan and cook for 3 minutes per side or until golden brown. Transfer the chicken to a plate and set aside.

2. Add the remaining 2 teaspoons oil to the skillet and heat over moderate heat. Add the onion, sugar, and ¼ teaspoon of the salt. Cover and cook, stirring occasionally, for 10 minutes or until very soft. Uncover and cook for 10 minutes or until golden brown.

3. Add the broth, ⅓ cup of water, the rosemary, pepper, and the remaining ¼ teaspoon salt to the pan. Bring to a boil. Reduce to a simmer, return the chicken to the pan, cover, and cook for 5 minutes or until the chicken is cooked through. Serve the chicken topped with the onions and parsley. Serves 4.

Per serving: Calories 242; Fiber 3g; Protein 29g; Total Fat 6g; Saturated Fat 1g; Cholesterol 66mg; Sodium 450mg

Scallion Pancakes
PREP: 1 HOUR 20 MINUTES
COOK: 15 MINUTES

- **1½ cups flour**
- **¾ teaspoon salt**
- **¾ teaspoon sugar**
- **½ teaspoon baking powder**
- **¾ cup boiling water**
- **2 teaspoons sesame oil**
- **8 scallions, thinly sliced**
- **4 teaspoons peanut oil**

1. In a medium bowl, combine the flour, salt, sugar, and baking powder. With a fork, stir in the boiling water until the dough forms a ball. Transfer to a floured surface and knead for 5 minutes or until smooth. Cover with plastic wrap and let rest 1 hour.

2. Transfer the dough to a floured surface and knead again until smooth. Roll out to an 11 x 8-inch rectangle. Brush the dough with the sesame oil, sprinkle with the scallions, and press them into the dough. Roll up the dough jelly-roll style, then slice into 4 pieces. Cover and let rest for 10 minutes.

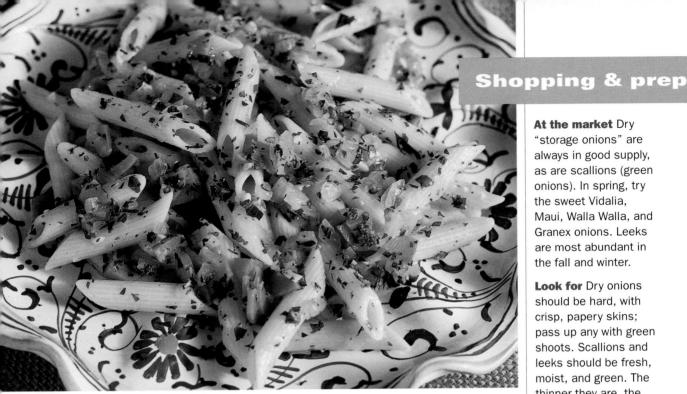

Pasta with Golden Onion Sauce is made with sweet Spanish onions and garlic.

At the market Dry "storage onions" are always in good supply, as are scallions (green onions). In spring, try the sweet Vidalia, Maui, Walla Walla, and Granex onions. Leeks are most abundant in the fall and winter.

Look for Dry onions should be hard, with crisp, papery skins; pass up any with green shoots. Scallions and leeks should be fresh, moist, and green. The thinner they are, the more tender they'll be.

3. Preheat the oven to 250°F. Roll out each piece of dough to a 5-inch round. In a small nonstick skillet, cook 1 pancake in 1 teaspoon of the peanut oil for 3 minutes per side or until light golden. Transfer to a baking sheet. Repeat with the remaining 3 teaspoons oil and pancakes. Bake for 5 minutes. Serves 4.

Per serving: Calories 251; Fiber 2g; Protein 6g; Total Fat 7g; Saturated Fat 1g; Cholesterol 0mg; Sodium 478mg

Pasta with Golden Onion Sauce

PREP: 25 MINUTES / COOK: 35 MINUTES

- 2 teaspoons vegetable oil
- 2 Spanish onions (1½ pounds total), finely chopped
- 3 cloves garlic, minced
- 1 teaspoon sugar
- ¾ teaspoon salt
- 1 carrot, quartered lengthwise and thinly sliced
- 12 ounces penne rigate pasta
- 3 tablespoons Marsala or water
- ¾ cup chicken broth
- 2 teaspoons unsalted butter
- ¼ cup chopped parsley

1. In a large nonstick skillet, heat the oil over moderate heat. Add the onions and garlic, and sprinkle with the sugar and salt. Cover and cook, stirring frequently, for 20 minutes or until the onion is very soft. Stir in the carrot and cook, uncovered, for 7 minutes or until the onions are golden and the carrot is very soft.

2. Meanwhile, in a large pot of boiling water, cook the pasta according to package directions until firm-tender. Reserving ¾ cup of the cooking liquid, drain the pasta and transfer to a large serving bowl.

3. Stir the Marsala into the skillet and cook for 1 minute or until evaporated. Add the broth and the reserved pasta cooking water, and cook, stirring frequently, for 5 minutes or until the liquid is reduced by half.

4. Add the onion sauce, butter, and chopped parsley to the hot pasta, tossing well to combine. Serves 4.

Per serving: Calories 460; Fiber 6g; Protein 14g; Total Fat 6g; Saturated Fat 2g; Cholesterol 5mg; Sodium 642mg

Prep To peel a dry onion, cut off the stem (not the root) end, and peel downward. Then cut off the root end and slice or chop the onion. Rinse scallions and cut off roots. Cut off the dark green tops of leeks, then trim roots, split stems lengthwise, and rinse thoroughly: Grit is often trapped in the base of the leaves.

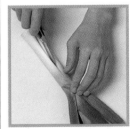

Splitting the stem of a leek lengthwise is the first step in washing it free of grit.

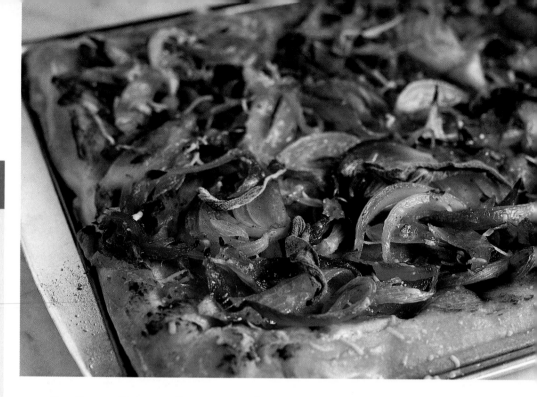

Double-Onion Pizza *is topped with savory sautéed onions and garlic, and flavored with Parmesan cheese and sage.*

Healthy Highlights

Leeks

PER 1 CUP COOKED

Calories	32
Fiber	1.0g
Protein	1g
Total Fat	0.2g
Saturated Fat	0g
Cholesterol	0mg
Sodium	10mg

Did you know? . . .
Saponins, as well as sulfur compounds called allyl sulfides, are cancer-fighting substances found in onions, leeks, and scallions. Saponins also have a heart-protective effect.

A study of Dutch men and their intake of flavonoids (antioxidants found in produce, tea, and wine) showed that those who consumed the most flavonoids had the lowest heart-disease risk. Onions, apples, and tea were the main flavonoid sources in the subjects' diets.

In the part of the state of Georgia where Vidalia onions are grown, the stomach cancer mortality rate is far lower than the national level.

Onion-Orzo Pilaf

PREP: 15 MINUTES / COOK: 35 MINUTES

This recipe uses orzo (a grain-shaped pasta) in place of rice for a pilaf that will dress up a simple meal of grilled chicken or fish.

- 2 teaspoons vegetable oil
- 1½ pounds onions, finely chopped
- 6 scallions, thinly sliced
- 2 cloves garlic, finely chopped
- ¾ cup orzo
- 1 cup chicken broth
- ½ teaspoon each salt and pepper
- ⅓ cup grated Parmesan cheese

1. In a medium-size nonstick saucepan, heat the oil over moderate heat. Add the onions, scallions, and garlic. Cover and cook, stirring occasionally, for 7 minutes or until the onions are soft. Uncover and cook, stirring occasionally, for 5 minutes or until golden.

2. Stir in the orzo. Add the broth, 1 cup of water, the salt, and pepper. Bring to a boil, reduce to a simmer, cover, and cook for 20 minutes or until the orzo is tender. Stir in the Parmesan. Serves 6.

Per serving: Calories 166; Fiber 3g; Protein 6g; Total Fat 4g; Saturated Fat 1g; Cholesterol 4mg; Sodium 447mg

Double-Onion Pizza

PREP: 25 MINUTES / COOK: 30 MINUTES

- 4 teaspoons olive oil
- 3 red onions (1 pound total), halved and cut into ¼-inch-thick slices
- 3 yellow onions (1 pound total), halved and sliced ¼-inch-thick slices
- 2 cloves garlic, minced
- ½ teaspoon sugar
- ¼ teaspoon salt
- 1 teaspoon dried sage leaves, crumbled
- ¼ teaspoon pepper
- 1 pound purchased pizza dough
- ¼ cup no-salt-added tomato paste
- ⅓ cup grated Parmesan cheese

1. In a large nonstick skillet, heat 2 teaspoons of the oil over moderate heat. Add the onions and garlic, and sprinkle with the sugar and salt. Cover and cook, stirring occasionally, for 7 minutes or until the onions are soft. Uncover and cook, stirring frequently, for 5 minutes or until golden brown. Stir in the sage and pepper.

2. Preheat the oven to 500°F. Spray a 15 x 10-inch baking sheet with sides with nonstick cooking spray. Pat the dough into the prepared pan. With your fingers, make several indentations in the top of the dough. Cover loosely and let stand for 15 minutes.

3. In a small bowl, stir together the tomato paste, 3 tablespoons of water, and the remaining 2 teaspoons oil. Brush the mixture over the dough and bake on the lowest shelf for 10 minutes. Spread the onion mixture on top, sprinkle with the Parmesan, and bake for 7 minutes or until the dough is crisp and the onions are piping hot. Serves 6.

Per serving: Calories 312; Fiber 4g; Protein 11g; Total Fat 8g; Saturated Fat 2g; Cholesterol 4mg; Sodium 606mg

Braised Leeks with Tomato, Orange & Olives

PREP: **20** MINUTES / COOK: **25** MINUTES

- **8** medium leeks (3 pounds total), roots and dark green ends trimmed
- **1** tablespoon olive oil
- **3** cloves garlic, minced
- **1** large tomato, diced
- **½** cup orange juice
- **1** tablespoon no-salt-added tomato paste
- **¼** cup coarsely chopped Gaeta, Calamata, or Spanish green olives
- **¼** teaspoon salt

1. With a sharp paring knife, starting 1 inch above the root end of each leek, make 4 lengthwise cuts. Soak the leeks in several changes of warm water until thoroughly clean. Pat dry.

2. In a large nonstick skillet, heat the oil over moderate heat. Add the leeks, turning until well coated. Add the garlic and cook for 2 minutes or until tender.

3. Add the tomato, orange juice, tomato paste, olives, and salt, and bring to a boil. Reduce to a simmer, cover, and cook for 10 minutes or until the leeks are fork-tender. Serve warm, at room temperature, or chilled. Serves 4.

Per serving: Calories 179; Fiber 3g; Protein 3g; Total Fat 6g; Saturated Fat 1g; Cholesterol 0mg; Sodium 325mg

Red Onion & Pepper Relish In a nonstick skillet, sauté 3 cups diced red onions, 1 cup diced red bell pepper, and 2 cloves minced garlic in 2 tsp. olive oil until tender. Add ¼ cup red wine vinegar, 1 tbsp. tomato paste, and 2 tsp. honey. Simmer 2 minutes. Serve chilled. Makes 2 cups/ 8 servings. *[Cal 47; Fat 1g; Sod 23mg]*

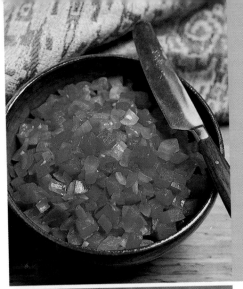

Creamy Onion & Scallion Soup In nonstick saucepan, heat 2 tsp. olive oil. Add 3 cups diced onions, 6 sliced scallions, and 3 cloves minced garlic. Sprinkle with 1 tsp. sugar, ½ tsp. thyme, and ¼ tsp. salt, and sauté until tender. Add ¾ cup each chicken broth and water, and simmer, covered, for 5 minutes. Purée with 1 cup reduced-fat (2%) milk. Heat through to serve. Serves 4. *[Cal 116; Fat 4g; Sod 370mg]*

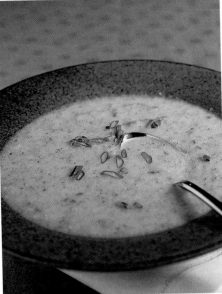

Sweet & Sour Pearl Onions In a nonstick skillet, bring ½ cup distilled white vinegar, ⅓ cup sugar, ½ tsp. salt, and ¼ tsp. thyme to a boil. Add two 10-oz. packages frozen pearl onions. Cover and simmer until tender. Uncover and cook until glazed. Stir in 2 tbsp. chopped parsley. Serves 4. *[Cal 118; Fat 0g; Sod 288mg]*

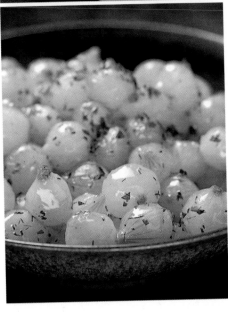

Parsnips

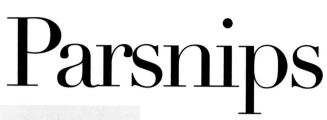

Nutritional power

This carrot cousin lacks beta carotene, but is a good source of vitamin C and is high in fiber, too. Parsnips also provide folate, as well as manganese.

Healthy Highlights

PER 1 CUP COOKED	
Calories	126
Fiber	6.2g
Protein	2g
Total Fat	0.5g
Saturated Fat	0.1g
Cholesterol	0mg
Sodium	16mg

NUTRIENTS	
	% Daily Value
Vitamin C	33%
Folate	23%
Manganese	23%

Did you know? . . .

Try young, tender parsnips raw in salad or slaw. You'll get every bit of their vitamin C.

Some of a parsnip's starch turns to sugar when the vegetable is chilled (making it tastier), so commercial growers place parsnips in cold storage for a few weeks. This does not diminish the nutritional value.

Honey-Glazed Parsnips

PREP: 10 MINUTES / COOK: 20 MINUTES

Like carrots, parsnips are right at home in a sweet, satiny sauce. The cooking liquid is reduced to make the glaze, so you don't lose nutrients.

1¼   **pounds parsnips, peeled and thinly sliced**
⅓   **cup honey**
2   **tablespoons lemon juice**
1   **tablespoon unsalted butter**
½   **teaspoon salt**
¼   **teaspoon pepper**
¼   **teaspoon dried rosemary, crumbled**
¼   **cup chopped parsley**

1. In a large skillet, combine the parsnips, honey, lemon juice, butter, salt, pepper, rosemary, and 1 cup of water. Bring to a boil over moderate heat. Cover and cook for 10 minutes or until crisp-tender.

2. Uncover and cook for 10 minutes or until the liquid has evaporated and the parsnips are richly glazed and tender. Stir in the parsley. Serves 4.

Per serving: Calories 204; Fiber 6g; Protein 2g; Total Fat 3g; Saturated Fat 2g; Cholesterol 8mg; Sodium 290mg

Parsnip-Apple Purée

PREP: 20 MINUTES / COOK: 30 MINUTES

Your first taste of this mashed-potato lookalike will be a happy surprise. The apples underscore the parsnips' natural sweetness; onions and garlic lend savory contrast.

2   **teaspoons vegetable oil**
1   **small onion, thinly sliced**
6   **cloves garlic, thinly sliced**
1½   **pounds parsnips, peeled and thinly sliced**
2   **McIntosh apples, peeled and coarsely chopped**
2   **tablespoons rice**
2   **cups reduced-fat (2%) milk**
½   **teaspoon each salt and pepper**

1. In a medium saucepan, heat the oil over moderate heat. Add the onion and garlic, and sauté for 7 minutes or until the onion is tender.

2. Add the parsnips, tossing to coat with the oil. Add the apples, rice, milk, salt, and pepper. Bring to a boil, reduce to a simmer, cover, and cook for 20 minutes or until the rice and parsnips are tender. (Don't worry if the mixture appears curdled.) Transfer to a food processor and process until smooth. Serves 6.

Per serving: Calories 181; Fiber 6g; Protein 5g; Total Fat 4g; Saturated Fat 1g; Cholesterol 7mg; Sodium 234mg

Parsnip Pancakes with Scallions

PREP: 20 MINUTES / COOK: 10 MINUTES

Parsnips and carrots complement one another in these delicately crusty pancakes. Take a cue from potato-pancake traditions and serve them with applesauce or sour cream.

- 1 **pound parsnips, peeled and shredded**
- 1 **large carrot, shredded**
- 2 **scallions, thinly sliced**
- 1 **egg**
- 1 **tablespoon flour**
- ½ **teaspoon baking powder**
- ½ **teaspoon salt**
- 1 **tablespoon vegetable oil**

1. Preheat the oven to 250°F. In a steamer or colander set over a pot of boiling water, steam the parsnips and carrot for 5 minutes or until softened but not mushy. Set aside to cool slightly.

2. Transfer the vegetables to a medium bowl and add the scallions, egg, flour, baking powder, and salt, stirring until well combined.

3. In a large nonstick skillet, heat 1½ teaspoons of the oil over moderate heat. Using a ¼-cup measure, spoon 6 pancakes into the pan, using half of the batter. Cook for 2 minutes per side or until golden brown. Transfer the first batch of parsnip pancakes to a large baking sheet.

4. Repeat with the remaining batter and 1½ teaspoons oil. Bake the parsnip pancakes for 7 minutes or until they are heated through and lightly crisped. Serves 4.

Per serving: Calories 141; Fiber 5g; Protein 3g; Total Fat 5g; Saturated Fat 1g; Cholesterol 53mg; Sodium 370mg

At the market
Parsnips are in best supply from the fall through early spring, but many markets offer them all year.

Look for Parsnips are often sold in bags, like carrots, so you can't select them individually. If you can pick and choose, look for firm, medium-size, uniformly shaped roots (large parsnips may have a tough, woody core).

Prep Peel parsnips and trim the top and bottom. Cook whole, or cut up for faster cooking.

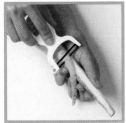

Peel parsnips with a vegetable peeler, just as you would carrots.

Basic cooking Steam sliced parsnips (or cook them in a small amount of liquid) for 5 to 15 minutes. Bake whole parsnips in a little liquid, covered, for 20 to 30 minutes at 350°F. To microwave 1 pound of cut-up parsnips, place in a dish with ¼ cup water. Cover and cook at high for 9 to 11 minutes.

Parsnip Pancakes with Scallions *A delightful change from rice or potatoes.*

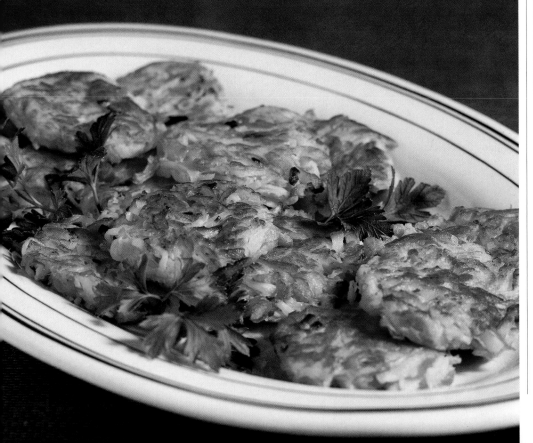

Peas

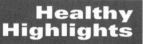

Nutritional power
Fresh peas are a good low-fat protein source. They are rich in vitamin C, folate, manganese, potassium, and thiamin, and also contain lutein.

Healthy Highlights

Green Peas
PER 1 CUP COOKED

Calories	134
Fiber	8.8g
Protein	9g
Total Fat	0.4g
Saturated Fat	0g
Cholesterol	0mg
Sodium	5mg

NUTRIENTS

	% Daily Value
Vitamin C	38%
Manganese	21%
Vitamin A	19%
Potassium	15%
Thiamin	14%
Folate	13%

Did you know? . . .
Peas contain lutein, a carotenoid that fights macular degeneration, the leading cause of blindness in older Americans.

Nutritionally, frozen green peas are very close to fresh, although added salt does raise the sodium content.

Peas & Cheese Salad

PREP: 20 MINUTES / CHILL: 4 HOURS

This is a lower-fat version of a classic American layered salad. Make it in a glass bowl to show off the layers.

- 1   cup plain nonfat yogurt
- ⅓   cup light mayonnaise
- ¾   teaspoon grated lemon zest
- 3   tablespoons lemon juice
- 2   cups shredded romaine lettuce
- 4   cups frozen peas, thawed
- 1   large red bell pepper, diced
- 1   large yellow bell pepper, diced
- 1   large red onion, diced
- ¾   cup shredded Cheddar cheese (3 ounces)

1. In a small bowl, combine the yogurt, mayonnaise, lemon zest, and lemon juice; set aside.

2. In an 8- to 10-cup glass bowl, arrange the remaining ingredients in layers as follows: the lettuce, peas, red and yellow bell peppers, and onion. Pour the yogurt mixture on top and sprinkle with the cheese. Cover well and refrigerate for at least 4 hours or up to 12 hours.

3. At serving time, toss the salad at the table. Serves 4.

Per serving: Calories 338; Fiber 8g; Protein 18g; Total Fat 15g; Saturated Fat 6g; Cholesterol 30mg; Sodium 500mg

Penne with Sugar Snaps & Smoked Salmon

PREP: 20 MINUTES / COOK: 15 MINUTES

Cook sugar snaps quickly to preserve their tempting color and "snap." A brief blanching does the trick, and conserves vitamins, too.

- 12   ounces penne or ziti pasta
- 1   pound sugar snap peas, strings removed
- ⅓   cup snipped fresh dill
- 3   scallions, thinly sliced
- ¾   cup chicken broth
- 3   tablespoons reduced-fat sour cream
- 1   tablespoon unsalted butter
- 1   teaspoon grated lemon zest
- 2   tablespoons lemon juice
- ½   teaspoon salt
- 4   ounces smoked salmon, slivered

1. In a large pot of boiling water, cook the pasta according to package directions until firm-tender. Add the sugar snaps to the water during the final 1 minute of cooking; drain.

2. Meanwhile, in a large bowl, combine the dill, scallions, broth, sour cream, butter, lemon zest, lemon juice, and salt. Add the hot pasta and sugar snaps, tossing well. Add the smoked salmon and toss again. Serves 4.

Per serving: Calories 453; Fiber 5g; Protein 20g; Total Fat 7g; Saturated Fat 3g; Cholesterol 18mg; Sodium 711mg

Sweet & Sour Shrimp with Snow Peas

PREP: 40 MINUTES / COOK: 10 MINUTES

Look for dried shiitake mushrooms in a specialty food store if they're not in your supermarket. Serve the shrimp and vegetables over rice to take advantage of the deliciously tangy sauce.

- ¼ cup dried shiitake or other imported dried mushrooms
- 1 cup boiling water
- ¼ cup ketchup
- 2 tablespoons lower-sodium soy sauce
- 2 tablespoons rice vinegar or cider vinegar
- 2 teaspoons light brown sugar
- 1 teaspoon cornstarch
- ½ teaspoon ground ginger
- 2 teaspoons vegetable oil
- 2 carrots, halved lengthwise and thinly sliced
- 2 cloves garlic, minced
- 1¼ pounds medium shrimp, peeled and deveined
- ¾ pound snow peas, strings removed, halved crosswise

1. In a small bowl, combine the dried mushrooms and the boiling water and let stand for 10 minutes or until softened. Reserving the soaking liquid, scoop out the dried mushrooms, rinse, and thinly slice; set aside.

2. Strain the mushroom soaking liquid through a coffee filter or a paper towel-lined sieve into a small bowl. Add the ketchup, soy sauce, vinegar, brown sugar, cornstarch, and ginger, whisking to combine.

3. In a large nonstick skillet, heat the oil over moderately high heat. Add the carrots and garlic, and sauté for 3 minutes or until crisp-tender. Add the shrimp, snow peas, sliced mushrooms, and ¼ cup of water. Cover the pan and cook for 5 minutes or until the shrimp are just cooked through and the snow peas are crisp-tender. Stir the ketchup mixture to recombine and pour into the skillet. Cook for 1 minute or until lightly thickened. Serves 4.

Per serving: Calories 227; Fiber 4g; Protein 27g; Total Fat 5g; Saturated Fat 1g; Cholesterol 174mg; Sodium 665mg

At the market Green peas are abundant from early spring through July; sugar snaps have a short season in late spring/early summer. Snow peas are sold all year.

Look for Shop where peas are kept refrigerated (this keeps their sugars from turning to starch). Choose plump, medium-size pods with satiny skins and good green color.

Prep Crack open green pea pods and push out peas with your thumb. Pinch tips off snow peas and zip off strings from snow peas and both edges of sugar snap peas.

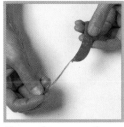

You need to remove the strings from both sides of sugar snap pea pods.

Basic cooking Cook green peas in a little liquid for 5 to 10 minutes; snow peas and sugar snaps, just 1 to 2 minutes. Or, steam snow peas or sugar snaps for 3 to 5 minutes. Microwave 1 cup shelled green peas with 1 tablespoon water. Cook at high for 5 minutes.

***Penne with Sugar Snaps & Smoked Salmon** partners emerald-green sugar snaps and luxurious smoked salmon in a creamy lemon-dill sauce.*

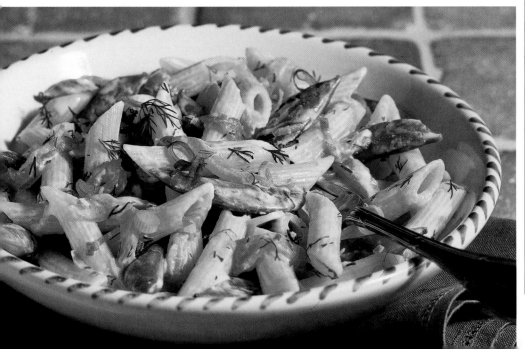

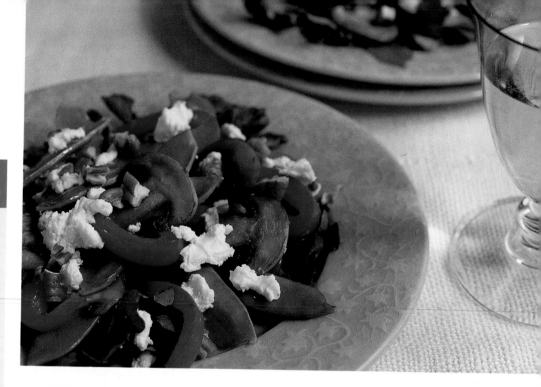

Warm Snow Pea Salad with Mushrooms & Goat Cheese is served slightly warm to enhance its flavors.

Healthy Highlights

Edible-Pod Peas
PER 1 CUP COOKED

Calories	67
Fiber	4.5g
Protein	5g
Total Fat	0.4g
Saturated Fat	0.1g
Cholesterol	0mg
Sodium	6mg

NUTRIENTS

	% Daily Value
Vitamin C	128%
Iron	17%
Manganese	13%
Thiamin	13%
Folate	12%
Vitamin B6	12%

Did you know? . . .
Cooked edible-pod peas contain three times as much vitamin C as green peas. If they are eaten raw or just barely cooked, their vitamin C levels are even higher.

Sugar snap peas, introduced in the 1970s, have a thin, edible pod enclosing good-sized peas; both pod and peas are super-sweet. Because their peas are more fully developed, sugar snaps are somewhat higher in protein than snow peas (the figures given above are an average).

Warm Snow Pea Salad with Mushrooms & Goat Cheese

PREP: 15 MINUTES / COOK: 10 MINUTES
MARINATE: 20 MINUTES

- 2 teaspoons olive oil
- ½ pound mushrooms, thinly sliced
- 2 cloves garlic, minced
- 1 pound snow peas, strings removed
- 1 small red bell pepper, cut into 2 x ¼-inch strips
- ½ teaspoon salt
- 3 tablespoons rice vinegar
- 2 teaspoons honey
- 4 cups watercress leaves
- 4 ounces mild goat cheese
- 2 tablespoons pecans, toasted and chopped

1. In a large nonstick skillet, heat 1 teaspoon of the oil over moderately high heat. Add the mushrooms and sauté for 4 minutes or until tender and lightly browned. Add the garlic and cook for 1 minute. Add the snow peas, bell pepper, and salt, and sauté for 4 minutes or until crisp-tender.

2. Transfer to a large bowl and add the vinegar, honey, and the remaining 1 teaspoon oil, tossing to combine. Let stand for 20 minutes before serving.

3. Divide the watercress among 4 salad plates and top with the snow pea mixture. Sprinkle with the goat cheese and pecans. Serves 4.

Per serving: Calories 225; Fiber 5g; Protein 12g; Total Fat 14g; Saturated Fat 6g; Cholesterol 22mg; Sodium 441mg

Sautéed Lamb & Sugar Snaps

PREP: 20 MINUTES / COOK: 15 MINUTES

- 2 teaspoons vegetable oil
- 3 scallions, thinly sliced
- 2 cloves garlic, minced
- 1 tablespoon minced fresh ginger
- 1 red bell pepper, cut into thin strips
- 1 pound well-trimmed leg of lamb, cut into 2 x ½-inch strips
- 1 pound sugar snap peas, strings removed
- ½ cup chicken broth
- ¼ cup chili sauce
- 1 tablespoon lower-sodium soy sauce
- 2 teaspoons honey
- ¼ teaspoon salt

1. In a large nonstick skillet, heat the oil over moderate heat. Add the scallions, garlic, and ginger, and sauté for 3 minutes or until the garlic is tender.

2. Add the bell pepper and sauté for 2 minutes or until crisp-tender. Add the lamb and sugar snaps, and sauté for 4 minutes or until the lamb is just cooked through but still juicy and the peas are crisp-tender.

3. In a small bowl, combine the broth, chili sauce, soy sauce, honey, and salt. Pour into the skillet and cook for 1 minute to heat through. Serves 4.

Per serving: Calories 251; Fiber 2g; Protein 26g; Total Fat 8g; Saturated Fat 2g; Cholesterol 73mg; Sodium 718mg

Risi e Bisi

Prep: 10 minutes / Cook: 40 minutes

Risi e bisi simply means "rice and peas" in Italian. In the springtime, you can substitute fresh peas for the frozen: Add the peas along with the rice in Step 2.

2	slices bacon (1 ounce), finely chopped
1	small onion, finely chopped
1	cup rice
1¾	cups chicken broth
½	teaspoon pepper
¼	teaspoon salt
3	cups frozen peas
¼	cup chopped parsley
¼	cup grated Parmesan cheese
2	teaspoons unsalted butter

1. In a large nonstick saucepan, combine the bacon and ¼ cup of water over moderate heat. Cook, stirring occasionally, for 5 minutes or until the bacon has rendered its fat. Add the onion and sauté for 7 minutes or until golden brown and tender.

2. Add the rice, stirring to coat. Add the broth, 1½ cups of water, the pepper, and salt, and bring to a boil. Reduce to a simmer, cover, and cook for 15 minutes. Stir in the peas and parsley, cover, and cook, stirring occasionally, for 10 minutes or until the rice is tender and the peas are heated through. Stir in the Parmesan and butter. Serves 4.

Per serving: Calories 355; Fiber 5g; Protein 13g; Total Fat 9g; Saturated Fat 4g; Cholesterol 14mg; Sodium 863mg

Sugar Snaps with Mint Remove strings from 1½ pounds sugar snap peas. In large steamer, cook sugar snaps until crisp-tender. Transfer to large bowl, add 1 tbsp. olive oil, ½ cup chopped fresh mint, and ¾ tsp. salt. Toss to combine. Serves 4. *[Cal 100; Fat 3g; Sod 412mg]*

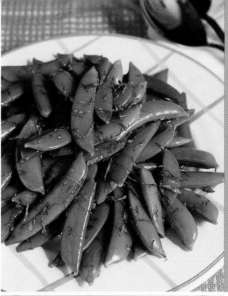

Snow Pea & Pepper Salad Remove strings from 1½ pounds snow peas. In large steamer, cook snow peas until crisp-tender. In large bowl, combine 2 tbsp. balsamic vinegar, 1 tbsp. olive oil, ½ tsp. brown sugar, and ½ tsp. salt. Add snow peas, 1 slivered small red onion, 1 slivered yellow bell pepper, and one 8-oz. can drained sliced water chestnuts. Toss well. Serves 4. *[Cal 137; Fat 4g; Sod 288mg]*

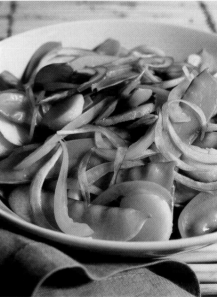

Mockamole In food processor, combine two 10-oz. packages thawed frozen peas, ½ cup cilantro leaves, 2 tbsp. lime juice, 2 tbsp. light mayonnaise, ½ tsp. ground coriander, and ½ tsp. salt. Process until smooth. Transfer to serving bowl and stir in ¾ cup chopped tomato and 2 sliced scallions. Serves 4. *[Cal 146; Fat 3g; Sod 496mg]*

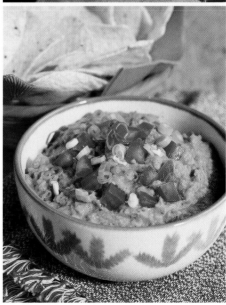

Potatoes

Nutritional power
Potatoes combine energy-giving complex carbohydrates, with plenty of vitamin C, fiber, and potassium. They're filling and, if sensibly prepared, low in fat.

Healthy Highlights

PER 1 LARGE BAKED*	
Calories	247
Fiber	5.4g
Protein	5g
Total Fat	0.2g
Saturated Fat	0.1g
Cholesterol	0mg
Sodium	18mg

NUTRIENTS	
	% Daily Value
Vitamin C	48%
Vitamin B6	40%
Copper	35%
Potassium	32%
Manganese	26%
Niacin	19%
Iron	17%
Thiamin	16%

*with skin

Did you know? . . .
Potatoes are the number-one source of vitamin C in the American diet, simply because they are the most consumed vegetable.

A baked potato supplies more than twice as much potassium as a banana.

Onion & Potato Pancakes

PREP: 15 MINUTES / COOK: 40 MINUTES

Sautéed onions bring robust flavor to these mashed-potato pancakes.

- 1½   **pounds baking potatoes, peeled and thinly sliced**
- 5   **teaspoons vegetable oil**
- 2   **onions, finely chopped**
- 3   **tablespoons reduced-fat sour cream**
- ¾   **teaspoon salt**
- ¼   **teaspoon pepper**
- ⅛   **teaspoon grated nutmeg**
- 3   **tablespoons flour**

1. In a pot of boiling water, cook the potatoes for 15 minutes or until tender. Drain and transfer to a large bowl.

2. Meanwhile, in a large nonstick skillet, heat 1 teaspoon of the oil over moderate heat. Add the onions and sauté for 7 minutes or until golden brown and tender.

3. Add the sour cream, salt, pepper, and nutmeg to the bowl with the potatoes and mash with a potato masher. Stir in the sautéed onions. Using a ⅓-cup measure, shape into 8 cakes.

4. In a 12-inch nonstick skillet, heat 2 teaspoons of the oil over moderate heat. Dredge the cakes in the flour, shaking off the excess. Sauté 4 of the cakes for 3 minutes per side or until golden brown and crusty. Repeat with the remaining 2 teaspoons oil and 4 potato cakes. Serves 4.

Per serving: Calories 225; Fiber 4g; Protein 5g; Total Fat 8g; Saturated Fat 2g; Cholesterol 4mg; Sodium 428mg

Potato Salad with Mustard Dressing

PREP: 20 MINUTES / COOK: 30 MINUTES

- 2   **pounds red potatoes, cut into ½-inch chunks**
- 1   **tablespoon olive oil**
- 1   **large onion, cut into ½-inch cubes**
- 1   **red bell pepper, cut into ½-inch squares**
- 1   **green bell pepper, cut into ½-inch squares**
- 1   **cup chicken broth**
- 3   **tablespoons distilled white vinegar**
- 1   **tablespoon Dijon mustard**
- ½   **teaspoon salt**
- 2   **ounces smoked turkey, cut into ½-inch cubes**

1. In a large pot of boiling water, cook the potatoes for 25 minutes or until tender. Drain well.

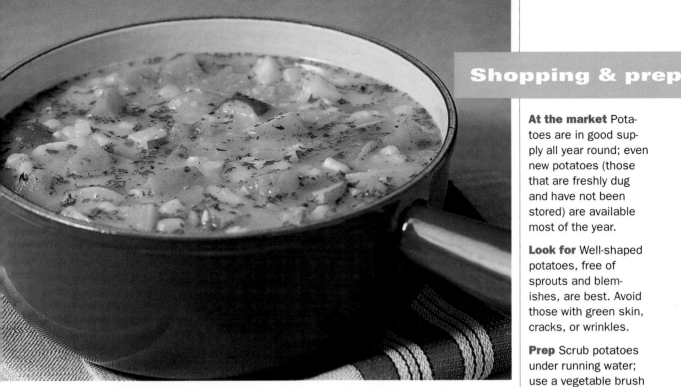

Mixed Potato Chowder Three kinds of potatoes go into this satisfying stew.

At the market Potatoes are in good supply all year round; even new potatoes (those that are freshly dug and have not been stored) are available most of the year.

Look for Well-shaped potatoes, free of sprouts and blemishes, are best. Avoid those with green skin, cracks, or wrinkles.

Prep Scrub potatoes under running water; use a vegetable brush if necessary.

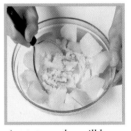

A potato masher will leave some texture in mashed potatoes. A food processor can turn them gluey.

2. Meanwhile, in a large skillet, heat the oil over moderate heat. Add the onion and bell peppers, and sauté for 5 minutes or until the peppers are crisp-tender. Transfer the vegetables to a large serving bowl.

3. Whisk the broth, vinegar, mustard, and salt into the bowl. Add the potatoes and turkey, tossing until well combined. Serve warm or chilled. Serves 6.

Per serving: Calories 181; Fiber 4g; Protein 6g; Total Fat 3g; Saturated Fat 1g; Cholesterol 5mg; Sodium 527mg

Mixed Potato Chowder

PREP: 20 MINUTES / COOK: 40 MINUTES

The red and sweet potatoes will hold their shape, but the baking potatoes will fall apart as they simmer, thickening the broth.

- 2 **teaspoons vegetable oil**
- 1 **onion, finely chopped**
- 3 **cloves garlic, minced**
- 1 **pound baking potatoes, peeled and thinly sliced**
- ¾ **pound red potatoes, cut into ½-inch chunks**
- ½ **pound sweet potatoes, peeled and cut into ½-inch chunks**
- 1 **cup chicken broth**
- ¾ **teaspoon salt**
- ½ **teaspoon dried sage**
- 1 **cup reduced-fat (2%) milk**
- ⅔ **cup frozen corn kernels**
- ½ **cup chopped parsley**

1. In a medium saucepan, heat the oil over moderate heat. Add the onion and garlic, and sauté for 7 minutes or until the onion is soft.

2. Add the baking potatoes, red potatoes, and sweet potatoes, stirring to coat. Add the broth, 2 cups of water, the salt, and sage, and bring to a boil. Reduce to a simmer, cover, and cook for 25 minutes or until the red potatoes and sweet potatoes are tender, and the baking potatoes are soft and creamy.

3. Stir in the milk and corn, and simmer for 4 minutes or until the corn is heated through. Stir in the parsley. Serves 4.

Per serving: Calories 282; Fiber 6g; Protein 8g; Total Fat 5g; Saturated Fat 1g; Cholesterol 5mg; Sodium 728mg

Basic cooking When boiling potatoes, start them in boiling water to preserve vitamin C. Whole small potatoes take 10 to 15 minutes, larger potatoes 20 to 40 minutes, depending on size. Boil cut-up potatoes for 15 to 20 minutes. Before baking or microwaving, pierce whole potatoes in several places. Oven-bake for 45 to 60 minutes at 375°F. Microwave 4 baking potatoes at high for 13 to 15 minutes.

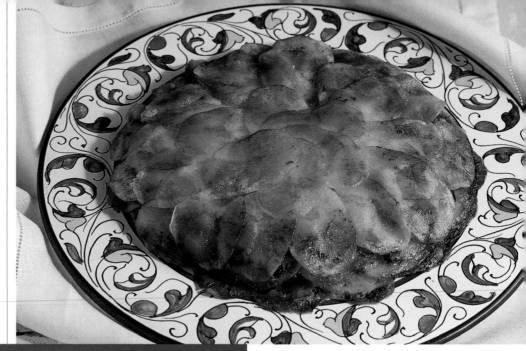

Potato Torte Made of thin layers of potatoes, this savory "cake" is actually very easy to prepare.

Did you know? . . .
Starting potatoes to cook in cold water increases the loss of vitamin C and may cause the potatoes to discolor. Instead, add the potatoes to already-boiling water, or place them in a pot and pour boiling water over them.

Starchy potatoes are best for baking, waxy ones are good for boiling and salads.

Greenish skin—or sprouts—on a potato signal elevated levels of solanine, a bitter-tasting compound that is a natural component of this vegetable. Bruising or improper storage encourages solanine to develop. It's best to discard any potatoes that have a greenish tinge or more than one or two sprouts. It would take a lot of solanine to make you ill, but it's best to avoid it.

Plain potatoes are virtually fat-free, but 2 ounces of commercial potato chips pack about 20 grams of fat.

Potato Torte
PREP: 10 MINUTES / COOK: 50 MINUTES

- **5** teaspoons olive oil
- **2** pounds baking potatoes, peeled and very thinly sliced
- **¾** teaspoon each salt and pepper
- **¼** cup grated Parmesan cheese
- **2** scallions, thinly sliced
- **3** tablespoons snipped fresh dill

1. Preheat the oven to 450°F. Brush a 9-inch pie plate with 1 teaspoon of the oil. Cover the bottom with an overlapping layer of potatoes, using one-fourth of the total. Sprinkle with 1 teaspoon of the oil, ¼ teaspoon each of the salt and pepper, 1 tablespoon of the Parmesan, one-third of the scallions, and 1 tablespoon of the dill.

2. Repeat for 2 more layers. Top with a final layer of potatoes and the remaining 1 teaspoon oil and 1 tablespoon Parmesan. Place an empty pie plate or round baking dish on top of the potatoes and bake in the lower third of the oven for 50 minutes or until the potatoes are crusty on the bottom (lift gently with a spatula to check) and tender throughout.

3. Cool in the pan for 5 minutes before loosening the bottom and sides with a small spatula and inverting onto a platter. Serves 4.

Per serving: Calories 212; Fiber 3g; Protein 6g; Total Fat 7g; Saturated Fat 2g; Cholesterol 4mg; Sodium 518mg

Scalloped Potatoes with Smoked Turkey
PREP: 20 MINUTES / COOK: 1 HOUR
The aroma of this casserole as it bakes ensures that nobody will be late for dinner. Serve it with a big green salad.

- **1** clove garlic, peeled and halved
- **2¼** pounds baking potatoes, peeled and thinly sliced
- **2** ounces smoked turkey, sliced and cut into ½-inch squares
- **¼** cup plus 2 tablespoons grated Parmesan cheese
- **3** tablespoons flour
- **½** teaspoon each salt and pepper
- **1** cup chicken broth
- **¼** cup reduced-fat sour cream

1. Preheat the oven to 400°F. Rub a 9-inch square glass or ceramic baking dish with the garlic; discard the garlic.

2. Dividing evenly, make alternating layers of potatoes, turkey, ¼ cup of the Parmesan, the flour, salt, and pepper.

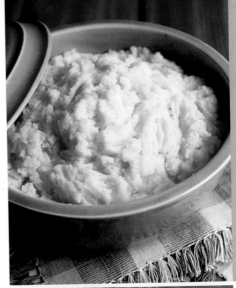

3. In a medium bowl, whisk together the broth and sour cream. Pour the mixture over the potatoes. Sprinkle the top with the remaining 2 tablespoons Parmesan, cover with foil, and bake for 45 minutes. Uncover and bake for 15 minutes or until the potatoes are tender. Serves 4.

Per serving: Calories 256; Fiber 3g; Protein 12g; Total Fat 5g; Saturated Fat 3g; Cholesterol 18mg; Sodium 839mg

Curried Cauliflower & Potato Stew

PREP: 15 MINUTES / COOK: 35 MINUTES

Indian spices enliven this unusual stew.

- 2 teaspoons olive oil
- 2 scallions, thinly sliced
- 2 tablespoons minced fresh ginger
- 2 pounds all-purpose potatoes, peeled and cut into 1-inch chunks
- 1 head of cauliflower, cut into florets
- 1 tablespoon curry powder
- 1 teaspoon each ground coriander and cumin
- ½ teaspoon salt
- 1 cup canned no-salt-added chopped tomatoes
- ⅓ cup plain low-fat yogurt
- 2 teaspoons flour

1. In a large nonstick skillet, heat the oil over moderate heat. Add the scallions and ginger, and sauté for 2 minutes or until the scallions are tender. Add the potatoes, cauliflower, curry powder, coriander, cumin, and salt, stirring to combine. Add 1½ cups of water and bring to a boil. Reduce to a simmer, cover, and cook for 15 minutes or until the potatoes are not quite tender.

2. Add the tomatoes, cover, and cook for 10 minutes or until the potatoes and cauliflower are tender. In a small bowl, combine the yogurt and flour. Whisk the yogurt mixture into the pan and cook for 1 minute or until lightly thickened. Serves 4.

Per serving: Calories 231; Fiber 8g; Protein 9g; Total Fat 4g; Saturated Fat 1g; Cholesterol 1mg; Sodium 331mg

Garlic-Cheddar Mashed Potatoes

In saucepan of boiling water, cook 2 lbs. peeled, thinly sliced baking potatoes and 6 peeled cloves garlic until tender. Drain and mash with ⅓ cup buttermilk, ¾ cup shredded Cheddar, ¾ tsp. salt, and ½ tsp. paprika. Serves 6.
[Cal 188; Fat 5g; Sod 379mg]

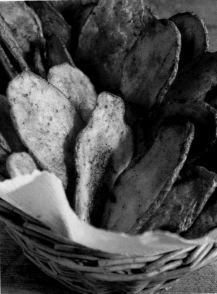

Cajun Oven Fries

Preheat oven to 425°F. Thinly slice lengthwise 2 lbs. unpeeled baking potatoes. In large bowl, combine 2 tbsp. vegetable oil, 2 tsp. chili powder, ½ tsp. thyme, ½ tsp. black pepper, and ¼ tsp. cayenne. Add potatoes, tossing to coat. Place on 2 baking sheets and bake for 30 to 45 minutes or until browned and crisp. Serves 4.
[Cal 233; Fat 7g; Sod 29mg]

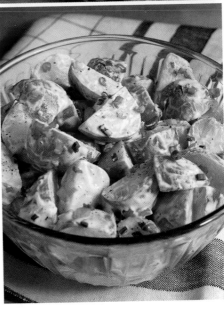

Deli-Style Potato Salad

In large bowl, combine ⅓ cup plain nonfat yogurt, ¼ cup light mayonnaise, ¼ cup chicken broth, 3 tbsp. red wine vinegar, 4 sliced scallions, ½ tsp. salt, and ½ tsp. pepper. In large pot of boiling water, cook 2 lbs. quartered small red potatoes until tender. Drain. Add to bowl and toss. Serves 4.
[Cal 253; Fat 6g; Sod 488mg]

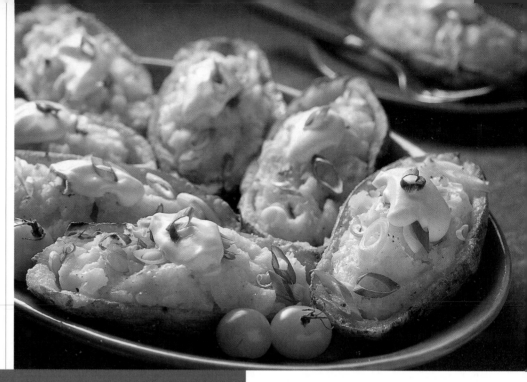

Crisp Potato Skins with Creamy Mashed Potato Stuffing rolls *two all-American favorites into one delicious side dish.*

Did you know? . . .
"Baking" potatoes in a microwave is a healthful way to cook them, and a great timesaver, too. But be sure to pierce the potatoes in several places with a fork or knife before microwaving, or the potatoes may explode.

For maximum nutrition, it's a good idea to eat baked potatoes skin and all.

It's a good idea to eat baked potatoes skin and all: Some of the nutrients (such as iron, phosphorus, and potassium) are concentrated in or just under the skin. You'll also get more dietary fiber by eating the skin.

To flavor potatoes without adding fat, toss a few garlic cloves, onion slices, or dried herbs into the cooking water.

Potatoes and onions shouldn't be stored together. A gas given off by the onions will speed up the spoilage of potatoes (and vice versa).

Spice Cake with Brown Sugar Frosting

PREP: 25 MINUTES / COOK: 45 MINUTES

10	ounces baking potatoes, peeled and thinly sliced
2	cups flour
1	teaspoon cinnamon
¾	teaspoon ground ginger
¾	teaspoon baking powder
½	teaspoon baking soda
¼	teaspoon salt
⅛	teaspoon each ground cloves and allspice
⅓	cup vegetable oil
1½	cups granulated sugar
1	egg
2	egg whites
8	ounces reduced-fat cream cheese (Neufchâtel), at room temperature
¼	cup firmly packed light brown sugar
1	teaspoon vanilla extract
½	cup apricot jam

1. Preheat the oven to 350°F. Spray a 9-inch springform pan with nonstick cooking spray. Line the bottom with a circle of wax paper and spray with nonstick cooking spray. Dust with flour, shaking off the excess.

2. In a large pot of boiling water, cook the potatoes for 12 minutes or until tender. Drain well. Mash with a potato masher; set aside.

3. On a sheet of wax paper, combine the flour, cinnamon, ginger, baking powder, baking soda, salt, cloves, and allspice. In a large bowl with an electric mixer, beat the oil and granulated sugar until well blended. Add the whole egg and egg whites, one at a time, beating well after each addition. Beat in the potatoes. Fold in the flour mixture.

4. Scrape the batter into the prepared pan, smoothing the top. Bake for 45 minutes or until a cake tester inserted in the center comes out just clean. Cool for 15 minutes in the pan on a rack, then invert onto the rack to cool completely. With a long serrated knife, cut the cake into 2 horizontal layers and place the bottom layer on a cake plate.

5. In a medium bowl with an electric mixer, cream the cream cheese with the brown sugar and vanilla. In a small saucepan, melt the jam over low heat. Spread the bottom layer with the jam.

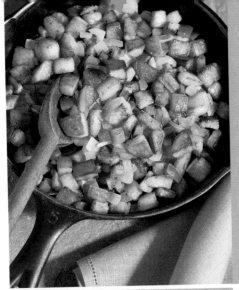

Top with the second layer and spread the frosting over the top and sides of the cake. Serves 10.

Per serving: Calories 413; Fiber 1g; Protein 7g; Total Fat 12g; Saturated Fat 4g; Cholesterol 32mg; Sodium 288mg

Crisp Potato Skins with Creamy Mashed Potato Stuffing

PREP: 15 MINUTES
COOK: 1 HOUR 10 MINUTES

- 4 large (8-ounce) baking potatoes
- 2 teaspoons vegetable oil
- ¼ cup grated Parmesan cheese
- ½ cup reduced-fat (2%) milk
- 3 tablespoons reduced-fat cream cheese (Neufchâtel)
- ¾ teaspoon salt
- ¼ teaspoon pepper
- ⅛ teaspoon grated nutmeg
- 4 teaspoons reduced-fat sour cream
- 2 scallions, thinly sliced

1. Preheat the oven to 450°F. Prick the potatoes in several places with a fork and bake for 1 hour or until firm-tender. Leave the oven on.

2. Halve the potatoes lengthwise and scoop out the flesh, leaving ¼ inch of flesh on the skin. Brush the insides of the potato skins with the oil and sprinkle with 2 tablespoons of the Parmesan cheese. Place the skins, cut-sides up, on a baking sheet and bake for 5 minutes or until they are crisp and golden. Leave the oven on.

3. Meanwhile, in a medium bowl, mash the potato flesh with the milk, cream cheese, salt, pepper, nutmeg, and the remaining 2 tablespoons Parmesan.

4. Spoon the mashed potato mixture into the crisped potato skins, return to the oven, and bake for 5 minutes or until piping hot. Top the potatoes with the sour cream and sprinkle with the scallions. Serves 4.

Per serving: Calories 262; Fiber 4g; Protein 8g; Total Fat 7g; Saturated Fat 3g; Cholesterol 14mg; Sodium 593mg

Hash Browns Cook 1½ lbs. all-purpose potatoes in boiling water; peel and dice. In skillet, sauté 1 large chopped onion, 1 chopped green pepper, and 1 clove chopped garlic in 1 tbsp. olive oil. Add potatoes to pan with ¾ tsp. salt and ½ tsp. pepper; cook until browned. Serves 4. *[Cal 193; Fat 4g; Sod 424mg]*

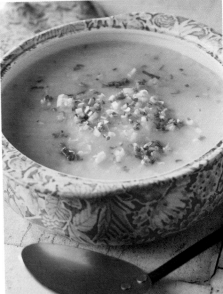

Potato-Cheese Soup In saucepan, combine 2 cups chicken broth, 2 cups water, 3 cloves garlic, and 4 sliced scallions. Bring to boil, add 1½ lbs. peeled and sliced all-purpose potatoes, and cook until tender. Partially mash with potato masher. Stir in 1 cup shredded white Cheddar until melted. Serve garnished with ¼ cup minced scallion. Serves 4. *[Cal 270; Fat 10g; Sod 715mg]*

Roasted New Potatoes Preheat oven to 425°F. Pour 2 tbsp. oil into 9 x 13-inch pan. Add 4 cloves garlic and ½ tsp. rosemary. Heat 5 minutes in oven. Add 2 lbs. quartered small red potatoes; cook, tossing occasionally, for 50 minutes or until done. Sprinkle with ½ teaspoon salt. Serves 4. *[Cal 249; Fat 7g; Sod 292mg]*

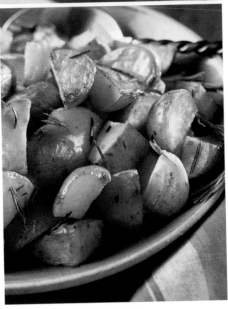

Salad greens

Nutritional power

Since we eat salad greens fresh and raw, they're a reliable source of vitamin C. Leafy greens also supply beta carotene, folate, and some minerals.

Healthy Highlights

Romaine Lettuce
PER 2 CUPS RAW

Calories	18
Fiber	1.9g
Protein	2g
Total Fat	0.2g
Saturated Fat	0g
Cholesterol	0mg
Sodium	9mg

NUTRIENTS

	% Daily Value
Vitamin A	58%
Vitamin C	45%
Folate	38%
Manganese	36%

Looseleaf Lettuce
PER 2 CUPS RAW

Calories	20
Fiber	2.1g
Protein	2g
Total Fat	0.3g
Saturated Fat	0g
Cholesterol	0mg
Sodium	10mg

NUTRIENTS

	% Daily Value
Vitamin A	43%
Manganese	42%
Vitamin C	33%
Folate	14%
Iron	11%

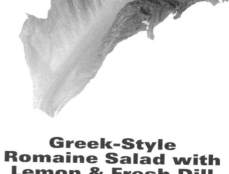

Tossed Salad with Pears, Pecans & Blue Cheese

PREP: 20 MINUTES

An elegant starter for a dinner party, this salad combines three salad greens plus chives for lots of beta carotene.

- **2** pears, halved, cored and sliced lengthwise
- **¾** cup low-fat (1.5%) buttermilk
- **2** tablespoons blue cheese, crumbled
- **1** tablespoon white wine vinegar
- **½** teaspoon salt
- **⅛** teaspoon pepper
- **2** tablespoons snipped fresh chives or scallion greens
- **4** cups torn Boston lettuce
- **6** cups torn red leaf or other looseleaf lettuce
- **2** cups watercress leaves
- **1½** cups thinly sliced cucumber half-rounds
- **3** tablespoons chopped toasted pecans

1. In a small bowl, toss the pears with 2 tablespoons of the buttermilk. In another small bowl, whisk together the remaining ½ cup plus 2 tablespoons buttermilk, the blue cheese, vinegar, salt, and pepper. Stir in the chives.

2. In a large bowl, toss together the Boston and red leaf lettuces, the watercress, and cucumber. Arrange the greens on plates and top with the sliced pears and toasted pecans. Drizzle with some of the dressing and serve the remainder alongside. Serves 6.

Per serving: Calories 102; Fiber 3g; Protein 4g; Total Fat 4g; Saturated Fat 1g; Cholesterol 4mg; Sodium 251mg

Greek-Style Romaine Salad with Lemon & Fresh Dill

PREP: 10 MINUTES

Sturdy but sweet, romaine stands up to zesty dressings and robust ingredients, such as the feta cheese in this salad.

- **¼** cup lemon juice
- **1** tablespoon olive oil
- **¼** teaspoon salt
- **6** cups shredded romaine lettuce
- **½** cup snipped fresh dill
- **4** scallions, thinly sliced
- **4** ounces feta cheese, crumbled

1. In a large bowl, whisk together the lemon juice, oil, and salt.

2. Add the lettuce, dill, and scallions, tossing well. Add the feta and toss again. Serves 4.

Per serving: Calories 130; Fiber 2g; Protein 6g; Total Fat 10g; Saturated Fat 5g; Cholesterol 25mg; Sodium 467mg

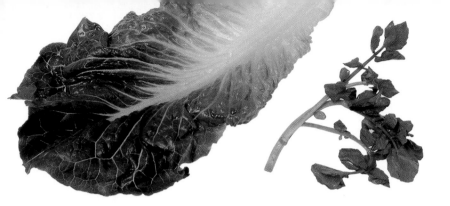

Romaine Salad with Avocado & Oranges

PREP: 15 MINUTES

The oranges and avocado team up to bestow a good portion of potassium on this sun-bright salad.

- 2   navel oranges
- 2   tablespoons lemon juice
- 2   teaspoons extra-virgin olive oil
- 1   teaspoon Dijon mustard
- ¼   teaspoon salt
- 6   cups shredded romaine lettuce
- 2   scallions, thinly sliced
- ½   cup diced avocado

1. With a paring knife, remove the skin and white pith from the oranges. Working over a large salad bowl to catch the juices, cut between the membranes to release the orange sections; set aside.

2. Add the lemon juice, oil, mustard, and salt to the orange juice in the bowl, whisking to blend. Add the lettuce and scallions, tossing well. Add the avocado and toss gently to combine. Serves 4.

Per serving: Calories 101; Fiber 4g; Protein 3g; Total Fat 6g; Saturated Fat 1g; Cholesterol 0mg; Sodium 177mg

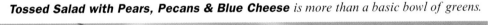

Tossed Salad with Pears, Pecans & Blue Cheese *is more than a basic bowl of greens.*

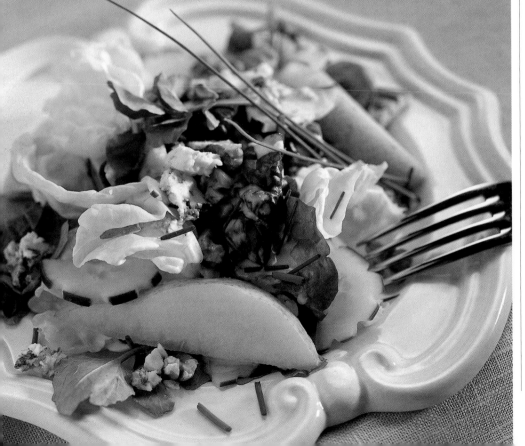

At the market Most salad greens are sold all year round. For a wider selection than your supermarket offers, shop at a greengrocer or farmers' market.

Look for It's easy to tell when salad greens are fresh: They're crisp, unbrowned, and moist but not wet.

Prep Don't wash or tear salad greens until shortly before you use them; this helps conserve their vitamin C. Rinse greens lightly but thoroughly in cool water, then shake or spin them dry. Blot any excess moisture with a kitchen towel. Tear greens rather than cutting them; contact with a steel knife causes the leaves to brown. The tough lower stems of watercress should be trimmed off. Some recipes call for watercress leaves, but this can easily include the more tender upper branches.

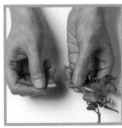

Remove the toughest, lower portions of watercress stems and use the rest of the sprigs.

Watercress
PER 1 CUP RAW

Calories	4
Fiber	0.5g
Protein	1g
Total Fat	0g
Saturated Fat	0g
Cholesterol	0mg
Sodium	14mg

NUTRIENTS

	% Daily Value
Vitamin A	32%
Vitamin C	25%

Arugula
PER 1 CUP RAW

Calories	5
Fiber	0.3g
Protein	1g
Total Fat	0.1g
Saturated Fat	0g
Cholesterol	0mg
Sodium	5mg

Did you know? . . .
As a rule, the darker the greens, the more nutritious the salad. Romaine, water-cress, and arugula, for instance, have more beta carotene and vitamin C than iceberg or Boston lettuce. For the same reason, it's a good idea to use—rather than toss out—the outer, darker leaves from a head of lettuce.

Wilted Greens with Bacon Dressing

PREP: 20 MINUTES / COOK: 10 MINUTES

Canadian bacon adds great smoky flavor to this salad—but with considerably less fat than regular bacon. For a bit of crunch and extra health benefits, we've added radishes, a cruciferous vegetable with the cancer-fighting potential of all members of this family.

- 2 tablespoons flour
- 1 tablespoon light brown sugar
- 1 teaspoon dry mustard
- ¼ teaspoon salt
- ⅓ cup cider vinegar
- 1 tablespoon vegetable oil
- 2 ounces Canadian bacon, diced
- 1 tablespoon reduced-fat sour cream
- 8 cups torn romaine lettuce
- 2 cups watercress leaves
- ½ cup thinly sliced radishes
- ½ pound cooked turkey breast, cut into 2 x ¼-inch matchsticks

1. In a small bowl, combine the flour, brown sugar, mustard, and salt. Add the vinegar and ⅔ cup of water, and whisk until blended.

2. In a small saucepan, heat the oil over moderate heat. Add the Canadian bacon and cook for 3 minutes or until lightly browned.

3. Remove from the heat and stir in the flour mixture. Return to the heat and cook, stirring, for 5 minutes or until thickened. Remove from the heat and stir in the sour cream.

4. In a salad bowl, toss together the romaine, watercress, and radishes. Pour the hot dressing over the salad, tossing to coat. Top with the turkey and serve warm. Serves 4.

Per serving: Calories 190; Fiber 3g; Protein 23g; Total Fat 6g; Saturated Fat 1g; Cholesterol 55mg; Sodium 387mg

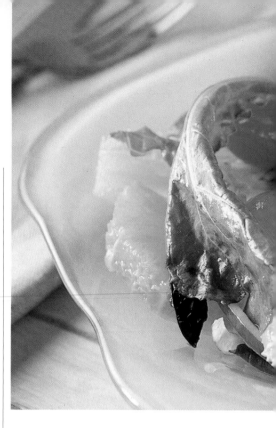

Arugula Salad with Spicy Vinaigrette

PREP: 25 MINUTES

- ½ cup orange juice
- 2 tablespoons red wine vinegar
- 2 teaspoons jalapeño pepper sauce
- 1 teaspoon olive oil
- ½ teaspoon salt
- ¼ teaspoon sugar
- ⅛ teaspoon pepper
- 8 cups arugula leaves
- 2 cups torn romaine lettuce
- 1 cup yellow and/or red cherry tomatoes, halved
- 1 navel orange, peeled and sliced into half-rounds
- 6 oil-cured black olives, slivered
- ½ small red onion, thinly sliced

1. In a small bowl, whisk together the orange juice, vinegar, jalapeño pepper sauce, oil, salt, sugar, and pepper.

2. In a salad bowl, combine the aru-gula, lettuce, tomatoes, orange, olives, and onion. Add the dressing, tossing to coat well. Serves 4.

Per serving: Calories 79; Fiber 4g; Protein 3g; Total Fat 3g; Saturated Fat 0g; Cholesterol 0mg; Sodium 461mg

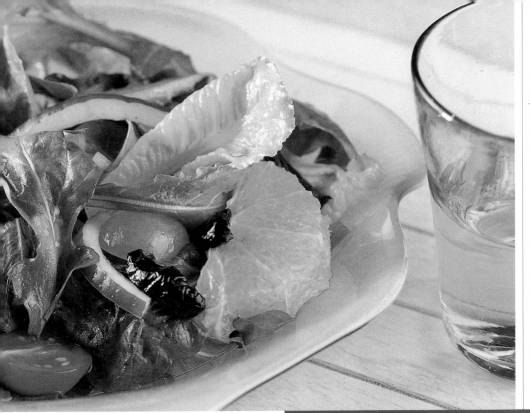

Arugula Salad with Spicy Vinaigrette *features the tang of citrus and the piquancy of hot pepper sauce.*

Did you know? . . . Arugula and watercress are both cruciferous vegetables, relatives of cabbage and broccoli. Vegetables in this family contain cancer-fighting nitrogen compounds called indoles.

Tuna Salad with Mixed Greens, Roasted Peppers & Potatoes

PREP: 25 MINUTES / COOK: 30 MINUTES

Inspired by the Provençal classic, salade niçoise, this great summer supper dish is made with a nutrition-packed variety of vegetables. Use light tuna rather than white, if you prefer its bolder flavor. You can also garnish the salad with ripe tomato wedges.

- 2 **red bell peppers, cut lengthwise into flat panels**
- 2 **cloves garlic, peeled**
- 1 **pound small red potatoes, quartered**
- 1 **red onion, halved and thinly sliced**
- ⅓ **cup chicken broth**
- 3 **tablespoons red wine vinegar**
- 2 **tablespoons light mayonnaise**
- ¼ **teaspoon salt**
- 4 **cups torn looseleaf lettuce**
- 4 **cups torn iceberg lettuce**
- 2 **cans (6½ ounces each) water-packed chunk white tuna, drained**

1. Preheat the broiler. Place the bell pepper pieces, skin-side up, on the broiler rack. Broil the peppers 4 inches from the heat for 10 minutes, or until the skin is blackened. When the peppers are cool enough to handle, peel them and cut into 2-inch-wide strips.

2. In a large pot of boiling water, cook the garlic for 3 minutes to blanch. Remove with a slotted spoon. Add the potatoes and cook for 12 minutes or until firm-tender. Meanwhile, place the onion in a small bowl and cover with ice water. Let stand at room temperature while the potatoes cook.

3. In a large bowl, whisk together the broth, vinegar, mayonnaise, and salt. Mash the garlic and add to the bowl. Drain the potatoes and onion, and add them to the bowl along with the peppers and lettuces. Toss well. Divide the vegetable mixture among 4 plates and top with the tuna. Serves 4.

Per serving: Calories 277; Fiber 4g; Protein 29g; Total Fat 4g; Saturated Fat 1g; Cholesterol 37mg; Sodium 596mg

It's a good idea to use—rather than toss out—the darker lettuce leaves.

A colorful salad mixture called *mesclun* is sold in many supermarkets. An authentic *mesclun* consists of young, tender leaves of a variety of lettuces and herbs. Torn leaves of more mature greens are sometimes sold as *mesclun,* but they'll be less nutritious: Tearing causes the leaves to lose water-soluble nutrients, including vitamin C.

Other greens to consider when making salads are chicory (curly endive) and escarole—both members of the same family. Chicory, with its dark green leaves, is the more nutritious of the two.

Snap beans

Nutritional power
Delightfully crisp, fresh snap beans offer vitamin C, folate, iron, and, in the case of green beans, some beta carotene.

Healthy Highlights

Snap Beans
PER 1 CUP COOKED

Calories	44
Fiber	4.0g
Protein	2g
Total Fat	0.4g
Saturated Fat	0.1g
Cholesterol	0mg
Sodium	4mg

NUTRIENTS

	% Daily Value
Vitamin C	20%
Manganese	18%
Potassium	13%
Iron	11%
Folate	10%

Did you know? . . .
Although most people associate beta carotene with orange vegetables and fruits, the chlorophyll in green vegetables often masks the orange color. Green beans, for example, have eight times as much beta carotene as yellow wax beans.

Lemony Snap Beans

PREP: 15 MINUTES / COOK: 10 MINUTES

Snap beans used to be called "string beans" because their pods had a fibrous string along the sides. The string has been bred out of modern varieties.

- 1½ **pounds green beans or yellow wax beans, halved crosswise**
- 2 **teaspoons olive oil**
- 3 **cloves garlic, minced**
- ¼ **cup chicken broth**
- 1 **teaspoon grated lemon zest**
- ¼ **cup lemon juice**
- ½ **teaspoon salt**
- ⅓ **cup snipped fresh dill**
- 2 **teaspoons unsalted butter**

1. In a steamer or colander set over a pot of boiling water, steam the beans for 6 minutes or until crisp-tender.

2. Meanwhile, in a large nonstick skillet, heat the oil over moderately low heat. Add the garlic and cook for 2 minutes or until soft. Add the broth, lemon zest, lemon juice, and salt, and bring to a boil. Add the beans and cook for 2 minutes or until heated through and well coated. Add the dill, remove from the heat, and stir in the butter until melted. Serves 4.

Per serving: Calories 101; Fiber 3g; Protein 4g; Total Fat 5g; Saturated Fat 2g; Cholesterol 5mg; Sodium 355mg

Green Beans with Pearl Onions, Fresh Tomatoes & Basil

PREP: 20 MINUTES / COOK: 15 MINUTES

Serving the beans in their cooking liquid ensures that you get all the available nutrients. You can substitute cubed yellow onions for the pearl onions.

- 1 **tablespoon olive oil**
- 1 **cup frozen pearl onions, thawed**
- 3 **cloves garlic, minced**
- 1½ **pounds green beans, halved crosswise**
- 2 **tomatoes, chopped**
- ½ **cup chopped fresh basil**
- 2 **tablespoons balsamic vinegar**
- ½ **teaspoon salt**

1. In a large nonstick skillet, heat the oil over moderate heat. Add the pearl onions and sauté for 4 minutes or until lightly browned.

2. Add the garlic, green beans, tomatoes, basil, vinegar, and salt, and bring to a boil. Reduce to a simmer, partially cover, and cook for 9 minutes or until the beans are crisp-tender. Serves 4.

Per serving: Calories 119; Fiber 4g; Protein 4g; Total Fat 4g; Saturated Fat 1g; Cholesterol 0mg; Sodium 295mg

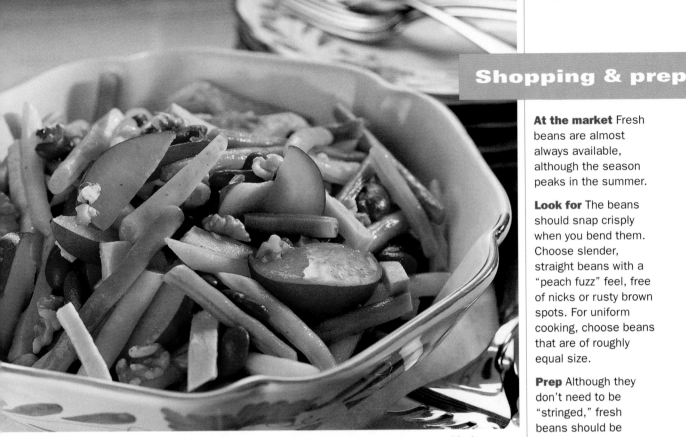

At the market Fresh beans are almost always available, although the season peaks in the summer.

Look for The beans should snap crisply when you bend them. Choose slender, straight beans with a "peach fuzz" feel, free of nicks or rusty brown spots. For uniform cooking, choose beans that are of roughly equal size.

Prep Although they don't need to be "stringed," fresh beans should be topped and tailed— their stem ends and pointed tips removed.

Multi-Bean Salad with Smoked Turkey, Plums & Walnuts Snap beans and kidney beans are combined with turkey, fruit, and nuts for a filling main dish.

Multi-Bean Salad with Smoked Turkey, Plums & Walnuts

PREP: 15 MINUTES / COOK: 15 MINUTES

Try this at your next picnic. The appealing sweet-tart dressing, made with chicken broth, lime juice, mustard, and plum jam, has just one tablespoon of oil.

- ¼ cup walnuts
- ⅓ cup chicken broth
- ¼ cup lime juice
- 3 tablespoons plum jam
- 1 tablespoon olive oil
- 1 tablespoon Dijon mustard
- ¼ teaspoon salt
- ½ pound green beans, halved on the diagonal
- ½ pound yellow wax beans, halved on the diagonal
- 1 can (8¾ ounces) red kidney beans, rinsed and drained
- 2 plums (½ pound total), halved and cut into thin wedges
- 6 ounces smoked turkey, cut into 2 x ¼-inch matchsticks

1. Preheat the oven to 375°F. Bake the walnuts until lightly crisped and fragrant, about 5 minutes. When cool enough to handle, coarsely chop.

2. In a small saucepan, combine the broth, lime juice, jam, oil, mustard, and salt. Stir over low heat until the jam is melted. Transfer the dressing to a large salad bowl.

3. In a steamer or colander set over a pot of boiling water, cook the green and yellow beans for 4 minutes or until just tender. Drain, rinse under cold water, and drain well.

4. Add the green and yellow beans to the bowl with the dressing. Add the kidney beans, plums, and turkey, tossing well to combine. Serve the salad at room temperature or chilled, sprinkled with the toasted walnuts. Serves 4.

Per serving: Calories 280; Fiber 6g; Protein 15g; Total Fat 10g; Saturated Fat 2g; Cholesterol 22mg; Sodium 835mg

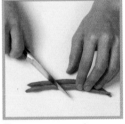

For a more attractive presentation, cut snap beans on the diagonal.

Basic cooking Steam snap beans, or cook them in a small amount of water, for 3 to 5 minutes; they should remain bright green and crisp-tender. Microwave 1 pound snap beans with ¼ cup liquid at high for 5 to 6 minutes.

Spinach

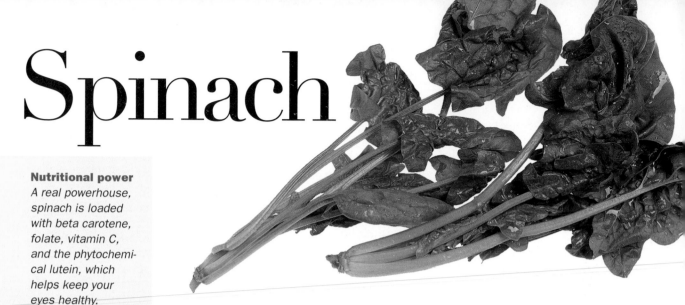

Nutritional power

A real powerhouse, spinach is loaded with beta carotene, folate, vitamin C, and the phytochemical lutein, which helps keep your eyes healthy.

Healthy Highlights

PER 2 CUPS RAW	
Calories	13
Fiber	1.6g
Protein	2g
Total Fat	0.2g
Saturated Fat	0g
Cholesterol	0mg
Sodium	47mg

NUTRIENTS	
	% Daily Value
Vitamin A	81%
Folate	29%
Vitamin C	28%
Manganese	27%
Potassium	11%

Did you know? . . .

Although spinach contains a lot of iron and a considerable amount of calcium, the oxalic acid in the spinach inhibits the body's absorption of these minerals.

Spinach is higher in protein than most vegetables—which may be why Popeye relied on it for his muscle-building.

Spinach Lasagne with Dill & Scallions

PREP: 20 MINUTES / COOK: 55 MINUTES

12	lasagne noodles (10 ounces)
4	teaspoons olive oil
8	scallions, thinly sliced
2	cloves garlic, minced
2	packages (10 ounces each) frozen chopped spinach, thawed and squeezed dry
1	teaspoon grated lemon zest
1	container (15 ounces) part-skim ricotta cheese
1	pound low-fat (1%) cottage cheese
¼	cup plus 2 tablespoons grated Parmesan cheese
2	eggs
⅔	cup snipped fresh dill
¼	cup chopped fresh mint
1	teaspoon salt
¾	teaspoon pepper

1. Preheat the oven to 350°F. In a large pot of boiling water, cook the lasagne noodles according to package directions until firm-tender. Drain well.

2. Meanwhile, in a large nonstick skillet, heat 2 teaspoons of the oil over moderate heat. Add the scallions and garlic, and sauté for 2 minutes or until the scallions are soft. Add the spinach and lemon zest, and cook for 4 minutes or until the spinach is heated through. Transfer to a large bowl. Stir in the ricotta, cottage cheese, ¼ cup of the Parmesan, the eggs, dill, mint, salt, and pepper.

3. Line the bottom of a 9 x 13-inch baking dish with a layer of lasagne noodles. Spoon one-third of the spinach mixture over and top with another layer of noodles. Make 2 more layers with the remaining spinach and noodles, ending with noodles. Cover with foil and bake for 30 minutes. Uncover, brush with the remaining 2 teaspoons oil, and sprinkle with the remaining 2 tablespoons Parmesan. Bake for 15 minutes or until the lasagne is piping hot and just set. Serves 6.

Per serving: Calories 437; Fiber 4g; Protein 32g; Total Fat 14g; Saturated Fat 6g; Cholesterol 100mg; Sodium 956mg

Sautéed Spinach & Red Peppers

PREP: 15 MINUTES / COOK: 15 MINUTES

2	teaspoons olive oil
1	small red onion, finely chopped
3	cloves garlic, minced
1	large red bell pepper, cut into ½-inch squares
8	cups packed fresh spinach leaves
¼	teaspoon salt
⅛	teaspoon sugar

1. In a large nonstick skillet, heat the oil over moderate heat. Add the onion and garlic, and sauté for 5 minutes. Add the bell pepper and sauté for 3 minutes or until crisp-tender.

2. Add the spinach, sprinkle with the salt and sugar, and cook, turning, for 4 minutes or until the spinach is wilted. Serves 4.

Per serving: Calories 91; Fiber 7g; Protein 7g; Total Fat 3g; Saturated Fat 0g; Cholesterol 0mg; Sodium 316mg

Wilted Spinach Salad with Garlic Croutons

PREP: 15 MINUTES / COOK: 15 MINUTES

- **4** ounces Italian bread, cut into ½-inch slices
- **1** clove garlic, peeled and halved
- **2** tablespoons olive oil
- **1** large red onion, cut into ½-inch chunks
- **½** pound mushrooms, thinly sliced
- **2** bunches of spinach (2¼ pounds total), torn into bite-size pieces
- **⅔** cup chicken broth
- **½** cup balsamic vinegar
- **2** teaspoons light brown sugar
- **¼** teaspoon salt
- **¾** teaspoon cornstarch blended with 1 tablespoon water

1. Preheat the oven to 375°F. Place the bread on a baking sheet and bake for 5 minutes or until golden brown and crisp. Rub the toast lightly with the cut garlic (discard the garlic). Cut the toast into cubes.

2. Meanwhile, in a large nonstick skillet, heat 2 teaspoons of the oil over moderate heat. Add the onion and sauté for 4 minutes or until crisp-tender. Add the mushrooms and cook, stirring occasionally, for 4 minutes or until the mushrooms are softened. Transfer to a large bowl. Add the spinach and toast cubes, tossing to combine.

3. Add the remaining 4 teaspoons oil to the skillet along with the broth, vinegar, brown sugar, and salt. Bring to a rolling boil and cook for 1 minute. Stir in the cornstarch mixture and cook, stirring, for 1 minute or until lightly thickened. Pour the hot dressing over the spinach mixture and toss. Serve immediately. Serves 4.

Per serving: Calories 250; Fiber 9g; Protein 12g; Total Fat 9g; Saturated Fat 1g; Cholesterol 0mg; Sodium 689mg

At the market Curly-leaf (Savoy) spinach, sold in bags, is always available. Spinach on the stem, either flat-leaf or curly, appears in the market in the spring. Look for local crops at farmers' markets.

Look for Choose emerald-green spinach with crisp but tender leaves and slender stems. Pass up wilted or yellowed spinach. Bagged spinach should feel springy when you squeeze the bag.

Prep Wash spinach carefully (even if labeled "prewashed"), as it is often sandy. Strip the coarse stems from curly-leaf spinach; the stems of flat-leaf spinach can be left on, but should be trimmed to about 2 inches.

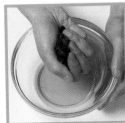

Be sure to squeeze excess liquid out of frozen spinach after thawing it.

Basic cooking Cook damp, washed spinach in a covered pan (or steam it over boiling water) for 3 to 5 minutes. Microwave ½ pound spinach for 2 to 3 minutes at high.

Spinach Lasagne with Dill & Scallions features a flavor innovation: fresh dill and mint.

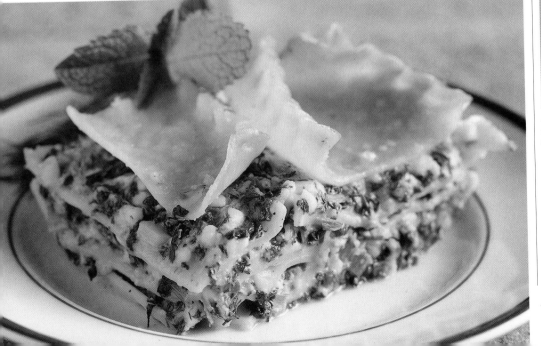

Sweet potatoes

Nutritional power

An outstanding source of beta carotene, sweet potatoes also have vitamin C, B vitamins, and a respectable amount of dietary fiber.

Healthy Highlights

PER 1 LARGE BAKED (WITH SKIN)

Calories	185
Fiber	5.4g
Protein	3g
Total Fat	0.2g
Saturated Fat	0g
Cholesterol	0mg
Sodium	18mg

NUTRIENTS

	% Daily Value
Vitamin A	786%
Vitamin C	73%
Manganese	50%
Vitamin B6	22%
Potassium	21%
Copper	19%
Riboflavin	14%
Folate	10%

Did you know? . . .

Sweet potatoes can be substituted for white potatoes in many recipes. It's an excellent way to increase your beta-carotene intake.

One cup of mashed sweet potatoes supplies eight times the Daily Value for vitamin A.

Moroccan Lamb & Sweet Potato Stew

PREP: 20 MINUTES
COOK: 1 HOUR 15 MINUTES

This subtly spiced stew was inspired by a North African dish called a tagine. Couscous is a traditional accompaniment for a tagine; the stew can also be served over rice.

- 2 teaspoons olive oil
- 1 pound well-trimmed boneless lamb shoulder, cut into ½-inch chunks
- 1 large onion, finely chopped
- 3 cloves garlic, minced
- 1 teaspoon ground coriander
- ¾ teaspoon paprika
- ¾ teaspoon salt
- ½ teaspoon pepper
- 2 tablespoons no-salt-added tomato paste
- 1½ pounds sweet potatoes, peeled and cut into 1-inch chunks
- ½ cup pitted prunes, coarsely chopped

1. Preheat the oven to 350°F. In a nonstick Dutch oven or flameproof casserole, heat the oil over moderately high heat. Add the lamb and sauté for 4 minutes or until lightly browned. With a slotted spoon, transfer the lamb to a plate. Add the onion and garlic to the pan, and sauté for 7 minutes or until the onion is tender.

2. Return the lamb to the pan. Add the coriander, paprika, salt, and pepper, stirring to coat. Add the tomato paste and 1 cup of water, and bring to a boil. Cover and transfer to the oven. Bake for 30 minutes.

3. Add the sweet potatoes, prunes, and ⅓ cup of water. Re-cover and bake for 30 minutes or until the lamb and sweet potatoes are tender. Serves 4.

Per serving: Calories 394; Fiber 7g; Protein 26g; Total Fat 11g; Saturated Fat 3g; Cholesterol 75mg; Sodium 516mg

Sweet Potato & Apple Bake

PREP: 20 MINUTES / COOK: 45 MINUTES

Unlike the familiar marshmallow topping, apples make a substantial nutritional contribution to a sweet-potato casserole.

- 1 tablespoon unsalted butter
- 1 onion, finely chopped
- 2 pounds sweet potatoes, peeled and thinly sliced
- 2 McIntosh apples, cut into ½-inch-thick wedges
- 3 tablespoons sugar
- 2 tablespoons lemon juice
- ¾ cup chicken broth
- ½ teaspoon salt
- ¼ teaspoon pepper

1. Preheat the oven to 450°F. In a very large nonstick skillet, heat the butter over moderate heat. Add the onion and sauté for 5 minutes or until tender.

2. Add the sweet potatoes, apples, 2 tablespoons of the sugar, and the lemon juice, and cook until the sugar has melted. Add the broth, salt, and pepper, and bring to a boil.

3. Transfer the mixture to a 7 x 11-inch glass baking dish. Cover with foil

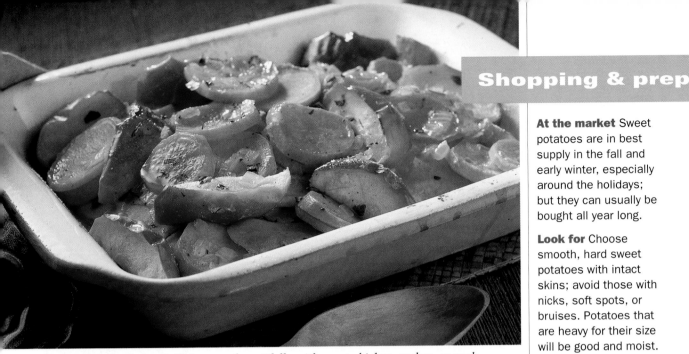

Sweet Potato & Apple Bake goes beautifully with roast chicken, turkey, or pork.

and bake for 25 minutes or until the sweet potatoes are tender. Uncover, sprinkle with the remaining 1 tablespoon sugar, and bake for 10 minutes or until lightly browned. Serves 4.

Per serving: Calories 307; Fiber 8g; Protein 4g; Total Fat 4g; Saturated Fat 2g; Cholesterol 8mg; Sodium 495mg

Thai Sweet Potato & Chicken Salad

PREP: 15 MINUTES / COOK: 30 MINUTES

Many Thai dishes incorporate a peanut butter sauce, its richness "cut" with hot pepper and lime juice. The use of several different herbs is also typical of Thai cuisine.

- 2 **pounds sweet potatoes, peeled and cut into ½-inch cubes**
- 2 **cloves garlic, peeled**
- 1 **pound skinless, boneless chicken breasts**
- 3 **tablespoons peanut butter**
- 2 **tablespoons lime juice**
- ¾ **teaspoon salt**
- ½ **teaspoon hot red pepper sauce**
- ½ **cup chopped fresh basil**
- ¼ **cup chopped fresh mint**
- 1 **pound tomatoes, cut into ½-inch-thick wedges**

1. In a large steamer or colander set over a pot of boiling water, steam the sweet potatoes for 30 minutes or until they are fork-tender.

2. Meanwhile, in a small skillet, bring 1¾ cups of water to a boil over moderate heat. Add the garlic and cook for 3 minutes or until softened. Remove the garlic from the pan with a slotted spoon; when cool enough to handle, finely chop the garlic.

3. Add the chicken to the skillet, reduce to a simmer, cover, and cook, turning the chicken over midway, for 10 minutes or until the chicken is just cooked through. Reserving the cooking liquid, transfer the chicken to a plate. When cool enough to handle, cut across the grain into ½-inch-thick slices.

4. In a large bowl, combine the peanut butter, lime juice, salt, and hot pepper sauce. Whisk in the garlic, ¾ cup of the reserved cooking liquid, the basil, and mint. Add the chicken, sweet potatoes, and tomatoes, tossing to combine. Serve at room temperature or chilled. Serves 4.

Per serving: Calories 399; Fiber 8g; Protein 34g; Total Fat 9g; Saturated Fat 2g; Cholesterol 66mg; Sodium 592mg

At the market Sweet potatoes are in best supply in the fall and early winter, especially around the holidays; but they can usually be bought all year long.

Look for Choose smooth, hard sweet potatoes with intact skins; avoid those with nicks, soft spots, or bruises. Potatoes that are heavy for their size will be good and moist.

Prep Scrub the potatoes gently, being careful not to nick the skin.

Basic cooking To bake, pierce with a fork in several places, then bake for 45 to 60 minutes. Boil whole, unpeeled potatoes for 20 to 40 minutes, cut-up potatoes for 10 to 20 minutes. Pierce whole potatoes before microwaving, then cook at high for 15 to 20 minutes (for 4 potatoes). Remove potatoes from microwave, wrap or cover, and let stand for 3 minutes.

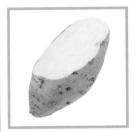

Most sweet potatoes are a deep orange, but you may also run across the yellow-fleshed variety (above), which is starchier and needs less cooking time.

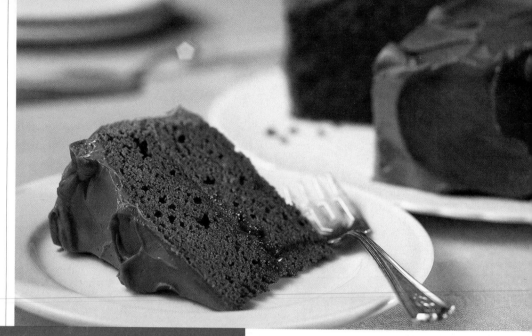

Layered Chocolate-Sweet Potato Cake *has a healthy amount of beta carotene concealed in every slice.*

Did you know? . . .
Their scrumptious flavor and lush texture are misleading: Ounce for ounce, sweet potatoes have no more calories than white potatoes.

A daily serving of sweet potatoes raised researchers' beta-carotene levels 116%.

Researchers studying carotenoids at the Beltsville Human Nutrition Research Center experimented on themselves by eating a high-carotenoid lunch every day for three weeks. They chose sweet potatoes as their beta-carotene source; eating just 5½ ounces per day raised their plasma levels of beta carotene by more than 100 percent.

Studies have shown that high doses of beta carotene *supplements* may be harmful to smokers, but there's no evidence that a diet rich in sweet potatoes, carrots, and other natural beta-carotene sources can be anything other than beneficial.

Layered Chocolate-Sweet Potato Cake

PREP: 30 MINUTES / COOK: 30 MINUTES

2	cups flour
¾	teaspoon baking soda
¾	teaspoon cinnamon
¼	teaspoon salt
¾	pound sweet potatoes, peeled and thinly sliced
¼	cup vegetable oil
¾	cup granulated sugar
¾	cup packed light brown sugar
2	eggs
3	egg whites
3	ounces unsweetened chocolate, melted
1½	teaspoons vanilla extract
½	cup low-fat (1.5%) buttermilk
1	package (8 ounces) reduced-fat cream cheese (Neufchâtel)
1	package (8 ounces) nonfat cream cheese
1	cup confectioners sugar
¼	cup unsweetened cocoa powder
½	cup apricot jam

1. Preheat the oven to 350°F. Spray two 8-inch round cake pans with non-stick cooking spray; set aside. In a medium bowl, stir together the flour, baking soda, cinnamon, and salt.

2. In a large steamer, cook the sweet potatoes for 20 minutes or until very tender. Transfer to a bowl and mash.

3. In a large bowl with an electric mixer, beat the oil, granulated sugar, and brown sugar until well combined. Beat in the whole eggs and egg whites, one at a time, beating well after each addition. Beat in the chocolate, vanilla, and mashed potato. Alternately fold in the flour mixture and buttermilk, beginning and ending with the flour mixture.

4. Divide the batter evenly between the prepared pans. Bake for 30 minutes or until a cake tester inserted in the center comes out clean. Cool 10 minutes in the pans on a wire rack, then turn out onto the rack to cool completely.

5. Meanwhile, in a medium bowl with an electric mixer, cream the nonfat and reduced-fat cream cheeses, the confectioners sugar, and cocoa together.

6. Place one layer on a cake plate. Spread the layer with the apricot jam. Top with the second layer and frost the top and sides with the cream cheese frosting. Serves 16.

Per serving: Calories 324; Fiber 2g; Protein 8g; Total Fat 10g; Saturated Fat 4g; Cholesterol 35mg; Sodium 260mg

Stir-Fried Sweet Potatoes

PREP: 30 MINUTES / COOK: 20 MINUTES

- 2 **pounds sweet potatoes, peeled and thinly sliced**
- 2½ **teaspoons sesame oil**
- 2½ **teaspoons vegetable oil**
- 3 **cloves garlic, minced**
- 2 **scallions, minced**
- 1 **tablespoon minced fresh ginger**
- ¾ **teaspoon sesame seeds**
- ¾ **teaspoon salt**

1. In a large steamer, cook the sweet potatoes for 12 minutes or until tender.

2. Meanwhile, in a large skillet, heat the sesame oil and vegetable oil over moderate heat. Add the garlic, scallions, and ginger, and sauté for 2 minutes or until the scallions are tender.

3. Add the sweet potatoes to the skillet, tossing until well coated and cooked through. Sprinkle with the sesame seeds and salt. Serves 4.

Per serving: Calories 232; Fiber 5g; Protein 3g; Total Fat 7g; Saturated Fat 1g; Cholesterol 0mg; Sodium 435mg

Candied Sweet Potatoes

PREP: 15 MINUTES / COOK: 25 MINUTES

- 2 **pounds sweet potatoes, peeled and thinly sliced**
- 4 **teaspoons unsalted butter**
- ¼ **cup firmly packed dark brown sugar**
- ¼ **cup lime juice**
- ¾ **teaspoon salt**
- ½ **teaspoon ground ginger**

1. In a large steamer, cook the sweet potatoes for 12 minutes or until tender.

2. In a large skillet, melt the butter over moderate heat. Add the sugar and lime juice, and bring to a boil. Add the sweet potatoes, salt, and ginger, and cook for 10 minutes or until the sweet potatoes are nicely glazed. Serves 4.

Per serving: Calories 261; Fiber 5g; Protein 3g; Total Fat 4g; Saturated Fat 3g; Cholesterol 10mg; Sodium 442mg

Twice-Baked Sweet Potatoes Bake four 8-oz. sweet potatoes at 425°F for 45 minutes or until firm-tender. Scoop out flesh, leaving ¼-inch shell. Mash flesh with ¼ cup Parmesan, 1 tbsp. butter, 1 tsp. salt, and ¼ tsp. pepper. Spoon into shells and bake 20 minutes or until shell is crispy. Serves 4. *[Cal 220; Fat 5g; Sod 694mg]*

Spiced Sweet Potato Soup Peel and thinly slice 1½ lbs. sweet potatoes. Combine in saucepan with 1¾ cups chicken broth, 1 cup water, 1 tsp. ground coriander, ¼ tsp. red pepper flakes, ½ tsp. sugar, and ½ tsp. salt. Simmer, covered, until tender. Purée in food processor. Stir in 2 tbsp. lime juice. Serves 4. *[Cal 144; Fat 1g; Sod 751mg]*

Oven-Roasted Sweet Potatoes & Garlic In large baking pan, combine 2 tbsp. olive oil, 8 cloves garlic (unpeeled), and ½ tsp. rosemary. Heat in 425°F oven for 5 minutes. Add 2 lbs. peeled, thinly sliced sweet potatoes. Bake, turning occasionally, for 40 minutes or until tender. Sprinkle with ½ tsp. salt. Serves 4. *[Cal 307; Fat 8g; Sod 304mg]*

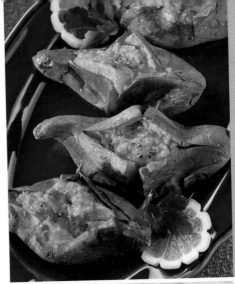

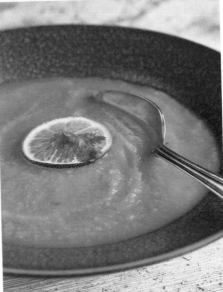

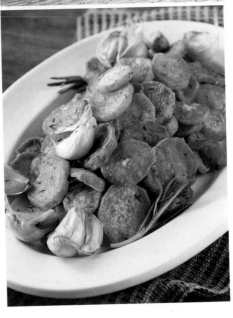

Tomatoes

Nutritional power

Low in calories and big on flavor, tomatoes are a treat. Along with vitamin C, they offer a tremendous amount of lycopene, a cancer-fighting carotenoid.

Healthy Highlights

PER 1 CUP RAW

Calories	38
Fiber	2.0g
Protein	2g
Total Fat	0.6g
Saturated Fat	0.1g
Cholesterol	0mg
Sodium	16mg

NUTRIENTS

	% Daily Value
Vitamin C	57%
Vitamin A	22%
Potassium	13%

Did you know? . . .
Tomatoes in all their forms—fresh, canned, dried, and as juice or pasta sauce—are loaded with lycopene. A large study done in 1995 revealed that men who ate lots of tomato products had a greatly reduced risk of prostate cancer; the researchers theorized that the lycopene in the tomatoes might be the protective factor.

Three-Tomato Marinara Sauce

PREP: 15 MINUTES / COOK: 40 MINUTES

This makes a big batch of sauce—enough for 20 servings. When the sauce is done, ladle it into 2-cup freezer containers, cool to room temperature, and refrigerate or freeze.

½	cup sun-dried tomatoes (not oil-packed)
2	tablespoons olive oil
2	large onions, finely chopped
8	cloves garlic, minced
10	cups no-salt-added canned tomatoes, chopped with their juice
3	tablespoons no-salt-added tomato paste
1½	teaspoons salt
½	teaspoon sugar

1. In a small bowl, soak the sun-dried tomatoes in boiling water to cover. Let stand for 15 minutes or until softened. Drain and finely chop.

2. Meanwhile, in a large saucepan, heat the oil over low heat. Add the onions and garlic, and sauté for 15 minutes or until the onions are very soft.

3. Add the sun-dried tomatoes, the canned tomatoes and their juice, the tomato paste, salt, and sugar. Bring to a boil, reduce to a simmer, cover, and cook for 20 minutes or until the sauce is richly flavored and lightly thickened. Makes 10 cups.

Per ½-cup serving: Calories 55; Fiber 2g; Protein 2g; Total Fat 2g; Saturated Fat 0g; Cholesterol 0mg; Sodium 185mg

Tomato Bruschetta

PREP: 20 MINUTES / COOK: 10 MINUTES

This delightful Italian appetizer makes brilliant use of fresh tomatoes. Plum tomatoes are less juicy than other types, so the topping won't "wilt" the bread.

24	slices (½-inch-thick) Italian bread (12 ounces total)
3	cloves garlic, peeled and halved
2	tablespoons olive oil
1½	pounds plum tomatoes, coarsely chopped
⅓	cup chopped fresh basil
1	tablespoon no-salt-added tomato paste
¾	teaspoon salt
½	teaspoon grated orange zest
¼	teaspoon pepper

1. Preheat the oven to 400°F. Rub the bread with one of the halved garlic cloves. Brush the bread with 1 tablespoon of the oil and bake for 7 minutes or until golden brown and crisp.

2. In a small pan of boiling water, cook the 2 remaining garlic cloves for 3 minutes to blanch. Finely chop.

3. In a medium bowl, combine the chopped garlic, tomatoes, basil, tomato paste, salt, orange zest, pepper, and the remaining 1 tablespoon oil. Spoon on top of the toasted garlic bread. Serves 4.

Per serving: Calories 335; Fiber 5g; Protein 9g; Total Fat 10g; Saturated Fat 2g; Cholesterol 0mg; Sodium 927mg

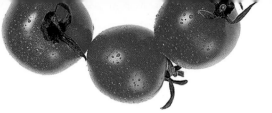
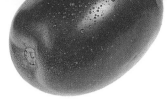

Manhattan Seafood Chowder

PREP: 25 MINUTES / COOK: 30 MINUTES

Manhattan-style chowder, made with tomatoes, has a distinct nutritional advantage over New England cream-based chowder: It's lower in fat and is high in lycopene.

1	onion, finely chopped
½	cup dry white wine or chicken broth
1	dozen little neck clams, well scrubbed
¾	pound all-purpose potatoes, peeled and cut into ½-inch cubes
1	red bell pepper, cut into ½-inch squares
1	stalk celery, cut into ¼-inch dice
3	cups no-salt-added canned tomatoes, chopped with their juice
1	cup chicken broth
½	teaspoon dried thyme
½	teaspoon salt
1	pound cod steak, cut into ½-inch cubes

1. In a Dutch oven or flameproof casserole, combine the onion, wine, and clams. Bring to a boil over moderate heat, cover, and cook for 5 minutes or until the clams have opened. Remove the clams from the pan (discard any that have not opened). Remove the clam meat from the shells and discard the shells.

2. Add the potatoes, bell pepper, celery, and 1 cup of water to the pan and bring to a boil. Reduce to a simmer, cover, and cook for 5 minutes. Add the tomatoes and their juice, the broth, thyme, and salt, and return to a boil. Reduce the heat to a simmer, cover, and cook for 15 minutes or until the potatoes are tender.

3. Add the cod to the pan, cover, and cook for 5 minutes or until the fish is almost cooked through. Return the clams to the pan and cook just until heated through. Serves 4.

Per serving: Calories 230; Fiber 4g; Protein 28g; Total Fat 2g; Saturated Fat 0g; Cholesterol 58mg; Sodium 652mg

At the market Seasonal local tomatoes are tastiest, but you'll find California and Florida tomatoes in stores all year round. If you can't buy vine-ripened tomatoes at a farmstand or farmers' market, do shop where the tomatoes are kept at room temperature (not chilled). Small, egg-shaped plum (Roma) tomatoes, are often flavorful when round tomatoes are pale and tasteless.

Look for Choose tomatoes that are heavy for their size, evenly colored, and unblemished. Even if unripe, they should be more pink than green.

Prep If the tomatoes are not fully ripe, keep them in a paper bag at room temperature for a few days. Don't store tomatoes in the refrigerator unless they're threatening to spoil.

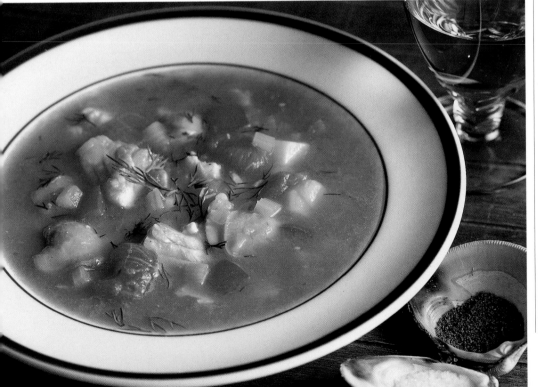

Manhattan Seafood Chowder boasts clams and chunks of cod in a tomato broth.

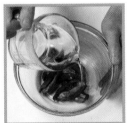

Dry-packed sun-dried tomatoes need to be soaked in boiling water to soften them before chopping.

Did you know? . . .

A university study indicates that lycopene may fight heart disease as well as cancer. The study results suggest that lycopene offers a greater protective effect than beta carotene. Based on their findings, the researchers recommend that people eat more dishes made with cooked tomatoes.

It takes about 17 pounds of fresh tomatoes to yield one pound of sun-dried. In the process, nutrients are greatly concentrated. So 3½ ounces of sun-dried tomatoes supply 110 milligrams of calcium—about 22 times as much as the same weight of fresh tomatoes.

Because it's concentrated, tomato paste has more vitamin C than fresh tomatoes.

Studies indicate that the disease-fighting lycopene in tomatoes is best absorbed when the tomatoes have been heat-processed (i.e., cooked or canned) using a small amount of oil.

Stir-Fried Beef with Cherry Tomatoes
Hot, juicy tomatoes enliven this beef and vegetable dish.

Gazpacho

PREP: 30 MINUTES / CHILL: 2 HOURS

To make gazpacho in a food processor, chop one vegetable at a time, using quick on-and-off pulses so that the vegetables are very coarsely chopped, not puréed. Add each vegetable in turn to a large bowl, then stir in the remaining ingredients.

- 2 pounds tomatoes, coarsely chopped
- 1 red bell pepper, cut into ¼-inch dice
- 1 green bell pepper, cut into ¼-inch dice
- 1 small red onion, finely chopped
- 1 stalk celery, cut into ¼-inch dice
- ¼ cup red wine vinegar
- ¾ teaspoon salt
- ½ teaspoon ground coriander
- ½ teaspoon hot red pepper sauce

1. In a large bowl, combine the tomatoes, peppers, onion, celery, vinegar, salt, coriander, and hot pepper sauce.

2. Refrigerate the gazpacho for 2 hours or until well chilled. Ladle into soup bowls. Serves 4.

Per serving: Calories 73; Fiber 4g; Protein 3g; Total Fat 1g; Saturated Fat 0g; Cholesterol 0mg; Sodium 461mg

Stir-Fried Beef with Cherry Tomatoes

PREP: 20 MINUTES / COOK: 15 MINUTES

- 1 tablespoon cornstarch
- 1 tablespoon lower-sodium soy sauce
- ½ teaspoon ground ginger
- 1 teaspoon sugar
- 1 pound well-trimmed flank steak, halved lengthwise and thinly sliced across the grain, on the diagonal
- 1 tablespoon vegetable oil
- 3 scallions, cut into 1-inch lengths
- 3 cloves garlic, minced
- 6 ounces sugar snap peas, strings removed
- 2 pints cherry tomatoes, halved

1. In a medium bowl, combine the cornstarch, soy sauce, ginger, and ½ teaspoon of the sugar. Add the beef, tossing well to coat.

2. In a large nonstick skillet, heat 1½ teaspoons of the oil over moderately high heat. Add half of the beef and sauté for 2 minutes or until no longer pink. With a slotted spoon, transfer the beef to a plate. Repeat with the remaining 1½ teaspoons oil and the remaining beef.

3. Add the scallions and garlic to the skillet and sauté for 1 minute or until the scallions are crisp-tender. Add the sugar snap peas, tomatoes, and the

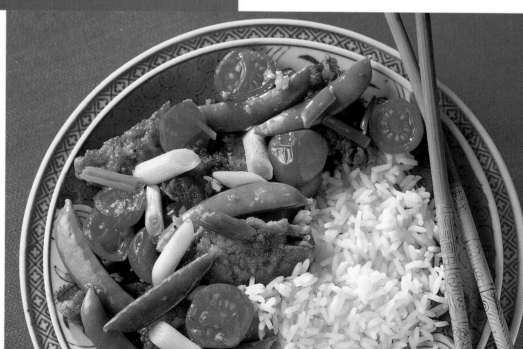

114

remaining ½ teaspoon sugar, and cook for 2 minutes or until the tomatoes just begin to collapse. Return the beef to the skillet and cook until heated through. Serves 4.

Per serving: Calories 265; Fiber 3g; Protein 26g; Total Fat 12g; Saturated Fat 4g; Cholesterol 57mg; Sodium 244mg

Chicken Cacciatore

PREP: 15 MINUTES / COOK: 40 MINUTES

You can make this a day ahead and reheat it: It will taste even better the second day.

- 4 skinless, bone-in chicken breast halves (8 ounces each)
- 3 tablespoons flour
- 1 tablespoon olive oil
- 1 red onion, finely chopped
- 4 cloves garlic, minced
- 1 red bell pepper, cut into ½-inch squares
- ½ pound small mushrooms, quartered
- 1 pound tomatoes, finely chopped
- ¼ cup chicken broth
- ¾ teaspoon salt
- ½ teaspoon dried rosemary, crumbled
- ½ teaspoon black pepper

1. Dredge the chicken in the flour, shaking off the excess. In a large non-stick skillet, heat the oil over moderate heat. Add the chicken and cook for 3 minutes per side or until golden brown. Transfer the chicken to a plate.

2. Reduce the heat to moderately low, add the onion and garlic, and sauté for 7 minutes or until the onion is tender. Add the bell pepper and cook for 4 minutes or until crisp-tender. Add the mushrooms and cook, stirring, for 3 minutes or until softened.

3. Add the tomatoes, broth, salt, rosemary, and black pepper, and bring to a boil. Return the chicken to the pan, reduce the heat to a simmer, cover, and cook, turning the chicken over midway, for 20 minutes or until the chicken is cooked through. Serves 4.

Per serving: Calories 312; Fiber 4g; Protein 44g; Total Fat 6g; Saturated Fat 1g; Cholesterol 101mg; Sodium 609mg

Caprese Salad In medium bowl, combine 2 pints halved cherry tomatoes, 4 oz. part-skim mozzarella cut into ¼-inch cubes, ⅓ cup slivered green olives, ⅓ cup chopped fresh basil, 2 tbsp. balsamic vinegar, 1 tbsp. olive oil, and ½ tsp. salt. Toss. Serves 4. *[Cal 139; Fat 10g; Sod 685mg]*

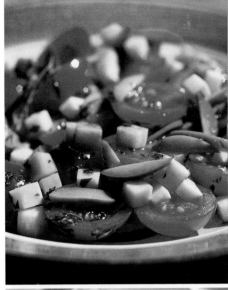

Baked Herbed Tomatoes Slice off and discard top quarter of four large (9-oz.) tomatoes. Scoop out and discard the seeds. In small bowl, mix ½ cup chopped parsley, ¼ cup sliced scallions, ¼ cup seasoned dried bread crumbs, and 1 tbsp. olive oil. Spoon into tomatoes. Bake at 400°F for 20 to 30 minutes or until piping hot. Serves 4. *[Cal 111; Fat 4g; Sod 224mg]*

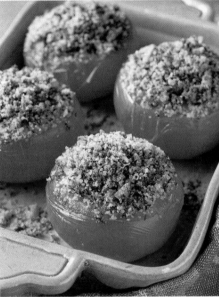

Fresh Tomato Salsa In bowl, combine 1 lb. chopped tomatoes, 4 sliced scallions, ½ cup chopped cilantro, 2 minced jalapeño peppers (fresh or pickled), 2 tbsp. red wine vinegar, ½ tsp. each ground coriander and cumin, and ¼ tsp. salt. Makes 3 cups/½ cup per serving. *[Cal 23; Fat 0g; Sod 100mg]*

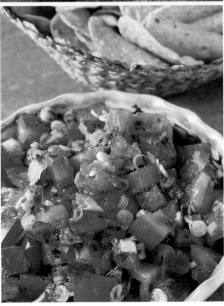

Turnips

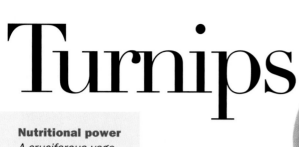

Nutritional power

A cruciferous vege-table, turnips con-tain cancer-fighting indoles and also supply vitamin C. Rutabagas (yellow-fleshed turnips) have beta carotene, too.

Healthy Highlights

White Turnip
PER 1 CUP COOKED

Calories	28
Fiber	3.1g
Protein	1g
Total Fat	0.1g
Saturated Fat	0g
Cholesterol	0mg
Sodium	78mg

NUTRIENTS

	% Daily Value
Vitamin C	30%

Rutabaga
PER 1 CUP COOKED

Calories	94
Fiber	4.3g
Protein	3g
Total Fat	0.5g
Saturated Fat	0.1g
Cholesterol	0mg
Sodium	48mg

NUTRIENTS

	% Daily Value
Vitamin C	75%
Vitamin A	27%
Potassium	26%
Manganese	21%
Thiamin	13%
Calcium	12%
Vitamin B6	12%

Pan-Roasted Turnips with Garlic

PREP: 10 MINUTES / COOK: 35 MINUTES

Crusty and golden, these pan-roasted turnips are every bit as tasty as roasted potatoes.

- 2 **pounds white turnips, peeled and cut into ½-inch-thick wedges**
- 1 **tablespoon olive oil**
- 5 **cloves garlic, peeled and halved**
- 1 **tablespoon sugar**
- ½ **cup chicken broth**
- ½ **teaspoon each crumbled dried rosemary and salt**
- ¼ **cup chopped parsley**

1. In a steamer or colander set over a pot of boiling water, steam the turnips for 10 minutes or until crisp-tender.

2. In a large nonstick skillet, heat the oil over low heat. Add the garlic and cook, turning it as it colors, for 2 minutes or until light golden. Add the turnips and sugar, and cook for 7 minutes or until the turnips are golden.

3. Add the broth, rosemary, and salt, and bring to a boil. Cook for 10 minutes or until the liquid has evaporated and the turnips are tender. Add the parsley, tossing to combine. Serves 4.

Per serving: Calories 102; Fiber 4g; Protein 2g; Total Fat 4g; Saturated Fat 1g; Cholesterol 0mg; Sodium 530mg

Mashed Rutabaga with Carrots & Potatoes

PREP: 15 MINUTES / COOK: 35 MINUTES

- 1¾ **pounds rutabaga, peeled, quartered, and thinly sliced**
- ½ **pound all-purpose potatoes, peeled and thinly sliced**
- ½ **pound carrots, thinly sliced**
- 5 **cloves garlic, peeled**
- 1 **bay leaf**
- ¾ **teaspoon salt**
- ½ **teaspoon dried thyme**
- ¼ **teaspoon pepper**
- 1 **tablespoon olive oil**
- ¼ **cup grated Parmesan cheese**

1. In a large saucepan, combine the rutabaga, potatoes, carrots, garlic, bay leaf, ¼ teaspoon of the salt, the thyme, pepper, and 4 cups of water. Bring to a boil over moderate heat, reduce to a simmer, cover, and cook for 30 minutes or until tender. Reserving ½ cup of the cooking liquid, drain the vegetables and garlic. Remove and discard the bay leaf.

2. With a potato masher, mash the vegetables and garlic along with the reserved cooking liquid and the oil. Stir in the Parmesan and the remaining ½ teaspoon salt. Serves 4.

Per serving: Calories 179; Fiber 7g; Protein 6g; Total Fat 5g; Saturated Fat 2g; Cholesterol 4mg; Sodium 562mg

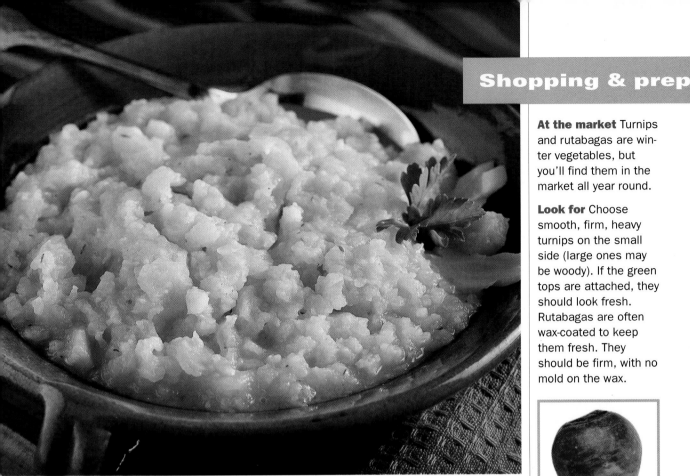

Mashed Rutabaga with Carrots & Potatoes *Serve this mellow golden vegetable blend instead of mashed potatoes; it's perfect with poultry, pork, or beef.*

At the market Turnips and rutabagas are winter vegetables, but you'll find them in the market all year round.

Look for Choose smooth, firm, heavy turnips on the small side (large ones may be woody). If the green tops are attached, they should look fresh. Rutabagas are often wax-coated to keep them fresh. They should be firm, with no mold on the wax.

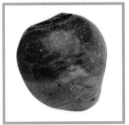

Softball-size or larger, rutabagas are sold trimmed of their tops and waxed.

Prep Cut off and reserve turnip greens, which can be prepared like other cooking greens. Using a vegetable peeler, peel turnips very thinly; remove the waxed skin from rutabagas with a sturdy paring knife.

Basic cooking Steam cut-up turnips for about 15 minutes; cut-up rutabaga will take 25 to 35 minutes. Microwave 1 pound cubed turnip or rutabaga with 3 tablespoons water, covered, for 7 to 9 minutes.

Braised Pork with Turnips

PREP: 20 MINUTES / COOK: 25 MINUTES

When braising, brown the meat and vegetables, then cook them, covered, in a small amount of liquid; the cooking liquid becomes a sauce. This conserves all the flavor and a substantial amount of the nutrients.

- 1   tablespoon cornstarch
- 1   tablespoon lower-sodium soy sauce
- ½   teaspoon sugar
- 1   pound well-trimmed pork tenderloin, cut into ½-inch chunks
- 4½ teaspoons vegetable oil
- 2   pounds white turnips, peeled and cut into ½-inch-thick wedges
- 6   cloves garlic, minced
- 1⅓ cups chicken broth
- ½   teaspoon dried rosemary, crumbled
- ¼   teaspoon each salt and pepper

1. In a medium bowl, combine the cornstarch, soy sauce, and sugar. Add the pork, tossing until well coated.

2. In a large nonstick skillet, heat 1½ teaspoons of the oil over moderately high heat. Add half of the pork and cook for 3 minutes or until lightly browned. Transfer the pork to a plate. Repeat with another 1½ teaspoons oil and the remaining pork.

3. Add the turnips and the remaining 1½ teaspoons oil to the pan and cook, stirring frequently, for 4 minutes or until lightly browned. Add the garlic and cook for 1 minute.

4. Add the broth, rosemary, salt, and pepper, and bring to a boil. Reduce to a simmer, cover, and cook for 10 minutes or until the turnips are tender. Add the pork to the pan and cook for 2 minutes or until just cooked through. Serves 4.

Per serving: Calories 259; Fiber 3g; Protein 26g; Total Fat 10g; Saturated Fat 2g; Cholesterol 74mg; Sodium 816mg

Winter squash

Nutritional power

Sweet and meaty, these sturdy squashes boast lots of beta carotene if their flesh is deep orange. Pumpkin is the clear leader in this category.

Healthy Highlights

Pumpkin

PER ½ CUP CANNED

Calories	42
Fiber	3.6g
Protein	1g
Total Fat	0.3g
Saturated Fat	0.2g
Cholesterol	0mg
Sodium	6mg

NUTRIENTS

	% Daily Value
Vitamin A	542%
Iron	11%

Did you know? . . .
Canned pumpkin purée is nearly as nutritious as raw pumpkin, however canned pumpkin-pie filling has about 100 more calories per cup.

The Great Pumpkin would not make good eating: Large "field" pumpkins are stringy and dry. For cooking, choose small "sugar" pumpkins weighing no more than 5 pounds.

Pumpkin-Date Muffins with Almonds

PREP: 20 MINUTES / COOK: 35 MINUTES

The dates and almonds account for a good portion of the dietary fiber in these tender, lightly sweet muffins.

1½ cups flour
⅓ cup packed light brown sugar
2 teaspoons baking powder
½ teaspoon baking soda
¼ teaspoon salt
½ cup chopped dates
¼ cup chopped almonds
1 cup canned solid-pack pumpkin purée
2 eggs, lightly beaten
½ cup low-fat (1.5%) buttermilk
½ cup reduced-fat sour cream

1. Preheat the oven to 350°F. Line a 2½-inch muffin tin with paper liners. In a large bowl, stir together the flour, brown sugar, baking powder, baking soda, and salt. Stir in the dates and almonds.

2. In a medium bowl, combine the pumpkin, eggs, buttermilk, and sour cream. Make a well in the center of the

dry ingredients and pour in the pumpkin mixture. Stir just until combined. Spoon into the prepared muffin cups and bake for 30 to 35 minutes or until a cake tester inserted in the center comes out clean. Makes 12 muffins.

Per muffin: Calories 157; Fiber 2g; Protein 5g; Total Fat 4g; Saturated Fat 1g; Cholesterol 39mg; Sodium 204mg

Fresh Pumpkin Stew with Chick-Peas

PREP: 25 MINUTES / COOK: 35 MINUTES

This tasty combination of squash, potatoes, tomatoes, and chick-peas is thickened with peanut butter—a West African technique.

1 tablespoon olive oil
1 large onion, finely chopped
3 cloves garlic, minced
2½ pounds fresh pumpkin or butternut squash, peeled and cut into 1-inch chunks
¾ pound small red potatoes, halved
1 cup chicken broth
1 can (14½ ounces) no-salt-added stewed tomatoes, chopped with their juice

¾ teaspoon each dried oregano and salt

1 can (16 ounces) chick-peas, rinsed and drained

2 tablespoons creamy peanut butter

1. In a nonstick Dutch oven, flame-proof casserole, or large saucepan, heat the oil over moderate heat. Add the onion and garlic, and sauté for 5 minutes or until the onion is soft.

2. Add the pumpkin and potatoes, stirring to coat. Add the broth, tomatoes and their juice, oregano, and salt. Bring to a boil, reduce to a simmer, cover, and cook for 20 minutes.

3. Add the chick-peas, stir in the peanut butter, and cook for 10 minutes or until the pumpkin and potatoes are tender. Serves 4.

Per serving: Calories 334; Fiber 8g; Protein 12g; Total Fat 10g; Saturated Fat 2g; Cholesterol 0mg; Sodium 866mg

Pumpkin-Date Muffins with Almonds *make a tempting breakfast or snack; they freeze beautifully if well wrapped.*

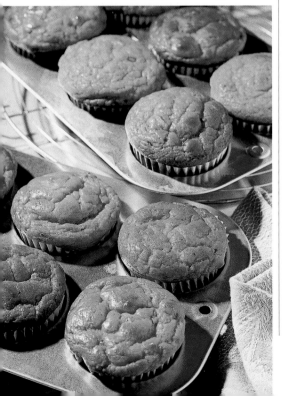

Pumpkin Cheesecake

PREP: 20 MINUTES / COOK: 2 HOURS
CHILL: 4 HOURS

3 ounces gingersnaps (about 12 cookies)

1 tablespoon vegetable oil

¾ cup plus 1 tablespoon sugar

2 packages (8 ounces each) reduced-fat cream cheese (Neufchâtel)

1 package (8 ounces) nonfat cream cheese

1 can (15 ounces) solid-pack pumpkin purée

2 eggs

4 egg whites

½ cup plain nonfat yogurt

1 teaspoon vanilla extract

¼ teaspoon salt

1. Preheat the oven to 300°F. Spray a 9-inch springform pan with nonstick cooking spray.

2. In a food processor, combine the gingersnaps, oil, and 1 tablespoon of the sugar. Process until the crumbs are evenly moistened. Press the crumb mixture into the bottom of the prepared pan; set aside.

3. In a medium bowl, with an electric mixer, beat the cream cheeses and the remaining ¾ cup sugar until well combined. Beat in the pumpkin until well combined. Beat in the whole eggs and egg whites, one at a time, beating well after each addition. Beat in the yogurt, vanilla, and salt until blended.

4. Pour the batter into the prepared crust and bake for 1 hour and 30 minutes or until set. Turn the oven off and let the cake stand in the oven for 30 minutes; then cool on a wire rack and refrigerate for 4 hours or until well chilled. Serves 12.

Per serving: Calories 228; Fiber 1g; Protein 10g; Total Fat 9g; Saturated Fat 5g; Cholesterol 55mg; Sodium 396mg

At the market You can buy winter squash all year round, but fall and winter are the times of peak availability for most varieties.

Look for The rind of a winter squash should be dry and clean, with a dull, almost velvety-looking finish and clear, uniform color.

Prep If you're not cooking a squash whole, use a heavy chef's knife to split it (notch the rind first to give the blade a secure hold). If necessary, use a mallet to tap the knife through the squash.

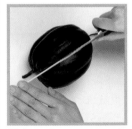

If the rind is not too tough, you can gradually "rock" the knife through it.

Basic cooking Bake squash halves or quarters in a foil-lined pan at 400°F for 40 to 45 minutes. Steam peeled squash chunks for 15 to 20 minutes. Because of its thick skin, winter squash may explode if microwaved whole. Instead, microwave squash halves or quarters, covered, for 7 to 10 minutes.

Chicken Stew with Butternut Squash

Winter squash takes the place of potatoes in this hearty stew.

Healthy Highlights

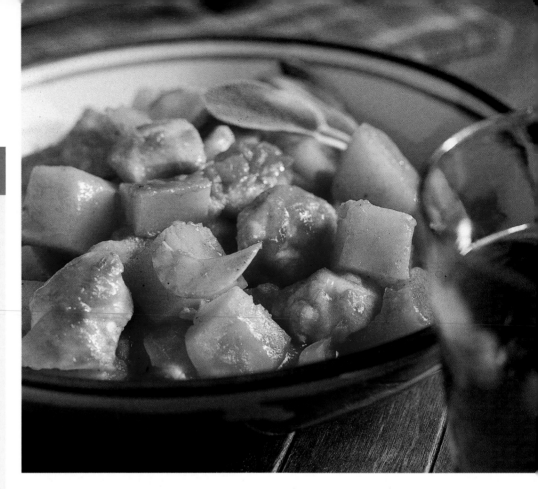

Acorn Squash

PER 1 CUP COOKED	
Calories	115
Fiber	9.0g
Protein	2g
Total Fat	0.3g
Saturated Fat	0.1g
Cholesterol	0mg
Sodium	8mg

NUTRIENTS	
	% Daily Value
Vitamin C	37%
Potassium	30%
Manganese	25%
Thiamin	23%
Vitamin B6	20%
Vitamin A	18%

Butternut Squash

PER 1 CUP COOKED	
Calories	82
Fiber	2.6g
Protein	2g
Total Fat	0.2g
Saturated Fat	0g
Cholesterol	0mg
Sodium	8mg

NUTRIENTS	
	% Daily Value
Vitamin A	287%
Vitamin C	52%
Potassium	19%
Manganese	18%
Vitamin B6	13%
Folate	10%
Niacin	10%

Did you know? . . .
Winter squash that has been stored for several months has a higher beta carotene content than fresh-picked.

Chicken Stew with Butternut Squash

PREP: 25 MINUTES / COOK: 35 MINUTES
An appealing autumn dinner.

- 1 tablespoon vegetable oil
- 1¼ pounds skinless, boneless chicken breasts, cut into 1-inch chunks
- 3 tablespoons flour
- 1 onion, cut into ½-inch chunks
- 4 cloves garlic, slivered
- 1 large butternut squash (2½ pounds), peeled and cut into 1-inch chunks
- 2 cups canned no-salt-added chopped tomatoes
- 1 cup chicken broth
- ½ cup apple juice
- 2 tablespoons no-salt-added tomato paste
- ½ teaspoon each dried sage and salt
- ¼ teaspoon pepper

1. In a large nonstick Dutch oven or flameproof casserole, heat 1½ teaspoons of the oil over moderate heat.

Dredge the chicken in the flour, shaking off the excess. Add half of the chicken to the pan and sauté for 3 minutes or until lightly browned on both sides. Transfer the chicken to a plate. Repeat with the remaining chicken and 1½ teaspoons oil.

2. Add the onion and garlic to the pan and sauté for 7 minutes or until the onion is soft. Add the squash, stirring to coat. Add the chopped tomatoes, broth, apple juice, tomato paste, sage, salt, and pepper, and bring to a boil. Reduce to a simmer, cover, and cook for 7 minutes.

3. Return the chicken to the pan, bring to a simmer, cover, and cook for 10 minutes or until the chicken is cooked through and the squash is tender. Serves 4.

Per serving: Calories 388; Fiber 7g; Protein 38g; Total Fat 6g; Saturated Fat 1g; Cholesterol 82mg; Sodium 662mg

Butternut Squash Tea Bread

PREP: 15 MINUTES
COOK: 1 HOUR 30 MINUTES

Cornmeal adds a lovely texture to this not-too-sweet bread. For best results, don't overmix after adding the dry ingredients.

- 1 **small butternut squash (1½ pounds), halved lengthwise and seeded**
- 1¼ **cups flour**
- ½ **cup yellow cornmeal**
- 1 **teaspoon baking powder**
- ¾ **teaspoon cinnamon**
- ½ **teaspoon each ground ginger, baking soda, and salt**
- ¼ **teaspoon pepper**
- ½ **cup packed light brown sugar**
- ¼ **cup vegetable oil**
- 1 **egg**
- 2 **egg whites**

1. Preheat the oven to 400°F. Spray an 8½ x 4½ x 3-inch loaf pan with non-stick cooking spray; set aside. Place the squash, cut-sides down, in a small baking pan. Add ½ cup water, cover, and bake for 30 minutes or until the squash is tender. When cool enough to handle, scoop the flesh into a bowl and mash with a fork. Measure out 1¼ cups (save any remainder for another use). Reduce the oven temperature to 350°F.

2. In a medium bowl, stir together the flour, cornmeal, baking powder, cinnamon, ginger, baking soda, salt, and pepper; set aside.

3. In another medium bowl, with an electric mixer, beat together the brown sugar and oil until well combined. Add the whole egg and egg whites, one at a time, beating well after each addition. Beat in the 1¼ cups mashed squash. Fold in the dry ingredients.

4. Spoon the batter into the prepared pan and bake for 1 hour or until a cake tester inserted in the center comes out clean. Serves 12.

Per serving: Calories 175; Fiber 2g; Protein 3g; Total Fat 5g; Saturated Fat 1g; Cholesterol 18mg; Sodium 204mg

Pumpkin-Cheese Soup In saucepan, sauté 1 small onion and 2 cloves garlic in 2 tsp. oil until tender. Add 15-oz. can solid-pack pumpkin purée, 1½ cups low-fat (1%) milk, ¾ tsp. salt, and ½ tsp. pepper. Boil 1 minute. Add 1 cup shredded Cheddar and stir until melted. Serves 4. *[Cal 223; Fat 13g; Sod 640mg]*

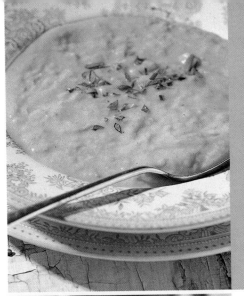

Sweet Spiced Pumpkin Butter In heavy-bottomed saucepan, combine 15-oz. can solid-pack pumpkin, ⅔ cup packed light brown sugar, ⅓ cup granulated sugar, ¼ cup orange juice, 1 tsp. ground ginger, and ¾ tsp. cinnamon. Cook over moderate heat, stirring, for 25 minutes or until thick enough to spread like jam. Keep refrigerated. Makes 2 cups/16 servings. *[Cal 62; Fat 0g; Sod 5mg]*

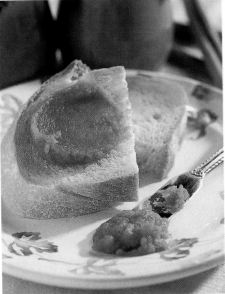

Apricot-Maple Acorn Squash Halve and seed two 1-lb. acorn squash. Place cut-sides down in baking pan, add ⅓ cup water, cover with foil, and bake for 25 minutes at 400°F. Drain. Turn cut-sides up. Stir together ¼ cup apricot jam and 2 tbsp. maple syrup. Spoon into squash. Bake for 35 minutes or until tender. Serves 4. *[Cal 143; Fat 0g; Sod 14mg]*

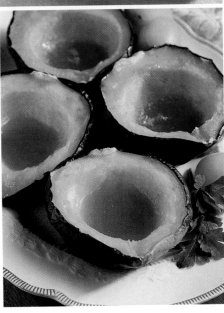

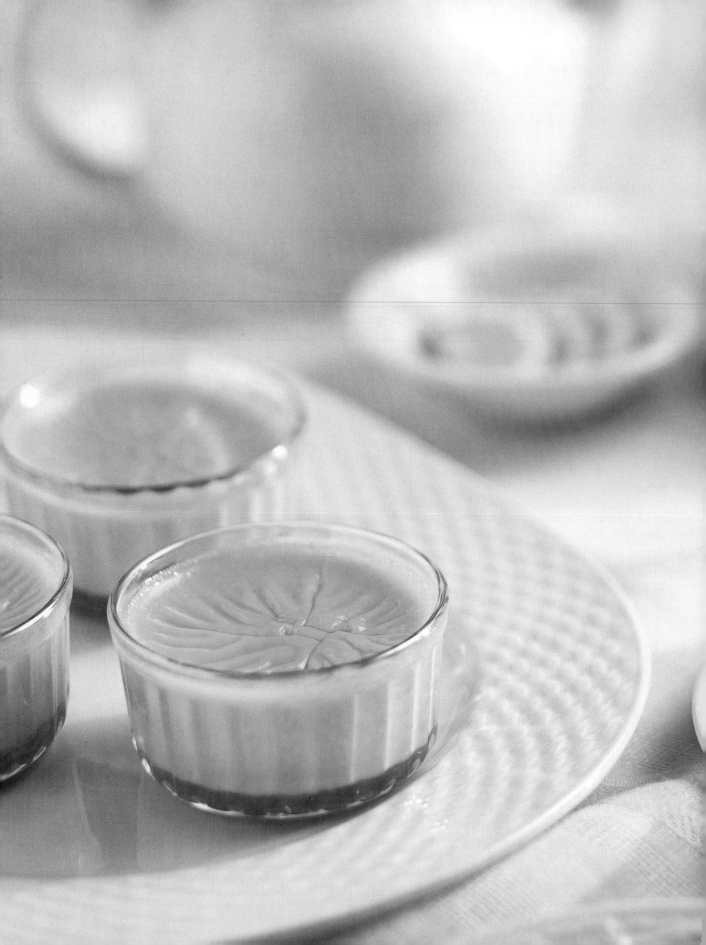

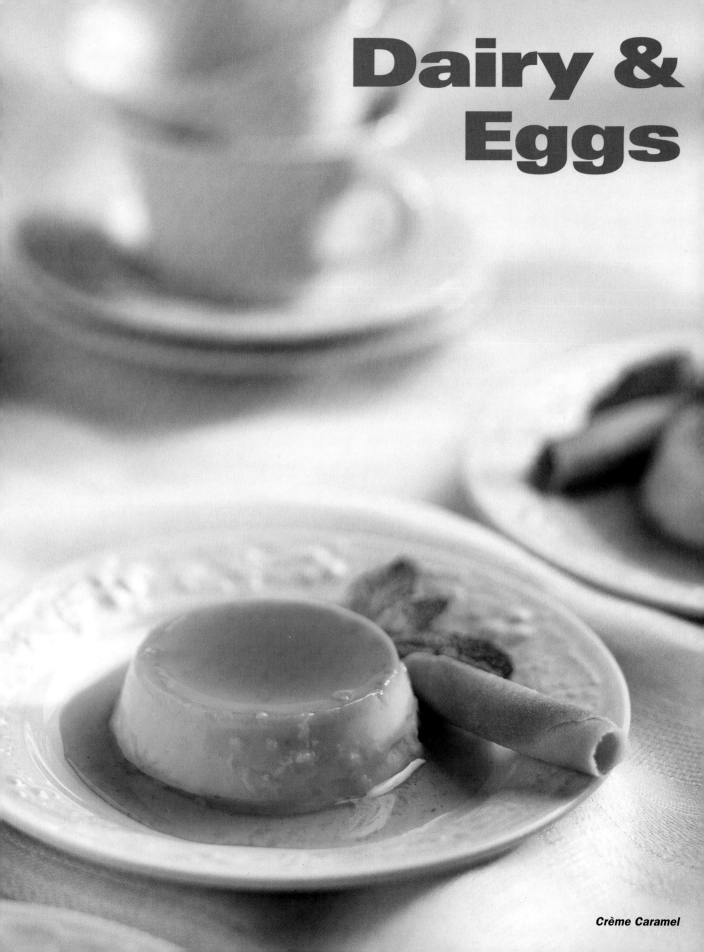

Dairy & Eggs

Crème Caramel

Milk

Nutritional power
Our main calcium source, milk is fortified with vitamin D, which enhances calcium absorption. And drinking low-fat milk may lower blood pressure.

Healthy Highlights

Low-Fat (1%) Milk
PER 1 CUP

Calories	102
Fiber	0g
Protein	8g
Total Fat	2.6g
Saturated Fat	1.6g
Cholesterol	10mg
Sodium	123mg

NUTRIENTS

	% Daily Value
Calcium	30%
Vitamin D	25%
Riboflavin	24%
Vitamin B12	15%
Potassium	13%
Vitamin A	10%

Did you know? . . .
A study called DASH—Dietary Approaches to Stop Hypertension—found that a diet rich in fruits, vegetables, and low-fat dairy products could substantially reduce blood pressure. The same diet, minus the dairy products, was not as effective.

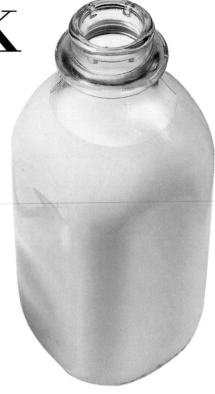

Creamy Espresso Milkshake

PREP: 5 MINUTES / COOK: 5 MINUTES

For a really thick shake, place the milk in the freezer for about 10 minutes before blending. If possible, chill the espresso mixture, too.

- ¼ cup sugar
- 2 tablespoons instant espresso powder
- 1 teaspoon unsweetened cocoa powder
- 4 cups ice-cold low-fat (1%) milk
- 8 ice cubes
- ½ teaspoon vanilla extract

1. In a small saucepan, combine the sugar, espresso powder, cocoa powder, and ¼ cup of water. Bring to a boil over low heat. Remove from the heat; set aside to cool to room temperature.

2. Pour half of the espresso mixture into a blender. Add 2 cups of the milk, 4 of the ice cubes, and ¼ teaspoon of the vanilla, and blend until thick and foamy. Pour into 2 tall (16-ounce) glasses. Repeat with the remaining espresso mixture, milk, ice, and vanilla. Serves 4.

Per serving: Calories 157; Fiber 0g; Protein 8g; Total Fat 3g; Saturated Fat 2g; Cholesterol 10mg; Sodium 123mg

Butterscotch Pudding

PREP: 10 MINUTES / COOK: 10 MINUTES

Although packaged pudding mixes are temptingly convenient, they usually contain artificial colors and flavors. But with just six ingredients (and in just 20 minutes), you can produce a delicious, all-natural dessert.

- 4 teaspoons unsalted butter
- ¾ cup packed dark brown sugar
- 2 cans (12 ounces each) evaporated skimmed milk
- ⅓ cup flour
- ¼ teaspoon salt
- 1½ teaspoons vanilla extract

1. In a medium-size heavy-bottomed saucepan, melt the butter over moderate heat. Add ½ cup of the brown sugar and cook, stirring, until well blended. Gradually stir in all but ½ cup of the evaporated milk, bring to a boil, and stir until the brown sugar has melted.

2. In a small bowl, whisk together the flour and the remaining ¼ cup brown sugar. Stir in the remaining ½ cup evaporated milk until blended. Gradually whisk some of the hot milk mixture into the flour mixture, then whisk the flour mixture back into the saucepan. Whisk in the salt. Bring to a boil and cook for 5 minutes or until no floury taste remains and the pudding is thick.

3. Remove the pudding from the heat. Cool to room temperature and stir in the vanilla. Spoon into 4 dessert bowls, cover, and chill until serving time. Serves 4.

Per serving: Calories 380; Fiber 0g; Protein 16g; Total Fat 4g; Saturated Fat 3g; Cholesterol 18mg; Sodium 372mg

---

White Borscht

PREP: 15 MINUTES / COOK: 10 MINUTES
CHILL: 3 HOURS

A cool purée that includes potatoes, cucumber, onion, radishes, and walnuts.

- ¾ **pound small red potatoes, thinly sliced**
- 3 **cups low-fat (1.5%) buttermilk**
- 1 **large cucumber, peeled, seeded, and thinly sliced**
- 1 **small red onion, thinly sliced**
- ⅓ **cup walnuts**
- ¾ **teaspoon salt**
- ½ **teaspoon pepper**
- ¾ **cup thinly sliced radishes, cut into thin matchsticks**
- ¼ **cup snipped fresh dill**

1. In a medium pot of boiling water, cook the potatoes for 10 minutes or until tender. Drain well and set aside to cool to room temperature.

2. Meanwhile, in a food processor, combine 2 cups of the buttermilk, the cucumber, onion, walnuts, salt, and pepper. Process until well blended.

3. Transfer the mixture to a large bowl and whisk in the remaining 1 cup buttermilk. Add the potatoes, radishes, and dill. Cover and refrigerate for 3 hours or until well chilled. Serves 4.

Per serving: Calories 250; Fiber 3g; Protein 11g; Total Fat 10g; Saturated Fat 2g; Cholesterol 11mg; Sodium 527mg

White Borscht *Tangy buttermilk is the perfect foil for potatoes, dill, and crisp radishes.*

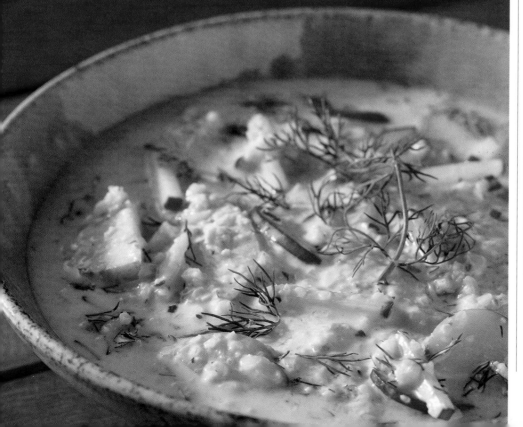

At the market Low-fat (1%) milk has about one-quarter the fat of whole milk. Milk also comes in fat-free (skim) and reduced-fat (2%) forms. Our recipes call for low-fat buttermilk, which has a 1.5% fat content.

Look for Studies suggest that milk in translucent plastic jugs loses riboflavin and vitamin D when exposed to fluorescent light, so buy milk in cardboard cartons if you can.

Basic cooking When a recipe says to "scald" milk, bring it nearly to the boiling point: Heat the milk over low heat just until small bubbles begin to form around the edge.

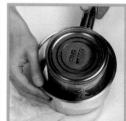

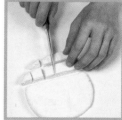

To make fresh cheese (page 126), curdle milk with lemon juice, pour off the whey, and compress the drained curds with a weight (here, a can placed in a saucepan). The firmed cheese will cut cleanly.

Buttermilk
PER 1 CUP

Calories	99
Fiber	0g
Protein	8g
Total Fat	2.2g
Saturated Fat	1.3g
Cholesterol	9mg
Sodium	257mg

NUTRIENTS

	% Daily Value
Calcium	29%
Riboflavin	22%
Potassium	12%

Evaporated Skimmed Milk
PER ½ CUP

Calories	100
Fiber	0g
Protein	10g
Total Fat	0.3g
Saturated Fat	0.2g
Cholesterol	5mg
Sodium	147mg

NUTRIENTS

	% Daily Value
Calcium	37%
Riboflavin	24%
Potassium	14%
Vitamin A	10%

Did you know? . . .
To appreciate the healthy advantage of evaporated skimmed milk, just compare it with cream. A half cup of heavy cream supplies only 8% of the Daily Value for calcium—and has 44g fat and 163mg cholesterol.

Curried Spinach & Fresh Cheese

**PREP: 15 MINUTES / DRAIN: 2 HOURS
COOK: 30 MINUTES**

This cheese (called "panir" in India) is also served with other curry-sauced vegetables, such as potatoes, green beans, or peas.

- 2 quarts low-fat (1%) milk
- ⅓ cup lemon juice
- 4 teaspoons vegetable oil
- 1 onion, finely chopped
- 4 cloves garlic, minced
- 1 teaspoon ground coriander
- ¾ teaspoon turmeric
- ¼ teaspoon salt
- 1 package (10 ounces) frozen chopped spinach, thawed and squeezed dry
- 1 cup chicken broth
- 2 tablespoons no-salt-added tomato paste
- 2 teaspoons jalapeño pepper sauce

1. In a large saucepan, bring the milk to a boil over moderate heat. Remove from the heat and stir in the lemon juice. Let stand until the curds and whey separate. Line a sieve with a double layer of cheesecloth. Place the sieve in the sink and pour in the curdled milk, draining off the whey. Place the sieve over a bowl and let stand for 20 minutes. Tie the cheesecloth up and gently squeeze to remove any remaining liquid. Flatten the cheese into a disk, place a weight on top (see photo, page 125), and let stand at room temperature for 2 hours or until firm enough to cut.

2. In a large nonstick skillet, heat 2 teaspoons of the oil over moderate heat. Add the onion and garlic, and sauté for 7 minutes or until tender. Add the coriander, turmeric, and salt, stirring to combine. Add the spinach, broth, tomato paste, and jalapeño sauce, and bring to a boil. Reduce to a simmer, cover, and cook for 5 minutes or until the spinach is flavorful. Transfer the mixture to a bowl and wipe out the skillet.

3. Cut the cheese into ½-inch chunks. Add the remaining 2 teaspoons oil to the skillet and heat over moderate heat. Add the cheese and cook, stirring frequently, for 4 minutes or until lightly browned and crusty on all sides. Gently stir in the spinach mixture and cook for 4 minutes or until heated through. Serves 4.

Per serving: Calories 302; Fiber 3g; Protein 20g; Total Fat 11g; Saturated Fat 4g; Cholesterol 20mg; Sodium 741mg

Orange Buttermilk Sherbet

**PREP: 10 MINUTES / COOK: 5 MINUTES
FREEZE: 1 TO 4 HOURS**

A noteworthy dessert with emphatic orange flavor and 225mg calcium per serving.

- ⅔ cup sugar
- ⅓ cup light corn syrup
- 6 strips (3 x ½ inch) of orange zest
- ⅛ teaspoon salt
- 1 quart low-fat (1.5%) buttermilk
- 1 can (12 ounces) frozen orange juice concentrate

1. In a medium saucepan, combine the sugar, corn syrup, orange zest, salt, and ½ cup of water. Bring to a boil over moderate heat and cook for 2 minutes. Cool to room temperature. Discard the orange zest.

2. In a medium bowl, combine the buttermilk, orange juice concentrate, and sugar syrup. Transfer to the canister of an ice cream machine and freeze according to the manufacturer's directions. Alternatively, to still-freeze, pour into a shallow 9 x 13 x 2-inch pan and

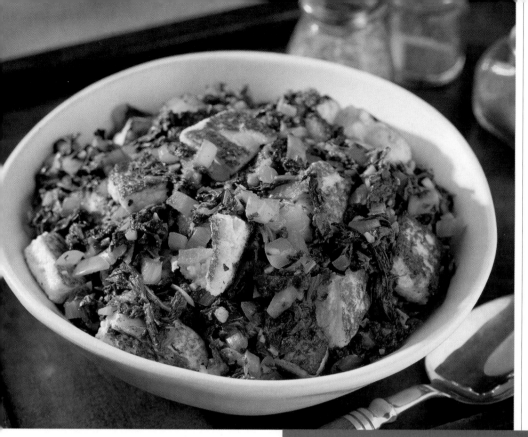

Curried Spinach & Fresh Cheese *This Indian dish features fresh cheese made from low-fat milk, combined with spinach and lively seasonings.*

Did you know? . . .
Some dairy products, such as yogurt, contain more calcium than milk. But the vitamin D added to milk enables your body to absorb more of the calcium.

freeze for 2 to 3 hours or until almost frozen. Cut into chunks and process in a food processor until smooth. Serve immediately. Serves 6.

Per serving: Calories 331; Fiber 1g; Protein 8g; Total Fat 3g; Saturated Fat 2g; Cholesterol 10mg; Sodium 154mg

Chocolate Latte Cotto

PREP: 15 MINUTES / COOK: 10 MINUTES
CHILL: 4 HOURS

This "latte cotto" (cooked milk) is a lightened version of the Italian classic "panna cotta" (cooked cream). It's a chilled chocolate pudding made in individual cups.

- 3 **tablespoons unsweetened cocoa powder**
- 1 **envelope unflavored gelatin**
- 3 **cups low-fat (1%) milk**
- ½ **cup packed light brown sugar**
- 1 **ounce semisweet chocolate, coarsely chopped**
- ⅛ **teaspoon grated nutmeg**

1. In a small bowl, combine the cocoa powder and 3 tablespoons of water, stirring until the cocoa is moistened. In a separate bowl, sprinkle the gelatin over 1 cup of the milk and let stand for 5 minutes or until softened.

2. Meanwhile, in a medium saucepan, combine the remaining 2 cups milk, the brown sugar, semisweet chocolate, and nutmeg. Bring to a simmer and cook just until the chocolate has melted. Remove from the heat and stir in the cocoa mixture.

3. Stir in the softened gelatin, return to the heat, and cook for 3 minutes or just until the gelatin has dissolved. Divide the mixture among six 6-ounce custard cups and cool to room temperature. Refrigerate for at least 4 hours or until set and well chilled. Serves 6.

Per serving: Calories 153; Fiber 1g; Protein 6g; Total Fat 3g; Saturated Fat 2g; Cholesterol 5mg; Sodium 72mg

Milk's advantage over other dairy products is that it is fortified with vitamin D.

Prescription drugs, including certain antacids, blood-pressure medications, and corticosteroids, can cause calcium deficiencies. (Coffee, tea, and carbonated drinks also contribute to calcium loss.) If you take such drugs (or drink a lot of coffee, tea, or soda), ask your doctor about adding calcium to your diet—perhaps by drinking more milk.

Check your store's dairy case for calcium-fortified low-fat milk, which supplies 500 mg of additional calcium per cup.

Yogurt

Nutritional power
A top calcium source, and high in protein, yogurt is a versatile food that you can substitute for cream and other high-fat ingredients.

Healthy Highlights

Low-Fat Yogurt
PER 1 CUP

Calories	155
Fiber	0g
Protein	13g
Total Fat	3.8g
Saturated Fat	2.5g
Cholesterol	15mg
Sodium	172mg

NUTRIENTS

	% Daily Value
Calcium	45%
Riboflavin	31%
Vitamin B12	23%
Potassium	19%
Zinc	15%

Nonfat Yogurt
PER 1 CUP

Calories	137
Fiber	0g
Protein	14g
Total Fat	0.4g
Saturated Fat	0.3g
Cholesterol	4mg
Sodium	187mg

NUTRIENTS

	% Daily Value
Calcium	49%
Riboflavin	34%
Vitamin B12	25%
Potassium	21%
Zinc	16%

Fruit-Topped Yogurt Cheese Tart

PREP: 25 MINUTES / CHILL: 1 HOUR
COOK: 40 MINUTES

This splendid dessert is rich in vitamin C, thanks to the kiwifruit and strawberries.

- 1 cup flour
- 1 tablespoon plus ⅓ cup sugar
- ¼ teaspoon salt
- 4 tablespoons unsalted butter, cut up
- 2 tablespoons reduced-fat sour cream
- 2 cups Yogurt Cheese (at right)
- ¾ teaspoon vanilla extract
- 1 pint strawberries, halved
- 2 kiwifruit, peeled and thinly sliced
- ¼ cup apricot jam

1. In a large bowl, combine the flour, 1 tablespoon of the sugar, and the salt. With a pastry blender or two knives, cut in the butter until the mixture resembles coarse meal. In a small bowl, combine the sour cream and 1 tablespoon of ice water. Stir into the flour mixture until just combined. Flatten the dough into a disk, wrap in plastic wrap, and refrigerate for at least 1 hour.

2. Preheat the oven to 350°F. On a lightly floured surface, roll the dough out to a 13-inch round. Fit into a 9-inch tart pan with a removable bottom. With a fork, prick the bottom of the tart shell in several places. Line with foil and weight down with pie weights or dried beans. Bake for 20 minutes or until the crust is beginning to set. Remove the pie weights and foil and bake for 15 minutes or until the crust is cooked through. Transfer the shell to a wire rack to cool completely.

3. In a medium bowl, combine the Yogurt Cheese, the remaining ⅓ cup sugar, and the vanilla. Spread in the bottom of the baked and cooled shell. Arrange the strawberries and kiwi slices in concentric circles on top of the tart.

4. In a small saucepan, melt the jam over low heat. Brush the jam over the fruit. Let cool until set. Serves 8.

Per serving: Calories 255; Fiber 2g; Protein 8g; Total Fat 8g; Saturated Fat 4g; Cholesterol 20mg; Sodium 112mg

Fruity Yogurt Parfait

PREP: 1 HOUR 15 MINUTES

- 1 quart plain low-fat yogurt
- 1 cup part-skim ricotta cheese
- ¼ cup plus 2 tablespoons sugar
- ½ teaspoon almond or vanilla extract
- 4 cups mixed fruit, such as sliced peaches, cubed bananas, and raspberries
- 4 teaspoons chopped toasted almonds

1. Place the yogurt in a cheesecloth- or paper towel-lined sieve set over a bowl and drain at room temperature for 1 hour.

2. In a food processor, process the ricotta and sugar for 1 minute or until very smooth. Transfer to a medium bowl and stir in the drained yogurt and almond extract.

3. Dividing evenly, spoon one-third of the yogurt mixture into each of 6 parfait glasses. Divide half the fruit among the glasses. Spoon in another one-third of the yogurt mixture; top with the remaining fruit. Spoon the remaining yogurt mixture on top and sprinkle with the toasted almonds. Serves 6.

Per serving: Calories 264; Fiber 3g; Protein 14g; Total Fat 7g; Saturated Fat 4g; Cholesterol 22mg; Sodium 159mg

Yogurt Cheese

PREP: 5 MINUTES / DRAIN: 12 HOURS

Draining the whey from plain yogurt produces nutritious, creamy yogurt cheese, which can stand in for cream cheese, sour cream, or even mayonnaise. Offer one of the variations as a spread for crackers or toast, or as a dip, with vegetable sticks or sliced fruit.

1 quart plain low-fat yogurt

Line a fine-mesh sieve with dampened cheesecloth. Spoon the yogurt into the sieve and set it over a bowl. Place in the refrigerator and let stand overnight. Makes about 2 cups.

Per ¼ cup: Calories 50; Fiber 0g; Protein 6g; Total Fat 2g; Saturated Fat 0g; Cholesterol 3mg; Sodium 36mg

SCALLION-PEPPER YOGURT CHEESE
In a small skillet, heat 2 teaspoons vegetable oil over moderate heat. Add 4 thinly sliced scallions and 2 diced red bell peppers and cook, stirring occasionally, for 4 minutes or until tender. Cool, then stir into the Yogurt Cheese. Cover and refrigerate. Serve chilled. Makes about 2½ cups.

GARLIC-DILL YOGURT CHEESE
In a small pot of boiling water, cook 8 cloves of garlic for 3 minutes to blanch. Mash with the flat side of a knife. Stir the garlic and ⅔ cup snipped fresh dill into the Yogurt Cheese. Cover and refrigerate. Serve chilled. Makes about 2 cups.

RASPBERRY YOGURT CHEESE
Reserving 2 tablespoons of the syrup, drain two 12-ounce packages frozen raspberries in syrup. In a food processor, process the raspberries, the reserved syrup, and 2 teaspoons sugar until smooth. Stir into the Yogurt Cheese. Cover and refrigerate. Serve chilled. Makes about 2½ cups.

At the market Most supermarkets offer a wide variety of yogurts. Health-food stores and farmers' markets may yield variations such as organic or goat's-milk yogurt.

Look for For maximum health benefits, choose a carton with the words "active yogurt cultures" on it.

Prep If store-bought yogurt is slightly separated, stir the liquid (whey) back in, as the whey contains nutrients, including calcium. When making yogurt cheese (see below), reserve the whey for use in such recipes as muffins or pancakes.

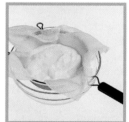

To make yogurt cheese, drain yogurt in a sieve lined with dampened cheesecloth or paper towels, or through a coffee filter. You can also buy a fine-mesh "funnel" specially designed for making yogurt cheese.

Basic cooking Yogurt used in cooked dishes will curdle if subjected to high heat. Combining the yogurt with flour before adding it will help, but keep the heat moderate.

Fruit-Topped Yogurt Cheese Tart A pretty pattern of fruit tops a vanilla-scented filling.

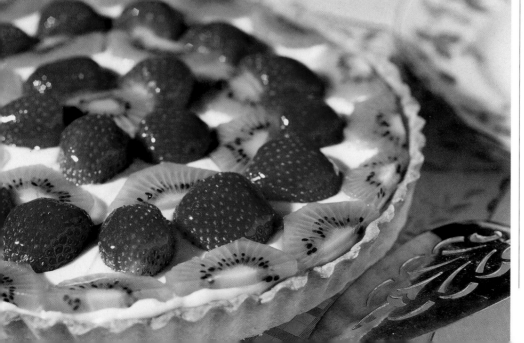

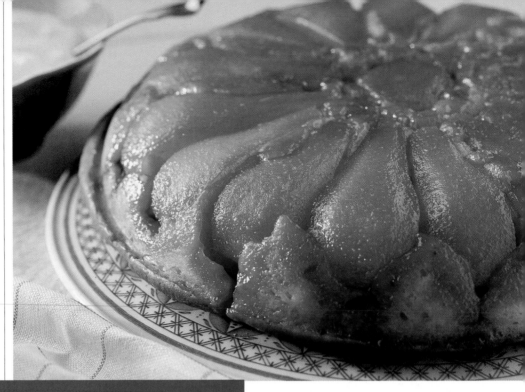

Pear-Yogurt Cake with Yogurt Topping
A crowning glory for any meal, this upside-down cake is served with sweet, lemony yogurt "cream."

Did you know? . . .
Subjects in a study who ate two cups of yogurt a day for four months had notably higher levels of interferon, a chemical vital to immune function.

Eating yogurt with active cultures helps maintain a healthy digestive system.

The bacteria used to culture yogurt—either *Lactobacillus bulgaricus* or *Streptococcus thermophilus*—are good for your digestive system. They help you digest the milk protein in the yogurt, and there is good evidence that they help maintain a healthy balance of "friendly" bacteria in your intestines.

The "fruit" in store-bought yogurt is usually jam or preserves—more sugar than fruit. Nutritionally speaking, you're better off stirring your favorite fresh or dried fruit into plain yogurt. A touch of vanilla or almond extract will enhance the flavor of the fruit.

Pear-Yogurt Cake with Yogurt Topping
PREP: 20 MINUTES
COOK: 1 HOUR 5 MINUTES

- 1¾ cups plus 2 tablespoons sugar
- ⅓ cup plus 1 tablespoon unsalted butter
- 1 tablespoon lemon juice
- 2 pounds pears, peeled, cored, and quartered
- 2½ cups flour
- 1½ teaspoons baking powder
- ½ teaspoon baking soda
- ¼ teaspoon salt
- 1 egg
- 2 egg whites
- 1½ teaspoons grated lemon zest
- 3¼ cups plain low-fat yogurt

1. Preheat the oven to 350°F. In a 10-inch nonstick ovenproof skillet, combine ¼ cup of the sugar, 1 tablespoon of the butter, and the lemon juice. Cook over moderate heat for 5 minutes or until the sugar has melted and is beginning to brown. Remove from the heat and cover the bottom of the skillet with the pears, arranging them spoke fashion, with the narrow ends of the pears toward the center. Set the skillet aside.

2. In a medium bowl, stir together the flour, baking powder, baking soda, and salt; set aside.

3. In a large bowl, with an electric mixer, cream the remaining ⅓ cup butter with 1½ cups of the sugar. Beat in the whole egg and egg whites, one at a time, beating well after each addition. Beat in 1 teaspoon of the lemon zest. Alternately fold in the flour mixture and 1¼ cups of the yogurt, beginning and ending with the flour mixture. Spoon the batter over the pears. Bake for 1 hour and 5 minutes or until a cake tester inserted in the center of the cake portion comes out clean.

4. Meanwhile, place the remaining 2 cups yogurt in a fine-mesh sieve set over a bowl; drain at room temperature while the cake bakes. Just before serving, stir in the remaining 2 tablespoons sugar and ½ teaspoon lemon zest.

5. Cool the cake in the pan on a rack for 5 minutes. Cover the pan with a heatproof plate, then invert the skillet and plate together. Leave the skillet upside down until the pears release, then carefully remove the pan. Serve warm or at room temperature with the sweetened yogurt topping. Serves 12.

Per serving: Calories 359; Fiber 3g; Protein 7g; Total Fat 8g; Saturated Fat 5g; Cholesterol 38mg; Sodium 218mg

Tandoori-Style Chicken

PREP: 25 MINUTES / MARINATE: 2 HOURS / COOK: 20 MINUTES

- 3 **cloves garlic, peeled and crushed**
- 1 **teaspoon paprika**
- ¾ **teaspoon each salt, ground cumin, and coriander**
- ½ **teaspoon cinnamon**
- ¼ **teaspoon pepper**
- 2 **cups plain low-fat yogurt**
- 4 **skinless, bone-in chicken breast halves (about 2 pounds total)**
- 1 **small red onion, finely chopped**
- 1 **cucumber, seeded and diced**
- ½ **cup chopped cilantro**

1. In a shallow glass or ceramic baking dish, combine the garlic, paprika, salt, cumin, coriander, cinnamon, and pepper. Stir in 1 cup of the yogurt until well blended. With a sharp knife, make several slashes in the flesh of the chicken, cutting almost to the bone. Place the chicken, cut-sides down, in the yogurt mixture. Cover and refrigerate for at least 2 hours or overnight, turning the chicken several times.

2. Preheat the oven to 500°F. Lift the chicken from its marinade and place on a broiler pan; discard any leftover marinade. Bake the chicken for 20 minutes or until cooked through but still juicy.

3. Meanwhile, in a medium bowl, combine the onion, cucumber, cilantro, and the remaining 1 cup yogurt. Serve the chicken with the yogurt mixture on the side. Serves 4.

Per serving: Calories 348; Fiber 1g; Protein 60g; Total Fat 5g; Saturated Fat 2g; Cholesterol 139mg; Sodium 645mg

Tropical Smoothie In blender, combine 1 cup plain low-fat yogurt, ¾ cup mango chunks, ½ cup banana slices, 1 tbsp. lime juice, 2 tsp. sugar, and 4 ice cubes. Blend until smooth and thick. Garnish with a mint sprig and slices of mango and lime. Serves 2. *[Cal 156; Fat 1g; Sod 89mg]*

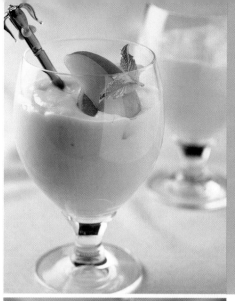

Green Goddess Salad Dressing In food processor, combine 2 cups plain nonfat yogurt, ½ cup packed parsley leaves, 2 tsp. anchovy paste, 1 tbsp. lemon juice, 2 tsp. dried tarragon, ½ tsp. salt, and 1 small garlic clove; process until smooth. Makes 2 cups. Use ½ cup dressing and 6 cups mixed greens to serve 4. *[Per 2-tablespoon serving: Cal 19; Fat .1g; Sod 106mg]*

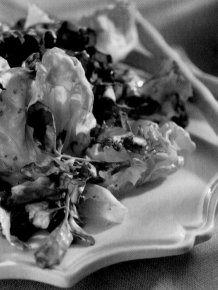

Two-Berry Yogurt Pops In food processor, process 6 oz. frozen unsweetened strawberries, ¼ cup seedless raspberry jam, and 2 tbsp. honey until smooth. Add 2 cups plain nonfat yogurt; process to combine. Freeze in ice pop molds. Serves 6. *[Cal 106; Fat 0g; Sod 64mg]*

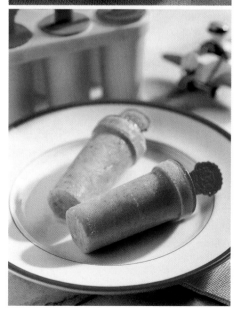

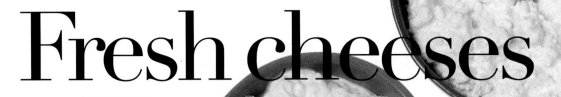

Fresh cheeses

Nutritional power
You get lots of high-quality protein in these delicate-tasting cheeses. They also make healthful substitutes for sour or heavy cream in recipes.

Healthy Highlights

Part-Skim Ricotta Cheese
PER ½ CUP

Calories	171
Fiber	0g
Protein	14g
Total Fat	9.8g
Saturated Fat	6.1g
Cholesterol	38mg
Sodium	155mg

NUTRIENTS

	% Daily Value
Calcium	34%
Riboflavin	14%
Vitamin A	11%
Zinc	11%

Low-Fat (1%) Cottage Cheese
PER ½ CUP

Calories	82
Fiber	0g
Protein	14g
Total Fat	1.2g
Saturated Fat	0.7g
Cholesterol	5mg
Sodium	459mg

NUTRIENTS

	% Daily Value
Vitamin B12	12%
Riboflavin	11%

Liptauer Cheese

PREP: 10 MINUTES / CHILL: 1 HOUR

Serve this Hungarian specialty with toasted rye bread or whole-grain crackers.

- **1** package (8 ounces) reduced-fat cream cheese (Neufchâtel)
- **4** ounces nonfat cream cheese
- **2** tablespoons low-fat (1%) milk
- **⅓** cup finely chopped red onion
- **4** anchovies, rinsed and mashed, or 2 teaspoons anchovy paste
- **2** tablespoons capers, rinsed and drained
- **¾** teaspoon grated lemon zest

1. In a bowl, with an electric mixer, beat together the cream cheeses and milk. Fold in the onion, anchovies, capers, and lemon zest.

2. Line a small (2- to 3-cup) bowl with plastic wrap, leaving a 2-inch overhang, and spoon the cheese mixture into it, smoothing the top. Fold the plastic wrap over and refrigerate for 1 hour or until well chilled and firm. Unmold onto a serving plate and remove the plastic wrap. Makes 1¾ cups.

Per ¼ cup: Calories 96; Fiber 0g; Protein 6g; Total Fat 5g; Saturated Fat 4g; Cholesterol 18mg; Sodium 424mg

Fettuccine Alfredo with Green Noodles

PREP: 10 MINUTES / COOK: 15 MINUTES

- **12** ounces spinach fettuccine
- **1** tablespoon unsalted butter
- **1** cup low-fat (1%) milk
- **2** tablespoons flour
- **4** ounces reduced-fat cream cheese (Neufchâtel)
- **⅓** cup grated Parmesan cheese
- **½** teaspoon each salt and pepper

1. In a large pot of boiling water, cook the pasta according to package directions until firm-tender. Reserving ½ cup of the cooking liquid, drain the pasta and transfer to a large bowl. Add the butter, tossing well to coat.

2. Meanwhile, in a medium saucepan, whisk the milk into the flour until well combined. Whisk over low heat for 3 minutes or until lightly thickened. Whisk in the cream cheese, Parmesan, salt, pepper, and reserved pasta cooking liquid. Pour the sauce over the pasta, tossing well to coat. Serves 4.

Per serving: Calories 474; Fiber 8g; Protein 19g; Total Fat 11g; Saturated Fat 7g; Cholesterol 29mg; Sodium 587mg

Coeur à la Crème

PREP: 10 MINUTES
DRAIN: 4 TO 6 HOURS

This French "cream heart" is traditionally made in a special mold (see photo, right), but a cheesecloth-lined sieve will work as well.

- **1   package (8 ounces) reduced-fat cream cheese (Neufchâtel)**
- **1   package (8 ounces) nonfat cream cheese**
- **1   cup low-fat (1%) cottage cheese**
- **⅔   cup confectioners sugar**
- **½   teaspoon vanilla extract**
- **2   cups frozen strawberries, thawed**
- **2   tablespoons honey**
- **1   tablespoon lime juice**

1. In a food processor, combine the cream cheeses and cottage cheese, and process until smooth. Add the sugar and vanilla, and pulse until combined.

2. Line a heart-shaped ceramic coeur à la crème mold (or a 4- to 6-cup sieve set over a bowl) with a double layer of dampened cheesecloth. Spoon the cream cheese mixture into the mold, wrap the cheesecloth over, and place the mold on a plate to drain. Refrigerate 4 to 6 hours or overnight.

3. Before serving, in a food processor or blender, combine the strawberries, honey, and lime juice. Process until smooth. At serving time, unwrap the cheesecloth mold and invert the mold onto a large plate. Remove the mold and peel off the cheesecloth. Serve with the strawberry sauce. Serves 6.

Per serving: Calories 236; Fiber 0g; Protein 14g; Total Fat 6g; Saturated Fat 4g; Cholesterol 23mg; Sodium 512mg

At the market

Cottage cheese, ricotta, and cream cheese come in full-fat, low-fat, and fat-free versions. There is also a variation on cottage cheese called pot cheese, which is cottage cheese that's been pressed to make it firmer and drier. Neufchâtel is another name for reduced-fat cream cheese, which has one-third less fat than regular cream cheese.

Prep Some recipes may call for cottage cheese and ricotta to be drained before you use them in cooking. Draining a "creamed" cottage cheese will also help remove some of the fat. To drain, place the cheese in a fine-mesh sieve and shake it gently to drain off some of the liquid.

Coeur à la Crème Berry sauce is the ideal accompaniment for this charming dessert.

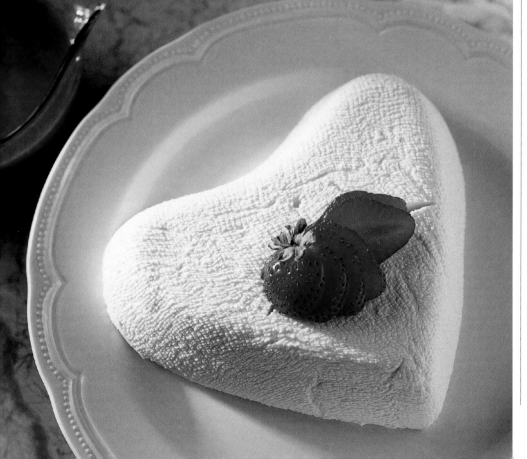

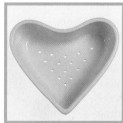

The porcelain mold for coeur à la crème measures about 6 x 7 inches; holes in the bottom allow liquid to drain off. The mold is lined with cheesecloth, which leaves the surface of the finished dessert with a rustic "woven" texture.

Neufchâtel Cream Cheese
PER OUNCE

Calories	74
Fiber	0g
Protein	3g
Total Fat	6.6g
Saturated Fat	4.2g
Cholesterol	22mg
Sodium	113mg

Nonfat Cream Cheese
PER OUNCE

Calories	27
Fiber	0g
Protein	4g
Total Fat	0.4g
Saturated Fat	0.3g
Cholesterol	2mg
Sodium	155mg

Did you know? . . .
The lower the fat content of milk, the higher its calcium content. Thus, since nonfat cream cheese is made from skim milk, it supplies a modest amount of calcium; full-fat cream cheese, which is made from whole milk and cream, does not. One ounce of nonfat cream cheese provides 8% of the Daily Value for calcium; Neufchâtel cheese (a reduced-fat cream cheese) provides 2% of the Daily Value.

Lemon-Lime Cheesecake

PREP: 20 MINUTES
COOK: 1 HOUR 5 MINUTES

If you don't tell, no one will know that this fabulous cake is made with low-fat cheeses.

- 3 ounces vanilla wafers
- 2 tablespoons unsalted butter, melted
- 1½ cups low-fat (1%) cottage cheese
- 1 package (8 ounces) reduced-fat cream cheese (Neufchâtel)
- 1 package (8 ounces) nonfat cream cheese
- 1 cup plus 1 tablespoon sugar
- 2 eggs
- 4 egg whites
- 2 tablespoons flour
- 1½ teaspoons grated lemon zest
- 1½ teaspoons grated lime zest
- 1 tablespoon lemon juice
- 1 tablespoon lime juice
- ¼ teaspoon salt
- ½ cup reduced-fat sour cream

1. Preheat the oven to 350°F. In a food processor, process the vanilla wafers until finely ground. Add the butter and pulse until moistened. Spoon the mixture into a 9-inch springform pan, patting it into the bottom. Bake for 10 minutes or until lightly browned; set aside. Leave the oven on.

2. In a food processor (you can use the same bowl), process the cottage cheese for 1 minute or until smooth.

3. In a medium bowl, with an electric mixer, beat the cream cheeses and 1 cup of the sugar until light and fluffy. Beat in the whole eggs and egg whites, one at a time, beating well after each addition. Beat in the puréed cottage cheese, the flour, lemon zest, lime zest, lemon juice, lime juice, and salt until well blended. Pour the batter into the prepared pan and bake for 50 minutes or until the center is set and the top is golden.

4. Meanwhile, in a small bowl, combine the sour cream and the remaining 1 tablespoon sugar. Spread over the top of the hot cake and bake for 5 minutes. Remove from the oven to a wire rack to cool. Refrigerate until serving time. Serves 12.

Per serving: Calories 240; Fiber 0g; Protein 11g; Total Fat 8g; Saturated Fat 5g; Cholesterol 56mg; Sodium 395mg

Cannoli Pudding with Chocolate Chips & Pistachios

PREP: 10 MINUTES / COOK: 10 MINUTES
CHILL: 2 HOURS

Enjoy "cannoli" without the deep-fried shell.

- ½ cup sugar
- 3 tablespoons quick-cooking tapioca
- ⅛ teaspoon salt
- 1 cup low-fat (1%) milk
- 1½ cups part-skim ricotta cheese
- 1 teaspoon vanilla extract
- ¼ cup mini chocolate chips
- ¼ cup shelled pistachios

1. In a medium saucepan, combine the sugar, tapioca, and salt. Gradually add the milk until well moistened. Cook over moderate heat, stirring constantly, until the mixture comes to a full boil. Reduce to a simmer and cook, stirring frequently, for 5 minutes or until the tapioca is tender.

2. Remove from the heat and stir in the ricotta. Let cool to room temperature, then stir in the vanilla. Fold in the chocolate chips and pistachios. Spoon into 6 serving bowls, cover, and refrigerate for 2 hours or until well chilled. Serves 6.

Per serving: Calories 250; Fiber 1g; Protein 10g; Total Fat 10g; Saturated Fat 5g; Cholesterol 21mg; Sodium 167mg

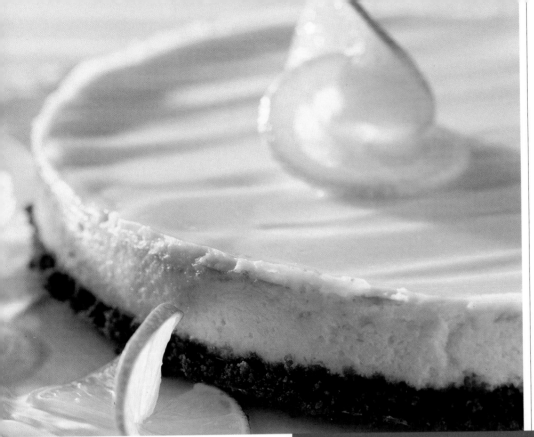

Lemon-Lime Cheesecake *A topping of sweetened sour cream crowns this elegant cake.*

Did you know? . . . Sodium content can vary by as much as 450mg among different brands of cottage cheese. If you're concerned about sodium intake, read the label.

Sweet Noodle Kugel with Apricots

PREP: 10 MINUTES / COOK: 30 MINUTES

In Eastern Europe, noodles go into desserts as well as main dishes. This old-fashioned noodle-cheese pudding, studded with apricots and sprinkled with cinnamon-sugar, is a pleasing way to round out a family dinner.

8	ounces wide egg noodles
1½	cups low-fat (1%) cottage cheese
½	cup low-fat (1%) milk
2	tablespoons unsalted butter, melted
1	egg
2	egg whites
⅓	cup plus 1 tablespoon sugar
¼	cup frozen orange juice concentrate, thawed
½	teaspoon vanilla extract
¼	teaspoon salt
½	cup dried apricots, chopped
¼	teaspoon cinnamon

1. Preheat the oven to 350°F. Butter a 7 x 11-inch baking dish; set aside. In a large pot of boiling water, cook the noodles according to package directions until firm-tender. Drain well.

The protein in fresh cheese is just as good as the protein in meat, poultry, or fish.

2. Meanwhile, in a food processor, combine the cottage cheese, milk, butter, whole egg, egg whites, ⅓ cup of the sugar, the orange juice concentrate, vanilla, and salt. Process to a smooth purée. Transfer the purée to a large bowl and add the drained noodles and the apricots, tossing well to combine. Spoon the noodle mixture into the prepared pan.

3. In a small bowl, combine the remaining 1 tablespoon sugar and the cinnamon. Sprinkle over the top of the noodle mixture.

4. Bake, uncovered, for 30 minutes or until the kugel is set and the top is slightly crusty. Serve warm, at room temperature, or lightly chilled. Serves 8.

Per serving: Calories 261; Fiber 2g; Protein 12g; Total Fat 6g; Saturated Fat 3g; Cholesterol 65mg; Sodium 276mg

A half-cup serving of low-fat cottage cheese supplies about 14g of protein—about one-quarter of an adult's daily protein requirement. And the protein in cottage cheese is as high in quality as that found in meat or fish.

Ricotta cheese, also an excellent protein source, has an additional advantage over meat: Ricotta supplies 337mg of calcium, while meat contains negligible amounts of this important mineral.

Goat & Feta

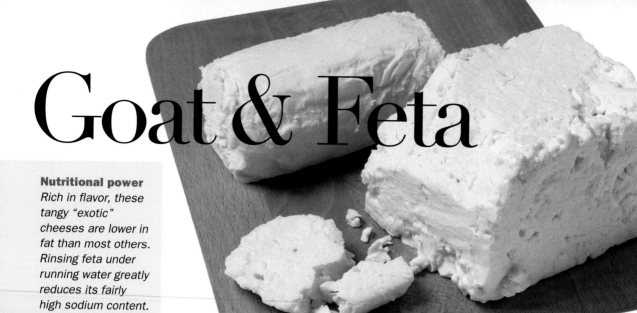

Nutritional power
Rich in flavor, these tangy "exotic" cheeses are lower in fat than most others. Rinsing feta under running water greatly reduces its fairly high sodium content.

Healthy Highlights

Goat Cheese
PER OUNCE

Calories	76
Fiber	0g
Protein	5g
Total Fat	6.0g
Saturated Fat	4.1g
Cholesterol	13mg
Sodium	104mg

NUTRIENTS

	% Daily Value
Copper	10%

Feta Cheese
PER OUNCE

Calories	75
Fiber	0g
Protein	4g
Total Fat	6.0g
Saturated Fat	4.2g
Cholesterol	25mg
Sodium	316mg

NUTRIENTS

	% Daily Value
Calcium	14%
Riboflavin	14%

Did you know? . . .
Many people who are allergic to cow's milk can tolerate goat's milk with no adverse reaction.

Crustless Mini-Quiches with Broccoli & Feta

PREP: 15 MINUTES / COOK: 35 MINUTES

Cheese, milk, and broccoli make this a calcium-rich main dish. Serve the tartlets with a green salad and whole-grain bread.

- 1 teaspoon olive oil
- 2 scallions, thinly sliced
- 2 cloves garlic, minced
- 1 package (10 ounces) frozen chopped broccoli, thawed and squeezed dry
- ⅓ cup low-fat (1%) cottage cheese
- ⅔ cup low-fat (1%) milk
- 2 eggs
- 3 egg whites
- 3 tablespoons flour
- ½ teaspoon pepper
- 6 ounces feta cheese or mild goat cheese

1. Preheat the oven to 350°F. Spray four 8-ounce custard cups or ramekins with nonstick cooking spray; set aside. In a medium nonstick skillet, heat the oil over moderate heat. Add the scallions and garlic, and sauté for 1 minute or until the garlic is tender. Stir in the broccoli and cook for 1 minute.

2. In a food processor, process the cottage cheese until smooth. Add the milk, whole eggs, egg whites, flour, and pepper, and process until well combined. Transfer the custard to a large bowl. Add the broccoli mixture and crumble in the feta cheese, stirring to combine. Spoon into the prepared cups, place on a baking sheet, and bake for 30 minutes or until the mini-quiches are puffy and set. Serves 4.

Per serving: Calories 251; Fiber 2g; Protein 18g; Total Fat 14g; Saturated Fat 8g; Cholesterol 147mg; Sodium 662mg

Creamy Polenta with Cheese

PREP: 10 MINUTES / COOK: 20 MINUTES

A staple food in Northern Italy, polenta is simply cornmeal mush. Our hearty polenta side dish is enlivened with tangy cheese.

- 1 cup yellow cornmeal
- 1½ cups low-fat (1%) milk
- ¼ teaspoon salt
- ⅛ teaspoon cayenne pepper
- 6 ounces feta cheese or mild goat cheese

1. In a small bowl, stir the cornmeal and 1 cup of the milk together until blended and smooth.

2. In a medium-size heavy-bottomed saucepan, bring 1½ cups of water, the

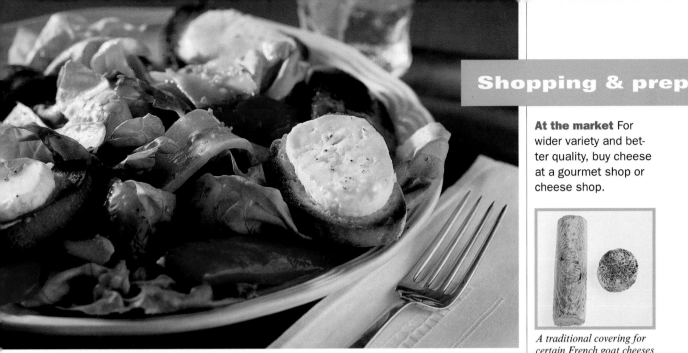

Composed Salad with Grilled Goat Cheese A sophisticated salad-and-sandwich meal.

At the market For wider variety and better quality, buy cheese at a gourmet shop or cheese shop.

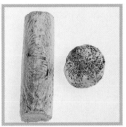

A traditional covering for certain French goat cheeses is a fine layer of ash (left). Other coatings—for both domestic and imported goat cheese—include such things as dried herbs or crushed peppercorns (right).

Look for The flavor of goat cheese ranges from gently tangy to sharply pungent; ask for a taste and choose a cheese that suits your taste. Young goat cheese is quite mild. Montrachet, which comes in slender 11-ounce logs, is ideal for these recipes, as are the generic "bûches" (thicker logs). Bûcheron and Ste.-Maure are somewhat more flavorful alternatives.

Prep Small goat cheese logs need no preparation, but if you're cooking with a slice from a thicker log, such as Bûcheron, you'll want to remove the rind. Feta should be rinsed under cold running water and drained well.

remaining ½ cup milk, the salt, and cayenne to a simmer over low heat. Stirring constantly, gradually pour in the cornmeal-milk mixture. Cook over low heat, stirring constantly, for 10 minutes or until thick and creamy.

3. Crumble in the feta and cook, stirring, for 3 to 4 minutes or until the cheese is melted. Serves 4.

Per serving: Calories 277; Fiber 2g; Protein 12g; Total Fat 11g; Saturated Fat 7g; Cholesterol 42mg; Sodium 656mg

Composed Salad with Grilled Goat Cheese

PREP: 20 MINUTES / COOK: 15 MINUTES

Roasted summer squash and bell peppers bring rich flavor to this contemporary classic.

- ¼ cup chicken broth
- 1 clove garlic, minced
- 1 yellow summer squash, thinly sliced
- 1 red bell pepper, cut lengthwise into flat panels
- 1 green bell pepper, cut lengthwise into flat panels
- 12 slices (2 x 2½ inches) Italian bread (5 ounces total)
- 8 ounces mild goat cheese, cut into 12 slices

- 3 tablespoons red wine vinegar
- 1 tablespoon olive oil
- 1 teaspoon Dijon mustard
- ½ teaspoon light brown sugar
- ¼ teaspoon salt
- 8 cups torn Boston lettuce

1. Preheat the broiler. In a small bowl, combine the broth and garlic. Add the squash, tossing to coat. Place the squash on the broiler rack. Place the bell pepper pieces, skin-side up, on the rack. Broil the vegetables 6 inches from the heat for 10 minutes or until the squash is tender and the pepper skin is blackened. Leave the broiler on. When the peppers are cool enough to handle, peel them and cut into 1-inch-wide strips.

2. Top each slice of bread with the cheese and broil for 1 minute or until the cheese is slightly melted and the bread is toasted.

3. In a small bowl, whisk together the vinegar, oil, mustard, brown sugar, and salt. Place the lettuce on 4 plates and arrange the peppers and squash on top. Drizzle the dressing over the salads and place 3 cheese toasts on each. Serves 4.

Per serving: Calories 323; Fiber 3g; Protein 16g; Total Fat 17g; Saturated Fat 9g; Cholesterol 26mg; Sodium 658mg

Provolone & Mozzarella

Nutritional power
These indispensable Italian cheeses are especially rich in calcium. In its part-skim form, mozzarella is lower in fat and cholesterol than most other cheeses.

Healthy Highlights

Provolone
PER OUNCE

Calories	100
Fiber	0g
Protein	7g
Total Fat	7.5g
Saturated Fat	4.8g
Cholesterol	20mg
Sodium	248mg

NUTRIENTS

	% Daily Value
Calcium	21%

Part-Skim Mozzarella
PER OUNCE

Calories	72
Fiber	0g
Protein	7g
Total Fat	4.5g
Saturated Fat	2.9g
Cholesterol	16mg
Sodium	132mg

NUTRIENTS

	% Daily Value
Calcium	18%

Did you know? . . .
"Low moisture" mozzarella is slightly higher in calories and fat than regular mozzarella.

Mozzarella Salad with Balsamic Dressing

PREP: 10 MINUTES / COOK: 10 MINUTES
MARINATE: 1 HOUR

What a luxurious way to get your calcium!

- 2 red bell peppers, cut lengthwise into flat panels
- 3 cloves garlic, peeled
- ¼ cup balsamic vinegar
- 1 tablespoon olive oil, preferably extra-virgin
- 1 teaspoon light brown sugar
- ½ teaspoon salt
- ¼ teaspoon black pepper
- ¼ cup chopped fresh basil
- 1 small red onion, halved and thinly sliced
- 8 ounces part-skim mozzarella cheese, cut into 16 slices
- 1 pound tomatoes, cut into 16 slices

1. Preheat the broiler. Place the bell pepper pieces, skin-side up, on a broiler pan and broil 4 inches from the heat for 10 minutes, or until the skin is blackened. When the peppers are cool enough to handle, peel them and cut into ½-inch-wide strips.

2. Meanwhile, in a small pan of boiling water, cook the garlic for 3 minutes to blanch. Drain, finely chop, and transfer to a large bowl. Whisk in the vinegar, oil, brown sugar, salt, and black pepper. Add the bell peppers, basil, and onion, tossing well. Cover

and refrigerate for 1 hour. Arrange the cheese and tomatoes on a platter, and spoon the pepper mixture on top. Serves 4.

Per serving: Calories 231; Fiber 3g; Protein 16g; Total Fat 13g; Saturated Fat 6g; Cholesterol 33mg; Sodium 554mg

Italian-Style Enchiladas with Provolone

PREP: 20 MINUTES / COOK: 45 MINUTES

Here's a favorite Mexican dish restyled with Italian seasonings. Thanks to the bounty of vegetables, these enchiladas are rich in beta carotene and vitamin C.

- 1 teaspoon olive oil
- 1 small onion, finely chopped
- 2 cloves garlic, minced
- 1 red bell pepper, cut into ½-inch squares
- 2 zucchini, halved lengthwise and thinly sliced
- ⅓ cup chicken broth
- 2 cups canned no-salt-added chopped tomatoes
- ½ cup chopped fresh basil
- ¼ teaspoon crushed red pepper flakes
- 8 corn tortillas (6-inch diameter)
- 1 can (8 ounces) no-salt-added tomato sauce
- 6 ounces provolone cheese, shredded

1. Preheat the oven to 375°F. Spray a 7 x 11-inch baking pan with nonstick cooking spray.

2. In a large nonstick skillet, heat the oil over moderate heat. Add the onion and garlic, and sauté for 5 minutes. Add the bell pepper, zucchini, and broth. Reduce to a simmer, cover, and cook for 3 minutes or until the zucchini is firm-tender. Stir in the chopped tomatoes, basil, and red pepper flakes, and bring to a boil. Reduce to a simmer, cover, and cook for 7 minutes or until the vegetable mixture is flavorful.

3. Place the tortillas on a baking sheet, cover with foil, and bake for 5 minutes or until just hot. Spoon one-third of the vegetable mixture over the warmed tortillas. Top with half the cheese. Stir the tomato sauce into the remaining vegetable mixture. Spoon half of the remaining vegetable mixture into the bottom of the prepared baking pan. Roll the tortillas up and place them, seam-side down, in the pan. Top with the remaining vegetable mixture.

4. Cover the pan with foil and bake for 15 minutes. Uncover, sprinkle the

Mushroom-Pepper Pizza A snap to prepare with ready-made pizza dough.

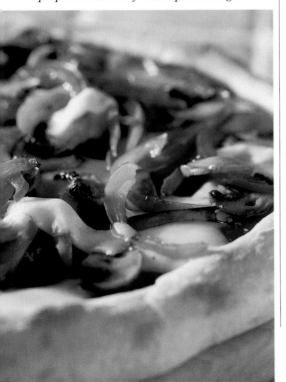

remaining cheese on top, and bake for 5 minutes or until the cheese has melted and the enchiladas are hot. Serves 4.

Per serving: Calories 351; Fiber 6g; Protein 18g; Total Fat 15g; Saturated Fat 8g; Cholesterol 29mg; Sodium 572mg

---

Mushroom-Pepper Pizza

PREP: 20 MINUTES / RISE: 25 MINUTES
COOK: 30 MINUTES

- 1 teaspoon olive oil
- 1 red bell pepper, thinly sliced
- 1 green bell pepper, thinly sliced
- ½ pound mushrooms, thinly sliced
- ½ teaspoon dried oregano
- ¼ teaspoon salt
- 1 pound purchased or homemade pizza dough
- 1 cup canned no-salt-added tomato sauce
- ⅛ teaspoon cinnamon
- 8 ounces part-skim mozzarella cheese, thinly sliced

1. In a large nonstick skillet, heat the oil over moderate heat. Add the bell peppers and sauté for 5 minutes or until crisp-tender. Add the mushrooms, oregano, and salt, and cook for 4 minutes or until the mushroom liquid has evaporated. Set aside.

2. Preheat the oven to 450°F. Spray a 12-inch pizza pan or large baking sheet with nonstick cooking spray. Pat the dough into a 12-inch round. Cover and let stand in a warm spot for 25 minutes or until doubled. Bake for 5 minutes.

3. In a small bowl, combine the tomato sauce and cinnamon. Spoon over the pizza. Top with the pepper mixture and the mozzarella. Bake for 15 minutes or until the cheese has melted and the crust is browned. Serves 6.

Per serving: Calories 326; Fiber 3g; Protein 17g; Total Fat 10g; Saturated Fat 5g; Cholesterol 22mg; Sodium 693mg

At the market Packaged factory-made mozzarella, in full-fat, part-skim, "light," and fat-free forms, is widely available, as is provolone in slices or chunks. (For a different, robust flavor, try smoked mozzarella and provolone.) Freshly made mozzarella, which has a deliciously delicate, milky flavor, can be found in gourmet shops and Italian groceries.

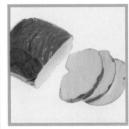

Smoked mozzarella has a rich, tangy taste. Try to find a cheese that's been smoked naturally (in a smokehouse) rather than treated with an artificial smoke flavoring.

Prep These cheeses are easier to grate or slice if well chilled.

Basic cooking Unlike factory mozzarella, fresh mozzarella softens and melts (rather than turning stringy) when heated. But like other cheeses, any type of mozzarella or provolone will turn rubbery if cooked too long or at too high a temperature.

Muenster & Jack

Nutritional power
Rich in calcium, mellow Muenster and tangy Monterey jack melt beautifully in sandwiches and casseroles.

Healthy Highlights

Muenster
PER OUNCE

Calories	104
Fiber	0g
Protein	7g
Total Fat	8.5g
Saturated Fat	5.4g
Cholesterol	27mg
Sodium	178mg

NUTRIENTS

	% Daily Value
Calcium	20%

Monterey Jack
PER OUNCE

Calories	106
Fiber	0g
Protein	7g
Total Fat	8.6g
Saturated Fat	5.4g
Cholesterol	25mg
Sodium	152mg

NUTRIENTS

	% Daily Value
Calcium	21%

Did you know? . . .
One-and-a-half ounces of Muenster or Monterey jack cheese supplies as much calcium as a cup of low-fat milk.

Cheesy Rice Bake

PREP: 10 MINUTES / COOK: 40 MINUTES

This baked rice-and-cheese dish makes a fine meatless main course: Serve it with a salad of sliced tomatoes. For a more substantial main dish, add 8 ounces of cubed cooked turkey or chicken in Step 2.

- 1 teaspoon vegetable oil
- 1 small onion, finely chopped
- 3 cloves garlic, minced
- 1 red bell pepper, diced
- 1 cup rice
- 1¼ cups chicken broth
- 1 cup low-fat (1%) milk
- ½ teaspoon salt
- ¼ teaspoon black pepper
- 6 ounces Muenster or Monterey jack cheese, shredded
- ⅓ cup chopped parsley or cilantro

1. Preheat the oven to 350°F. In a nonstick Dutch oven or flameproof casserole, heat the oil over moderate heat. Add the onion and garlic, and sauté for 5 minutes or until the onion is soft. Add the bell pepper and cook, stirring frequently, for 4 minutes or until firm-tender.

2. Stir in the rice. Add the broth, milk, salt, and black pepper, and bring to a boil. Stir in the cheese, cover tightly, and place in the oven for 25 minutes or until the rice is tender. Stir in the parsley and serve. Serves 4.

Per serving: Calories 390; Fiber 2g; Protein 16g; Total Fat 15g; Saturated Fat 9g; Cholesterol 43mg; Sodium 905mg

Mashed Potatoes with Pepper Jack

PREP: 10 MINUTES / COOK: 20 MINUTES

Highly preferable to potatoes whipped with butter and cream, this super side dish includes disease-fighting garlic, tomatoes, and chili powder as well as plenty of calcium.

- 2 pounds baking potatoes, peeled and thinly sliced
- ¼ cup sun-dried tomato halves (not oil-packed), cut into quarters
- 2 cloves garlic, peeled
- ¾ teaspoon chili powder
- ½ teaspoon salt
- 6 ounces pepper jack cheese, cut up

1. In a large pot of boiling water, cook the potatoes, sun-dried tomatoes, and garlic for 15 minutes or until the potatoes are tender. Reserving ⅓ cup of the cooking liquid, drain and transfer the potatoes, sun-dried tomatoes, and garlic to a large bowl.

2. Add the reserved cooking liquid, the chili powder, and salt to the bowl. With a potato masher or fork, mash the potatoes until well combined.

3. Add the pepper jack and mash for 3 to 4 minutes or until the cheese is melted. Serves 6.

Per serving: Calories 212; Fiber 3g; Protein 10g; Total Fat 9g; Saturated Fat 5g; Cholesterol 30mg; Sodium 386mg

Chicken & Cheese Tostadas

PREP: 15 MINUTES / COOK: 15 MINUTES

A tostada is an open-faced "sandwich" based on a crisp fried tortilla; baking the tortillas makes for a lighter tostada. The chilies in the topping supply cancer-fighting capsaicin.

2	teaspoons vegetable oil
4	scallions, thinly sliced
2	cloves garlic, minced
10	ounces skinless, boneless chicken breasts, cut into ½-inch chunks
1	cup frozen corn kernels, thawed
1	can (4 ounces) chopped mild green chilies
½	cup chopped cilantro
1	pickled jalapeño, halved, seeded, and finely chopped
2	tablespoons lime juice
8	corn tortillas (6-inch diameter)
6	ounces Monterey jack, pepper jack, or Muenster cheese, diced

1. In a large nonstick skillet, heat the oil over moderate heat. Add the scallions and garlic, and sauté for 2 minutes or until the scallions are tender. Add the chicken and sauté for 5 minutes or until just cooked through. Transfer to a large bowl. Add the corn, green chilies, cilantro, jalapeño, and lime juice, tossing to combine.

2. Meanwhile, preheat the oven to 400°F. Place the tortillas on a baking sheet and bake for 2 minutes.

3. Sprinkle half of the cheese over the tortillas. Top with the chicken mixture and the remaining cheese. Bake for 5 minutes or until the cheese is melted and bubbling. Serves 4.

Per serving: Calories 422; Fiber 4g; Protein 32g; Total Fat 18g; Saturated Fat 8g; Cholesterol 86mg; Sodium 610mg

At the market The mild, pale-yellow Muenster cheese used in these recipes is sometimes called American Muenster (or Munster) to distinguish it from a softer, more aromatic French cheese. The Monterey jack used here is a moist, ivory-colored, sliceable cheese, not to be confused with Dry Jack, an aged cheese more suitable for grating.

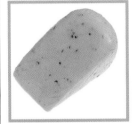

The bits of jalapeño in pepper jack add authentic flavor to Mexican and Tex-Mex dishes. Monterey jack also comes flavored with onion, chives, or herbs.

Prep Monterey jack and Muenster tend to be quite soft, so to shred them more easily, keep them refrigerated until ready for use. Or, if it doesn't matter to the recipe, dice the cheese instead of shredding it.

Cheesy Rice Bake is an easy oven main dish with the rich flavor of cheese.

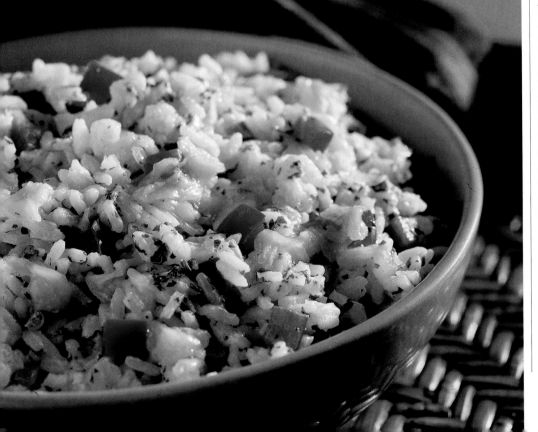

Cheddar & Swiss

Nutritional power
Potent flavorings, even in modest amounts, Cheddar and Swiss are rIch in calcium and protein. And they're usually not a problem for the lactose-intolerant.

Healthy Highlights

Cheddar
PER OUNCE

Calories	114
Fiber	0g
Protein	7g
Total Fat	9.4g
Saturated Fat	6.0g
Cholesterol	30mg
Sodium	176mg

NUTRIENTS

	% Daily Value
Calcium	20%

Swiss
PER OUNCE

Calories	107
Fiber	0g
Protein	8g
Total Fat	7.8g
Saturated Fat	5.0g
Cholesterol	26mg
Sodium	74mg

NUTRIENTS

	% Daily Value
Calcium	27%

Did you know? . . .
A number of studies have shown that cheese—especially Cheddar cheese—is an impressive cavity fighter.

Chicken Cheddar Chowder

PREP: 20 MINUTES / COOK: 20 MINUTES

You can enjoy Cheddar's robust bite in many dishes, but it's best if the other ingredients are low in fat. Here, skinless chicken breast, vegetables, and low-fat milk do the trick.

- 1½ cups chicken broth
- ¾ pound red potatoes, cut into ½-inch chunks
- 1 large carrot, thinly sliced
- 1 green bell pepper, cut into ½-inch squares
- 1 teaspoon paprika
- ½ teaspoon black pepper
- ¼ teaspoon salt
- ¾ pound skinless, boneless chicken breasts, cut into 1-inch chunks
- ½ cup low-fat (1%) milk
- 2 tablespoons flour
- 6 ounces Cheddar cheese, shredded

1. In a large saucepan, bring the broth and 2½ cups of water to a boil over moderate heat. Add the potatoes, carrot, bell pepper, paprika, black pepper, and salt. Reduce to a simmer, cover, and cook for 10 minutes or until the potatoes are firm-tender. Add the chicken and cook for 5 minutes or until it is cooked through.

2. In a small bowl, whisk the milk into the flour until smooth. Whisk the milk mixture into the soup and simmer for 3 minutes or until the soup is lightly thickened. Remove from the heat and stir in the cheese until melted. Serves 4.

Per serving: Calories 388; Fiber 3g; Protein 34g; Total Fat 16g; Saturated Fat 10g; Cholesterol 95mg; Sodium 880mg

Dijon Cheese Tart

PREP: 1 HOUR 25 MINUTES
COOK: 1 HOUR 10 MINUTES

- 1 cup flour
- ½ teaspoon sugar
- ¼ teaspoon each salt and cayenne pepper
- 2 ounces reduced-fat cream cheese (Neufchâtel), cut up
- 2 tablespoons unsalted butter, cut up
- 2 tablespoons reduced-fat sour cream
- 1 cup low-fat (1%) milk
- 1 egg
- 3 egg whites
- 1 tablespoon Dijon mustard
- 6 ounces Gruyère or other Swiss-style cheese, shredded

1. In a large bowl, combine the flour, sugar, salt, and cayenne. With a pastry blender or two knives, cut in the cream cheese and butter until the mixture resembles coarse meal. In a small bowl, combine the sour cream and 1 tablespoon of ice water. Stir into the flour mixture until just combined. Flatten into a disk, wrap in plastic wrap, and refrigerate at least 1 hour or overnight.

2. Preheat the oven to 350°F. On a lightly floured surface, roll the dough out to a 13-inch round. Fit into a 9-inch tart pan with a removable bottom. With a fork, prick the bottom of the shell in several places. Line with foil and weight down with pie weights or dried beans. Bake for 20 minutes or until the crust is beginning to set.

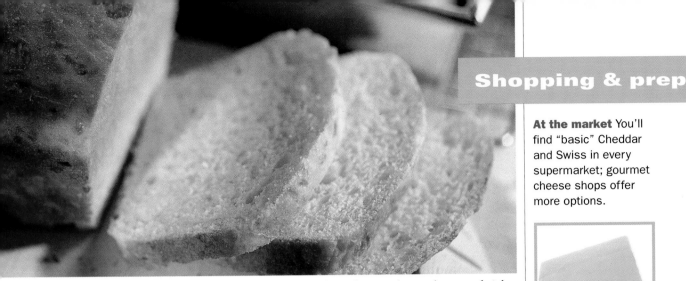

Cheddar-Potato Bread *is tasty with meals, or as the base for a turkey or ham sandwich.*

Remove the pie weights and foil and bake for 15 minutes or until the crust is cooked through. Leave the oven on.

3. In a medium bowl, whisk together the milk, whole egg, egg whites, and mustard. Stir in the Gruyère. Place the tart pan on a baking sheet with sides. Pour the cheese mixture into the crust and bake for 35 minutes or until puffed and golden brown. Serve warm or at room temperature. Serves 8.

Per serving: Calories 227; Fiber 1g; Protein 12g; Total Fat 12g; Saturated Fat 7g; Cholesterol 64mg; Sodium 264mg

Cheddar-Potato Bread

PREP: 15 MINUTES / RISE: 1 HOUR
COOK: 35 MINUTES

10	ounces baking potatoes (1 or 2 medium), peeled and thinly sliced
2	cloves garlic, peeled
2	tablespoons olive oil
1	package (¼ ounce) active dry yeast
1	teaspoon sugar
3¾	cups flour
1¼	teaspoons salt
¼	teaspoon cayenne pepper
2	cups shredded medium-sharp Cheddar cheese (8 ounces)

1. In a medium pot of boiling water, cook the potato and garlic for 15 minutes or until the potato is tender.

Reserving 1¼ cups of the liquid, drain the potatoes and garlic, and transfer to a large bowl. Add the oil and mash with a potato masher until smooth.

2. Place ¼ cup of the reserved cooking liquid in a small bowl and set aside to cool to lukewarm (105° to 115°F). Sprinkle the yeast and sugar over the lukewarm liquid and let stand for 5 minutes or until foamy.

3. Add the flour, salt, and cayenne to the potatoes, stirring until well combined. Stir in the remaining 1 cup reserved cooking liquid. Stir in the Cheddar. Add the yeast mixture and stir until well combined.

4. Turn the dough out onto a lightly floured surface and knead for 5 minutes or until smooth and elastic. Spray a large bowl with nonstick cooking spray; add the dough, turning to coat. Cover and let rise in a warm draftfree spot for 45 minutes or until doubled in bulk.

5. Preheat the oven to 400°F. Spray two 8½ x 4½-inch loaf pans with nonstick cooking spray. Punch the dough down, divide in half, form each portion into a loaf shape, and place in the prepared pans. Cover and let rise in a warm draftfree spot for 15 minutes. Bake for 30 to 35 minutes or until browned. Makes 2 loaves/16 servings.

Per serving: Calories 194; Fiber 1g; Protein 7g; Total Fat 7g; Saturated Fat 3g; Cholesterol 15mg; Sodium 261mg

At the market You'll find "basic" Cheddar and Swiss in every supermarket; gourmet cheese shops offer more options.

White Cheddar is made without the (natural) coloring that goes into yellow and orange Cheddars.

Look for Young Cheddars are moist and easily sliced; well-aged, slightly crumbly Cheddar (at least 6 months old), is more flavorful. Fine Cheddars are made in Great Britain, Canada, New York, and Vermont, among other places. English Cheshire and Double Gloucester are Cheddar relatives to sample. Among Swiss-style cheeses, Emmentaler (from Switzerland) is one of the best. Try nutty Swiss Gruyère, fruity French Comté, and mild Norwegian Jarlsberg, too.

Basic cooking Grated or shredded and added to hot food, these cheeses will melt quickly and smoothly. When subjected to high or prolonged heat, they will turn tough and rubbery.

Eggs

Nutritional power
The protein content is high and the price is right—eggs are a nutrition bargain. You also get riboflavin, folate, iron, B vitamins, phosphorus, and vitamin E.

Healthy Highlights

PER 1 LARGE	
Calories	75
Fiber	0g
Protein	6g
Total Fat	5.0g
Saturated Fat	1.6g
Cholesterol	213mg
Sodium	63mg

NUTRIENTS	
	% Daily Value
Riboflavin	15%

Did you know? . . .
New methods of analysis have shown eggs to be lower in cholesterol than previously thought (213 rather than 275mg). At any rate, saturated fat in the diet has a much greater effect on blood cholesterol, and an egg contains less than 2mg of saturated fat.

All of an egg's fat and cholesterol is in the yolk, but so is the lion's share of the B vitamins and minerals.

Asparagus & Red Pepper Frittata

PREP: 10 MINUTES / COOK: 20 MINUTES

- ½ pound asparagus, trimmed and cut into ½-inch lengths
- 1 red bell pepper, cut into ½-inch squares
- 3 eggs
- 4 egg whites
- 2 teaspoons flour
- ½ cup grated Parmesan cheese
- ½ teaspoon salt
- ¼ teaspoon black pepper
- 2 teaspoons olive oil
- 1 teaspoon unsalted butter

1. In a medium pot of boiling water, cook the asparagus and bell pepper for 2 minutes to blanch; drain well.

2. In a medium bowl, whisk together the whole eggs and egg whites. Whisk in the flour until well combined. Whisk in the Parmesan, salt, and black pepper. Stir in the asparagus and bell pepper.

3. In a 10-inch cast-iron or other broilerproof skillet, heat the oil and butter over low heat until the butter has melted. Pour in the egg mixture and cook without stirring for 15 minutes or until the eggs are set around the edges and almost set in the center. Meanwhile, preheat the broiler.

4. Broil the frittata 6 inches from the heat for 1 to 2 minutes or until the top is just set. Cut into wedges and serve hot, warm, at room temperature, or chilled. Serves 4.

Per serving: Calories 167; Fiber 1g; Protein 14g; Total Fat 10g; Saturated Fat 4g; Cholesterol 170mg; Sodium 563mg

Souffléed Omelet with Apple Topping

PREP: 10 MINUTES / COOK: 10 MINUTES

- 3 egg yolks
- 3 tablespoons flour
- ½ cup low-fat (1%) milk
- 1 tablespoon sugar
- 1 teaspoon grated lemon zest
- ¼ teaspoon salt
- 6 egg whites
- 1 tablespoon unsalted butter
- 3 tablespoons frozen apple juice concentrate
- 1 tablespoon lemon juice
- 2 large McIntosh apples, peeled and cut into thin wedges

1. Preheat the oven to 400°F. In a large bowl, whisk together the egg yolks, flour, milk, sugar, lemon zest, and salt. In a separate bowl, whisk the egg whites until stiff peaks form. Gently fold the whites into the yolk mixture.

2. In a deep, 10-inch ovenproof skillet, melt the butter over moderate heat. Pour in the egg mixture, place in the oven, and bake for 10 minutes or until set, puffed, and lightly browned.

3. Meanwhile, in a medium skillet, bring the apple juice concentrate and lemon juice to a boil over moderate heat. Add the apples and cook, tossing occasionally, for 4 minutes or until the apples are tender. Top the hot souffléed omelet with the apples. Serves 4.

Per serving: Calories 206; Fiber 2g; Protein 9g; Total Fat 7g; Saturated Fat 3g; Cholesterol 169mg; Sodium 243mg

Crème Caramel

PREP: 15 MINUTES / COOK: 50 MINUTES

Since the orange zest is used only for flavoring, cut it off the orange in broad strips.

- ¾ cup plus ⅔ cup sugar
- 2 cups low-fat (1%) milk
- 1 cup evaporated skimmed milk
- 6 strips of orange zest
- ¼ teaspoon salt
- 4 eggs
- 2 egg whites
- ½ teaspoon vanilla extract

1. In a small saucepan, combine ¾ cup of the sugar and ½ cup of water. Bring to a boil over moderately high heat and cook, without stirring, for 5 minutes or until amber-colored. Pour the caramel into eight 6-ounce custard cups, tilting them to cover the bottom and partway up the sides. Place the cups in a roasting pan and set aside.

2. In a medium saucepan, combine the milk, evaporated milk, ⅓ cup of the sugar, the orange zest, and salt. Bring to a simmer over moderate heat. Re-move from the heat, cover, and let stand for 30 minutes at room temperature. Discard the orange zest.

3. Preheat the oven to 325°F. In a large bowl, whisk together the whole eggs, egg whites, vanilla, and the remaining ⅓ cup sugar until well combined. Strain the milk mixture into the egg mixture and whisk to combine.

4. Pour the custard into the prepared custard cups. Pour boiling water into the roasting pan to come halfway up the sides of the cups. Bake for 45 minutes or until a knife inserted in the center of a custard comes out clean.

5. Remove the cups from the water bath and cool on a rack. When cool, refrigerate until ready to serve. Run a knife around the outside edge of the custard cups and invert the crème caramel onto dessert plates. Serves 8.

Per serving: Calories 231; Fiber 0g; Protein 8g; Total Fat 3g; Saturated Fat 1g; Cholesterol 110mg; Sodium 180mg

At the market Markets offer Medium, Large, and Extra-large eggs. Most published recipes—including ours—are developed with Large eggs.

Look for Buy eggs only in stores where they're kept refrigerated. Check the freshness date, then open the carton to see if the shells are intact.

Prep The easiest way to separate eggs is to use a gadget called an egg separator (see below). Or you can crack the egg into your (clean) hand, letting the white run between your fingers.

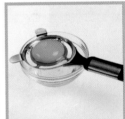

Unless you've had lots of practice, an egg separator is an indispensable tool.

Basic cooking Although salmonella is becoming less of a problem, it's best to cook eggs thoroughly: Cook soft-boiled eggs for at least 3½ minutes, scrambled eggs, omelets, and fried eggs past the runny stage.

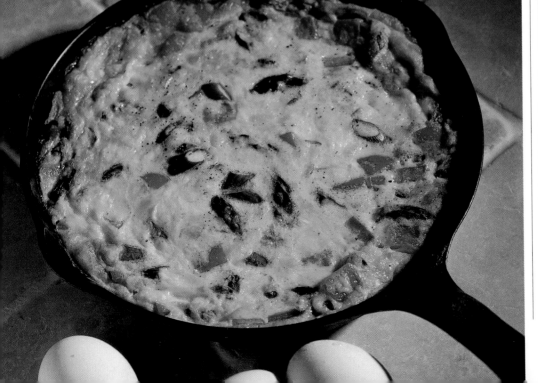

Asparagus & Red Pepper Frittata *A typically quick, easy egg dish with Italian flair.*

145

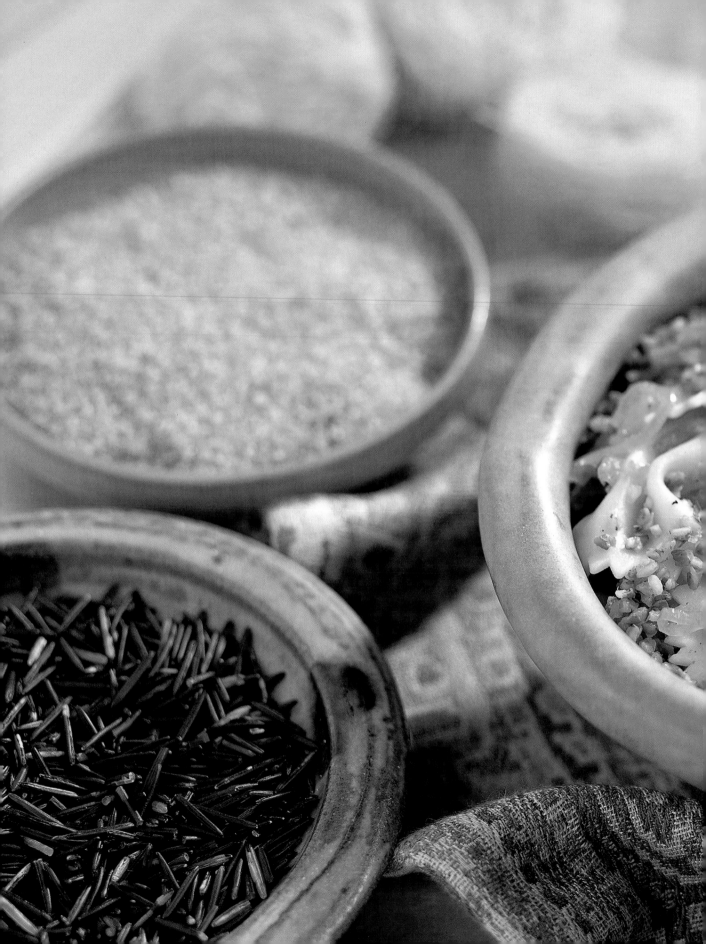

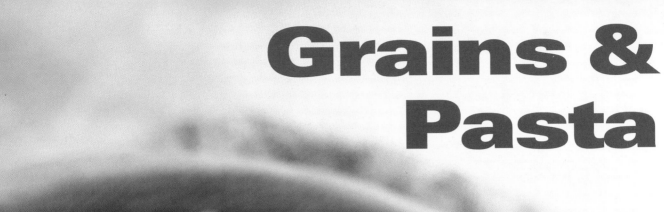

Grains & Pasta

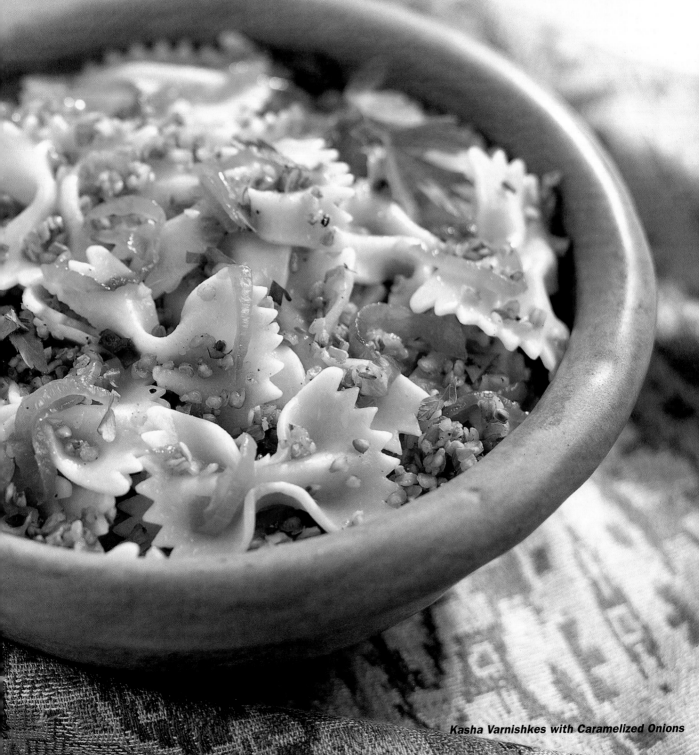

Kasha Varnishkes with Caramelized Onions

Pasta

Nutritional power
The inspiration for countless quick, healthful meals, pasta is a low-fat protein source. And most dried pastas are enriched with B vitamins and iron.

Healthy Highlights

PER 2 OUNCES UNCOOKED

Calories	211
Fiber	1.4g
Protein	7g
Total Fat	0.9g
Saturated Fat	0.1g
Cholesterol	0mg
Sodium	4mg

NUTRIENTS

	% Daily Value
Thiamin	39%
Niacin	22%
Manganese	20%
Riboflavin	17%
Iron	11%

Did you know? . . .
The most nutritious pastas are made from semolina, a coarse flour ground from durum wheat. Durum is a hard grain that has a higher protein content than other types of wheat.

Fettuccine alla Giardiniera

PREP: 20 MINUTES / COOK: 25 MINUTES
"Gardener's-style" pasta with a light sauce.

- 2 cups small cauliflower florets
- 2 cups small broccoli florets
- 10 ounces spinach fettuccine
- 1 tablespoon olive oil
- 1 red onion, diced
- 3 cloves garlic, minced
- ½ pound mushrooms, thinly sliced
- ¾ teaspoon salt
- ½ teaspoon dried rosemary, crumbled
- 1 large tomato, cut into ½-inch-thick wedges
- 1 tablespoon flour
- 1½ cups low-fat (1%) milk
- ⅓ cup grated Parmesan cheese
- ¼ cup chopped parsley

1. In a large pot of boiling water, cook the cauliflower and broccoli for 2 minutes to blanch. With a slotted spoon, transfer the vegetables to a plate.

2. Add the fettuccine to the boiling water and cook according to package directions until firm-tender. Drain and transfer to a large serving bowl.

3. Meanwhile, in a large nonstick skillet, heat 2 teaspoons of the oil over moderate heat. Add the onion and garlic, and sauté for 5 minutes or until tender. Add the mushrooms and sauté for 3 minutes or until softened.

4. Add the remaining 1 teaspoon oil to the pan. Return the cauliflower and broccoli to the pan, sprinkle with the salt and rosemary, and sauté for 1 minute or until the vegetables are heated through. Add the tomato and cook for 3 minutes or until softened.

5. Sprinkle the flour over the vegetables, stirring to coat. Add the milk and bring to a boil. Reduce to a simmer and cook, stirring, for 3 minutes or until slightly thickened. Stir in the Parmesan and parsley. Add to the hot pasta, tossing until combined. Serves 4.

Per serving: Calories 450; Fiber 13g; Protein 21g; Total Fat 8g; Saturated Fat 3g; Cholesterol 9mg; Sodium 655mg

Linguine with Creamy Garlic-Mint Sauce

PREP: 15 MINUTES / COOK: 15 MINUTES

- 12 ounces linguine
- ½ cup packed fresh mint leaves
- 8 cloves garlic, minced
- 1¾ cups chicken broth
- 4 teaspoons flour
- 4 tablespoons reduced-fat cream cheese (Neufchâtel)
- ¾ teaspoon salt
- ½ cup reduced-fat sour cream

1. Bring a large pot of water to a boil for the pasta. Place the mint in a strainer and place the strainer in the boiling water for 10 seconds to blanch the mint. Drain the mint well, transfer to a food processor, and process until smooth.

2. Return the water to a boil, add the linguine, and cook according to package directions until firm-tender. Drain and transfer to a large serving bowl.

3. Meanwhile, in a large skillet, cook the garlic in ¾ cup of the broth over low heat for 5 minutes or until the garlic is very soft. Whisk in the flour and stir until well combined. Add the remaining 1 cup broth, the mint purée, the cream cheese, and salt, and cook, stirring, for 4 minutes or until the sauce is lightly thickened and no floury taste remains. Remove from the heat and stir in the sour cream. Add to the hot pasta, tossing well. Serves 4.

Per serving: Calories 433; Fiber 2g; Protein 16g; Total Fat 9g; Saturated Fat 4g; Cholesterol 18mg; Sodium 970mg

Baked Macaroni with Vegetables & Cheese

PREP: 20 MINUTES / COOK: 40 MINUTES

- 10 ounces elbow macaroni
- 2 teaspoons olive oil
- 1 yellow summer squash (9 ounces), halved lengthwise and thinly sliced
- 4 scallions, thinly sliced
- 1 bottled roasted red pepper, diced
- 3 cloves garlic, minced
- 3 tablespoons flour
- 2½ cups low-fat (1%) milk
- ¾ teaspoon salt
- 1 cup grated sharp Cheddar cheese (4 ounces)
- ¼ cup grated Parmesan cheese

1. In a large pot of boiling water, cook the pasta according to package directions until firm-tender. Drain and transfer to a large bowl. Preheat the oven to 400°F.

2. Meanwhile, in a large nonstick skillet, heat the oil over moderate heat. Add the squash, scallions, roasted pepper, and garlic to the pan and sauté for 5 minutes or until the squash is crisp-tender. Add the flour and stir until well combined. Gradually add the milk, stirring until combined. Stir in the salt and cook, stirring, for 5 minutes or until the sauce is lightly thickened and no floury taste remains.

3. Add the hot white sauce to the pasta along with the Cheddar, tossing until well coated. Transfer to a 7 x 11-inch baking dish, sprinkle with the Parmesan, and bake for 25 minutes or until crusty and piping hot. Serves 4.

Per serving: Calories 531; Fiber 3g; Protein 25g; Total Fat 16g; Saturated Fat 8g; Cholesterol 40mg; Sodium 796mg

At the market There are hundreds of different pasta shapes, but all dried pastas (except egg noodles) are very similar in nutritional value.

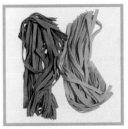

Pastas colored with vegetable extracts (these are spinach and tomato) add color to your favorite pasta dishes. Note, however, that they offer little or no nutritional advantage over regular pasta.

Look for For the best texture, choose a brand of pasta made from pure semolina. This includes most imported and many domestic brands.

Basic cooking Cook pasta in plenty of boiling water to keep it from sticking together. Add the pasta all at once, stir briefly, and return the water to a boil. Time the cooking from the second boil. Test the pasta for doneness a little sooner than the package directions recommend (overcooking ruins pasta), and drain it immediately when it is firm-tender to the bite.

Baked Macaroni with Vegetables & Cheese powers up the nutrition in a classic dish.

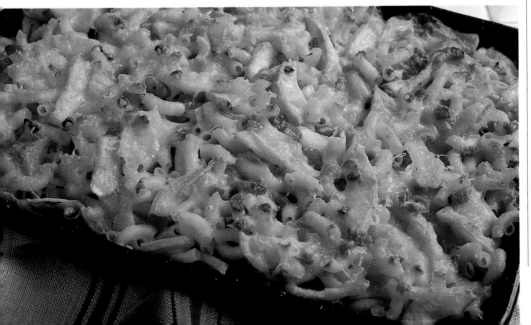

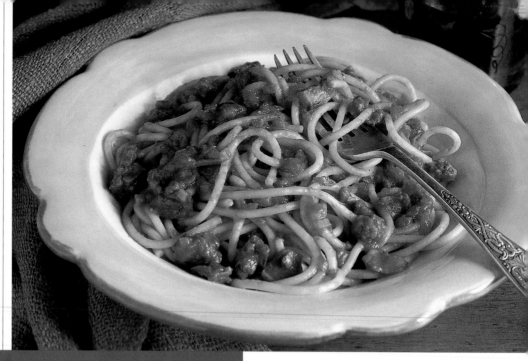

Spaghetti Bolognese
Even a creamy meat sauce can be healthful when made with lean beef and low-fat milk.

Did you know? . .
Pasta with tomato sauce is not just a tradition, it's a smart nutritional choice: The tomatoes' vitamin C helps your body absorb the pasta's iron.

The rich supply of vitamin C in tomatoes will help your body absorb the iron in pasta.

People used to think that pasta was fattening, but only the sauce can make it a high-fat dish: A cup of plain cooked pasta contains less than 1g of fat.

"High-protein" pastas are fortified with protein (in the form of soy flour, wheat germ, or dairy products, for instance). Such pastas may have up to 100 percent more protein than plain pasta.

Egg noodles (and some fresh pastas) contain more cholesterol than regular pasta: A cup of cooked egg noodles has about 50mg cholesterol. If this concerns you, look for "yolkless" noodles, which are cholesterol-free (and fat-free, too).

Mushroom-Stuffed Lasagne Rolls

PREP: **30** MINUTES / COOK: **40** MINUTES
A new twist—literally—on a pasta classic.

- **1** pound mushrooms, trimmed
- **12** lasagne noodles (10 ounces)
- **2** teaspoons olive oil
- **1** small onion, finely chopped
- **3** cloves garlic, minced
- **½** teaspoon salt
- **¼** teaspoon each dried sage and pepper
- **1** cup part-skim ricotta cheese
- **2** egg whites
- **1½** cups chicken broth
- **1½** cups low-fat (1%) milk
- **3** tablespoons flour
- **¼** cup grated Parmesan cheese

1. Preheat the oven to 375°F. Spray a 9 x 13-inch glass baking dish with non-stick cooking spray; set aside. In a food processor or by hand, coarsely chop the mushrooms.

2. In a large pot of boiling water, cook the lasagne noodles according to package directions until firm-tender; drain.

3. Meanwhile, in a large nonstick skillet, heat the oil over moderate heat. Add the onion and garlic, and sauté for 5 minutes or until the onion is tender. Add the mushrooms, ¼ teaspoon of the salt, the sage, and pepper, and sauté for 7 minutes or until the mushrooms are tender and their liquid has evaporated. Transfer the mushroom mixture to a medium bowl and stir in the ricotta cheese and egg whites.

4. Lay the lasagne noodles on a work surface. Spread ¼ cup of the mushroom mixture over each noodle and roll up. Place the rolls, seam-sides down, in the prepared baking dish.

5. In a medium saucepan, whisk the broth and milk into the flour. Stir in the remaining ¼ teaspoon salt and bring to a boil over moderate heat. Reduce to a simmer and cook, stirring constantly, for 5 minutes or until the sauce is lightly thickened. Pour the sauce over the lasagne rolls and sprinkle with the Parmesan. Bake, uncovered, for 25 minutes or until the filling is piping hot and the sauce is bubbling. Serves 4.

Per serving: Calories 513; Fiber 4g; Protein 27g; Total Fat 12g; Saturated Fat 5g; Cholesterol 27mg; Sodium 923mg

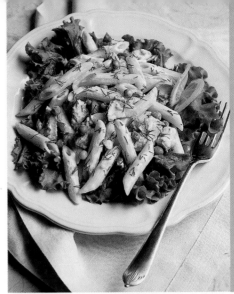

Spaghetti Bolognese

PREP: 15 MINUTES / COOK: 30 MINUTES

Italians call this type of sauce a "ragù."

- ¼ **ounce dried porcini or other dried mushrooms**
- ¾ **cup boiling water**
- 2 **ounces bacon, coarsely chopped (2 slices)**
- 1 **onion, finely chopped**
- 1 **carrot, finely chopped**
- 1 **stalk celery, finely chopped**
- ½ **pound extra-lean ground beef**
- 1 **can (6 ounces) no-salt-added tomato paste**
- ½ **cup dry red wine**
- ½ **teaspoon each salt and pepper**
- 1¼ **cups low-fat (1%) milk**
- 12 **ounces spaghetti**

1. In a small heatproof bowl, combine the dried mushrooms and the boiling water and let stand for 10 minutes or until softened. Reserving the soaking liquid, scoop out the mushrooms, rinse, and finely chop. Strain the soaking liquid through a coffee filter or a paper towel-lined sieve.

2. In a large skillet, combine the bacon and 2 tablespoons of water over low heat. Cook for 4 minutes or until the bacon has rendered its fat but is not crisp. Add the onion, carrot, and celery, and cook for 5 minutes or until the onion is soft.

3. Crumble in the beef and add the reserved soaking liquid, chopped mushrooms, tomato paste, wine, salt, and pepper. Bring to a boil, reduce to a simmer, and cook for 5 minutes or until the liquid has almost evaporated. Add half of the milk and cook until it has been absorbed. Add the remaining milk and simmer for 12 minutes or until the sauce is thick and richly flavored.

4. Meanwhile, in a large pot of boiling water, cook the pasta according to package directions until firm-tender. Drain and toss with the sauce. Serves 4.

Per serving: Calories 630; Fiber 6g; Protein 28g; Total Fat 20g; Saturated Fat 8g; Cholesterol 52mg; Sodium 498mg

Pasta-Salmon Salad

In large bowl, combine ½ cup plain low-fat yogurt, ¼ cup light mayonnaise, ¼ cup snipped fresh dill, 2 tbsp. lemon juice, and ¼ tsp. salt. Add 14¾-oz. can salmon, drained, and 1 cup thawed frozen peas. Cook 10 oz. penne, drain, add to bowl, and toss. Serves 4. *[Cal 484; Fat 12g; Sod 741mg]*

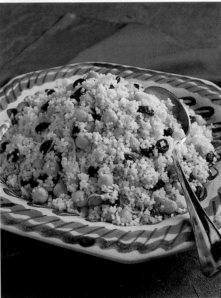

Moroccan Couscous

Bring 1¼ cups water, 1 cup chicken broth, 1 tbsp. vegetable oil, 1½ tsp. grated lemon zest, and ½ tsp. salt to a boil. Add 10-oz. box couscous, remove from heat, cover, and let stand 5 minutes. Fluff the couscous with a fork; add 19-oz. can rinsed canned chickpeas and 1 cup raisins. Toss. Serves 4. *[Cal 504; Fat 7g; Sod 696mg]*

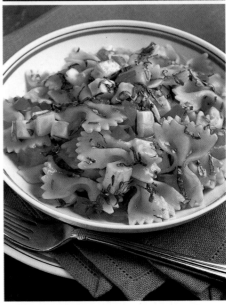

Bow-Ties with Mozzarella & Fresh Tomatoes

Cook 12 oz. bow-tie pasta. Drain. Meanwhile, in large skillet, bring 1 cup no-salt-added tomato sauce to a boil. Add 1 cup chopped fresh tomatoes, ¼ cup chopped fresh basil, and ½ tsp. each sugar and salt. Transfer to bowl, add hot pasta and 6 oz. diced part-skim mozzarella. Serves 4. *[Cal 456; Fat 9g; Sod 494mg]*

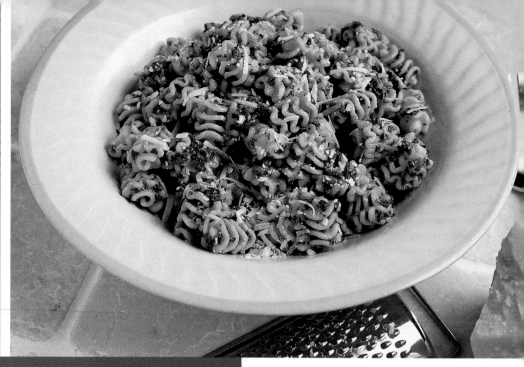

Radiatore with Pesto

These ruffled pasta shapes—modeled after Italian radiators—are uniquely suited to creamy sauces such as this basil-garlic purée.

Did you know? . . .
In 1920, Americans ate hardly any pasta at all; predictions for the year 2000 estimate annual pasta consumption at 30 pounds per person.

Pasta sold in cardboard boxes retains more riboflavin than pasta packed in plastic bags.

A University of Minnesota study revealed that enriched pasta loses considerable riboflavin when exposed to light. So choose pasta packed in cardboard boxes (those with a small transparent "window" are fine) rather than in clear plastic bags. At home, store pasta in an opaque container rather than a glass jar.

If you like whole-wheat pasta, with its earthy flavor and chewy texture, you reap a healthful bonus: Whole-wheat pasta has much more fiber than semolina pasta. But enriched semolina pasta and whole-wheat pasta are roughly comparable in terms of nutrients.

Pasta with Butternut Squash Sauce
PREP: 10 MINUTES / COOK: 55 MINUTES

- 1   **butternut squash (2 pounds), halved lengthwise and seeded**
- 12   **ounces fusilli or rotelle pasta**
- 2   **teaspoons olive oil**
- 2   **cloves garlic, minced**
- ⅓   **cup almonds**
- ⅓   **cup grated Parmesan cheese**
- 2   **tablespoons sugar**
- 2   **teaspoons yellow mustard**
- ¾   **teaspoon each dried sage and salt**
- ½   **teaspoon pepper**

1. Preheat the oven to 400°F. Place the squash, cut-sides down, in a small baking pan. Add ½ cup water, cover, and bake for 45 minutes or until the squash is tender. When cool enough to handle, scoop the flesh into a food processor.

2. Meanwhile, in a large pot of boiling water, cook the pasta according to package directions until firm-tender. Reserving ⅔ cup of the pasta cooking water, drain the pasta and transfer to a large bowl.

3. In a small nonstick skillet, heat the oil over low heat. Add the garlic and cook for 2 minutes or until softened.

4. Transfer the garlic to the food processor along with the reserved pasta cooking water, the almonds, Parmesan, sugar, mustard, sage, salt, and pepper. Process until smooth and add to the pasta, tossing to coat. Serves 4.

Per serving: Calories 544; Fiber 7g; Protein 18g; Total Fat 12g; Saturated Fat 2g; Cholesterol 5mg; Sodium 583mg

Radiatore with Pesto
PREP: 15 MINUTES / COOK: 15 MINUTES

- 3   **cloves garlic, peeled**
- 12   **ounces radiatore pasta**
- 2   **cups packed fresh basil leaves**
- 6   **tablespoons chicken or vegetable broth**
- 1   **tablespoon olive oil**
- 1   **tablespoon reduced-fat cream cheese (Neufchâtel)**
- ½   **teaspoon salt**
- ¼   **teaspoon pepper**
- ½   **cup grated Parmesan cheese**

1. In a large pot of boiling water, cook the garlic for 2 minutes to blanch. With a slotted spoon, transfer the garlic to a food processor.

2. Bring the water to a boil, add the pasta, and cook according to package directions until firm-tender. Drain and transfer to a large bowl.

3. Meanwhile, add the basil, broth, oil, cream cheese, salt, and pepper to the garlic, and process to a smooth purée. Add the Parmesan and process briefly just to combine. Add to the hot pasta, tossing well. Serves 4.

Per serving: Calories 440; Fiber 7g; Protein 19g; Total Fat 9g; Saturated Fat 3g; Cholesterol 10mg; Sodium 587mg

Angel Hair with Asparagus & Lemon Cream Sauce

PREP: 15 MINUTES / COOK: 15 MINUTES

12	ounces angel hair pasta
1	pound asparagus, trimmed and thinly sliced on the diagonal
1	cup chicken broth
4	teaspoons flour
2½	teaspoons grated lemon zest
¾	teaspoon salt
¼	teaspoon each dried marjoram and pepper
½	cup reduced-fat sour cream

1. In a large pot of boiling water, cook the pasta according to package directions until firm-tender. Add the asparagus for the last 1 minute of cooking. Drain; transfer to a large serving bowl.

2. Meanwhile, in a large nonstick skillet, combine the broth with ¼ cup of water; whisk in the flour and bring to a boil over moderate heat. Whisk in the lemon zest, salt, marjoram, and pepper. Reduce to a simmer and cook, stirring frequently, for 3 minutes or until lightly thickened. Remove the sauce from the heat and whisk in the sour cream.

3. Add the lemon cream sauce to the hot pasta and asparagus, tossing well to combine. Serves 4.

Per serving: Calories 402; Fiber 3g; Protein 16g; Total Fat 6g; Saturated Fat 2g; Cholesterol 10mg; Sodium 970mg

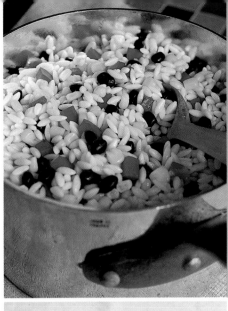

Mexican Confetti Orzo In large bowl, toss together 1 diced red bell pepper, 10-oz. can rinsed black beans, 1 cup frozen thawed corn kernels, 1 tbsp. olive oil, ¾ tsp. salt, and ¼ tsp. cayenne. Cook 10 oz. orzo, drain, add to bowl, and toss. Serves 4. *[Cal 373; Fat 5g; Sod 533mg]*

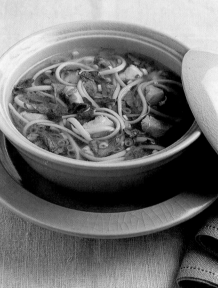

Chinese Chicken-Noodle Soup Bring 2 cups chicken broth, 3 cups water, 2 tsp. soy sauce, 1 tbsp. sesame oil, and 1 tbsp. rice vinegar to a boil. Add ½ lb. diced chicken breast and cook 2 minutes. Add 6 oz. fresh linguine, 2 cups watercress leaves, and 1 minced scallion, and cook for 2 minutes or until pasta is done. Serves 4. *[Cal 232; Fat 6g; Sod 753mg]*

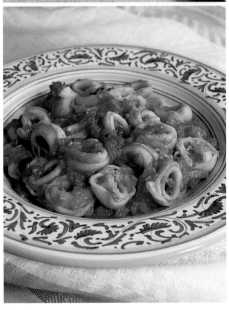

Tortellini with Zesty Tomato Sauce In large nonstick skillet, sauté 1 diced onion and 3 minced cloves garlic in 2 tsp. olive oil until tender. Add 14½-oz. can no-salt-added stewed tomatoes, 8-oz. can no-salt-added tomato sauce, ½ tsp. salt, and ¼ tsp. red pepper flakes. Simmer 10 minutes. Meanwhile, cook 15-oz. package cheese tortellini. Toss with sauce. Serves 4. *[Cal 412; Fat 10g; Sod 668mg]*

Bulghur

Nutritional power
Bulghur—parboiled wheat kernels that have been dried and cracked—gives you dietary fiber, B vitamins, and a healthy helping of minerals, including iron.

Healthy Highlights

PER ½ CUP RAW

Calories	239
Fiber	13g
Protein	9g
Total Fat	0.9g
Saturated Fat	0.2g
Cholesterol	0mg
Sodium	12mg

NUTRIENTS

	% Daily Value
Manganese	107%
Magnesium	29%
Niacin	18%
Copper	12%
Vitamin B6	12%
Iron	11%
Thiamin	11%

Did you know? . . .
The bone-building manganese in bulghur helps to prevent osteoporosis.

Although a small percentage of the fiber-rich bran is removed from bulghur during processing, plenty remains: A 1½-cup serving of cooked bulghur supplies half of your daily fiber requirement.

Mushroom-Bulghur Pilaf

PREP: 15 MINUTES / COOK: 30 MINUTES

Bulghur has a delicate nutlike flavor and cooks far more quickly than brown rice.

- 1 **tablespoon olive oil**
- 4 **scallions, thinly sliced**
- 2 **cloves garlic, minced**
- 1 **carrot, thinly sliced**
- 1 **stalk celery, thinly sliced**
- ½ **pound mushrooms, thinly sliced**
- 1 **cup coarse bulghur**
- 1½ **cups chicken broth**
- ¼ **teaspoon each crumbled dried rosemary, salt, and pepper**

1. Preheat the oven to 350°F. In a Dutch oven or flameproof casserole, heat the oil over moderate heat. Add the scallions and garlic, and sauté for 2 minutes or until the scallions are soft. Stir in the carrot and celery, and sauté for 4 minutes or until the carrot is crisp-tender. Add the mushrooms and sauté for 3 minutes or until the mushrooms are softened.

2. Stir in the bulghur, broth, 1 cup of water, the rosemary, salt, and pepper, and bring to a boil. Cover and bake for 20 minutes or until the bulghur is tender and the liquid has been absorbed. Serves 4.

Per serving: Calories 190; Fiber 8g; Protein 7g; Total Fat 5g; Saturated Fat 1g; Cholesterol 0mg; Sodium 555mg

Mexican-Style Tabbouleh

PREP: 15 MINUTES / SOAK: 1 HOUR
STAND: 1 HOUR

Tabbouleh, a refreshing grain salad, is Middle Eastern in origin. We've adapted the recipe with corn, bell pepper, cilantro, and other south-of-the-border seasonings.

- 1 **cup fine or coarse bulghur**
- 3 **cups boiling water**
- ¼ **cup lime juice**
- 1 **tablespoon olive oil**
- ¾ **teaspoon salt**
- ½ **teaspoon cumin**
- ¼ **teaspoon dried oregano**
- ⅛ **teaspoon allspice**
- 2 **cups cherry tomatoes, halved**
- 1 **cup frozen corn kernels, thawed**
- 1 **green bell pepper, diced**
- 3 **scallions, thinly sliced**
- ½ **cup chopped cilantro or parsley**

1. In a large bowl, combine the bulghur and boiling water. Let stand 1 hour at room temperature. Drain and squeeze the bulghur dry.

2. Meanwhile, in a large bowl, whisk together the lime juice, oil, salt, cumin, oregano, and allspice. Stir in the tomatoes, corn, bell pepper, scallions, and cilantro. Add the drained bulghur and toss to combine. Let stand for at least 1 hour. Serve chilled or at room temperature. Serves 4.

Per serving: Calories 210; Fiber 9g; Protein 6g; Total Fat 4g; Saturated Fat 1g; Cholesterol 0mg; Sodium 429mg

Bean & Bulghur Chili

PREP: 15 MINUTES / COOK: 40 MINUTES

One of the smartest meatless-chili tricks is using bulghur in place of ground beef—the texture is distinctly meaty. And this spicy chili is remarkably low in fat.

- 1 **tablespoon olive oil**
- 1 **large onion, finely chopped**
- 3 **cloves garlic, minced**
- 1 **red bell pepper, diced**
- 1 **pickled jalapeño pepper, seeded and finely chopped**
- 1 **cup coarse bulghur**
- 1 **can (14½ ounces) no-salt-added stewed tomatoes, chopped with their juice**
- 1 **teaspoon mild chili powder**
- 1 **teaspoon ground coriander**
- ¾ **teaspoon salt**
- 1 **can (15½ ounces) pinto beans, rinsed and drained**

1. In a Dutch oven, heat the oil over moderate heat. Add the onion and garlic, and sauté for 7 minutes or until the onion is tender. Add the bell pepper and jalapeño, and cook for 5 minutes or until the bell pepper is tender.

2. Stir in the bulghur, stewed tomatoes, chili powder, coriander, salt, and 2 cups of water, and bring to a boil. Reduce to a simmer, cover, and cook for 15 minutes or until most of the water has evaporated.

3. Stir in the beans and cook, uncovered, for 10 minutes or until the beans are heated through and the flavors have blended. Serves 4.

Per serving: Calories 270; Fiber 13g; Protein 10g; Total Fat 5g; Saturated Fat 1g; Cholesterol 0mg; Sodium 677mg

At the market Bulghur (which is sometimes spelled "bulgur") comes in three granulations: coarse, medium, and fine. Coarse bulghur is good for chilis, stuffings, and pilafs; medium is usually cooked as a cereal; and fine bulghur is traditional for tabbouleh and other salads. At the supermarket, bulghur may be on a shelf near the rice, or it may be with the Middle Eastern food products.

Basic cooking To cook bulghur by steeping, use a 1-to-3 ratio of bulghur to water: For 1 cup dry bulghur, place the grain in a heatproof bowl or a saucepan; add 3 cups boiling water and let stand for 1 hour. Drain off any excess liquid and squeeze the bulghur dry.

Mexican-Style Tabbouleh *is a light and tempting main dish for warm-weather dining.*

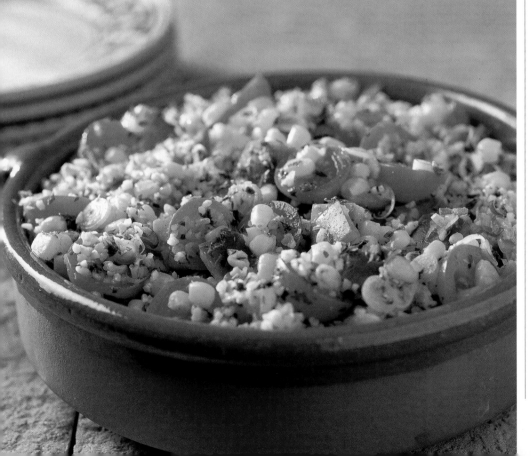

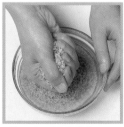

After steeping bulghur, pour off any water that remains, and then squeeze the bulghur with your hands until it's quite dry, transferring the bulghur to a clean bowl as you work.

155

Wheat

Nutritional power
*Whole-wheat flour
contains the grain's
bran and its germ,
too. The germ is rich
in protein, vitamin E
and B vitamins,
while wheat bran is
packed with fiber.*

Healthy Highlights

Whole-Wheat Flour
PER ½ CUP

Calories	203
Fiber	7.3g
Protein	8g
Total Fat	1.1g
Saturated Fat	0.2g
Cholesterol	0mg
Sodium	3mg

NUTRIENTS

	% Daily Value
Magnesium	21%
Niacin	19%
Thiamin	18%
Zinc	12%

Wheat Germ
PER ¼ CUP

Calories	104
Fiber	3.8g
Protein	7g
Total Fat	2.8g
Saturated Fat	0.5g
Cholesterol	0mg
Sodium	3mg

NUTRIENTS

	% Daily Value
Magnesium	17%
Thiamin	36%
Zinc	23%
Folate	20%
Vitamin B6	19%

Mushroom Roll-Ups

PREP: 30 MINUTES / CHILL: 1 HOUR
COOK: 35 MINUTES

A rich-tasting yet healthful appetizer.

- 1 cup minus 2 tablespoons whole-wheat flour
- ¼ cup all-purpose flour
- ¾ teaspoon salt
- ½ teaspoon dried rosemary, crumbled
- ¼ teaspoon baking soda
- 3 tablespoons unsalted butter
- 3 tablespoons honey
- 1 whole egg plus 1 egg white
- ½ cup chicken broth
- 2 scallions, thinly sliced
- 3 cloves garlic, minced
- ½ pound button mushrooms, minced
- ½ pound fresh shiitake mushrooms, trimmed and coarsely chopped
- ⅓ cup part-skim ricotta cheese

1. In a small bowl, combine both flours, ½ teaspoon of the salt, ¼ teaspoon of the rosemary, and the baking soda. In a medium bowl, cream the butter and honey. Beat in the whole egg. Stir in the dry ingredients until the mixture forms a dough. Divide in half, flatten into rectangles, wrap in plastic wrap, and refrigerate for at least 1 hour.

2. Meanwhile, in a large skillet, heat the broth over moderately low heat. Add the scallions and garlic, and cook for 4 minutes. Add both mushrooms, the remaining ¼ teaspoon each salt and rosemary, and cook, stirring, for 9 minutes or until the mushrooms are dry. Transfer to a bowl to cool slightly. Stir in the ricotta and egg white.

3. Preheat the oven to 350°F. Spray a baking sheet with nonstick cooking spray. On a floured surface, roll one piece of dough out to a 7 x 11-inch rectangle. Spoon half of the mushroom mixture down the center, leaving a 2-inch border on each long side and a ½-inch border at each short end. Fold the ends over the filling, then fold in the sides; pinch together to seal. Place seam-side down on the baking sheet. Repeat with the remaining dough and filling. Bake for 35 minutes. Cut each roll into 6 slices. Serves 6.

Per serving: Calories 226; Fiber 4g; Protein 8g; Total Fat 9g; Saturated Fat 5g; Cholesterol 55mg; Sodium 471mg

Crunchy Dessert Topping

PREP: 5 MINUTES / COOK: 25 MINUTES

This crisp, toasty topping has less than one-third the fat of jarred "nuts in syrup."

- ½ cup packed dark brown sugar
- 2 teaspoons lemon juice
- 1½ cups toasted wheat germ
- 1 tablespoon vegetable oil
- ¼ cup chopped pecans

1. In a large skillet, combine the brown sugar and lemon juice. Cook over low heat, stirring frequently, for 2 minutes or until the sugar has melted. Stir in the wheat germ and oil, and cook, stirring frequently, for 9 minutes or until richly browned.

2. Stir in the pecans and cook for 1 minute. Cool to room temperature,

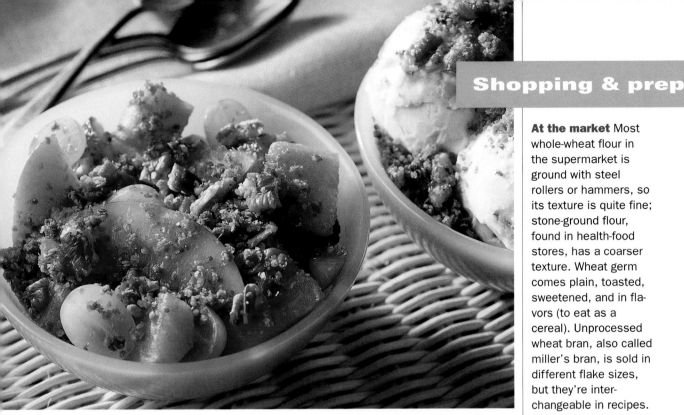

Crunchy Dessert Topping adds a sweet and crunchy fillip to frozen yogurt and sorbet.

At the market Most whole-wheat flour in the supermarket is ground with steel rollers or hammers, so its texture is quite fine; stone-ground flour, found in health-food stores, has a coarser texture. Wheat germ comes plain, toasted, sweetened, and in flavors (to eat as a cereal). Unprocessed wheat bran, also called miller's bran, is sold in different flake sizes, but they're interchangeable in recipes. Store all whole-wheat flour, wheat germ, and wheat bran in tightly covered containers in the refrigerator or freezer.

transfer to an airtight container, and store at room temperature for up to 3 days. Freeze for longer storage. Makes 2 cups/16 servings.

Per serving: Calories 85; Fiber 2g; Protein 3g; Total Fat 3g; Saturated Fat 0g; Cholesterol 0mg; Sodium 3mg

Banana Bran Muffins

**PREP: 15 MINUTES / COOK: 35 MINUTES
COOL: 10 MINUTES**

Tops as a fiber source, wheat bran has other nutritional benefits as well: It's a good source of niacin, iron, potassium, and magnesium. This recipe calls for more bran than flour—a healthy switch from the usual formula.

1½	cups unprocessed wheat bran
½	cup whole-wheat flour
1½	teaspoons baking soda
½	teaspoon salt
¼	cup vegetable oil
¼	cup packed light brown sugar
1	egg
1	egg white
1	cup low-fat (1.5%) buttermilk
1	banana, diced
½	cup crunchy bran nugget cereal

1. Preheat the oven to 400°F. Line a 2½-inch muffin tin with paper liners. On a baking sheet with sides, bake the bran for 15 minutes or until lightly toasted. Leave the oven on.

2. In a medium bowl, stir together the toasted bran, the flour, baking soda, and salt. In another medium bowl, with an electric mixer, beat the oil and sugar until well combined. Add the egg and egg white, 1 at a time, beating well after each addition. Alternately fold the flour mixture and the buttermilk into the egg mixture, beginning and ending with the flour mixture. Fold in the banana and cereal.

3. Spoon the batter into the prepared muffin cups and bake for 20 minutes or until a cake tester inserted in the center of a muffin comes out clean. Cool for 10 minutes in the pan on a rack, then transfer to the rack to cool completely. Serve warm or at room temperature. Makes 12.

Per muffin: Calories 133; Fiber 4g; Protein 4g; Total Fat 6g; Saturated Fat 1g; Cholesterol 19mg; Sodium 300mg

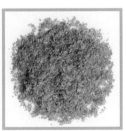

You can up your fiber intake by substituting unprocessed wheat bran for some of the flour in your favorite muffin and quick-bread recipes. You may need to add a little extra liquid, as bran absorbs more liquid than flour does.

Barley

*Cholesterol-lowering
soluble fiber is bar-
ley's biggest feature.
The plump, pearly
grains are also rich
in minerals and
B vitamins.*

Healthy Highlights

PER ½ CUP RAW	
Calories	326
Fiber	16g
Protein	12g
Total Fat	2.1g
Saturated Fat	0.4g
Cholesterol	0mg
Sodium	11mg

NUTRIENTS	
% Daily Value	
Thiamin	39%
Magnesium	31%
Copper	23%
Niacin	21%
Iron	17%
Zinc	17%
Riboflavin	15%
Vitamin B6	15%
Potassium	14%

Did you know? . . .
Barley contains the
same kind of soluble
fiber found in oats.
One study divided
subjects into two
groups: One of the
groups got daily
servings of oats,
while the other got
barley. The choles-
terol levels in both
groups dropped
about 5 percent.

Summery Barley-Vegetable Salad

PREP: 20 MINUTES / COOK: 10 MINUTES
*Lemon juice and mint make this a super-cool
supper. Let the salad stand a while before
serving so the grain can absorb the dressing.*

- 1½ cups quick-cooking barley
- ¾ teaspoon salt
- 1 tablespoon olive oil
- 1 yellow or red bell pepper, cut into ½-inch squares
- 1 zucchini or yellow summer squash, cut into ½-inch chunks
- 3 cloves garlic, minced
- ⅓ cup chopped fresh mint
- ¼ cup lemon juice
- ½ pound plum tomatoes (about 3), cut into thin wedges
- 1 cucumber, peeled, seeded, and cut into ¼-inch-thick slices
- ½ teaspoon black pepper
- 6 ounces mild goat cheese or feta cheese, crumbled

1. In a large saucepan, bring 3 cups of
water to a boil. Add the barley and
¼ teaspoon of the salt, and cook for
10 minutes or until tender. Drain well.

2. Meanwhile, in a large nonstick skillet, heat 2 teaspoons of the oil over
moderate heat. Add the bell pepper,
squash, garlic, and the remaining
½ teaspoon salt. Cook, stirring frequently, for 5 minutes or until the pepper is crisp-tender.

3. In a large bowl, whisk together the
mint, lemon juice, and the remaining

1 teaspoon oil. Add the barley, sautéed
vegetables, the tomatoes, cucumber, and
black pepper, tossing to combine. Add
the goat cheese and toss gently. Serve at
room temperature or lightly chilled.
Serves 4.

*Per serving: Calories 376; Fiber 7g;
Protein 16g; Total Fat 13g; Saturated Fat 7g;
Cholesterol 20mg; Sodium 582mg*

Old-Fashioned Mushroom-Barley Soup

PREP: 20 MINUTES / COOK: 1 HOUR
*The only thing "new-fashioned" about this
homey soup is the shiitake mushrooms, which
add a special depth of flavor. However, you
could make the soup with button mushrooms
alone (use a total of 1 pound).*

- 2 teaspoons olive oil
- 1 onion, finely chopped
- 2 cloves garlic, minced
- 2 carrots, halved lengthwise and thinly sliced
- ¾ pound button mushrooms, sliced
- ¼ pound shiitake mushrooms, trimmed and thinly sliced
- ½ cup pearled barley
- 1 cup chicken broth
- 1 cup no-salt-added tomato sauce
- ¾ teaspoon each ground ginger and salt
- ½ teaspoon pepper

1. In a large saucepan, heat the oil
over moderate heat. Add the onion and
garlic, and sauté for 5 minutes or until

tender. Add the carrots and cook, stirring frequently, for 4 minutes or until crisp-tender. Add the button and shiitake mushrooms, and cook, stirring frequently, for 5 minutes or until tender.

2. Stir in the barley, broth, 2 cups of water, the tomato sauce, ginger, salt, and pepper. Bring to a boil, reduce to a simmer, cover, and cook for 45 minutes or until the barley is tender. Serves 4.

Per serving: Calories 198; Fiber 8g; Protein 7g; Total Fat 4g; Saturated Fat 1g; Cholesterol 0mg; Sodium 707mg

Spiced Barley & Corn

PREP: 15 MINUTES / COOK: 55 MINUTES

You might guess by the flavorings—fresh ginger, cilantro, and garlic—that this dish has Indian roots. The technique of creating a seasoning paste, which is then sautéed, is also distinctly Indian. The blender whirls up the seasoning paste in seconds.

- 4 **scallions, thinly sliced**
- ½ **cup packed cilantro or flat-leaf parsley sprigs**
- 2 **tablespoons chopped fresh ginger**
- 3 **cloves garlic, peeled**
- 1 **tablespoon olive oil**
- 1 **green bell pepper, diced**
- 1 **cup pearled barley**
- 1 **cup chicken broth**
- 1 **cup canned no-salt-added tomatoes, chopped with their juice**
- ½ **teaspoon each ground coriander and salt**
- 1¼ **cups frozen corn kernels, thawed**

1. In a blender, combine the scallions, cilantro, ginger, garlic, and 3 tablespoons of water, and purée.

2. In a large saucepan, heat the oil over moderate heat. Add the bell pepper and sauté for 4 minutes or until crisp-tender. Add the scallion purée and sauté for 2 minutes. Add the barley, stirring to coat.

3. Add the broth, ½ cup of water, the tomatoes, coriander, and salt, and bring to a boil. Reduce to a simmer, cover, and cook for 45 minutes or until the barley is tender. Remove from the heat and stir in the corn. Serves 4.

Per serving: Calories 285; Fiber 10g; Protein 8g; Total Fat 5g; Saturated Fat 1g; Cholesterol 0mg; Sodium 555mg

At the market
Pearled (or pearl) barley is the most common type; it has been milled several times to completely remove the hull, leaving the grain pearly and smooth. Quick-cooking or instant barley is precooked by steaming, with no loss of nutritional value. Hulled barley retains its complete bran layer, while pot, or Scotch, barley has about half the bran left on the grain. Both Scotch and hulled barley take longer to cook than pearled barley.

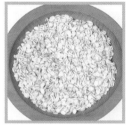

Quick-cooking barley, a real timesaver, is just as nutritious as regular pearled barley.

Basic cooking For pearled barley, use three times as much water as grain; for instant barley, use twice as much. Stir the barley into boiling water, cover, and simmer until tender. Pearled barley takes about 50 minutes; for quick-cooking barley, cook for 10 minutes, then let stand, covered, for 5 minutes.

Old-Fashioned Mushroom-Barley Soup brims with vegetables in a smooth tomato broth.

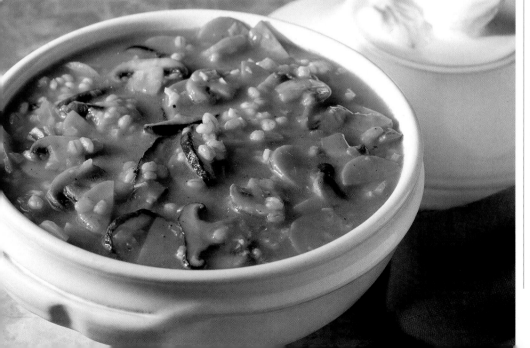

Buckwheat

Nutritional power
It's used as a grain, but buckwheat is actually the fruit of a rhubarb-like plant. Like true grains, buckwheat offers some B vitamins and iron.

Healthy Highlights

Roasted Buckwheat Groats
PER ¼ CUP RAW

Calories	142
Fiber	4.2g
Protein	5g
Total Fat	1.1g
Saturated Fat	0.2g
Cholesterol	0mg
Sodium	5mg

NUTRIENTS

	% Daily Value
Magnesium	23%
Copper	13%

Buckwheat Flour
PER ¼ CUP

Calories	101
Fiber	3.0g
Protein	4g
Total Fat	0.9g
Saturated Fat	0.2g
Cholesterol	0mg
Sodium	3mg

NUTRIENTS

	% Daily Value
Magnesium	19%

Did you know? . . .
Buckwheat contains more lysine (an essential amino acid) than do true grains.

Chicken & Soba Noodle Salad

PREP: 20 MINUTES / COOK: 15 MINUTES

Japanese soba noodles are chewy and robustly flavorful.

- ¾ cup chicken broth
- 2 cloves garlic, minced
- ½ teaspoon ground ginger
- ¼ teaspoon crushed red pepper flakes
- ¾ pound skinless, boneless chicken breasts
- 10 ounces soba noodles (buckwheat noodles)
- ½ pound green beans, halved lengthwise
- 2 carrots, cut into 2-inch matchsticks
- 2 tablespoons dark brown sugar
- 1 tablespoon lower-sodium soy sauce
- 1 tablespoon peanut or other vegetable oil
- 2 cups finely shredded cabbage

1. In a large skillet, bring the broth, garlic, ginger, and red pepper flakes to a boil over moderate heat. Reduce to a simmer, add the chicken, cover, and cook, turning the chicken over once, for 10 minutes or until the chicken is cooked through. Reserving the cooking liquid, transfer the chicken to a plate. When cool enough to handle, shred the chicken.

2. Meanwhile, in a large pot of boiling water, cook the noodles according to package directions until firm-tender. Add the green beans and carrots for the last 1 minute of cooking time; drain.

3. In a large bowl, whisk together the brown sugar, soy sauce, oil, and the reserved chicken cooking liquid. Add the shredded chicken, noodles, green beans, carrots, and cabbage, tossing to combine. Serve at room temperature or chilled. Serves 4.

Per serving: Calories 439; Fiber 6g; Protein 32g; Total Fat 5g; Saturated Fat 1g; Cholesterol 49mg; Sodium 989mg

Kasha Varnishkes with Caramelized Onions

PREP: 15 MINUTES / COOK: 50 MINUTES

This savory buckwheat-and-noodle combination is an old-fashioned dish.

- 1 tablespoon vegetable oil
- 4 cups thinly sliced onions
- 1 teaspoon sugar
- 1 teaspoon salt
- 1 cup kasha (buckwheat groats)
- 1 egg white
- 1 cup chicken broth
- ¼ teaspoon each dried sage and pepper
- 10 ounces bow-tie pasta

1. In a large nonstick skillet, heat the oil over moderate heat. Add the onions, sugar, and ¼ teaspoon of the salt, and cook, stirring occasionally, for 25 minutes or until the onions are golden brown and caramelized.

2. Meanwhile, in a medium bowl, combine the kasha and egg white until the kasha is well coated. Stir the kasha

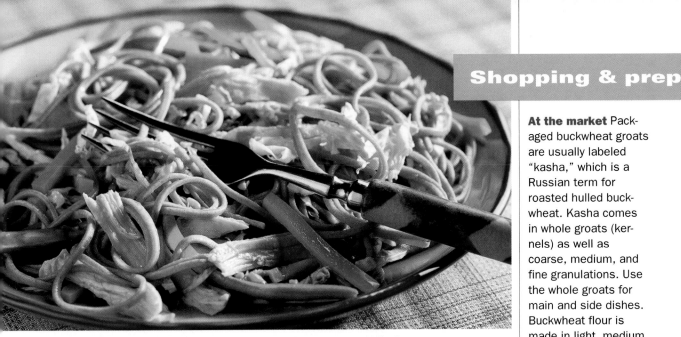

Chicken & Soba Noodle Salad is tossed with a tangy Asian-style dressing.

At the market Packaged buckwheat groats are usually labeled "kasha," which is a Russian term for roasted hulled buckwheat. Kasha comes in whole groats (kernels) as well as coarse, medium, and fine granulations. Use the whole groats for main and side dishes. Buckwheat flour is made in light, medium, and dark versions. The dark flour has the highest fiber content. Dried soba noodles are sold in many supermarkets; fresh soba noodles can sometimes be found in Asian markets.

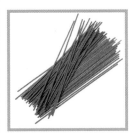

Soba noodles may be made from buckwheat flour alone, or from buckwheat and wheat flours.

Basic cooking Old-fashioned kasha recipes have you stir a whole egg into kasha before toasting it in a pan. You can reduce cholesterol by toasting the kasha with egg white instead, or toasting it in a dry pan. Stir constantly, though, as kasha can burn quickly.

into another large (ungreased) nonstick skillet and cook over moderate heat until the kasha is lightly toasted.

3. In a medium saucepan, bring the broth and 1 cup of water to a boil. Add the broth mixture to the kasha along with the sage, pepper, and the remaining ¾ teaspoon salt, and cook, stirring occasionally, for 20 minutes or until the kasha is tender but not mushy.

4. Meanwhile, in a large pot of boiling water, cook the pasta according to package directions until firm-tender. Drain and add to the kasha along with the onions. Cook until heated through. Serves 4.

Per serving: Calories 511; Fiber 10g; Protein 17g; Total Fat 6g; Saturated Fat 1g; Cholesterol 0mg; Sodium 841mg

Buckwheat Griddle Cakes

PREP: 10 MINUTES / COOK: 10 MINUTES

- 1 **cup low-fat (1.5%) buttermilk**
- 1 **egg yolk**
- 2 **tablespoons vegetable oil**
- 2 **egg whites**
- ¾ **cup buckwheat flour**
- ¼ **cup all-purpose flour**
- 1 **tablespoon light brown sugar**
- 1 **teaspoon baking powder**
- ½ **teaspoon each baking soda and salt**
- ¼ **cup honey**

1. In a small bowl, combine the buttermilk, egg yolk, and oil. In a separate bowl, beat the egg whites until stiff peaks form.

2. Preheat the oven to 250°F. In a medium bowl, combine the buckwheat flour, all-purpose flour, brown sugar, baking powder, baking soda, and salt. Stir the buttermilk mixture into the flour mixture. Fold in the egg whites.

3. Spray a large nonstick skillet with nonstick cooking spray and heat over moderate heat. Spoon the batter, a scant ¼ cup at a time, into the skillet. Cook for 2 minutes or until the pancakes are bubbly on one side, then turn them over and cook for 1 minute or until cooked through. Place on a baking sheet and keep warm in the oven while you prepare the remaining pancakes, re-spraying the pan with cooking spray (off the heat) for each batch.

4. Serve the pancakes drizzled with the honey. Serves 4.

Per serving: Calories 302; Fiber 3g; Protein 8g; Total Fat 11g; Saturated Fat 2g; Cholesterol 57mg; Sodium 615mg

Cornmeal

Nutritional power

Whole cornmeal is a good source of B vitamins and iron. Degerminated corn-meal is enriched with these nutrients to make up for their loss in processing.

Healthy Highlights

PER ½ CUP RAW	
Calories	253
Fiber	5.1g
Protein	6g
Total Fat	1.1g
Saturated Fat	0.2g
Cholesterol	0mg
Sodium	2mg

NUTRIENTS	
	% Daily Value
Thiamin	33%
Niacin	18%
Iron	17%
Riboflavin	16%

Did you know? . . .
The color of cornmeal (yellow or white) is determined by the type of corn used to make it. There's virtually no nutritional difference between the two types, except that yellow cornmeal contains minute amounts of beta carotene, alpha-carotene, lutein, and zeaxanthin—all disease-fighting carotenoids.

Mushroom-Topped Polenta

PREP: 15 MINUTES / COOK: 40 MINUTES

Polenta—Italian-style cornmeal mush—is as versatile as mashed potatoes. Here's a dressy way of serving it—topped with a garlicky tomato-mushroom sauce.

- ¾ cup yellow cornmeal
- 1 teaspoon salt
- 1 tablespoon olive oil
- 1 red onion, finely chopped
- 4 cloves garlic, minced
- 1 carrot, finely chopped
- ½ pound mushrooms, thinly sliced
- 2 cups canned no-salt-added tomatoes, chopped with their juice
- ¼ teaspoon dried rosemary, crumbled
- ⅛ teaspoon crushed red pepper flakes
- 3 tablespoons grated Parmesan cheese

1. Preheat the oven to 375°F. Spray an 8-inch square glass baking dish with nonstick cooking spray.

2. In a medium bowl, combine the cornmeal and 1 cup of cold water. In a large saucepan, bring 1½ cups of water to a boil. Reduce to a simmer, add ½ teaspoon of the salt and the corn-meal mixture. Cook, stirring constantly, for 5 minutes or until the mixture is thick and cooked through. Spoon the cornmeal mixture into the prepared baking dish and set aside.

3. In a large nonstick skillet, heat the oil over moderate heat. Add the onion and garlic, and sauté for 5 minutes or until the onion is tender. Add the carrot

and cook for 4 minutes or until tender. Add the mushrooms and cook, stirring occasionally, for 4 minutes or until ten-der. Add the tomatoes, rosemary, red pepper flakes, and the remaining ½ tea-spoon salt, and bring to a boil. Reduce to a simmer, cover, and cook for 5 min-utes or until the flavors have blended.

4. Pour the mushroom mixture over the cornmeal. Sprinkle with the Parmesan and bake for 15 minutes or until piping hot. Serves 4.

Per serving: Calories 211; Fiber 4g; Protein 7g; Total Fat 6g; Saturated Fat 1g; Cholesterol 3mg; Sodium 650mg

Lemon Poppy Seed Tea Bread

PREP: 10 MINUTES / COOK: 1 HOUR

- 2 tablespoons poppyseeds
- ¼ cup vegetable oil
- 2 tablespoons unsalted butter
- 1 cup sugar
- 1 egg
- 2 egg whites
- 1 tablespoon grated lemon zest
- 1 teaspoon baking soda
- 1 cup plain low-fat yogurt
- 1 cup yellow cornmeal
- 1 cup flour

1. Preheat the oven to 350°F. Place the poppyseeds in a small baking pan and bake for 5 minutes or until lightly toast-ed and crunchy. Spray an 8½ x 4½-inch loaf pan with nonstick cooking spray.

2. In a medium bowl, with an electric mixer, blend the oil, butter, and sugar. Add the whole egg and egg whites, one at a time, beating well after each addition. Beat in the lemon zest.

3. In a small bowl, stir the baking soda into the yogurt. Stir together the cornmeal and flour. Alternately fold the cornmeal mixture and the yogurt mixture into the egg mixture, beginning and ending with the cornmeal mixture. Fold in the poppyseeds.

4. Spoon the batter into the prepared pan and bake for 55 minutes or until a cake tester inserted in the center comes out clean. Cool for 10 minutes in the pan on a rack, then turn out onto the rack to cool completely. Serves 12.

Per serving: Calories 231; Fiber 1g; Protein 4g; Total Fat 8g; Saturated Fat 2g; Cholesterol 24mg; Sodium 134mg

Lemon Poppy Seed Tea Bread *The cornmeal gives it a distinctive texture.*

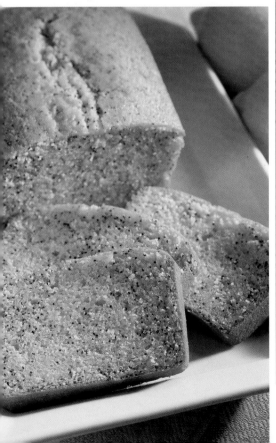

Corn Muffins with Fennel & Bacon

PREP: 10 MINUTES / COOK: 30 MINUTES
Serve these hearty muffins warm to accompany tomato soup or chili.

- 3 **ounces bacon, coarsely chopped**
  Vegetable oil (optional)
- ¼ **cup packed light brown sugar**
- 1 **egg**
- 1 **cup yellow cornmeal**
- 1 **cup flour**
- 1 **tablespoon baking powder**
- 1½ **teaspoons fennel seeds**
- ½ **teaspoon salt**
- 1 **cup low-fat (1%) milk**
- ½ **cup golden raisins**

1. In a small skillet, cook the bacon over low heat for 5 minutes or until it is crisp and has rendered its fat. Drain the bacon on paper towels. Pour the bacon fat into a measuring cup. If you don't have ¼ cup, add enough vegetable oil to make up the difference.

2. Preheat the oven to 400°F. Line a 2½-inch muffin tin with paper liners or spray with nonstick cooking spray. In a medium bowl, with an electric mixer, beat the bacon fat and brown sugar until well combined. Add the egg and beat until well combined.

3. In a small bowl, stir together the cornmeal, flour, baking powder, fennel seeds, and salt. Alternately fold the cornmeal mixture and the milk into the egg mixture, beginning and ending with the cornmeal mixture. Fold in the raisins and bacon.

4. Spoon the batter into the prepared muffin cups and bake for 25 minutes or until a cake tester inserted in the center of a muffin comes out clean. Cool for 10 minutes in the pan, then transfer the muffins to a rack to cool completely. Makes 12.

Per muffin: Calories 171; Fiber 1g; Protein 4g; Total Fat 5g; Saturated Fat 2g; Cholesterol 23mg; Sodium 280mg

At the market Cornmeal can be bought in several forms. Whole cornmeal includes both the bran and germ; stone-ground meal retains some of both components. (Both of these types of cornmeal should be kept in a tightly covered container in the refrigerator or freezer, as the oil in the germ can become rancid fairly quickly.) Degerminated meal lacks both the germ and bran, but it has a longer shelf life and is enriched to compensate for some of the lost nutrients.

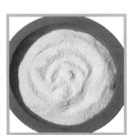

White cornmeal is available both whole and degerminated. It is traditionally favored in the South for such dishes as spoonbread, while Northerners have long preferred yellow cornmeal.

Oats

Nutritional power
High in protein and rich in iron and B vitamins, oats are also a renowned source of a type of soluble fiber that helps to lower blood cholesterol.

Healthy Highlights

PER ½ CUP RAW	
Calories	303
Fiber	8.3g
Protein	13g
Total Fat	5.4g
Saturated Fat	0.9g
Cholesterol	0mg
Sodium	2mg

NUTRIENTS

	% Daily Value
Manganese	192%
Thiamin	40%
Magnesium	35%
Copper	24%
Iron	22%
Zinc	21%
Folate	11%

Did you know? . . .
Although many foods contain soluble fiber, oats (like barley) contain beta glucan, a type of fiber particularly effective in lowering cholesterol.

One study compared oat bran with two cholesterol-lowering drugs, and found that the oat bran was just as effective —and far cheaper.

Granola Macaroons

PREP: 15 MINUTES / COOK: 25 MINUTES

For these cookies, you mix up your own granola rather than using commercial cereal, which can have up to 5 grams of fat per ounce.

- 2 cups old-fashioned rolled oats
- ½ cup chopped dried apples or raisins
- ⅓ cup sliced almonds (1¼ ounces)
- ½ cup granulated sugar
- ¼ cup packed light brown sugar
- ¼ teaspoon salt
- 3 egg whites
- 1 teaspoon vanilla extract

1. Preheat the oven to 350°F. Spray 2 baking sheets with nonstick cooking spray; set aside. Place the oats in a small baking pan and toast, stirring them occasionally, for 7 minutes or until lightly golden. Transfer to a large bowl and cool to room temperature.

2. Add the apples, almonds, granulated sugar, brown sugar, and salt, stirring to combine. Add the egg whites and vanilla, and mix until well combined.

3. With moistened hands, roll walnut-size pieces of dough into rounds and place them 1 inch apart on the prepared baking sheets. Flatten slightly and bake for 18 minutes or until golden brown and slightly firm, but not hard. Cool the cookies for 5 minutes on the pans, then transfer to a wire rack to cool completely. Makes 2½ dozen.

Per cookie: Calories 54; Fiber 1g; Protein 2g; Total Fat 1g; Saturated Fat 0g; Cholesterol 0mg; Sodium 26mg

Cream of Oats Brûlée

PREP: 5 MINUTES / COOK: 10 MINUTES

Here is oatmeal's elegant cousin. Because the oats are finely ground in a food processor, the texture of this hot cereal is smooth and creamy. As a delicious finishing touch, the cream of oats is topped with brown sugar and butter, and broiled.

- 2 cups old-fashioned rolled oats
- 1 can (12 ounces) evaporated skimmed milk
- 1¾ cups low-fat (1%) milk
- 3 tablespoons granulated sugar
- ½ teaspoon each salt and cinnamon
- ½ cup raisins
- 4 teaspoons light brown sugar
- 2 teaspoons unsalted butter

1. In a food processor, pulse the oats on and off until finely ground. In a medium saucepan, bring the evaporated milk, low-fat milk, granulated sugar, salt, and cinnamon to a boil over moderate heat. Reduce to a simmer, stir in the oats, and cook, stirring occasionally, for 5 minutes or until the cereal is thick and creamy. Remove from the heat and stir in the raisins.

2. Preheat the broiler. Transfer the oatmeal to an 8-inch square broiler-proof pan. Sprinkle the top of the cereal with the brown sugar and dot with the butter. Broil 6 inches from the heat for 2 minutes or until the sugar is melted. Cool slightly and serve. Serves 4.

Per serving: Calories 401; Fiber 5g; Protein 18g; Total Fat 6g; Saturated Fat 3g; Cholesterol 13mg; Sodium 443mg

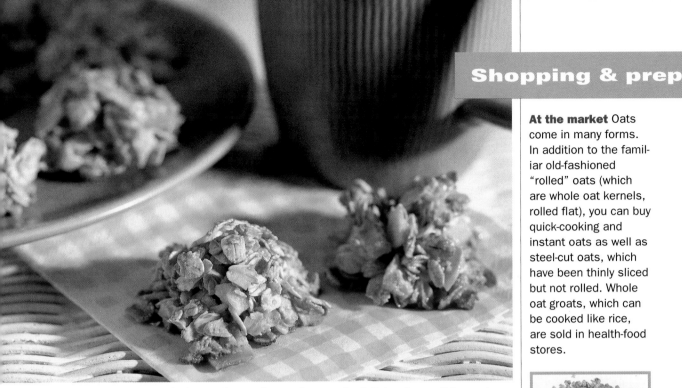

Granola Macaroons With the goodness of oats, these make deliciously sensible snacks.

Double-Oat Batter Bread

PREP: 15 MINUTES / RISE: 1 HOUR
30 MINUTES / COOK: 1 HOUR

These satisfying loaves are made with a combination of oat "flour" (you grind it in a food processor) and regular flour. Because oats have no gluten, they require some added flour to enable the dough to rise.

½	**cup pecans**
4	**cups old-fashioned rolled oats**
1	**package (¼ ounce) active dry yeast**
2¼	**cups lukewarm (105° to 115°F) water**
1	**teaspoon sugar**
2½	**cups flour**
⅓	**cup molasses**
1	**tablespoon vegetable oil**
2	**teaspoons salt**

1. Preheat the oven to 350°F. Place the pecans in a small baking pan and bake for 7 minutes or until crisp and fragrant. When the pecans are cool enough to handle, coarsely chop.

2. At the same time, on a baking sheet, toast the oats, stirring occasionally, for 7 minutes or until lightly browned, crisp, and fragrant. (Turn the oven off.) Place 2 cups of the oats in a food processor and process until the consistency of flour.

3. In a large bowl, combine the yeast, ¼ cup of the water, and the sugar. Let stand for 5 minutes or until foamy. Stir in the remaining 2 cups warm water, the flour, molasses, oil, and salt. Stir in the oat "flour," rolled oats, and pecans. With a wooden spoon, stir well for 3 minutes. Cover with plastic wrap and let stand in a warm draftfree spot for 1 hour or until doubled in bulk.

4. Spray two 8½ x 4½-inch loaf pans with nonstick cooking spray. Punch the dough down and transfer to the prepared pans. Cover with plastic wrap and let stand in a warm draftfree spot for 30 minutes or until doubled in bulk.

5. Preheat the oven to 350°F. Bake the bread for 1 hour or until golden brown and crusty. Cool for 10 minutes in the pans on a rack, then transfer to the rack to cool completely. Makes 2 loaves/16 servings.

Per serving: Calories 200; Fiber 3g; Protein 6g; Total Fat 5g; Saturated Fat 1g; Cholesterol 0mg; Sodium 279mg

At the market Oats come in many forms. In addition to the familiar old-fashioned "rolled" oats (which are whole oat kernels, rolled flat), you can buy quick-cooking and instant oats as well as steel-cut oats, which have been thinly sliced but not rolled. Whole oat groats, which can be cooked like rice, are sold in health-food stores.

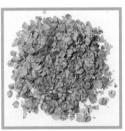

Quick-cooking oats, which have been sliced before rolling, can be substituted for old-fashioned oats in many recipes. However, the finished product may have less textural "character."

Basic cooking For basic oatmeal, stir ½ cup old-fashioned or quick oats into 1 cup boiling water in a small saucepan. Simmer old-fashioned oats for 5 minutes; cook quick oats for 1 minute, then cover and let stand for a few minutes, until the oatmeal is the desired consistency. Cook ½ cup steel-cut oats in 2 cups boiling water for 20 to 30 minutes.

Rice

Nutritional power
Half the world's people rely on rice as their staple starch. Rice offers B vitamins and minerals; its protein features a good balance of amino acids.

Healthy Highlights

Long-Grain White Rice
PER 1 CUP COOKED

Calories	205
Fiber	0.6g
Protein	4g
Total Fat	0.4g
Saturated Fat	0.1g
Cholesterol	0mg
Sodium	2mg

NUTRIENTS

	% Daily Value
Manganese	37%
Thiamin	17%
Iron	11%
Niacin	12%

Did you know? . . .
When rice kernels are milled to produce white rice, the bran and germ are polished away. But in the United States, white rice is enriched with thiamin, niacin, and iron to compensate for some of the nutrients that are lost in the process.

Pork Fried Rice

PREP: 10 MINUTES / COOK: 20 MINUTES

Here's how to turn leftover rice into a hearty main dish. You'll get the best results if the rice is cool; if you cook a fresh pot of rice for this dish, spread it out on a platter and quick-chill it in the freezer.

- 1 tablespoon cornstarch
- 2 teaspoons lower-sodium soy sauce
- ¾ pound well-trimmed pork tenderloin, cut into ½-inch-wide strips
- 1 tablespoon vegetable oil
- 1 red bell pepper, cut into ½-inch squares
- 1 large carrot, thinly sliced
- 3 scallions, thinly sliced
- 1 tablespoon minced fresh ginger
- 2 cloves garlic, minced
- ¾ teaspoon salt
- 3 cups Napa cabbage, cut into ½ x 2-inch strips
- 4 cups cooked brown or white rice
- 2 tablespoons rice vinegar
- 1 teaspoon sesame oil

1. In a medium bowl, combine the cornstarch and soy sauce. Add the pork and toss well. In a large nonstick skillet, heat the oil over moderately high heat. Add the pork and stir-fry for 5 minutes or until lightly browned. With a slotted spoon, transfer the pork to a plate.

2. Add the bell pepper, carrot, scallions, ginger, garlic, and salt, and stir-fry for 3 minutes or until the carrot is crisp-tender. Add the Napa cabbage and stir-fry for 2 minutes or until the cabbage is crisp-tender.

3. Add the rice and cook, stirring, for 5 minutes or until the rice is lightly browned. Return the pork to the pan and cook for 2 minutes or until heated through. Add the vinegar and sesame oil, tossing to combine. Serves 4.

Per serving: Calories 400; Fiber 5g; Protein 24g; Total Fat 9g; Saturated Fat 2g; Cholesterol 55mg; Sodium 581mg

Baked Chicken & Rice

PREP: 15 MINUTES / COOK: 40 MINUTES

- 1 tablespoon olive oil
- 8 skinless, bone-in chicken thighs (2½ pounds total)
- 1 onion, finely chopped
- 4 cloves garlic, minced
- 1 pound mushrooms, quartered
- 1¼ cups rice
- 1¼ cups chicken broth
- ½ teaspoon each crumbled dried rosemary and salt
- ¼ teaspoon pepper
- 1 cup frozen peas

1. Preheat the oven to 350°F. In a large skillet, heat the oil over moderate heat. Add the chicken and cook for 4 minutes or until lightly browned on both sides. Remove and set aside.

2. Add the onion and garlic to the skillet and cook, stirring occasionally, for 5 minutes or until soft. Add the mushrooms and cook for 3 minutes. Add the rice, stirring to coat. Add the broth, 1½ cups of water, the rosemary, salt, and pepper, and bring to a boil. Stir in the peas.

3. Pour the rice mixture into a 9 x 13-inch glass baking dish. Place the chicken on top, cover with foil, and bake for 25 to 30 minutes, or until the chicken is cooked through and the rice is tender. Serves 4.

Per serving: Calories 573; Fiber 4g; Protein 50g; Total Fat 13g; Saturated Fat 3g; Cholesterol 172mg; Sodium 830mg

Indian Biryani

PREP: 10 MINUTES / COOK: 30 MINUTES

Basmati is an aromatic rice grown in India and Pakistan. American-grown Texmati, which is less expensive, can be used instead.

- **1 tablespoon vegetable oil**
- **½ teaspoon each cinnamon, ground cardamom, and turmeric**
- **1 pinch of ground cloves**
- **1 onion, finely chopped**
- **1 cup basmati rice, well rinsed**
- **2 tablespoons plain low-fat yogurt**
- **¾ teaspoon salt**
- **½ cup golden raisins**
- **¼ cup coarsely chopped pistachios**

1. Preheat the oven to 350°F. In a small Dutch oven or flameproof casserole, heat the oil over moderate heat. Add the cinnamon, cardamom, turmeric, and cloves, and cook for 30 seconds or until the spices are fragrant. Add the onion and sauté for 7 minutes or until tender.

2. Stir in the rice, yogurt, 2½ cups of water, and the salt, and bring to a boil. Cover and bake for 25 minutes or until the rice is tender. Stir in the raisins and pistachios. Serves 4.

Per serving: Calories 308; Fiber 3g; Protein 8g; Total Fat 8g; Saturated Fat 1g; Cholesterol 0mg; Sodium 441mg

At the market In addition to long-grain brown and white rice, try medium- and short-grain types such as Arborio (see photo below), which cook up softer and stickier. Converted rice is specially treated to conserve nutrients. Quick-cooking rice is precooked. Fragrant rices, such as basmati, Texmati, Wehani, jasmine, and wild pecan rice, have a delicately sweet, nutlike aroma and flavor.

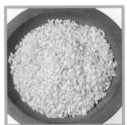

Plump and pearly grains of Italian Arborio rice are used to make traditional creamy risottos (see recipe, next page).

Basic cooking Add the rice to boiling water (use about twice as much water as rice), cover, and cook for 15 to 20 minutes (white rice) or 40 minutes (brown). You can add more boiling water if the water is absorbed before the rice is done, but be quick about re-covering the pot.

Pork Fried Rice *This favorite Chinese-restaurant dish makes an appealing centerpiece for an informal supper. A bounty of colorful vegetables rounds out the dish.*

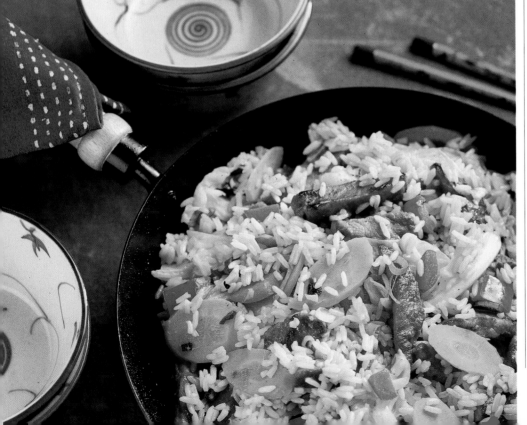

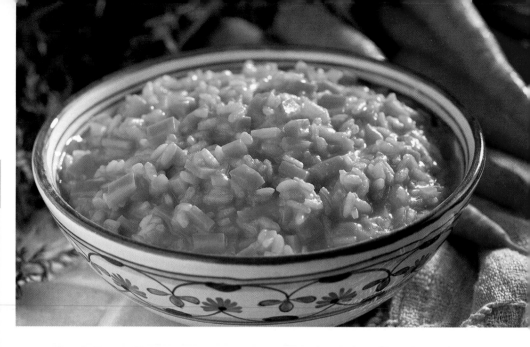

Golden Risotto with Carrots is gloriously colorful and delightfully creamy.

Healthy Highlights

Long-Grain Brown Rice
PER 1 CUP COOKED

Calories	216
Fiber	3.5g
Protein	5g
Total Fat	1.8g
Saturated Fat	0.4g
Cholesterol	0mg
Sodium	10mg

NUTRIENTS

	% Daily Value
Manganese	88%
Magnesium	21%
Thiamin	13%
Niacin	15%
Vitamin B6	14%
Copper	10%

Did you know? . . .
The main advantage of brown rice over white is that it retains its bran, which gives brown rice a superior fiber content.

Soaking brown rice overnight can cut cooking time in half. The key to conserving the B vitamins is to soak the rice in the measured amount of cold water, and then to cook the rice in the same water.

People with multiple food allergies are rarely allergic to rice.

Golden Risotto with Carrots
PREP: 15 MINUTES / COOK: 35 MINUTES

Carrot juice replaces some of the wine here, blessing the risotto with ample beta carotene.

- 2 teaspoons olive oil
- 1 small onion, finely chopped
- 2 large carrots, cut into ¼-inch dice
- 1 cup Arborio rice
- ½ cup dry white wine
- 1½ cups chicken broth
- 1 cup carrot juice
- ¼ teaspoon salt
- ¼ cup grated Parmesan cheese
- ¼ teaspoon pepper

1. In a medium nonstick saucepan, heat the oil over moderate heat. Add the onion and sauté for 5 minutes or until tender. Add the carrots and sauté for 4 minutes or until crisp-tender. Add the rice, stirring to coat.

2. Add the wine and cook, stirring occasionally, for 2 minutes or until evaporated by half. In a medium bowl, combine the broth, carrot juice, ½ cup of water, and the salt. Add 1½ cups of the broth mixture to the rice and cook, stirring, until absorbed. Add ¾ cup of the broth mixture and cook, stirring, until absorbed. Then add the remaining ¾ cup broth mixture and stir until absorbed. (The total time will be about 20 minutes.)

3. Remove from the heat. Stir in the Parmesan and pepper. Serves 4.

Per serving: Calories 308; Fiber 3g; Protein 7g; Total Fat 5g; Saturated Fat 2g; Cholesterol 4mg; Sodium 661mg

Shrimp Jambalaya
PREP: 25 MINUTES / COOK: 30 MINUTES

- 1 tablespoon olive oil
- 5 scallions, thinly sliced
- 3 cloves garlic, minced
- 1 stalk celery, thinly sliced
- 1 green bell pepper, cut into ½-inch squares
- 1 red bell pepper, cut into ½-inch squares
- 4 ounces fresh chorizo sausage, thinly sliced
- 1¼ cups rice
- 1 cup chicken broth
- ½ teaspoon each dried thyme, salt, and black pepper
- 1 pound medium shrimp, peeled and deveined

1. In a large saucepan, heat the oil over moderate heat. Add the scallions and garlic, and sauté for 1 minute or until soft. Add the celery and bell peppers, and sauté for 5 minutes or until the peppers are crisp-tender. Stir in the chorizo.

2. Add the rice, stirring to coat. Add the broth, 1¾ cups of water, the thyme, salt, and black pepper, and bring to a boil. Reduce to a simmer, cover, and cook for 17 minutes or until the rice is tender. Stir in the shrimp, cover, and cook for 3 to 4 minutes or until the shrimp are firm and pink. Serves 4.

Per serving: Calories 493; Fiber 2g; Protein 31g; Total Fat 17g; Saturated Fat 5g; Cholesterol 165mg; Sodium 1037mg

Italian Rice & Cheese Torte

PREP: 15 MINUTES
COOK: 1 HOUR 5 MINUTES

With three kinds of cheese, this rice "cake" provides 222mg of calcium per serving.

- 1½   **cups rice**
- 4   **cloves garlic, minced**
- ⅓   **cup sun-dried tomato halves (not oil-packed), chopped**
- ½   **teaspoon salt**
- ¾   **cup chopped fresh basil**
- 4   **ounces shredded Fontina cheese**
- 4   **ounces shredded part-skim mozzarella**
- 3   **tablespoons grated Parmesan cheese**
- 3   **egg whites, lightly beaten**

1. In a medium saucepan, bring 3¼ cups of water to a boil. Add the rice, garlic, sun-dried tomatoes, and salt. Reduce to a simmer, cover, and cook for 17 minutes or until the rice is tender. Transfer the rice to a large bowl.

2. Preheat the oven to 400°F. Spray an 8½-inch springform pan with nonstick cooking spray. Stir the basil, Fontina, mozzarella, and Parmesan into the rice until well combined. Stir in the egg whites. Transfer to the prepared pan, smoothing the top. Cover with foil and bake for 20 minutes. Uncover and bake for 25 minutes or until the rice is set. Remove the sides of the pan, cut into wedges, and serve hot or at room temperature. Serves 8.

Per serving: Calories 248; Fiber 1g; Protein 13g; Total Fat 8g; Saturated Fat 5g; Cholesterol 26mg; Sodium 377mg

Lemony Rice Salad

Toss 2 cups cooked rice with 1 large diced tomato, 1 cup thawed frozen peas, 2 sliced scallions, 2 tbsp. light mayonnaise, 1 tbsp. lemon juice, and ½ tsp. grated lemon zest. Pack mixture into custard cups sprayed with nonstick spray. Chill. Unmold to serve. Serves 4. *[Cal 204; Fat 4g; Sod 107mg]*

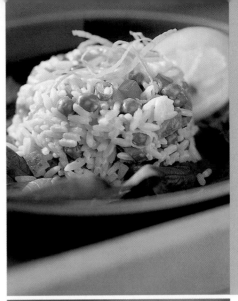

Rice & Beans

In medium saucepan, cook 1 small chopped onion, 1 diced green bell pepper, and 4 cloves minced garlic in 1 tbsp. olive oil until soft. Add ⅔ cup rice, 1½ cups chicken broth, ¼ tsp. oregano, and ¼ tsp. black pepper. Cover and cook 17 minutes or until tender. Add 19-oz. can pinto beans, rinsed and drained, and cook until heated through. Serves 4. *[Cal 248; Fat 5g; Sod 615mg]*

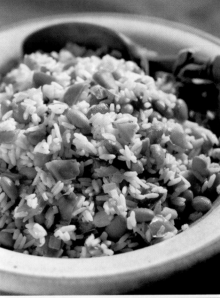

Spicy Tomato-Rice Soup

In large saucepan, combine 14½-oz. can no-salt-added stewed tomatoes, 1 cup chicken broth, 1 cup water, 2 tbsp. tomato paste, ¾ tsp. ground ginger, ½ tsp. salt, and ¼ tsp. cayenne. Bring to a boil. Stir in 2 cups cooked rice and heat through. Serves 4. *[Cal 174; Fat 1g; Sod 621mg]*

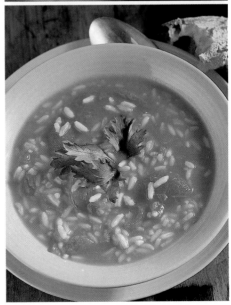

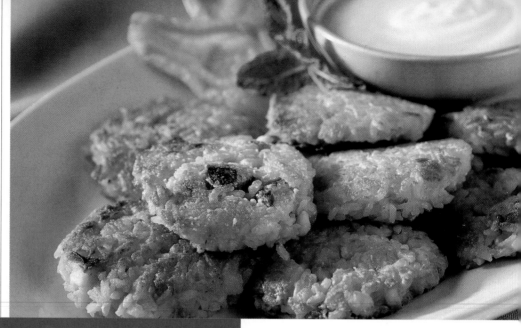

Sweet Rice Cakes
Surprise the family with a novel dessert: Plump little rice patties served with a sweet yogurt sauce.

Did you know? . . .
It's not necessary or desirable to wash domestic packaged rice before or after you cook it; doing so will rinse away vitamins and minerals.

Washing rice before cooking it, or rinsing it afterward, will wash away nutrients.

Several studies have shown rice bran to lower blood cholesterol. It's believed that the oil found in the rice germ (which ends up in the bran when rice is milled) is the key component. Brown rice includes some of the germ, but pure rice bran is a far more concentrated source. You can sprinkle rice bran over your breakfast cereal or add it to baked goods.

Converted rice is white rice that has been steamed under pressure to force the nutrients deeper into the grain so that they are not lost when the rice is milled. It takes slightly longer to cook than regular white rice.

Sweet Rice Cakes

PREP: 15 MINUTES / COOK: 10 MINUTES
These tender pancakes are dotted with fruit and pine nuts. You can make them with white rice or brown, plain or aromatic.

- 1 **cup plain low-fat yogurt**
- ⅔ **cup low-fat (1%) milk**
- ⅓ **cup plus 1 tablespoon sugar**
- ½ **cup plus 2 tablespoons flour**
- 3 **cups cooked rice**
- ½ **cup mixed dried fruit, chopped**
- 2 **tablespoons pine nuts, toasted**
- 1 **teaspoon vanilla extract**
- ¼ **teaspoon salt**
- 4 **teaspoons vegetable oil**
- 2 **teaspoons unsalted butter**

1. Place the yogurt in a fine-meshed sieve and let drain while you prepare the rice patties.

2. In a medium saucepan, whisk the milk and ⅓ cup of the sugar into 2 tablespoons of the flour and cook over moderate heat, stirring, until combined. Transfer to a medium bowl and stir in the rice, fruit, pine nuts, vanilla, and salt. Shape into 8 patties.

3. Dredge the patties in the remaining ½ cup flour, shaking off the excess. In a large nonstick skillet, heat the oil

and butter over moderate heat until the butter has melted. Add the patties and cook for 3 minutes per side or until the rice cakes are golden brown and heated through.

4. Stir the remaining 1 tablespoon sugar into the yogurt and serve with the rice cakes. Serves 4.

Per serving: Calories 528; Fiber 3g; Protein 12g; Total Fat 11g; Saturated Fat 3g; Cholesterol 10mg; Sodium 203mg

Southern Rice Bread

PREP: 10 MINUTES / COOK: 20 MINUTES
This is traditionally made with white rice, but brown rice is fine, too. Serve the bread fresh and hot, with preserves or fruit butter.

- 1 **cup flour**
- 2 **tablespoons white or yellow cornmeal**
- ½ **teaspoon each salt, baking powder, and baking soda**
- 1 **cup cooked white or brown rice**
- ½ **cup low-fat (1.5%) buttermilk**
- ¼ **cup reduced-fat sour cream**
- 1 **egg**

1. Preheat the oven to 425°F. Spray an 8-inch cast-iron skillet or metal cake pan with nonstick cooking spray and place in the oven to preheat.

2. In a small bowl, stir together the flour, cornmeal, salt, baking powder, and baking soda. In a medium bowl, mash the rice with a potato masher until almost smooth. Stir in the buttermilk, sour cream, and egg until well combined. Fold in the flour mixture.

3. Pour the batter into the hot pan and bake for 20 minutes or until lightly golden and a cake tester inserted in the center comes out clean. Serves 4.

Per serving: Calories 256; Fiber 1g; Protein 9g; Total Fat 5g; Saturated Fat 2g; Cholesterol 60mg; Sodium 532mg

---

Cherry-Almond Rice Pudding

PREP: 10 MINUTES / COOK: 40 MINUTES
CHILL: 2 HOURS

- 1 cup rice
- ½ teaspoon salt
- 1 can (12 ounces) evaporated skimmed milk
- ⅓ cup packed light brown sugar
- ½ teaspoon grated orange zest
- ½ cup low-fat (1%) milk
- ½ teaspoon vanilla extract
- ⅛ teaspoon almond extract
- ½ cup dried cherries, sweetened dried cranberries, or raisins
- ¼ cup slivered almonds, toasted

1. In a medium saucepan, bring 2¼ cups of water to a boil. Add the rice and salt, reduce to a simmer, cover, and cook for 17 minutes or until the rice is tender.

2. Add the evaporated milk, brown sugar, and orange zest; cover and cook for 10 minutes. Uncover and cook, stirring frequently, for 10 minutes or until the rice is very creamy and most of the liquid has been absorbed.

3. Stir in the milk, vanilla, and almond extract, and remove from the heat. Cool to room temperature, stir in the cherries and almonds, and refrigerate for 2 hours or until chilled. Serves 4.

Per serving: Calories 419; Fiber 1g; Protein 13g; Total Fat 5g; Saturated Fat 1g; Cholesterol 5mg; Sodium 410mg

Green Rice In medium saucepan, sauté 4 sliced scallions and 2 cloves minced garlic in 1 tbsp. olive oil until tender. Add 1 cup rice, 2¼ cups water, and ½ tsp. salt, and cook until tender. Stir in ½ cup chopped cilantro or parsley. Serves 4. *[Cal 206; Fat 4g; Sod 279mg]*

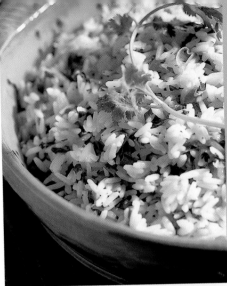

Rice Frittata In 9-inch broilerproof skillet, heat 1 tbsp. olive oil over moderately low heat. In large bowl, combine 2 cups cooked rice, 4 egg whites, 3 eggs, ⅓ cup grated Parmesan cheese, ½ tsp. salt, and ¼ tsp. pepper. Pour into pan and sprinkle with ⅓ cup diced roasted red pepper. Cook until bottom is set. Broil for 2 to 3 minutes to brown top. Serves 4. *[Cal 269; Fat 9g; Sod 524mg]*

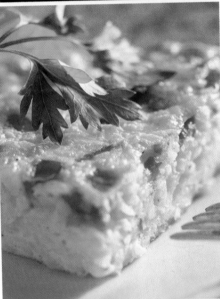

Brown Rice & Nut Pilaf In medium saucepan, cook 1 large chopped onion and 3 cloves minced garlic in 1 tbsp. olive oil until soft. Add 1 cup brown rice, 1¼ cups chicken broth, 1¼ cups water, ½ tsp. salt, and ¼ tsp. rosemary. Bring to a boil. Cover and simmer 45 minutes or until tender. Stir in ¼ cup toasted slivered almonds. Serves 4. *[Cal 284; Fat 10g; Sod 608mg]*

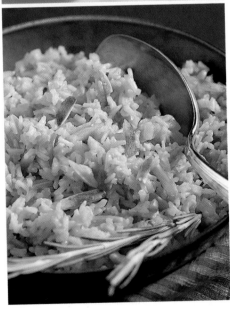

Wild rice

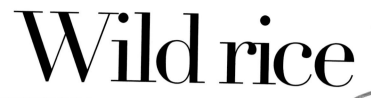

Nutritional power

Not a true grain, but the seed of a wild grass, wild rice supplies more protein, potassium, and B vitamins than brown rice—and it's lower in calories.

Healthy Highlights

PER 1 CUP COOKED	
Calories	166
Fiber	3.0g
Protein	7g
Total Fat	0.6g
Saturated Fat	0.1g
Cholesterol	0mg
Sodium	5mg

NUTRIENTS	
	% Daily Value
Manganese	23%
Zinc	15%
Magnesium	13%
Folate	11%
Niacin	11%
Vitamin B6	11%
Copper	10%

Did you know? . . .
Wild rice is a very good source of zinc, which might be called the "food-lover's mineral," because it keeps your sense of taste working properly. In addition, some studies have shown that zinc (in the form of lozenges) helps fight the common cold.

Wild Rice-Brown Rice Pilaf

PREP: 5 MINUTES / COOK: 55 MINUTES

Wild rice is relatively expensive (although the fact that it quadruples in volume when cooked is a saving grace). Wild rice is often cooked along with white or brown rice to make this luxury ingredient go further.

- 2 teaspoons vegetable oil
- 1 large onion, finely chopped
- ¾ cup wild rice (about 4 ounces)
- ½ cup brown rice
- 1½ cups chicken broth
- ½ teaspoon dried sage
- ¼ teaspoon each salt and pepper
- ¼ cup grated Parmesan cheese
- 1 cup frozen peas, thawed
- ¼ cup chopped cashews

1. In a medium saucepan, heat the oil over moderate heat. Add the onion and sauté for 5 minutes or until crisp-tender. Add the wild rice and brown rice, stirring to combine. Stir in the broth, 2 cups of water, the sage, salt, and pepper. Bring to a boil, reduce to a simmer, cover, and cook for 45 minutes or until the rice is tender.

2. Stir in the Parmesan, peas, and cashews. Serves 6.

Per serving: Calories 225; Fiber 3g; Protein 8g; Total Fat 6g; Saturated Fat 2g; Cholesterol 3mg; Sodium 452mg

Wild Rice & Pecan Stuffing

PREP: 10 MINUTES / COOK: 1 HOUR

This sophisticated "stuffing," cooked in a casserole in the oven, is a dressy accompaniment to any kind of poultry, from game hens to turkey. The pecans and water chestnuts are added at the last minute so that they keep their crunch.

- 2 teaspoons vegetable oil
- 1 large onion, finely chopped
- 3 cloves garlic, minced
- 1 carrot, halved lengthwise and thinly sliced
- 1 stalk celery, halved lengthwise and thinly sliced
- 1 cup wild rice (5¼ ounces)
- 1 cup chicken broth
- ¾ teaspoon salt
- ½ teaspoon each crumbled dried rosemary and pepper
- 1 cup canned sliced water chestnuts
- ⅓ cup chopped pecans

1. Preheat the oven to 350°F. In a Dutch oven or flameproof casserole, heat the oil over moderate heat. Add the onion and garlic, and sauté for 5 minutes or until soft. Add the carrot and celery, and sauté for 4 minutes or until the carrot is crisp-tender.

2. Stir in the wild rice, broth, 2 cups of water, the salt, rosemary, and pepper. Bring to a boil. Cover, transfer to the oven, and bake for 50 minutes or until the wild rice is tender. Stir in the water chestnuts and pecans. Serves 6.

Per serving: Calories 184; Fiber 4g; Protein 5g; Total Fat 6g; Saturated Fat 1g; Cholesterol 0mg; Sodium 483mg

Wild Rice Salad

PREP: **10** MINUTES / COOK: **45** MINUTES

A Granny Smith apple is just one option here; feel free to use another firm, crisp apple, such as Macoun, Winesap, or Empire.

- **1 cup wild rice (5¼ ounces)**
- **½ teaspoon each dried thyme and salt**
- **3 tablespoons sherry wine vinegar or cider vinegar**
- **1 tablespoon olive oil**
- **2 teaspoons Dijon mustard**
- **6 ounces smoked turkey, cut into ½-inch cubes**

- **2 cups cubed plum tomatoes**
- **1 Granny Smith apple, cut into ½-inch chunks**
- **1 cucumber, peeled, halved lengthwise, seeded, and cut into ¼-inch-thick slices**

1. Bring 3 cups of water to a boil. Add the wild rice, thyme, and ¼ teaspoon of the salt. Reduce to a simmer, cover, and cook for 45 minutes or until the wild rice is tender. Drain well.

2. Meanwhile, in a large bowl, whisk together the vinegar, oil, mustard, and the remaining ¼ teaspoon salt. Add the wild rice, tossing to coat. Add the turkey, tomatoes, apple, and cucumber, and toss again. Serve at room temperature or chilled. Serves 4.

Per serving: Calories 262; Fiber 4g; Protein 15g; Total Fat 6g; Saturated Fat 1g; Cholesterol 22mg; Sodium 794mg

At the market Wild rice is sold at most supermarkets; it is also available at gourmet shops and by mail order from growers.

Prep Unlike most packaged rice, wild rice must be thoroughly rinsed before cooking to eliminate any chaff or debris that may remain after the rice is hulled. (Wild rice is not milled like regular rice.)

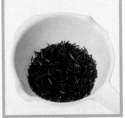

Place wild rice in a colander or strainer and rinse it under running water until the water runs clear.

Basic cooking Use a 1-to-3 ratio of rice to water. For 1 cup of raw rice (which will yield about 4 cups cooked), bring 3 cups of water to a boil. Stir in the rice, reduce the heat, and simmer, covered, for 45 minutes, or until the rice is tender and most of the water has been absorbed.

Wild Rice Salad *Half portions of this autumnal salad could be served as a first course.*

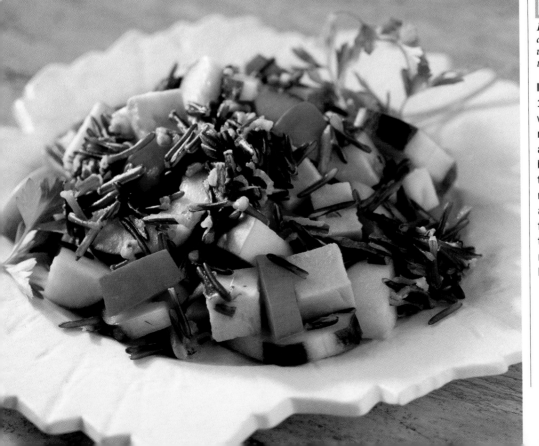

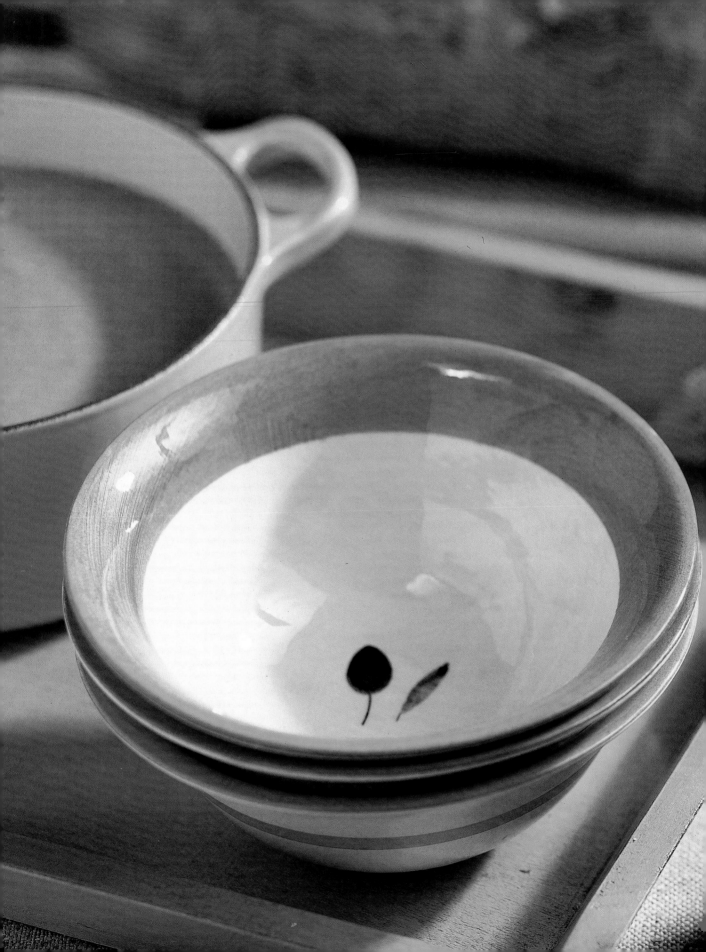

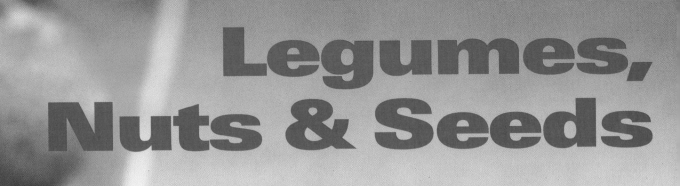

Legumes, Nuts & Seeds

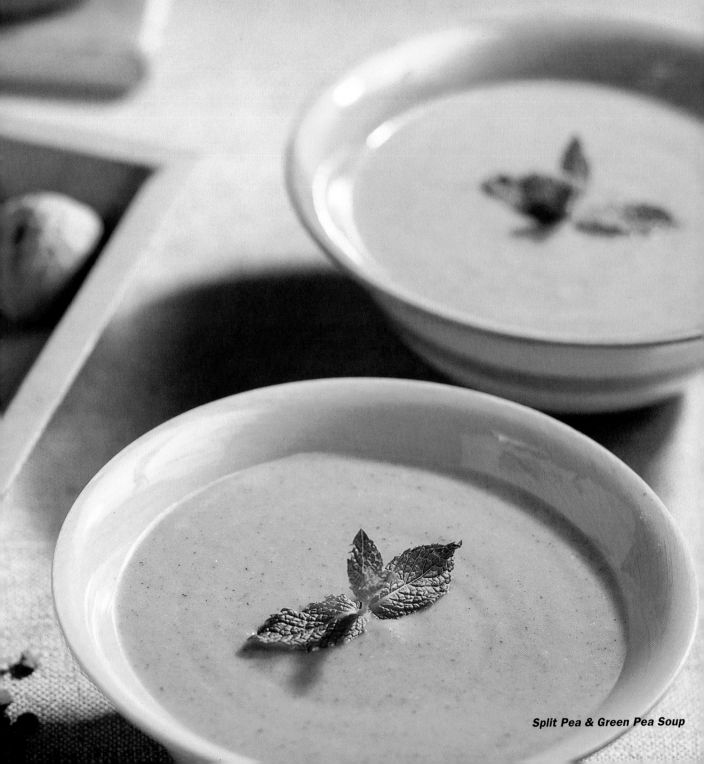

Split Pea & Green Pea Soup

Beans

Nutritional power
The unbeatable bean is a great low-fat, high-fiber protein source that's rich in folate (and other B vitamins) as well as minerals, including iron and potassium.

Healthy Highlights

Pinto Beans

PER 1 CUP COOKED	
Calories	234
Fiber	14.7g
Protein	14g
Total Fat	0.9g
Saturated Fat	0.2g
Cholesterol	0mg
Sodium	3mg

NUTRIENTS

	% Daily Value
Folate	74%
Manganese	48%
Potassium	27%
Magnesium	24%
Copper	22%
Iron	22%
Thiamin	21%
Vitamin B6	14%
Zinc	12%

Did you know? . . .
Beans provide substantial amounts of both insoluble fiber (the kind that helps prevent colon cancer) and soluble fiber (which helps lower blood cholesterol, thereby helping to prevent heart disease and stroke).

Bean & Cheese Burritos

PREP: 10 MINUTES / COOK: 20 MINUTES
Some of the beans are mashed to give the filling a thick, meaty texture.

- 8 flour tortillas (8-inch diameter)
- 2 teaspoons vegetable oil
- 3 scallions, thinly sliced
- 2 cloves garlic, minced
- 1 pickled jalapeño pepper, seeded and finely chopped
- 3 cups cooked red kidney beans
- 1 teaspoon ground coriander
- ¼ teaspoon salt
- ½ cup chopped cilantro or parsley
- 1 cup shredded Monterey jack cheese (4 ounces)
- ¼ cup reduced-fat sour cream
- ½ cup mild or medium bottled salsa

1. Preheat the oven to 350°F. Wrap the tortillas in foil and bake until heated through, but not crisp.

2. Meanwhile, in a large nonstick skillet, heat the oil over moderate heat. Add the scallions, garlic, and jalapeño, and sauté for 2 minutes or until the scallions are soft. Stir in the beans, coriander, salt, and ¼ cup of water, and bring to a boil. Reduce to a simmer, cover, and cook for 5 minutes or until the flavors have blended and the beans are hot. With a potato masher or the back of a spoon, mash about half of the beans. Stir in the cilantro.

3. Spoon the bean mixture down the center of each tortilla. Sprinkle the cheese over the beans and roll up. Place, seam-side down, on a baking sheet and bake for 3 minutes or until heated through. Serve the burritos topped with the sour cream and salsa. Serves 4.

Per serving: Calories 564; Fiber 7g; Protein 26g; Total Fat 19g; Saturated Fat 7g; Cholesterol 35mg; Sodium 1018mg

Southwestern Pork & Bean Stew

PREP: 20 MINUTES / COOK: 20 MINUTES
This Tex-Mex treat is not highly spiced, but you can add more chili powder (or hotter chilies) if you wish. Warm corn bread is the ideal accompaniment for the stew.

- 1 tablespoon vegetable oil
- ½ pound well-trimmed pork tenderloin, cut into ½-inch chunks
- 2 tablespoons flour
- 1 large onion, finely chopped
- 3 cloves garlic, minced
- 1 green bell pepper, cut into ½-inch squares
- 1 can (14½ ounces) no-salt-added tomatoes, chopped with their juice
- 1 can (4 ounces) chopped mild green chilies
- 1½ teaspoons mild chili powder
- ½ teaspoon each dried oregano and salt
- 3 cups cooked black beans
- 1 tablespoon lime juice

1. In a large nonstick skillet, heat the oil over moderately high heat. Dust the pork with the flour, shaking off the excess. Add to the pan and sauté for 2 minutes or until lightly browned. With a slotted spoon, transfer the pork to a plate.

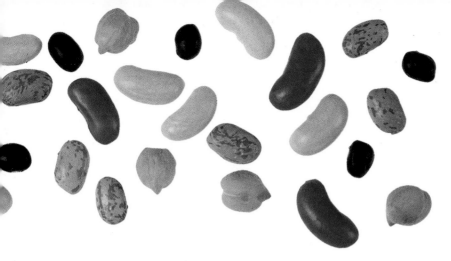

2. Add the onion and garlic to the pan and sauté for 5 minutes or until soft. Add the bell pepper and sauté for 4 minutes or until soft.

3. Add ¼ cup of water, the tomatoes, green chilies, chili powder, oregano, and salt, and bring to a boil. Reduce to a simmer, return the pork to the pan; add the beans, cover, and cook for 7 minutes or until the pork is tender. Stir in the lime juice. Serves 4.

Per serving: Calories 341; Fiber 5g; Protein 26g; Total Fat 7g; Saturated Fat 1g; Cholesterol 37mg; Sodium 518mg

Vegetarian Burgers *You can "hold the beef" and still serve up a hearty, juicy burger.*

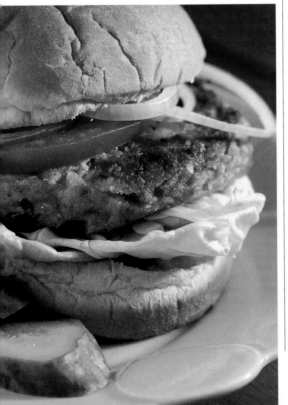

Vegetarian Burgers

PREP: 15 MINUTES / COOK: 15 MINUTES

The original veggie burger was a high-fat patty made from nuts and cheese. These bean-based burgers are far more healthful.

2	cloves garlic, peeled
3	cups cooked pinto beans
2	tablespoons light mayonnaise
1	tablespoon chili sauce
2	teaspoons lime juice
2	tablespoons plain dry bread crumbs
2	scallions, thinly sliced
½	teaspoon pepper
¼	teaspoon salt
2	tablespoons flour
4	teaspoons vegetable oil
4	hamburger buns, toasted
4	Boston lettuce leaves
4	slices each of tomato and red onion

1. In a small pan of boiling water, cook the garlic for 4 minutes to soften. In a large bowl, mash the garlic, beans, mayonnaise, chili sauce, and lime juice with a potato masher or fork. Stir in the bread crumbs, scallions, pepper, and salt. Shape into 4 patties.

2. Dredge the patties in the flour, shaking off the excess. In a large non-stick skillet, heat the oil over moderate heat. Sauté the patties for 3 minutes per side or until browned and crisp on the outside and heated through.

3. Place the burgers on hamburger buns and top each with lettuce, tomato, and onion. Serves 4.

Per serving: Calories 406; Fiber 7g; Protein 16g; Total Fat 10g; Saturated Fat 2g; Cholesterol 3mg; Sodium 534mg

At the market Dried and canned beans are widely available. For a good selection, check the Latin and Italian food sections of your supermarket.

Prep Before cooking dried beans, spread them out and pick through them, removing any dirt or damaged beans; then rinse the beans in cold water. Drain and rinse canned beans to remove excess sodium.

Basic cooking Soaking dried beans shortens their cooking time: Place beans in a large pot and add cold water to cover. Let stand 8 to 12 hours. (For a quicker soak, bring the water slowly to a boil and simmer the beans 2 minutes. Cover the pot, remove from the heat, and let stand 1 to 2 hours.) After soaking, drain the beans, add fresh water to cover, bring to a boil, and simmer about 1 hour, or until tender.

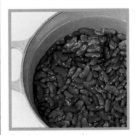

Soak beans in a large pot— they double in volume when soaked. First place the beans in the pot, then add water to cover by 2 inches.

Red Kidney Beans

PER 1 CUP COOKED

Calories	225
Fiber	13.1g
Protein	15g
Total Fat	0.9g
Saturated Fat	0.1g
Cholesterol	0mg
Sodium	4mg

NUTRIENTS

	% Daily Value
Potassium	71%
Folate	57%
Manganese	42%
Iron	28%
Copper	21%
Magnesium	20%
Thiamin	19%
Zinc	13%
Vitamin B6	11%

White Kidney Beans

PER 1 CUP COOKED

Calories	249
Fiber	11.3g
Protein	17g
Total Fat	0.6g
Saturated Fat	0.2g
Cholesterol	0mg
Sodium	11mg

NUTRIENTS

	% Daily Value
Manganese	57%
Iron	39%
Folate	36%
Potassium	34%
Magnesium	28%
Copper	26%
Zinc	17%
Calcium	16%
Thiamin	14%

Pasta e Fagioli

PREP: 15 MINUTES / COOK: 40 MINUTES

The Italian name of this nourishing soup simply means "pasta and beans."

1 tablespoon olive oil
1 onion, diced
1 carrot, halved lengthwise and cut into ¼-inch-thick slices
1 red bell pepper, cut into ½-inch squares
3 cloves garlic, minced
1 cup canned no-salt-added tomatoes, chopped with their juice
½ cup chopped fresh basil
½ teaspoon salt
¼ teaspoon black pepper
3 cups cooked red kidney beans
1½ cups chicken broth
2 cups wagon wheel pasta (4 ounces)
3 ounces smoked turkey, cut into ¼-inch dice
½ cup grated Parmesan cheese

1. In a medium saucepan, heat the oil over moderate heat. Add the onion, carrot, bell pepper, and garlic, and sauté for 7 minutes or until the onion is soft. Stir in the tomatoes, basil, salt, and black pepper, and cook for 5 minutes or until some of the tomato liquid has evaporated.

2. Stir in the beans, broth, and 3 cups of water. Bring to a boil, reduce to a simmer, cover, and cook for 15 minutes or until the beans are beginning to break up and thicken the liquid. With the back of a spoon, mash one-fourth of the beans against the side of the pan.

3. Return to a boil, add the pasta and turkey; cook, uncovered, for 10 minutes or until the pasta is firm-tender. Serve topped with Parmesan. Serves 4.

Per serving: Calories 429; Fiber 8g; Protein 26g; Total Fat 9g; Saturated Fat 3g; Cholesterol 19mg; Sodium 1106mg

Sweet Bean Pie

PREP: 20 MINUTES / CHILL: 1 HOUR
COOK: 1 HOUR 15 MINUTES

A pie made out of beans might seem odd, but this variation on an African-American recipe makes smart use of chick-peas, which are puréed with evaporated milk, a whole egg, egg whites, and corn syrup to make a rich, smooth custard.

1 cup flour
1 tablespoon plus ¾ cup sugar
½ teaspoon salt
2 tablespoons unsalted butter, cut up
2 tablespoons solid vegetable shortening
3 tablespoons reduced-fat sour cream
3 cups cooked chick-peas
1 cup evaporated skimmed milk
1 egg
2 egg whites
2 tablespoons corn syrup
1½ teaspoons vanilla extract
1 teaspoon cinnamon
⅛ teaspoon nutmeg

1. In a large bowl, combine the flour, 1 tablespoon of the sugar, and ¼ teaspoon of the salt. With a pastry blender or two knives, cut in the butter and shortening until the mixture resembles coarse meal. In a small bowl, combine the sour cream and 1 tablespoon of ice water; stir into the flour mixture until just combined. Flatten the dough into a disk, wrap in plastic wrap, and refrigerate for at least 1 hour.

2. Preheat the oven to 350°F. On a lightly floured surface, roll the dough out to a 13-inch round. Fit into a 9-inch deep-dish pie plate and form a high fluted edge. Lightly prick the bottom of the shell with a fork and line with foil. Fill the foil with pie weights or dried beans. Place on a baking sheet and bake for 20 minutes. Remove the foil and beans and bake for 5 minutes or until lightly golden around the edges.

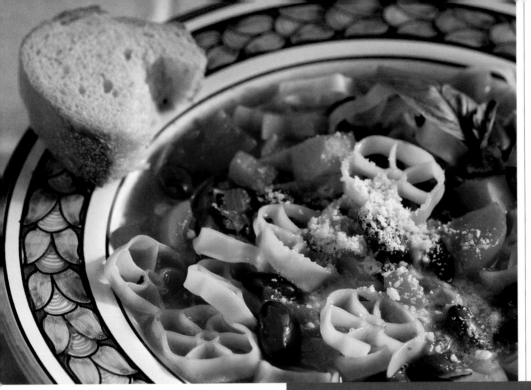

Pasta e Fagioli
Sautéing the vegetables adds extra flavor to this old-fashioned soup.

Did you know? . . .
To improve the digestibility of beans that are cooked from scratch, discard the soaking water and cook the beans in fresh water.

3. In a blender or food processor, combine the chick-peas, evaporated milk, whole egg, egg whites, corn syrup, vanilla, cinnamon, nutmeg, and the remaining ¼ teaspoon salt and ¾ cup sugar. Process until smooth. Pour into the prepared shell. Place on the baking sheet and bake for 50 minutes or until set. Serve warm or at room temperature. Serves 12.

Per serving: Calories 239; Fiber 2g; Protein 8g; Total Fat 6g; Saturated Fat 2g; Cholesterol 25mg; Sodium 145mg

Molasses Baked Beans

PREP: 10 MINUTES
COOK: 1 HOUR 45 MINUTES

The generous amount of tomatoes in this recipe adds lycopene, a disease-fighting phytochemical, to the already rich nutritional bounty of white beans.

3   ounces bacon, chopped (3 slices)
1   small onion, finely chopped
2   cloves garlic, minced
1   can (14½ ounces) no-salt-added stewed tomatoes, chopped with their juice
1   can (8 ounces) no-salt-added tomato sauce

Beans and other legumes are the best protein sources in the plant kingdom.

¼   cup molasses
1   tablespoon cider vinegar
1   tablespoon dark brown sugar
2   teaspoons yellow mustard
¾   teaspoon ground ginger
½   teaspoon salt
3   cups cooked white beans

1. Preheat the oven to 350°F. In a medium Dutch oven or ovenproof saucepan, cook the bacon over low heat for 5 minutes or until it has rendered its fat. Add the onion and garlic, and sauté for 5 minutes or until soft. Add the stewed tomatoes, tomato sauce, molasses, vinegar, brown sugar, mustard, ginger, and salt. Bring to a boil and cook for 5 minutes.

2. Add the beans, cover, and transfer to the oven. Bake for 1½ hours or until the beans are richly flavored, well coated, and the cooking liquid is thick. Serves 6.

Per serving: Calories 290; Fiber 6g; Protein 11g; Total Fat 9g; Saturated Fat 3g; Cholesterol 10mg; Sodium 344mg

Studies done at the University of Kentucky, a major center for research into dietary fiber, showed that consuming at least 4 ounces of cooked beans each day can significantly reduce high cholesterol levels.

All beans supply some calcium: Great Northerns, navy beans, and chick-peas are among the best sources.

Beans cause a slow, steady rise in blood sugar rather than a rapid, abrupt one—good news for diabetics, who may be able to lower their insulin dosage if they add beans to their diets.

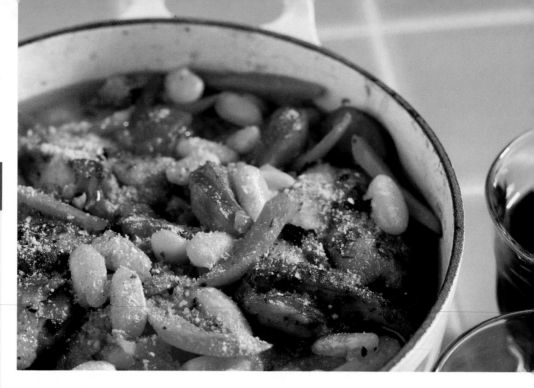

Cassoulet is a hearty French casserole made with white beans, chicken, and sausage.

Healthy Highlights

Black Beans

PER 1 CUP COOKED

Calories	227
Fiber	15.0g
Protein	15g
Total Fat	0.9g
Saturated Fat	0.2g
Cholesterol	0mg
Sodium	2mg

NUTRIENTS

	% Daily Value
Folate	64%
Manganese	38%
Magnesium	30%
Thiamin	28%
Iron	22%
Potassium	20%
Copper	18%
Zinc	13%

Chick-Peas

PER 1 CUP COOKED

Calories	269
Fiber	12.5g
Protein	15g
Total Fat	4.2g
Saturated Fat	0.4g
Cholesterol	0mg
Sodium	11mg

NUTRIENTS

	% Daily Value
Manganese	85%
Folate	71%
Copper	29%
Iron	28%
Magnesium	20%
Zinc	17%
Potassium	16%
Thiamin	13%
Vitamin B6	12%
Potassium	12%

Hummus

PREP: 10 MINUTES / COOK: 10 MINUTES

Serve this Middle Eastern dip with pita wedges or raw vegetable sticks.

- 4 cloves garlic, peeled
- 1 can (19 ounces) chick-peas, rinsed and drained
- ⅓ cup plain nonfat yogurt
- 2 tablespoons reduced-fat sour cream
- 1 tablespoon lemon juice
- 1 tablespoon sesame oil
- ½ teaspoon salt
- ½ teaspoon ground coriander
- ⅛ teaspoon each cayenne pepper and allspice
- ¼ cup chopped parsley or cilantro (optional)
- 1 teaspoon paprika (optional)

1. In a small pot of boiling water, cook the garlic for 2 minutes to blanch. Drain and transfer to a food processor.

2. Add the chick-peas, yogurt, sour cream, lemon juice, sesame oil, salt, coriander, cayenne, and allspice to the processor and purée. Transfer to a serving bowl and sprinkle with the parsley and paprika. Makes 2 cups.

Per ¼ cup: Calories 75; Fiber 2g; Protein 3g; Total Fat 3g; Saturated Fat 1g; Cholesterol 1mg; Sodium 229mg

Chick-Peas & Greens Soup with Carrots

PREP: 10 MINUTES / COOK: 15 MINUTES

For more variations, try Swiss chard or kale instead of the greens called for; or try a different bean, such as white kidney beans (cannellini) or pinto beans.

- ¾ cup chicken broth
- 2 carrots, quartered lengthwise and thinly sliced
- 3 cloves garlic, minced
- ½ teaspoon dried sage
- ¼ teaspoon pepper
- 2 cups cooked chick-peas, red kidney beans, or black beans
- 4 cups packed, torn spinach and/or watercress leaves

1. In a large saucepan, bring the broth to a boil over moderate heat. Add the carrots, garlic, sage, and pepper, and cook for 5 minutes or until the carrots are tender. Add ¾ cup of water and the chick-peas and return to a boil. Reduce to a simmer, cover, and cook for 7 minutes or until the soup is flavorful and the chick-peas are piping hot.

2. Stir in the greens and cook for 1 minute or just until wilted. Serves 4.

Per serving: Calories 183; Fiber 7g; Protein 11g; Total Fat 3g; Saturated Fat 0g; Cholesterol 0mg; Sodium 304mg

Cassoulet

PREP: 15 MINUTES
REFRIGERATE: 1 HOUR
COOK: 50 MINUTES

This French country dish traditionally takes several days to make and requires 20 or more different ingredients. We've composed a greatly simplified cassoulet for today's cook.

- **4** **skinless, boneless chicken thighs (3 ounces each)**
- **4** **cloves garlic, minced**
- **½** **teaspoon each dried thyme and salt**
- **¼** **teaspoon pepper**
- **2** **teaspoons olive oil**
- **1** **small onion, finely chopped**
- **2** **carrots, halved lengthwise and thinly sliced**
- **1** **cup canned no-salt-added tomatoes, chopped with their juice**
- **3** **cups cooked white kidney beans (cannellini)**
- **6** **ounces kielbasa or other fully cooked garlic sausage, thinly sliced**
- **3** **tablespoons plain dry bread crumbs**

1. In a large bowl, toss the chicken with the garlic, thyme, salt, and pepper. Cover and refrigerate for at least 1 hour.

2. In a small Dutch oven or flame-proof casserole, heat the oil over moderate heat. Add the chicken and cook for 4 minutes or until the chicken is very lightly browned on both sides. Transfer the chicken to a plate.

3. Preheat the oven to 400°F. Meanwhile, add the onion and carrots to the pan and sauté for 7 minutes or until the onion is soft. Add the tomatoes and their juice, the beans, and kielbasa. Bring to a boil, reduce to a simmer, and return the chicken to the pan. Cover, transfer to the oven, and bake for 20 minutes or until the chicken is cooked through.

4. Sprinkle the bread crumbs on top, drizzle with 3 tablespoons of the cooking liquid to moisten the crumbs, and bake for 20 minutes or until the crumbs are golden. Serves 4.

Per serving: Calories 485; Fiber 7g; Protein 36g; Total Fat 18g; Saturated Fat 6g; Cholesterol 99mg; Sodium 889mg

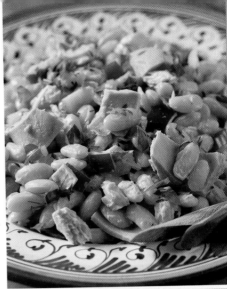

Tuscan White Bean & Tuna Salad In large bowl, toss together 19-oz. can rinsed and drained white kidney beans, two 6-oz. cans drained water-packed tuna, 1 diced red onion, ¼ cup light mayonnaise, 1 tbsp. lemon juice, and ½ tsp. sage. Sprinkle with chopped parsley. Serves 4. *[Cal 263; Fat 6g; Sod 557mg]*

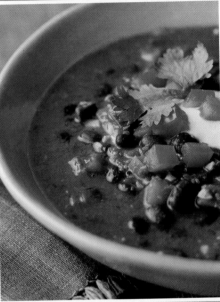

Black Bean Soup In saucepan, sauté 1 diced green bell pepper, 2 sliced scallions, and 3 cloves minced garlic in 2 tsp. oil until soft. Add 19-oz. can rinsed and drained black beans, 1½ cups chicken broth, and 1 tsp. each ground coriander and cumin. Simmer 5 minutes. Purée half the beans; reheat soup. Top with 2 tbsp. reduced-fat sour cream and ¼ cup diced tomato. Serves 4. *[Cal 161; Fat 5g; Sod 817mg]*

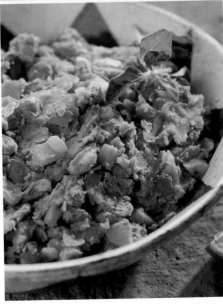

Refried Beans In large skillet, sauté 1 small diced onion and 1 diced carrot in 1 tbsp. olive oil over moderate heat until soft. Add two 15½-oz. cans rinsed and drained pinto beans, 2 tsp. tomato paste, ¼ cup water, ¼ tsp. dried oregano, ¼ tsp. salt, and ⅛ teaspoon cayenne. Cook, stirring and breaking up half of the beans. Serves 4. *[Cal 173; Fat 4g; Sod 527mg]*

Lentils

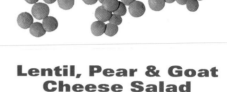

Nutritional power

Lentils offer an extraordinary amount of folate, along with plenty of protein and fiber. They're also a very good source of iron and potassium.

Healthy Highlights

PER 1 CUP COOKED	
Calories	230
Fiber	16g
Protein	18g
Total Fat	0.8g
Saturated Fat	0.1g
Cholesterol	0mg
Sodium	4mg

NUTRIENTS

	% Daily Value
Folate	90%
Manganese	49%
Iron	39%
Copper	25%
Potassium	24%
Thiamin	22%
Magnesium	18%
Vitamin B6	18%
Zinc	17%
Niacin	11%

Did you know? . . .

One cup of lentils supplies 7 mg of iron—more than twice as much as in a 3½-ounce serving of lean top round steak. The steak has nearly 8 grams of fat, while the lentils have less than 1 gram.

Country Ham & Lentil Salad

PREP: 25 MINUTES / COOK: 25 MINUTES

- 1 cup lentils
- 3 cloves garlic, minced
- ½ teaspoon each salt and black pepper
- ¼ teaspoon dried sage
- ¾ pound red potatoes (about 3 medium), cut into ½-inch cubes
- ⅓ cup red wine vinegar
- 4 teaspoons Dijon mustard
- 2 teaspoons olive oil
- 6 ounces smoked ham, cut into ½-inch cubes
- 2 stalks celery, halved lengthwise and thinly sliced
- 1 red bell pepper, cut into ½-inch squares
- ½ cup snipped fresh dill

1. In a medium saucepan of boiling water, cook the lentils, garlic, ¼ teaspoon each of the salt and black pepper, and the sage for 20 minutes or until the lentils are tender; drain any liquid remaining. Meanwhile, in a separate pan of boiling water, cook the potatoes for 7 minutes or until tender. Drain.

2. As the potatoes cook, in a large bowl, whisk together the vinegar, mustard, oil, and the remaining ¼ teaspoon each salt and black pepper.

3. Add the hot lentils, potatoes, ham, celery, bell pepper, and dill, tossing to combine. Serve warm, at room temperature, or chilled. Serves 4.

Per serving: Calories 327; Fiber 8g; Protein 24g; Total Fat 5g; Saturated Fat 1g; Cholesterol 20mg; Sodium 1048mg

Lentil, Pear & Goat Cheese Salad

PREP: 15 MINUTES / COOK: 20 MINUTES

While the lentils cook, you can toast the pecans for 8 to 10 minutes for extra flavor.

- 1½ cups lentils
- ¾ teaspoon salt
- ½ teaspoon pepper
- ¼ cup lime juice
- 2 tablespoons honey
- ½ teaspoon ground ginger
- 2 pears, cut into ½-inch chunks
- 1 bunch watercress, large stems trimmed
- 4 ounces mild goat cheese, crumbled
- 2 tablespoons coarsely chopped pecans

1. In a medium saucepan of boiling water, cook the lentils with ¼ teaspoon each of the salt and pepper for 20 to 25 minutes or until the lentils are tender. Drain.

2. Meanwhile, in a medium bowl, whisk together the lime juice, honey, ginger, and the remaining ½ teaspoon salt and ¼ teaspoon pepper. Add the lentils and cool to room temperature.

3. Add the pears and watercress, tossing to combine. Serve the salads sprinkled with the goat cheese and chopped pecans. Serves 4.

Per serving: Calories 487; Fiber 12g; Protein 28g; Total Fat 12g; Saturated Fat 6g; Cholesterol 22mg; Sodium 610mg

Hearty Chicken & Lentil Stew

PREP: 20 MINUTES / COOK: 1 HOUR

Even though the lentils simmer for about 45 minutes, they won't turn mushy, because the acid in the tomatoes slows the rate at which the lentils cook.

- 1 **tablespoon olive oil**
- 4 **large skinless, boneless chicken thighs (4 ounces each), quartered**
- 1 **onion, finely chopped**
- 1 **yellow or red bell pepper, diced**
- 4 **cloves garlic, minced**
- ¾ **cup lentils**
- 1¼ **cups chicken broth**
- ¾ **cup canned no-salt-added tomatoes, chopped with their juice**
- 1 **teaspoon each ground coriander and ginger**
- ½ **teaspoon salt**
- 10 **ounces red potatoes, cut into ½-inch chunks**

1. In a large nonstick skillet, heat the oil over moderate heat. Add the chicken and cook for 6 minutes or until browned on both sides. With a slotted spoon, transfer the chicken to a plate.

2. Add the onion, bell pepper, and garlic to the skillet and cook for 5 minutes or until soft. Add the lentils, broth, ½ cup of water, the tomatoes, coriander, ginger, and salt, and bring to a boil. Reduce to a simmer, cover, and cook for 20 minutes or until the lentils are just barely tender.

3. Return the chicken to the pan and add the potatoes. Return to a boil, reduce to a simmer, cover, and cook for 25 minutes or until the chicken is cooked through and the potatoes are tender. Serves 4.

Per serving: Calories 388; Fiber 7g; Protein 35g; Total Fat 9g; Saturated Fat 2g; Cholesterol 94mg; Sodium 733mg

At the market Brown lentils are a supermarket staple. For other varieties, such as red or green lentils, try a gourmet shop, health-food store, or Indian food shop. All Indian lentils (called "dals"), including red lentils, have been hulled, so they cook more quickly than whole lentils.

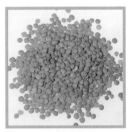

Because red lentils are hulled, they cook quickly. However, they have less fiber than whole lentils.

Prep Unlike dried beans, lentils do not need to be soaked before cooking. They should, however, be picked over and rinsed to remove any debris.

Basic cooking Lentils can be cooked in water or broth. Use three times as much liquid as lentils: Combine the lentils and liquid in a pot and bring to a boil. Cover, reduce the heat, and simmer until the lentils are tender but still hold their shape—20 to 25 minutes for brown lentils, 12 to 15 minutes for red lentils.

Lentil, Pear & Goat Cheese Salad Lentils are the foil for tart greens and tangy cheese.

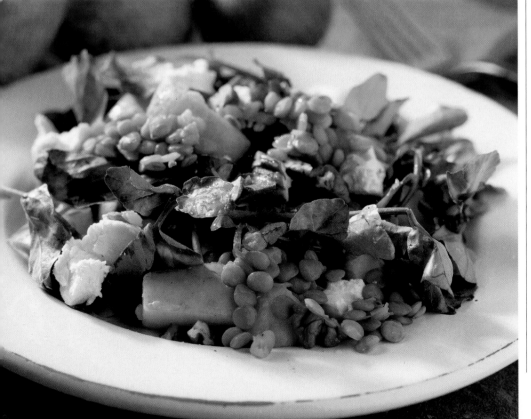

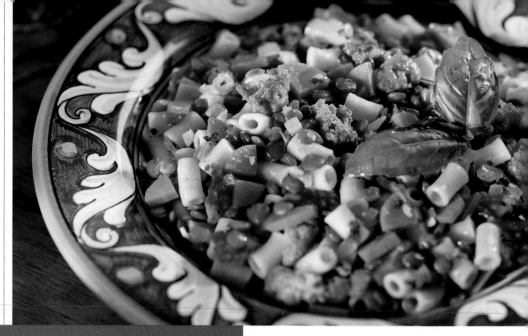

Ditalini with Lentils & Sausage *Sweet Italian sausage, redolent of garlic and fennel, combines beautifully with earthy lentils and pasta.*

Did you know? . . . Lentils contain protease inhibitors, a class of compounds that interfere with certain types of enzymatic action and thus may help fight cancer.

Lentils are a top non-meat source of the disease-fighting B vitamin, folate.

A 1-cup serving of lentils provides one-quarter of your daily requirement for copper, a mineral that may help lower blood cholesterol.

The iron in lentils is more easily absorbed by the body if you cook or serve the lentils with a food rich in vitamin C, such as tomatoes, bell peppers, cabbage, broccoli, or citrus juice.

On average, Americans eat less than 2½ ounces of lentils per person per year—a pity, since lentils supply so much of the vital nutrient folate. There is increasing evidence that folate may reduce the risk of heart disease and colon cancer.

Baked Lentil & Mushroom Stuffing
PREP: 15 MINUTES / COOK: 40 MINUTES

2   teaspoons vegetable oil
1   onion, finely chopped
3   cloves garlic, minced
1   pound mushrooms, quartered
1   cup lentils
1   cup chicken broth
½   teaspoon each dried sage, salt, and pepper
⅓   cup chopped walnuts

1. Preheat the oven to 350°F. In a small Dutch oven or ovenproof saucepan, heat the oil over moderate heat. Add the onion and garlic, and sauté for 5 minutes or until the onion is soft. Add the mushrooms and sauté for 5 minutes or until beginning to soften.

2. Add the lentils, broth, ½ cup of water, the sage, salt, and pepper. Bring to a boil. Cover, transfer to the oven, and bake for 30 minutes or until the lentils are tender. Remove from the oven and stir in the walnuts. Serves 4.

Per serving: Calories 301; Fiber 8g; Protein 18g; Total Fat 10g; Saturated Fat 1g; Cholesterol 0mg; Sodium 564mg

Ditalini with Lentils & Sausage
PREP: 20 MINUTES / COOK: 40 MINUTES
Ditalini are small pasta tubes named for their resemblance to thimbles. If you can't find them, elbow macaroni work perfectly well in this dish.

¾   pound sweet Italian-style turkey sausages, casings removed
1   large onion, finely chopped
3   cloves garlic, minced
1   large carrot, quartered lengthwise and thinly sliced
1   large tomato, finely chopped
¾   cup chicken broth
1   cup lentils
10 ounces ditalini, tubetti, or elbow macaroni
⅓   cup chopped fresh basil

1. Crumble the turkey sausage into a large nonstick skillet. Add ½ cup of water and cook over moderately high heat for 5 minutes or until the sausage has rendered its fat. With a slotted spoon, transfer the sausage to a plate.

2. Add the onion and garlic to the skillet and sauté for 5 minutes or until soft. Add the carrot and sauté for 4 minutes or until soft. Stir in the tomato, broth, and 1⅓ cups of water, and bring to a boil. Add the lentils, reduce to a simmer, cover, and cook for 25 minutes or until the lentils are tender.

3. Meanwhile, in a large pot of boiling water, cook the pasta according to package directions until firm-tender. Drain and transfer to a large bowl.

4. Return the sausage to the skillet, cover, and cook, stirring occasionally, for 5 minutes or until heated through. Add the lentil-sausage mixture to the pasta along with the basil, tossing to combine. Serves 4.

Per serving: Calories 621; Fiber 10g; Protein 39g; Total Fat 11g; Saturated Fat 3g; Cholesterol 46mg; Sodium 780mg

Curried Lentil Dip

PREP: 10 MINUTES / COOK: 25 MINUTES

You could use any kind of lentils here; just cook them until they're tender enough to make a smooth purée. And although we call for a Granny Smith apple, you could use another green apple, such as Newtown Pippin or Greening, or a tart red apple, such as Macoun.

1 cup lentils
1 tablespoon vegetable oil
1 Granny Smith apple, peeled and thinly sliced
1 small onion, diced
2 cloves garlic, minced
2 teaspoons curry powder
1/3 cup chicken broth
3/4 teaspoon salt

1. In a medium saucepan of boiling water, cook the lentils for 25 minutes or until tender. Drain the lentils and transfer to a food processor or blender.

2. Meanwhile, in a medium nonstick skillet, heat the oil over moderate heat. Add the apple, onion, garlic, and curry powder, and sauté for 10 minutes or until the apple, onion, and garlic are very tender.

3. Add the sautéed apple-onion mixture to the lentils in the food processor. Add the broth and salt, and process to a smooth purée. Serve at room temperature or chilled. Makes 3 cups.

Per 1/4 cup: Calories 76; Fiber 2g; Protein 5g; Total Fat 1g; Saturated Fat 0g; Cholesterol 0mg; Sodium 176mg

Cream of Red Lentil Soup In saucepan, combine 2½ cups water, 1 cup red lentils, 2 chopped red bell peppers, 3 sliced garlic cloves, ¾ tsp. each salt and cumin, and ⅛ tsp. cayenne; cook until lentils are soft. Purée with ½ cup evaporated milk. Top with diced red pepper. Serves 4. *[Cal 219; Fat 3g; Sod 476mg]*

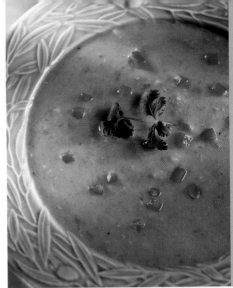

Warm Lentil & Tomato Salad Bring 3 cups water to a boil. Add 1 cup lentils, 1 diced carrot, ¾ tsp. dried thyme, ½ tsp. salt, and ½ tsp. pepper. Cover and simmer 25 minutes or until tender. Drain and toss with 3 tbsp. red wine vinegar, 1 tbsp. olive oil, 2 tsp. Dijon mustard, 2 cups diced plum tomatoes, and 2 tbsp. sliced scallions. Serves 4. *[Cal 225; Fat 4g; Sod 370mg]*

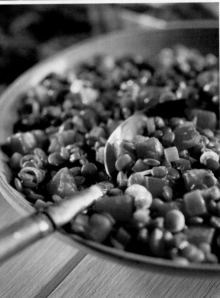

Lentils & Peas In medium saucepan, sauté 1 diced onion and 3 minced garlic cloves in 1 tbsp. oil. Add 1 cup lentils, 2 cups water, ¾ tsp. salt, ½ tsp. crumbled dried rosemary, and ¼ tsp. pepper. Bring to a boil, reduce to a simmer, cover, and cook 25 minutes or until tender. Add 1½ cups frozen peas and cook until hot. Serves 4. *[Cal 254; Fat 4g; Sod 503mg]*

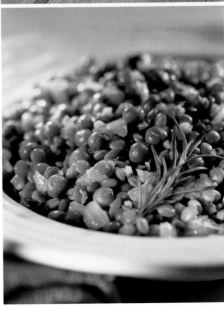

Split peas

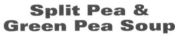

Nutritional power

An abundant source of fiber and protein, split peas also supply good amounts of minerals, including potassium, and the disease-fighting B-vitamin, folate.

Healthy Highlights

PER 1 CUP COOKED	
Calories	231
Fiber	16g
Protein	16g
Total Fat	0.8g
Saturated Fat	0.1g
Cholesterol	0mg
Sodium	4mg

NUTRIENTS	
	% Daily Value
Manganese	39%
Folate	32%
Thiamin	25%
Potassium	24%
Copper	18%
Iron	17%
Zinc	13%

Did you know? . . .

One cup of cooked split peas supplies more fiber than three slices of whole-wheat bread.

Split peas are a good dietary choice for diabetics, as their complex carbohydrates (starches) are metabolized relatively slowly into glucose (blood sugar).

Mexican Split Pea Salsa

PREP: 20 MINUTES / COOK: 35 MINUTES

Something like a salsa and a bit like guacamole, this nicely spiced appetizer is the perfect mate for oven-baked tortilla chips or warm tortilla triangles.

- 1½ cups split peas
- 3 cloves garlic, minced
- ¼ cup fresh mint sprigs
- ¾ teaspoon salt
- 1 tablespoon vegetable oil
- ¾ teaspoon ground coriander
- ½ teaspoon ground cumin
- ⅛ teaspoon cayenne pepper
- ⅓ cup lime juice
- ½ cup chopped cilantro
- 1 large tomato, diced

1. In a medium pot of boiling water, combine the split peas, garlic, mint, and ¼ teaspoon of the salt. Reduce to a simmer and cook, stirring occasionally, for 30 minutes or until the split peas are tender. Drain; discard the mint.

2. Meanwhile, in a small skillet, heat the oil over low heat. Add the coriander, cumin, and cayenne, and cook for 30 seconds or until fragrant.

3. Transfer the spiced oil to a medium bowl and whisk in the lime juice and the remaining ½ teaspoon salt. Add the hot split peas, the cilantro, and tomato, tossing well. Serve warm, at room temperature, or chilled. Makes 6 cups.

Per ¼ cup: Calories 51; Fiber 1g; Protein 3g; Total Fat 1g; Saturated Fat 0g; Cholesterol 0mg; Sodium 76mg

Split Pea & Green Pea Soup

PREP: 15 MINUTES / COOK: 35 MINUTES

When fresh peas are in season, you can substitute them for the frozen peas in this recipe. Add them to the soup about 5 minutes earlier than you would add the frozen peas.

- 2 teaspoons vegetable oil
- 6 scallions, thinly sliced
- 3 cloves garlic, minced
- 1¼ cups split peas
- 1 cup shredded iceberg lettuce
- ⅓ cup fresh mint leaves
- ¾ teaspoon salt
- ¼ teaspoon dried marjoram
- 1½ cups frozen green peas
- 1 can (12 ounces) evaporated skimmed milk

1. In a large saucepan, heat the oil over moderate heat. Add the scallions and garlic, and sauté for 2 minutes or until the scallions are tender. Add 3 cups of water, the split peas, lettuce, mint, salt, and marjoram, and bring to a boil. Reduce to a simmer, cover, and cook for 25 minutes. Stir in the green peas and cook for 5 minutes or until the split peas are tender.

2. Transfer the mixture to a food processor, add the evaporated milk, and

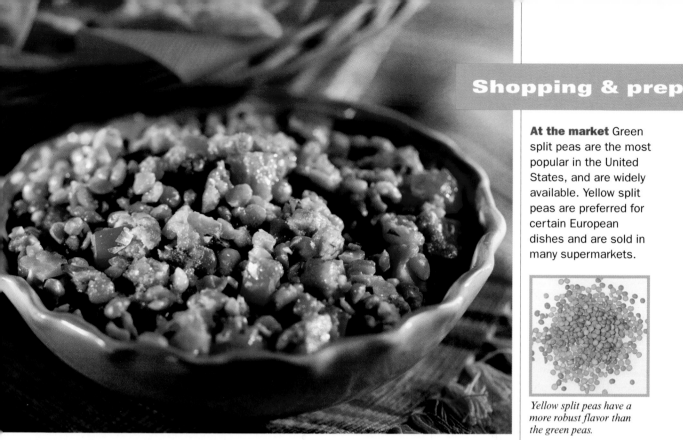

At the market Green split peas are the most popular in the United States, and are widely available. Yellow split peas are preferred for certain European dishes and are sold in many supermarkets.

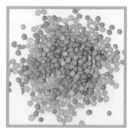

Yellow split peas have a more robust flavor than the green peas.

Mexican Split Pea Salsa is fragrant with fresh mint and cilantro.

purée. Return the soup to the pan and cook for 3 minutes or until heated through. Serves 4.

Per serving: Calories 363; Fiber 7g; Protein 26g; Total Fat 4g; Saturated Fat 1g; Cholesterol 4mg; Sodium 623mg

Pasta with Creamy Green Sauce

PREP: 15 MINUTES / COOK: 40 MINUTES

Although this dish is meatless, it provides plenty of protein, thanks to the split peas, pasta, skimmed milk, and cream cheese.

   2 **teaspoons olive oil**
   4 **cloves garlic, peeled**
   1 **cup split peas**
   1 **cup chicken broth**
   ½ **teaspoon each crumbled dried rosemary, salt, and sugar**
   10 **ounces medium pasta shells**
   ½ **cup frozen chopped spinach**
   1 **cup evaporated skimmed milk**
   3 **tablespoons reduced-fat cream cheese (Neufchâtel)**
   ¼ **cup grated Parmesan cheese**

1. In a medium saucepan, heat the oil over low heat. Add the garlic and cook for 4 minutes or until the oil is fragrant. Add the split peas, broth, ½ cup of water, the rosemary, salt, and sugar. Bring to a boil over moderate heat. Reduce to a simmer, cover, and cook for 30 minutes or until the split peas are tender.

2. Meanwhile, in a large pot of boiling water, cook the pasta according to package directions until firm-tender. Drain the pasta well and transfer to a large bowl.

3. Transfer the split-pea mixture to a food processor along with the spinach, evaporated milk, and cream cheese, and purée. Return the sauce to the pan and cook for 3 minutes or until heated through and creamy. Add the sauce to the pasta along with the Parmesan, tossing to combine. Serves 4.

Per serving: Calories 569; Fiber 5g; Protein 30g; Total Fat 8g; Saturated Fat 3g; Cholesterol 14mg; Sodium 797mg

Prep Split peas do not require presoaking, but they should be picked over and rinsed before cooking.

Basic cooking Use four times as much water as peas: For ½ cup of raw split peas, place the peas in a pot with 2 cups water and bring to a boil. Cover the pot, reduce the heat so that the water simmers, and cook for about 30 minutes, or until the peas are tender.

Tofu

Nutritional power

This versatile food is remarkably nutritious, supplying complete protein and important minerals. It also contains the cancer-fighting substance genistein.

Healthy Highlights

Tofu
PER ¼ POUND

Calories	86
Fiber	1.4g
Protein	9g
Total Fat	5.4g
Saturated Fat	0.8g
Cholesterol	0mg
Sodium	8mg

NUTRIENTS

	% Daily Value
Manganese	34%
Iron	33%
Magnesium	26%
Calcium	12%
Copper	11%

Did you know? . . .
Asian peoples, who eat soy products on a daily basis, have lower cancer rates than other populations; genistein, a phytochemical found in soybeans (and tofu), is one likely reason for this. Genistein is currently being studied in the U.S. as a potential anticancer drug.

Spicy Tofu with Pork

PREP: 15 MINUTES / COOK: 10 MINUTES

When people replace some of the meat in their diet with soy products such as tofu, their cholesterol levels drop significantly.

6	ounces pork shoulder, cut into chunks
3	tablespoons lower-sodium soy sauce
2¼	teaspoons red hot pepper sauce
1½	teaspoons sugar
1	tablespoon vegetable oil
4	scallions, thinly sliced
3	tablespoons minced fresh ginger
6	cloves garlic, minced
¾	cup chicken broth
1½	pounds silken tofu, cut into 1 x ½-inch chunks
2¼	teaspoons cornstarch blended with 2 tablespoons water
1½	teaspoons sesame oil

1. In a food processor, process the pork, 1½ tablespoons of the soy sauce, the hot pepper sauce, and the sugar until the pork is finely ground.

2. In a large nonstick skillet, heat the vegetable oil over moderately high heat. Add the pork and cook for 30 seconds, breaking up any clumps. Add the scallions, ginger, and garlic, and stir-fry for 2 minutes or until the garlic is tender.

3. Add the broth, tofu, and the remaining 1½ tablespoons soy sauce, and cook, stirring gently, for 2 minutes or until the tofu is heated through. Bring to a boil, stir in the cornstarch mixture, and cook, stirring gently, for 1 minute or until lightly thickened. Stir in the sesame oil and serve. Serves 4.

Per serving: Calories 257; Fiber 1g; Protein 24g; Total Fat 12g; Saturated Fat 2g; Cholesterol 29mg; Sodium 871mg

Hearty Vegetarian Lasagne

PREP: 15 MINUTES / COOK: 45 MINUTES

Tofu is a well-kept secret in this delicious and satisfying pasta bake.

6	lasagne noodles (5½ ounces total)
2	teaspoons olive oil
1	large onion, finely chopped
3	cloves garlic, minced
½	pound mushrooms, thinly sliced
2	packages (10 ounces each) frozen chopped spinach, thawed and squeezed dry
1½	teaspoons grated lemon zest
1½	teaspoons salt
½	teaspoon pepper
1	pound silken tofu
½	cup low-fat (1%) cottage cheese
½	cup part-skim ricotta cheese
½	cup grated Parmesan cheese
1	can (8 ounces) no-salt-added tomato sauce
4	tablespoons no-salt-added tomato paste
1	egg
2	egg whites

1. Preheat the oven to 350°F. In a large pot of boiling water, cook the lasagne noodles according to package directions until firm-tender. Drain.

2. Meanwhile, in a large nonstick skillet, heat the oil over moderate heat. Add the onion and garlic, and sauté for 5 minutes or until soft. Add the mushrooms and sauté for 4 minutes or until they begin to give up their juices. Add the spinach and cook, stirring, until no liquid remains. Transfer to a medium bowl and add the lemon zest, ¾ teaspoon of the salt, and ¼ teaspoon of the pepper. Toss well.

3. In a food processor, combine the tofu, cottage cheese, ricotta, 6 tablespoons of the Parmesan, the tomato sauce, tomato paste, whole egg, egg whites, the remaining ¾ teaspoon salt, and remaining ¼ teaspoon pepper, and process to a smooth purée.

4. Spray a 7 x 11-inch glass baking dish with nonstick cooking spray. Line the bottom with 2 of the lasagne noodles. Spoon half of the spinach mixture and one-third of the tofu mixture over the noodles. Make another layer of noodles, the remaining spinach mixture, and another one-third of the tofu mixture. Top with the remaining lasagne noodles and the remaining tofu mixture. Sprinkle the remaining 2 tablespoons Parmesan on top. Bake for 30 minutes or until hot. Serves 6.

Per serving: Calories 321; Fiber 5g; Protein 24g; Total Fat 9g; Saturated Fat 3g; Cholesterol 48mg; Sodium 977mg

Stir-Fried Vegetables with Tofu *Tofu has a miraculous ability to absorb flavors. Here, it tastes of soy sauce, ginger, and garlic.*

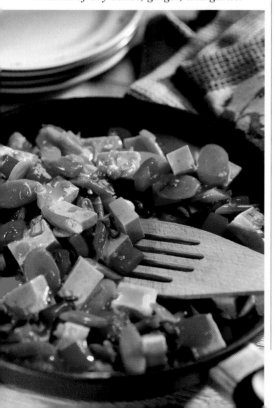

Stir-Fried Vegetables with Tofu

PREP: 15 MINUTES / MARINATE: 1 HOUR
COOK: 10 MINUTES

Very firm tofu has compressed edges; a block of it resembles a little sofa pillow. If you can't find this type, firm up regular (not silken) tofu as shown at right.

- **3 tablespoons lower-sodium soy sauce**
- **4 teaspoons dark brown sugar**
- **1 teaspoon ground ginger**
- **¼ teaspoon salt**
- **1 pound very firm tofu, halved horizontally**
- **¾ cup chicken broth**
- **2¼ teaspoons cornstarch**
- **1 tablespoon vegetable oil**
- **1 large red bell pepper, cut into ½-inch squares**
- **6 ounces green beans, cut into 1-inch lengths**
- **2 carrots, thinly sliced**
- **4 cloves garlic, minced**
- **2 scallions, thinly sliced**

1. In a shallow pan, combine the soy sauce, brown sugar, ginger, and salt. Add the tofu, cut-side down, and set aside to marinate for 1 hour. Reserving the marinade, remove the tofu and cut into 1 x ½-inch chunks. Stir the broth and cornstarch into the reserved marinade.

2. In a large nonstick skillet, heat the oil over moderate heat. Add the bell pepper, green beans, carrots, garlic, and scallions, and sauté for 5 minutes or until the pepper is crisp-tender. Stir the broth mixture well and pour into the skillet. Add the tofu and bring the mixture to a boil. Reduce to a gentle boil and cook for 4 minutes or until the sauce is lightly thickened and the tofu is heated through. Serves 4.

Per serving: Calories 183; Fiber 3g; Protein 12g; Total Fat 7g; Saturated Fat 1g; Cholesterol 0mg; Sodium 891mg

At the market Tofu is sold loose (displayed in tubs of water) in Asian markets, but it's best to buy it in sealed packages (tofu, like meat, is susceptible to bacterial contamination). Some packaged tofu must be refrigerated before opening, while silken tofu is available in aseptic packages and can be stored at room temperature.

Look for Choose tofu according to how you plan to use it. Delicate "silken" tofu can be simmered briefly, but it works best when puréed, in a shake, sauce, or dip. Regular and extra-firm tofu can be sliced, cubed, or crumbled.

Prep Pressing tofu renders it denser, drier and easier to slice. To press regular tofu, wrap, weight, and drain it as shown below for 30 minutes.

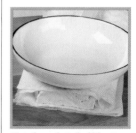

Cut the tofu in half horizontally, then sandwich it between several layers of paper towels. Place the tofu on a board, weight it and prop it at a slant near the sink to drain.

Chocolate-Hazelnut Cheesecake *Silken tofu is blended with cottage cheese for a luxuriously creamy texture.*

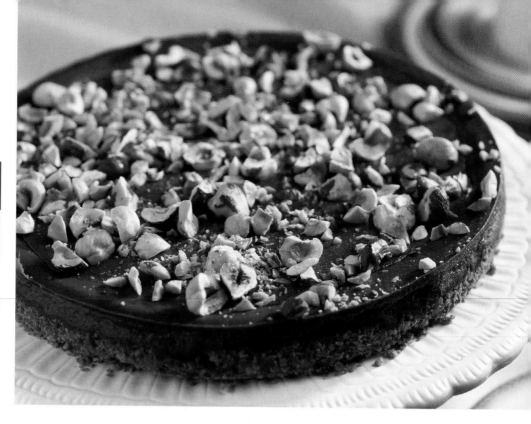

Healthy Highlights

Firm Tofu
PER ¼ POUND

Calories	164
Fiber	2.6g
Protein	18g
Total Fat	9.9g
Saturated Fat	1.4g
Cholesterol	0mg
Sodium	16mg

NUTRIENTS

	% Daily Value
Iron	67%
Manganese	67%
Magnesium	30%
Calcium	23%
Copper	21%
Thiamin	12%

Did you know? . . .
Tofu processed with calcium compounds (check the label for calcium chloride or calcium sulfate) is a good source of calcium. Firm tofu contains more calcium than soft tofu.

Two of the phytochemicals in soy—genistein and daidzein—seem to mimic the effect of estrogen in the body. In one study, adding soy protein to meals reduced the severity of hot flashes in menopausal women.

Although tofu is relatively high in fat, its saturated fat content is very low.

Chocolate-Hazelnut Cheesecake

PREP: 15 MINUTES / COOK: 50 MINUTES
CHILL: 2 HOURS

Crunchy toasted hazelnuts top this velvety cheesecake. For more of that heavenly hazelnut flavor, substitute 1 tablespoon Frangelico (hazelnut liqueur) for the vanilla.

⅓	cup hazelnuts
1	cup graham cracker crumbs (5 ounces)
1	tablespoon vegetable oil
¼	cup unsweetened cocoa powder
1	pound silken tofu
1	cup creamed (4%) cottage cheese
1	ounce semisweet chocolate, melted
½	cup granulated sugar
⅓	cup packed light brown sugar
2	tablespoons flour
1	egg
2	egg whites
1	teaspoon vanilla extract

1. Preheat the oven to 375°F. Toast the hazelnuts on a baking sheet for 7 minutes or until the skins begins to crinkle. (Leave the oven on.) Transfer the hazelnuts to a kitchen towel and rub to remove as much of the skin as possible (some skin will remain). When the hazelnuts are cool enough to handle, coarsely chop them; set aside.

2. In a small bowl, stir together the crumbs, oil, and 1 tablespoon of water. Press the mixture into the bottom and partway up the sides of a 9½-inch springform pan. Bake for 8 minutes or until the crust is set. Cool on a rack. Reduce the oven temperature to 350°F.

3. In a small bowl, combine the cocoa and ¼ cup of water until well moistened. In a food processor, combine the tofu, cottage cheese, melted semisweet chocolate, granulated sugar, brown sugar, flour, whole egg, egg whites, vanilla, and the cocoa mixture, and process until very smooth.

4. Pour the batter into the prepared crust and bake for 40 minutes. Reduce the oven temperature to 250°F, sprinkle the nuts on top, and bake for 10 minutes or until the cheesecake is just set. Cool to room temperature; refrigerate for 2 hours or until chilled. Serves 12.

Per serving: Calories 207; Fiber 1g; Protein 8g; Total Fat 7g; Saturated Fat 1g; Cholesterol 20mg; Sodium 189mg

Hot & Sour Soup

PREP: 40 MINUTES / COOK: 15 MINUTES

*This Chinese restaurant favorite
is surprisingly easy to make at home.*

- ¼ **cup dried porcini or other dried mushrooms**
- 1 **cup boiling water**
- 2 **tablespoons lower-sodium soy sauce**
- 1 **tablespoon cornstarch**
- 1 **teaspoon dark brown sugar**
- 6 **ounces well-trimmed pork tenderloin, thinly sliced and cut into ¼-inch-wide strips**
- 2 **teaspoons vegetable oil**
- ½ **pound fresh mushrooms, sliced**
- 4 **scallions, thinly sliced**
- 1½ **cups chicken broth**
- ¼ **cup rice vinegar or cider vinegar**
- 2 **tablespoons no-salt-added tomato paste**
- 1 **teaspoon ground ginger**
- ¼ **teaspoon cayenne pepper**
- 1 **pound firm tofu, cut into chunks**

1. In a medium bowl, combine the dried mushrooms and boiling water. Let stand for 20 minutes. Scoop the mushrooms out of the water, rinse, and thinly slice. Strain the liquid through a sieve lined with cheesecloth; reserve.

2. Meanwhile, in a bowl, combine the soy sauce, cornstarch, and brown sugar. Add the pork, tossing to coat.

3. In a large saucepan, heat the oil over moderate heat. Add the fresh mushrooms and scallions, and sauté for 4 minutes or until the mushrooms are soft. Stir in the broth, reserved mushroom soaking liquid, 1 cup of water, the vinegar, sliced porcini, tomato paste, ginger, and cayenne, and bring to a boil. Reduce to a simmer, cover, and cook for 7 minutes.

4. Return to a boil, add the pork mixture and tofu, and cook, stirring, for 2 minutes or until the pork is just cooked through and the soup is lightly thickened. Serves 4.

*Per serving: Calories 297; Fiber 2g;
Protein 30g; Total Fat 15g; Saturated Fat 2g;
Cholesterol 28mg; Sodium 742mg*

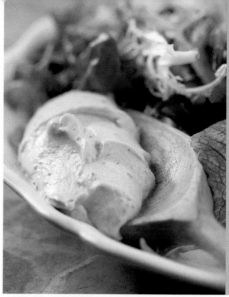

Creamy Basil-Parmesan Salad Dressing

In a food processor, purée 8 ounces silken tofu, ¼ cup Parmesan, ¼ cup fresh basil leaves, 1 tbsp. Dijon mustard, 2 tbsp. red wine vinegar, 1 tbsp. water, and ½ tsp. salt. Makes 1 cup/4 servings. *[Cal 65; Fat 3g; Sod 511mg]*

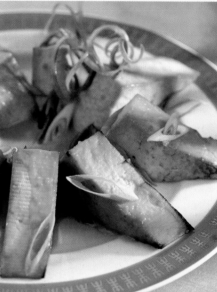

Grilled Tofu with Peanut Sauce

Cut 1 lb. firm tofu into eight ½-inch-thick triangles. Marinate for 1 hour in 2 tbsp. soy sauce, 2 tbsp. orange juice concentrate, and 1 tbsp. brown sugar. Grill or broil until browned. Purée ¼ cup chicken broth, 2 tbsp. peanut butter, ½ tsp. brown sugar, and ¼ tsp. ground ginger. Sprinkle tofu with sliced scallions; serve with the sauce. Serves 4. *[Cal 250; Fat 14g; Sod 635mg]*

Tofu-Vegetable Soup

In medium saucepan, bring 1½ cups chicken broth, 1½ cups water, 2 tbsp. rice vinegar, 2 tbsp. ketchup, 1 tbsp. sesame oil, ¾ tsp. salt, and ½ tsp. ground ginger to a boil. Add 1 lb. firm tofu cut into 1-inch chunks, 3 cups shredded Napa cabbage, 2 thinly sliced carrots, and 6 sliced scallions. Cook until the carrots are tender. Serves 4. *[Cal 245; Fat 14g; Sod 957mg]*

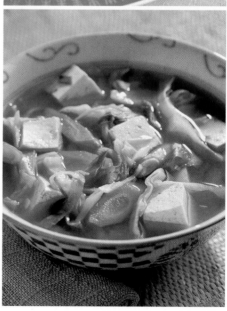

Soy milk

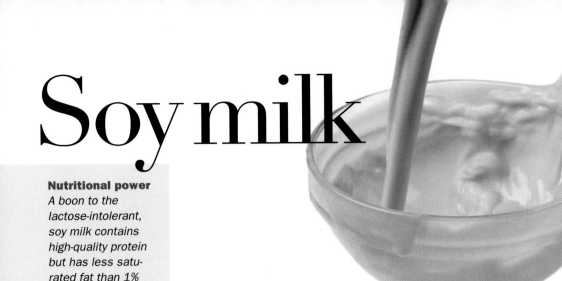

Nutritional power

A boon to the lactose-intolerant, soy milk contains high-quality protein but has less saturated fat than 1% low-fat milk—and no cholesterol.

Healthy Highlights

PER 1 CUP	
Calories	81
Fiber	3.2g
Protein	7g
Total Fat	4.7g
Saturated Fat	0.5g
Cholesterol	0mg
Sodium	29mg

NUTRIENTS	
	% Daily Value
Thiamin	26%
Manganese	21%
Copper	15%
Magnesium	12%
Potassium	12%
Riboflavin	10%

Did you know? . . .
Soy milk builds bones: In a university study, postmenopausal women given calcium-fortified soy milk gained significantly more bone density than women given protein and calcium in the form of milk powder.

Because it's made from a legume, soy milk—unlike dairy milk—contains fiber.

Piña Colada Pudding

PREP: 35 MINUTES / COOK: 10 MINUTES CHILL: 1 HOUR 20 MINUTES

Cooking the soy milk with coconut creates a "coconut milk" that's low in saturated fat.

- 3 **cups unflavored soy milk**
- ½ **cup sugar**
- ¼ **cup flaked coconut**
- ⅛ **teaspoon salt**
- 1 **package (¼ ounce) unflavored gelatin**
- 1 **cup canned juice-packed crushed pineapple, well drained**
- ½ **teaspoon coconut extract**

1. In a small saucepan, bring 2¾ cups of the soy milk, the sugar, coconut, and salt to a boil over moderate heat. Remove from the heat, cover, and let stand for 30 minutes at room temperature. Strain into a medium bowl, pushing on the solids to extract as much liquid as possible.

2. In a heatproof measuring cup, sprinkle the gelatin over the remaining ¼ cup soy milk. Let stand for 5 minutes to soften. Place the cup in a small pan of simmering water and heat for 2 minutes or until the gelatin is dissolved.

3. Stir the gelatin mixture into the soy-milk mixture. Set the bowl in a larger bowl of ice and water and let stand, stirring occasionally, for 20 minutes or until the mixture begins to set. Fold in the pineapple and coconut extract. Spoon the mixture into 4 dessert bowls, cover, and chill for 1 hour or until set. Serves 4.

Per serving: Calories 262; Fiber 1g; Protein 9g; Total Fat 4g; Saturated Fat 1g; Cholesterol 0mg; Sodium 175mg

Banana-Chocolate Shake

PREP: 5 MINUTES

A terrific snack, this ultra-thick shake is also a fine dessert; serve with crisp wafer cookies.

- 3 **tablespoons light brown sugar**
- 2 **tablespoons unsweetened cocoa powder**
- 1¾ **cups unflavored soy milk**
- 1 **large banana (8 ounces), peeled and thickly sliced**
- 2 **tablespoons chocolate syrup**
- 1 **teaspoon vanilla extract**
- 4 **ice cubes**

1. In a small bowl, combine the brown sugar and cocoa. Add ¼ cup of the soy milk and stir until well moistened and smooth.

2. Transfer the mixture to a blender along with the the remaining 1½ cups soy milk, the banana, chocolate syrup, vanilla, and ice cubes. Process until smooth, thick, and creamy. Serves 2.

Per serving: Calories 321; Fiber 3g; Protein 10g; Total Fat 5g; Saturated Fat 1g; Cholesterol 0mg; Sodium 127mg

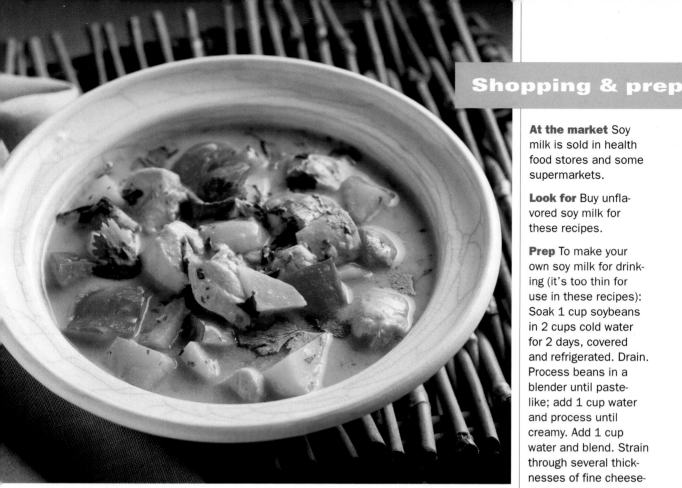

Thai Chicken Stew This fast, fresh main dish can be on the table in less than an hour.

Thai Chicken Stew

PREP: 25 MINUTES / COOK: 20 MINUTES

Thai cooking demands a careful balance of tastes and textures. Here, a creamy sauce, based on soy milk and peanut butter, is sparked with garlic, fresh ginger, and lime juice, as well as fresh basil and cilantro.

- 2 **teaspoons vegetable oil**
- 1 **red bell pepper, cut into ½-inch squares**
- 2 **cloves garlic, minced**
- 1 **tablespoon minced fresh ginger**
- ¾ **pound all-purpose potatoes (2 to 3 medium), peeled and cut into ½-inch chunks**
- 1 **cup chicken broth**
- 1 **pound skinless, boneless chicken breasts, cut into 1-inch chunks**
- 2 **cups unflavored soy milk**
- ⅓ **cup chopped fresh basil**
- ¼ **cup chopped cilantro**
- 2 **tablespoons lime juice**
- 2 **tablespoons lower-sodium soy sauce**
- 1 **tablespoon reduced-fat peanut butter**
- 2 **teaspoons dark brown sugar**
- ¼ **teaspoon coconut extract**

1. In a large nonstick skillet, heat the oil over moderate heat. Add the bell pepper, garlic, and ginger, and sauté for 4 minutes or until the pepper is crisp-tender. Add the potatoes and broth, and bring to a boil. Reduce to a simmer, cover, and cook for 7 minutes or until the potatoes are firm-tender.

2. Add the chicken, soy milk, basil, cilantro, lime juice, soy sauce, peanut butter, brown sugar, and coconut extract to the pan, and bring to a boil. Reduce to a simmer, cover, and cook for 5 minutes or until the chicken and potatoes are cooked through. Serves 4.

Per serving: Calories 317; Fiber 2g; Protein 34g; Total Fat 8g; Saturated Fat 1g; Cholesterol 66mg; Sodium 718mg

At the market Soy milk is sold in health food stores and some supermarkets.

Look for Buy unflavored soy milk for these recipes.

Prep To make your own soy milk for drinking (it's too thin for use in these recipes): Soak 1 cup soybeans in 2 cups cold water for 2 days, covered and refrigerated. Drain. Process beans in a blender until paste-like; add 1 cup water and process until creamy. Add 1 cup water and blend. Strain through several thicknesses of fine cheesecloth into a large saucepan. Bring to a simmer and cook, stirring, for 5 to 10 minutes. Cool; refrigerate in a covered container for up to 5 days.

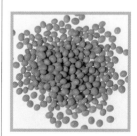

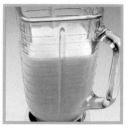

Soaked, dried soy beans (top) are puréed (bottom) to make soy milk.

Almonds & Walnuts

Nutritional power
These nuts supply good amounts of fiber and minerals. Almonds supply plenty of vitamin E; walnuts have omega-3 fatty acids, which lower triglycerides.

Healthy Highlights

Almonds
PER 1 OUNCE

Calories	167
Fiber	3.1g
Protein	6g
Total Fat	15g
Saturated Fat	1.4g
Cholesterol	0mg
Sodium	3mg

NUTRIENTS

	% Daily Value
Vitamin E	34%
Magnesium	21%
Copper	13%
Riboflavin	13%

Walnuts
PER 1 OUNCE

Calories	182
Fiber	1.4g
Protein	4g
Total Fat	18g
Saturated Fat	1.6g
Cholesterol	0mg
Sodium	3mg

NUTRIENTS

	% Daily Value
Manganese	41%
Copper	20%
Magnesium	12%

Did you know? . . .
Walnuts are a fair source of folate.

Walnut Bread
PREP: 15 MINUTES
RISE: 2 HOURS 15 MINUTES
COOK: 30 MINUTES

- 1 package (¼ ounce) active dry yeast
- 1¼ cups warm water
- 2 tablespoons honey
- ½ cup nonfat dry milk
- 2 tablespoons olive oil
- 3¾ cups flour
- 3 cups walnuts, coarsely chopped
- 2 teaspoons salt
- 2 tablespoons whole milk

1. In a large bowl, sprinkle the yeast over ¼ cup of the warm water. Add the honey and let stand for 5 minutes or until dissolved. Stir in the dry milk, oil, and the remaining 1 cup warm water.

2. In a food processor, combine 1 cup of the flour and 1 cup of the walnuts, and process until smooth. Stir the flour-nut mixture into the yeast mixture along with the remaining 2¾ cups flour and the salt. Turn out onto a lightly floured surface and knead for 5 minutes or until smooth and elastic. Spray a large bowl with nonstick cooking spray, add the dough and turn to coat. Cover with plastic wrap and let rise in a warm, draft-free spot for 1½ hours or until doubled in bulk.

3. Punch the dough down, transfer to a lightly floured work surface, and flatten. Place 1 cup of the walnuts on the dough and fold them in. Continue kneading and adding the remaining 1 cup nuts, pushing them into the dough as they pop out. Divide the dough in half, shape into balls, and flatten slightly. Place on 2 baking sheets, cover with plastic wrap, and let rise in a warm, draft-free spot for 45 minutes or until almost doubled in bulk.

4. Preheat the oven to 375°F. Brush the loaves with the milk; then, with a razor, small paring knife, or kitchen scissors, make 2 slashes in the top of each loaf. Bake for 30 minutes or until the bottoms of the loaves sound hollow when tapped and the tops are richly browned. Cool on a wire rack. Makes 2 loaves/24 servings.

Per serving: Calories 192; Fiber 1g; Protein 5g; Total Fat 11g; Saturated Fat 1g; Cholesterol 0mg; Sodium 205mg

Almond Brittle
PREP: 10 MINUTES / COOK: 15 MINUTES

- 1 cup whole natural almonds, coarsely chopped
- ⅓ cup slivered almonds
- 3 tablespoons sesame seeds
- ¾ cup sugar
- ½ cup light corn syrup
- 1 teaspoon vanilla extract
- ¼ teaspoon baking soda
- 1 tablespoon unsalted butter
- 1 cup air-popped popcorn

1. Preheat the oven to 350°F. Toast the chopped and slivered almonds for 5 minutes or until golden brown. In a separate pan, toast the sesame seeds for

5 minutes or until lightly browned. Spray a large baking sheet with nonstick cooking spray; set aside.

2. In a medium saucepan, combine the sugar, corn syrup, and ⅓ cup of water. Cook over moderately high heat, stirring until the sugar has dissolved. Continue to cook, without stirring, for 7 minutes or until the sugar mixture reaches 290°F on a candy thermometer.

3. Immediately remove from the heat and stir in the vanilla, baking soda, and butter. Working as quickly as possible, add the almonds, sesame seeds, and popcorn, stirring to coat. Quickly transfer to the prepared pan and use an oiled metal spatula to spread the brittle as flat as possible before it begins to harden. Cool to room temperature, then break the brittle into bite-size pieces. Makes 1 pound 2 ounces.

Per ounce: Calories 132; Fiber 1g; Protein 2g; Total Fat 7g; Saturated Fat 1g; Cholesterol 2mg; Sodium 30mg

Almond Brittle *This old-fashioned candy is made with sesame seeds as well as almonds.*

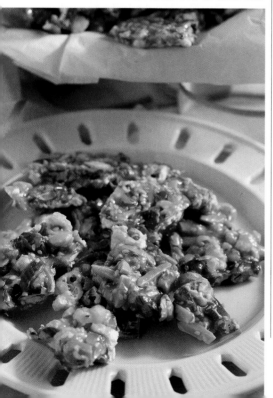

Chinese Walnut Chicken

PREP: 20 MINUTES / COOK: 20 MINUTES

The walnuts are coated in a sweet, crunchy glaze, then added to stir-fried chicken and vegetables.

- **1   tablespoon vegetable oil**
- **2½ tablespoons sugar**
- **1   cup walnut halves**
- **1   red bell pepper, cut into 1-inch squares**
- **4   scallions, cut into 1-inch lengths**
- **2   cloves garlic, minced**
- **1   tablespoon minced fresh ginger**
- **1   pound skinless, boneless chicken breasts, cut into 1-inch chunks**
- **1   cup chicken broth**
- **1   tablespoon soy sauce**
- **1   teaspoon sesame oil**
- **1½ teaspoons cornstarch**

1. In a medium skillet, heat 1 teaspoon of the vegetable oil over moderate heat. Add 2 tablespoons of the sugar, stirring to combine. Add the walnuts and cook, stirring constantly, for 7 minutes or until the walnuts are nicely coated and lightly crisped; set aside.

2. In a large nonstick skillet, heat the remaining 2 teaspoons vegetable oil over moderately high heat. Add the bell pepper and sauté for 2 minutes or until crisp-tender. Add the scallions, garlic, and ginger, and cook for 2 minutes. Add the chicken and sauté for 4 minutes or until no longer pink.

3. In a small bowl, whisk the broth, soy sauce, sesame oil, and the remaining 1½ teaspoons sugar into the cornstarch. Add to the pan, bring to a boil, and cook for 3 minutes or until the sauce is lightly thickened and the chicken is cooked through. Stir in the walnuts. Serves 4.

Per serving: Calories 382; Fiber 2g; Protein 31g; Total Fat 22g; Saturated Fat 3g; Cholesterol 66mg; Sodium 600mg

At the market
Almonds and walnuts are sold both in the shell and shelled. Whole shelled almonds are sold natural, blanched, or roasted; they also come slivered or sliced. Shelled walnuts are sold whole, in large pieces, or chopped.

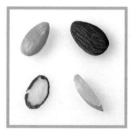

Top row: whole almonds, blanched and natural. Bottom row: sliced natural and slivered blanched almonds.

Look for When buying nuts in the shell, look for clean, uncracked shells. When buying shelled nuts in bulk, check for a pleasant smell; if left in the bin too long, nuts will turn rancid.

Basic cooking Toasting almonds and walnuts brings out their best flavor. Toast them in a heavy, ungreased skillet on the stovetop (or in a shallow baking pan in the oven) for 5 to 7 minutes, shaking the pan frequently; as soon as the nuts are lightly browned and fragrant, turn them out of the pan, or they will overcook from the heat retained by the pan.

Walnut-Crusted Snapper

Present this savory baked fish on a bed of steamed vegetables— perhaps a toss of zucchini, yellow squash, and carrots.

Did you know? . . .
Although walnuts and almonds are high in fat, most of it is unsaturated. Almonds are rich in monounsaturates; walnuts are highly polyunsaturated.

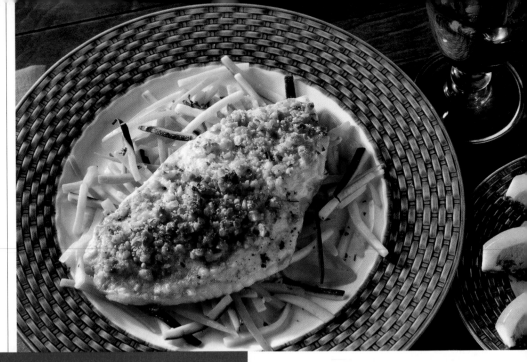

Research subjects who ate nuts frequently lowered their risk of heart disease.

A major study of Seventh-Day Adventists (who are vegetarians) revealed that those who ate walnuts, almonds, and peanuts almost every day increased their life expectancy and greatly reduced their risk of heart disease.

Almonds are the most nutritious nuts, providing more calcium and iron than other nuts. They also supply more dietary fiber than any other nut or seed.

Storing nuts in the freezer, in a tightly closed container, will help keep them from turning rancid.

Ounce for ounce, walnuts contain more potassium than bananas.

Walnut-Crusted Snapper

PREP: 10 MINUTES / COOK: 15 MINUTES
Light mayonnaise is the basis for the sauce, which puffs lightly as it bakes.

- 3 tablespoons light mayonnaise
- ½ teaspoon grated lemon zest
- 1 teaspoon lemon juice
- ¼ teaspoon each salt and pepper
- 4 red snapper fillets (6 ounces each), skinned
- ½ cup walnut halves
- 2 tablespoons grated Parmesan cheese

1. Preheat the oven to 450°F. Spray a large baking sheet with nonstick cooking spray; set aside.

2. In a small bowl, combine the mayonnaise, lemon zest, lemon juice, salt, and pepper. Place the fillets, skinned-side down, on the prepared baking sheet. Spread the mayonnaise mixture over the fish.

3. In a food processor, process the walnuts and Parmesan until finely ground (but not pasty). Sprinkle the nut mixture over the fish, patting it on. Bake for 15 minutes or until the nuts are lightly browned and the fish is just cooked through. Serves 4.

Per serving: Calories 302; Fiber 1g; Protein 38g; Total Fat 15g; Saturated Fat 2g; Cholesterol 69mg; Sodium 386mg

Pasta with Almond-Basil Pesto

PREP: 10 MINUTES / COOK: 15 MINUTES
Almonds make a more healthful pesto than the more traditional pine nuts.

- 4 cloves garlic, peeled
- 10 ounces fusilli, radiatore, or wagon wheel pasta
- 2 cups packed basil leaves
- ⅔ cup chicken broth
- ½ cup whole natural almonds, toasted
- ⅓ cup grated Parmesan cheese
- ½ teaspoon salt

1. In a large pot of boiling water, cook the garlic for 4 minutes to blanch. Scoop out with a slotted spoon and transfer to a food processor.

2. Add the pasta to the boiling water and cook according to package directions until firm-tender. Drain.

3. Meanwhile, to the garlic in the food processor, add the basil, broth, and

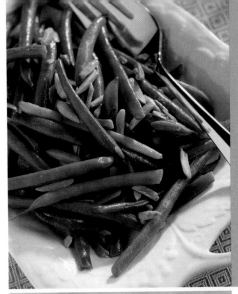

almonds, and purée. Transfer to a large bowl and stir in the Parmesan and salt. Add the hot pasta to the bowl, tossing to combine. Serves 4.

Per serving: Calories 420; Fiber 7g; Protein 18g; Total Fat 12g; Saturated Fat 2g; Cholesterol 5mg; Sodium 599mg

Chocolate-Almond Bars

PREP: 10 MINUTES / COOK: 15 MINUTES

A good amount of nutrition-packed almonds, rather than butter, makes these cookies rich.

- 1½ cups sliced almonds plus 30 almond slices for garnish
- ½ cup sugar
- 3 tablespoons unsweetened cocoa powder
- ¼ teaspoon salt
- 1 egg white
- 1 teaspoon vanilla extract
- ⅓ cup seedless red raspberry jam

1. Preheat the oven to 350°F. Spray a large baking sheet with nonstick cooking spray.

2. In a food processor, combine the 1½ cups almonds, the sugar, cocoa, and salt, and process until finely ground. Add the egg white and vanilla, and process until the mixture forms a very stiff dough.

3. Transfer the dough to the prepared baking sheet. With moistened hands, shape the dough into a log 15 inches long and ¾ inch in diameter. With moistened fingers, make an indentation down the center of the log. Bake for 15 minutes or until set.

4. Meanwhile, in a small saucepan, melt the jam over low heat. Spoon the hot jam into the indentation in the log. Transfer to a wire rack to cool completely. When cool, slice crosswise into 30 strips (about ½ inch wide). Place an almond slice on top of the jam in each bar. Makes 2½ dozen.

Per cookie: Calories 53; Fiber 0g; Protein 1g; Total Fat 3g; Saturated Fat 0g; Cholesterol 0mg; Sodium 23mg

Green Beans Amandine In large pot of boiling water, cook 1 lb. green beans until crisp-tender; drain. In large skillet, heat 2 tsp. olive oil and 2 tsp. unsalted butter until melted. Add ½ cup slivered almonds, tossing to coat. Add beans and ¼ tsp. salt and cook until heated through. Serves 4. *[Cal 172; Fat 13g; Sod 152mg]*

Chicken Salad with Almond Dressing In food processor, purée ⅓ cup whole almonds, ¼ cup light mayonnaise, 2 tbsp. lemon juice, and ½ tsp. salt. Transfer to large bowl. Add 2 cups diced cooked chicken, 2 sliced celery stalks, and 1 cup halved seedless red or green grapes; toss to coat. Serve on a bed of lettuce and garnish with sliced almonds. Serves 4. *[Cal 280; Fat 16g; Sod 486mg]*

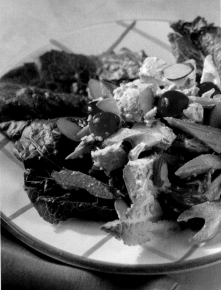

Spiced Walnuts In large heavy skillet, heat 1 tbsp. oil over moderate heat. Add 2 cups walnut halves, tossing to coat. Add 3 tbsp. sugar, ½ tsp. salt, and ½ tsp. cayenne, and cook, stirring constantly, for 8 minutes or until nuts are well coated and sugar has caramelized. Serve hot or at room temperature. Serves 12. *[Cal 129; Fat 12g; Sod 98mg]*

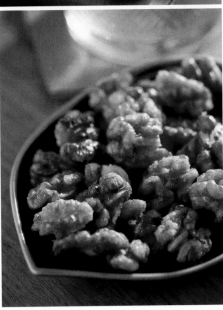

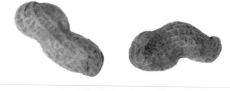

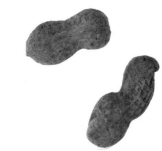

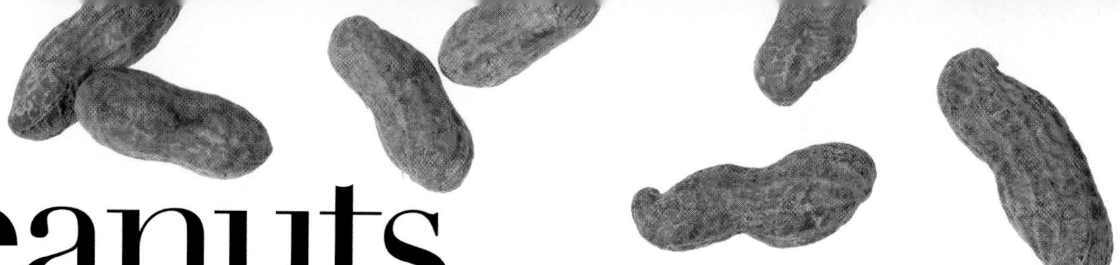

Peanuts

Nutritional power
Peanuts, which are legumes, provide more protein than any other nut. They also supply good amounts of fiber, vitamin E, and B vitamins, notably folate.

Healthy Highlights

PER 1 OUNCE DRY-ROASTED

Calories	166
Fiber	2.3g
Protein	7g
Total Fat	14g
Saturated Fat	2.0g
Cholesterol	0mg
Sodium	2mg

NUTRIENTS

	% Daily Value
Manganese	30%
Magnesium	13%
Vitamin E	11%
Folate	10%

Did you know? . . .
USDA researchers recently discovered that peanuts, like red wine, contain an antioxidant called resveratrol—a compound that has been associated with a lowered risk of heart disease. The red skin of the peanut (which most people usually discard) has a higher concentration of resveratrol than the nut itself.

Peanut Butter Blondies

PREP: 15 MINUTES / COOK: 25 MINUTES
Prune purée takes the place of most of the shortening in this recipe.

- **1** cup flour
- **½** teaspoon each baking powder and baking soda
- **¼** teaspoon salt
- **⅓** cup pitted prunes
- **¼** cup hot water
- **⅓** cup chunky peanut butter
- **2** tablespoons peanut or other vegetable oil
- **⅔** cup packed light brown sugar
- **2** tablespoons light corn syrup
- **1** egg
- **1** teaspoon vanilla extract

1. Preheat oven to 350°F. Spray a 9-inch square baking pan with nonstick cooking spray; set aside. In a small bowl, whisk together the flour, baking powder, baking soda, and salt. In a food processor, process the prunes and hot water until smooth.

2. In a medium bowl, with an electric mixer, beat the peanut butter, oil, and brown sugar until creamy. Beat in the prune purée and corn syrup until well combined. Beat in the egg and vanilla extract until well combined. Fold in the flour mixture.

3. Spoon the batter into the prepared pan. Bake for 25 minutes or until a cake tester inserted in the center comes out clean. Cool the cake in the pan on a rack. Cut into 16 squares. Makes 16.

Per blondie: Calories 130; Fiber 1g; Protein 3g; Total Fat 5g; Saturated Fat 1g; Cholesterol 13mg; Sodium 127mg

Banana, Apple & Peanut Salad

PREP: 15 MINUTES
You can make the dressing ahead of time, but don't mix the salad too far in advance, or the bananas will get mushy and the peanuts will lose their crunch.

- **⅓** cup honey
- **½** teaspoon grated lemon zest
- **3** tablespoons lemon juice
- **¼** teaspoon each salt and ground ginger
- **⅛** teaspoon nutmeg
- **1** pound bananas, cut into ½-inch-thick slices
- **1** pound apples, cut into ½-inch chunks
- **⅔** cup dry-roasted peanuts, coarsely chopped

1. In a large bowl, whisk together the honey, lemon zest, lemon juice, salt, ginger, and nutmeg.

2. Add the bananas, apples, and peanuts, tossing to combine. Serves 4.

Per serving: Calories 361; Fiber 5g; Protein 7g; Total Fat 13g; Saturated Fat 2g; Cholesterol 0mg; Sodium 149mg

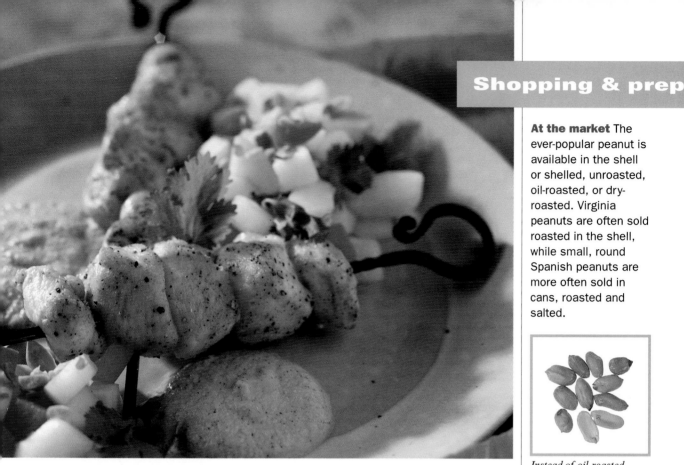

Chicken Satay with Peanut Sauce *Spicy chicken with a rich sauce and a cooling relish.*

Chicken Satay with Peanut Sauce

PREP: 25 MINUTES / COOK: 10 MINUTES

A savory peanut sauce is the traditional accompaniment for this Indonesian specialty. Garnish the dish with additional crushed peanuts and cilantro sprigs.

- 3 tablespoons rice vinegar
- 2 teaspoons sesame oil
- 2 teaspoons sugar
- ⅛ teaspoon crushed red pepper flakes
- 2 large cucumbers, peeled, seeded, and cut into ¼-inch dice
- 1 small red bell pepper, diced
- 1 pound skinless, boneless chicken breasts, cut into 1-inch chunks
- ½ teaspoon each ground coriander, salt, and black pepper
- 2 cloves garlic, peeled
- ½ cup dry-roasted peanuts
- ⅓ cup packed cilantro sprigs
- ½ cup chicken broth
- 2 tablespoons lime juice

1. In a medium bowl, whisk together the vinegar, sesame oil, 1 teaspoon of the sugar, and the red pepper flakes. Add the cucumbers and bell pepper, tossing to combine. Refrigerate until serving time.

2. Preheat the broiler. In a medium bowl, toss the chicken with the coriander, salt, and black pepper; set aside.

3. In a small pot of boiling water, cook the garlic for 4 minutes to blanch. Transfer to a food processor along with the peanuts, cilantro, broth, lime juice, and the remaining 1 teaspoon sugar. Purée.

4. Thread the chicken onto eight 8-inch skewers. Broil 6 inches from the heat, turning the skewers once, for 5 minutes or until cooked through. Serve 2 skewers of chicken per person, with the peanut sauce and cucumber salad alongside. Serves 4.

Per serving: Calories 292; Fiber 3g; Protein 32g; Total Fat 13g; Saturated Fat 2g; Cholesterol 66mg; Sodium 507mg

At the market The ever-popular peanut is available in the shell or shelled, unroasted, oil-roasted, or dry-roasted. Virginia peanuts are often sold roasted in the shell, while small, round Spanish peanuts are more often sold in cans, roasted and salted.

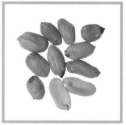

Instead of oil-roasted peanuts, which are very high in fat, use either unroasted peanuts (above) or dry-roasted peanuts for these recipes.

Look for If you're buying peanuts in the shell, choose nuts with clean, uncracked shells. If you're buying shelled peanuts in bulk, sniff them to be sure they're not rancid.

Prep You can toast shelled peanuts—on the stovetop in a heavy, ungreased pan, or in a 350° oven in a shallow baking dish—for 7 minutes, shaking the pan frequently. In-shell peanuts can be roasted in a shallow pan for about 15 minutes in a 350° oven.

Sunflower & Pumpkin seeds

Nutritional power
Packed with vitamin E, sunflower seeds also supply folate, a possible cancer-fighter. Pumpkin seeds are rich in zinc, an immune-system booster.

Healthy Highlights

Sunflower Seeds
PER 1 OUNCE

Calories	162
Fiber	3.0g
Protein	7g
Total Fat	14g
Saturated Fat	1.5g
Cholesterol	0mg
Sodium	1mg

NUTRIENTS

	% Daily Value
Vitamin E	71%
Copper	25%
Magnesium	25%
Thiamin	43%
Folate	16%
Iron	11%

Pumpkin Seeds
PER 1 OUNCE

Calories	153
Fiber	1.1g
Protein	7g
Total Fat	13g
Saturated Fat	2.5g
Cholesterol	0mg
Sodium	5mg

NUTRIENTS

	% Daily Value
Magnesium	38%
Copper	20%
Iron	22%
Zinc	14%

Sunflower Drop Biscuits

PREP: 10 MINUTES / COOK: 15 MINUTES

Buttermilk in the batter keeps these biscuits light and tender. They're a delicious addition to breakfast or brunch, and are also tasty with soup and salad as a lunch or light supper.

1½ cups flour
1¾ teaspoons baking powder
½ teaspoon each baking soda and salt
⅛ teaspoon cayenne pepper
2 tablespoons each unsalted butter and solid vegetable shortening
½ cup dry-roasted sunflower seeds
¾ cup low-fat (1.5%) buttermilk

1. Preheat the oven to 450°F. Spray a large baking sheet with nonstick cooking spray; set aside.

2. In a large bowl, combine the flour, baking powder, baking soda, salt, and cayenne. With a pastry blender or two knives, cut in the butter and shortening until the mixture resembles coarse meal. Stir in the sunflower seeds. Stir in the buttermilk until the mixture forms a soft dough. Do not overmix.

3. Drop the dough by well-rounded tablespoons 2 inches apart onto the prepared baking sheet. Bake for 12 minutes or until the biscuits are golden brown and crusty. Makes 1 dozen.

Per biscuit: Calories 132; Fiber 1g; Protein 3g; Total Fat 7g; Saturated Fat 2g; Cholesterol 6mg; Sodium 228mg

Mexican Chicken with Pumpkin Seed Sauce

PREP: 15 MINUTES / COOK: 25 MINUTES

The bell pepper, chilies, tomato, and lime juice in this dish combine to supply the daily adult requirement for vitamin C.

½ cup shelled pumpkin seeds
1 can (4 ounces) mild green chilies, drained
1 tomato, cut into large chunks
1 pickled jalapeño, stemmed
½ cup chicken broth
½ cup chopped cilantro or parsley
2 teaspoons olive oil
1 red bell pepper, cut into ½-inch squares
1 pound skinless, boneless chicken thighs, cut into 1-inch chunks
½ teaspoon salt
1 cup frozen corn kernels
1 tablespoon lime juice

1. In a small skillet, toast the pumpkin seeds over low heat for 3 minutes or until they begin to pop in the pan. Transfer to a blender or food processor. Add the mild green chilies, tomato, jalapeño, broth, and cilantro. Process until smooth.

2. In a large nonstick skillet, heat the oil over moderate heat. Add the bell pepper and cook for 4 minutes or until crisp-tender. Add the chicken and sauté for 4 minutes or until browned all over. Stir in the pumpkin-seed mixture and salt, and cook for 7 minutes or until the chicken is cooked through and the sauce is flavorful.

3. Stir in the corn and lime juice, and simmer for 5 minutes or until the corn is piping hot. Serves 4.

Per serving: Calories 251; Fiber 2g; Protein 26g; Total Fat 9g; Saturated Fat 2g; Cholesterol 94mg; Sodium 754mg

Crispy Seed-Topped Flat Breads

PREP: 1 HOUR 10 MINUTES
COOK: 15 MINUTES

These Near Eastern-style "crackers" are sprinkled with pumpkin seeds, sunflower seeds, and grated Parmesan.

2¼   **cups flour**
¾   **teaspoon salt**
¼   **teaspoon cayenne pepper**
1   **tablespoon each unsalted butter and solid vegetable shortening**
1   **egg white lightly beaten with 2 teaspoons water**
¼   **cup each shelled pumpkin seeds and shelled, dry-roasted sunflower seeds**
2   **tablespoons plus 2 teaspoons grated Parmesan cheese**

1. In a medium bowl, combine the flour, salt, and cayenne. With a pastry blender or two knives, cut in the butter and shortening until the mixture resembles coarse meal. Gradually add ⅔ cup of water to make a soft, smooth dough. Knead for 5 minutes or until smooth and elastic. Transfer to a bowl that has been sprayed with nonstick cooking spray, cover, and let rest for 1 hour.

2. Preheat the oven to 425°F. Spray 2 large baking sheets with nonstick cooking spray (or use nonstick pans); set aside. Cut the dough into 4 pieces. Roll each piece out to a 9-inch round (about ¹⁄₁₆ inch thick). Transfer to the prepared baking sheets. Brush the dough with the egg-white mixture. Sprinkle the pumpkin and sunflower seeds over the dough. Sprinkle each dough round with 2 teaspoons of the Parmesan. Bake for 12 minutes or until the bread is lightly puffed, golden brown, and crisp. Serves 12.

Per serving: Calories 133; Fiber 1g; Protein 4g; Total Fat 4g; Saturated Fat 1g; Cholesterol 4mg; Sodium 172mg

At the market Pumpkin and sunflower seeds are sold in and out of their shells, plain or roasted.

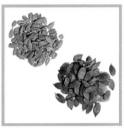

Shelled sunflower seeds (left) and pumpkin seeds should be plump and meaty. Those shown here are unroasted.

Look for When buying in-shell pumpkin and sunflower seeds in bulk, look for clean, unbroken shells; there should be a minimum of debris in the bin.

Prep When carving a pumpkin, don't throw out the seeds: Scoop them out, rinse them, and let them dry. Then toast the seeds in a 350° oven for 8 to 10 minutes, or until crisp. To enhance their flavor, toast shelled pumpkin-seeds in an ungreased skillet over very low heat for 3 minutes, or until they begin to pop.

Crispy Seed-Topped Flat Breads Serve these savory breads with dips or with dinner.

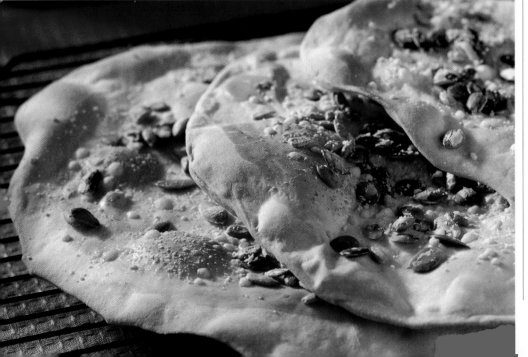

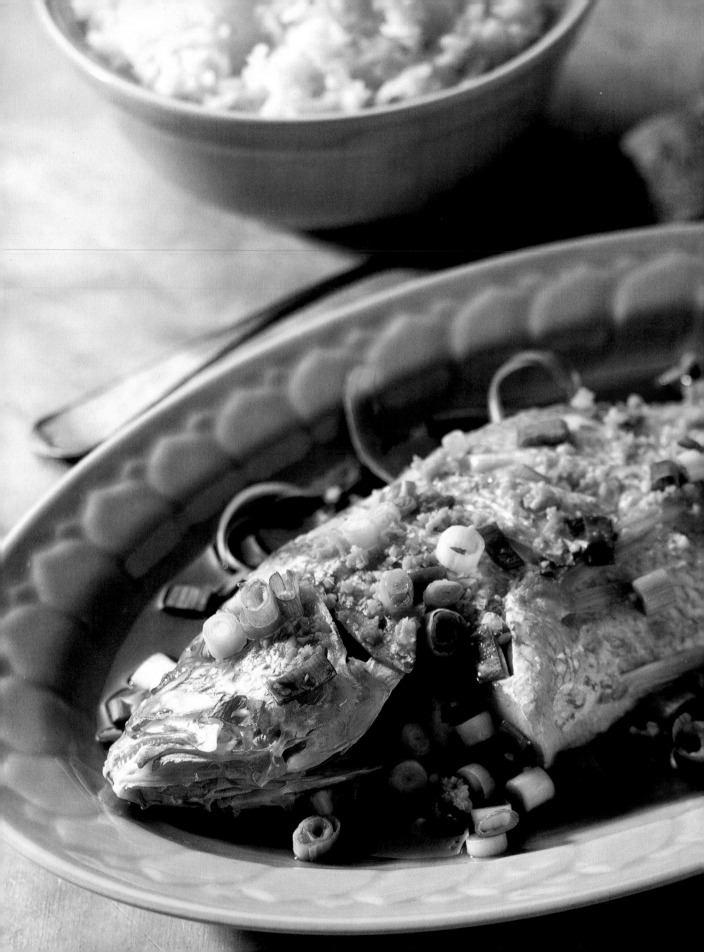

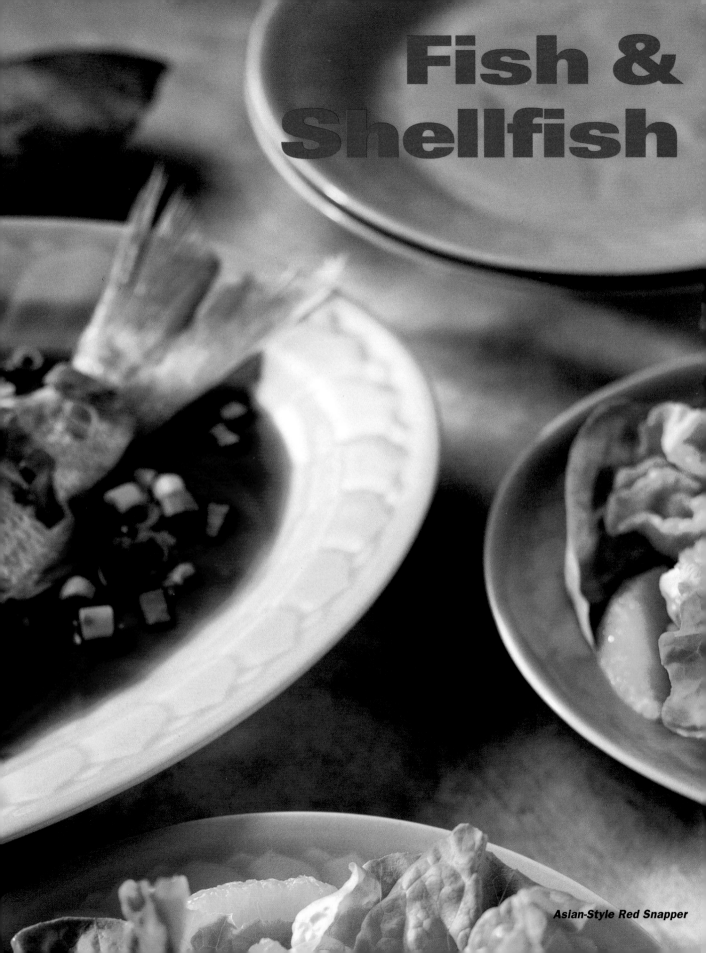

Fish &
Shellfish

Asian-Style Red Snapper

Salmon

Nutritional power
Salmon is one of the best sources of omega-3 fatty acids, which help lower triglycerides and may also fight cancer and reduce inflammation.

Healthy Highlights

Fresh Salmon

PER 3 OUNCES COOKED

Calories	151
Fiber	0g
Protein	21g
Total Fat	7.0g
Saturated Fat	1.7g
Cholesterol	54mg
Sodium	44mg

NUTRIENTS

	% Daily Value
Vitamin B12	45%
Niacin	32%
Vitamin B6	24%
Potassium	13%

Canned Salmon

PER 3 OUNCES

Calories	118
Fiber	0g
Protein	17g
Total Fat	5.1g
Saturated Fat	1.3g
Cholesterol	47mg
Sodium	471mg

NUTRIENTS

	% Daily Value
Vitamin B12	62%
Niacin	28%
Calcium	18%
Vitamin B6	13%

Salmon Steaks Veracruz-Style

PREP: 15 MINUTES / COOK: 55 MINUTES

A somewhat sharp tomato sauce, with the kick of capers and jalapeño, cuts the richness of the fish in this Mexican specialty.

- 2 teaspoons olive oil
- 1 small onion, finely chopped
- 2 cloves garlic, minced
- 1 teaspoon chili powder
- 1 can (14½ ounces) no-salt-added canned tomatoes, chopped with their juice
- 1 pickled jalapeño, finely chopped
- ¼ cup pitted green olives, coarsely chopped
- 1½ teaspoons capers, rinsed and drained
- ¼ teaspoon each dried oregano and thyme
- ⅛ teaspoon each cinnamon and salt
- 4 salmon steaks (8 ounces each)
- 2 tablespoons lime juice

1. In a large nonstick skillet, heat the oil over moderate heat. Add the onion and garlic, and sauté for 5 minutes or until soft. Add the chili powder, stirring to coat. Add the tomatoes, jalapeño, olives, capers, oregano, thyme, cinnamon, salt, and ¼ cup of water, and bring to a boil. Reduce to a simmer, cover, and cook for 30 minutes or until the sauce is richly flavored.

2. Preheat the oven to 350°F. Sprinkle the salmon with the lime juice and place in a 9 x 13-inch baking dish. Spoon ¾ cup of the sauce over the fish and bake for 15 to 20 minutes or until the salmon just flakes when tested with a fork. Reheat the remaining sauce and spoon over the fish before serving. Serves 4.

Per serving: Calories 353; Fiber 2g; Protein 41g; Total Fat 16g; Saturated Fat 2g; Cholesterol 110mg; Sodium 490mg

Cold Poached Salmon with Herbed Mayonnaise

PREP: 10 MINUTES / COOK: 15 MINUTES

This elegant presentation is ideal for a summer dinner party.

- 1 onion, sliced
- 1 carrot, thinly sliced
- 6 whole black peppercorns
- 1½ pounds salmon fillet, in one piece, skin on
- ¼ cup light mayonnaise
- 3 tablespoons reduced-fat sour cream
- 1 tablespoon lime juice
- ¼ cup chopped fresh basil
- 2 tablespoons snipped chives or scallion greens

1. In a large skillet, bring 3 cups of water to a boil over moderate heat. Add the onion, carrot, and peppercorns, and reduce to a simmer. Slip in the fish, skin-side up; cover and simmer for 10 minutes or until the salmon is just cooked through. Cool in the poaching liquid. Reserving 2 tablespoons of the poaching liquid, lift the fish out, transfer to a platter, cover, and refrigerate until chilled. Discard the remaining poaching liquid and the solids.

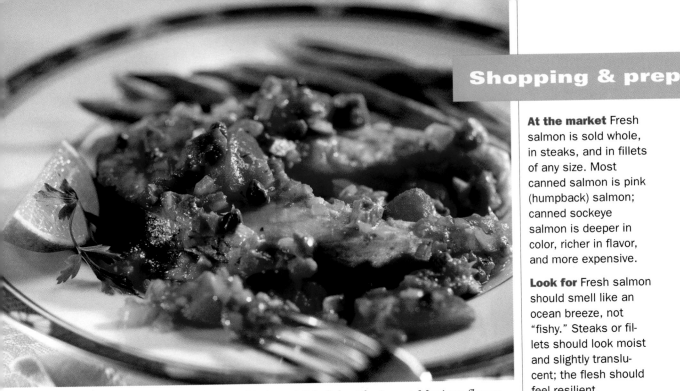

Salmon Steaks Veracruz-Style *A sophisticated fish dish with piquant Mexican flavors.*

At the market Fresh salmon is sold whole, in steaks, and in fillets of any size. Most canned salmon is pink (humpback) salmon; canned sockeye salmon is deeper in color, richer in flavor, and more expensive.

Look for Fresh salmon should smell like an ocean breeze, not "fishy." Steaks or fillets should look moist and slightly translucent; the flesh should feel resilient.

2. In a medium bowl, whisk together the reserved poaching liquid, the mayonnaise, sour cream, and lime juice. Stir in the basil and chives. Refrigerate until serving time.

3. At serving time, remove the salmon skin and cut the fillet into 4 portions. Serve the chilled salmon with the sauce spooned on top. Serves 4.

Per serving: Calories 309; Fiber 1g; Protein 33g; Total Fat 17g; Saturated Fat 3g; Cholesterol 96mg; Sodium 196mg

Roasted Salmon with Parsley-Lemon Dressing

PREP: 15 MINUTES / COOK: 15 MINUTES

The sauce, made with lemon zest and juice, red bell pepper, and parsley, supplies more than 40mg of vitamin C (67% of the RDA) per serving. Because the sauce is uncooked, the ingredients retain most of their vitamin C.

1/3   **cup chicken broth**
1   **teaspoon grated lemon zest**
1/4   **cup lemon juice**
4   **teaspoons olive oil**
1   **tablespoon Dijon mustard**
1   **teaspoon dried tarragon**

1/4   **teaspoon black pepper**
1   **red bell pepper, cut into 1/4-inch dice**
1/4   **cup chopped parsley**
1½   **pounds salmon fillet, in one piece, skin on**
1/4   **teaspoon salt**

1. Preheat the oven to 500°F. In a medium bowl, whisk together the broth, lemon zest, lemon juice, 3 teaspoons of the oil, the mustard, tarragon, and black pepper. Add the bell pepper and parsley. Set aside.

2. Spray a baking sheet with nonstick cooking spray. Place the salmon, skin-side down, on the baking sheet. Rub the remaining 1 teaspoon oil onto the salmon and sprinkle with the salt.

3. Bake for 12 to 15 minutes or until the salmon is medium-rare to medium. With a large spatula, lift the salmon off the baking sheet leaving the skin behind. Divide into 4 portions and serve with the sauce spooned on top. Serves 4.

Per serving: Calories 284; Fiber 1g; Protein 32g; Total Fat 15g; Saturated Fat 2g; Cholesterol 87mg; Sodium 395mg

Prep Salmon steaks and fillets sometimes contain "pin bones" firmly embedded in the flesh. Run your fingers over the surface of the fish to find them, then remove them with large tweezers or needle-nose pliers.

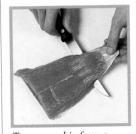

To remove skin from a salmon fillet, slip a knife between skin and flesh and "saw" it gently along, pulling the skin taut as you go.

Basic cooking Poach salmon in a large covered skillet of simmering water for 10 minutes, or until the fish barely flakes when tested with a knife.

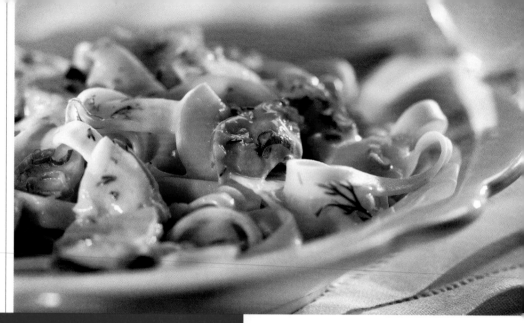

Fettuccine with Salmon *Lemon, fresh dill, and garlic flatter the flavor of salmon; you can use either fresh or canned fish.*

Did you know? . . .
Canned salmon is rich in calcium because during processing, the bones become soft enough to eat.

Salmon is rich in omega-3 fatty acids, which help lower blood triglyceride levels.

Studies have shown that the omega-3 fatty acids (polyunsaturated fats) found in some fish significantly reduce triglyceride levels. Triglycerides—blood fats—seem to be a contributing factor to heart disease, although the exact relationship is unclear.

The Center for Science in the Public Interest includes canned salmon—with its calcium-rich bones, vitamin D, and omega-3s—as one of five "super foods" for seniors.

A Michigan State University study showed that omega-3s suppressed breast tumor growth in laboratory animals.

Fettuccine with Salmon

PREP: 15 MINUTES / COOK: 25 MINUTES
You can substitute canned salmon for fresh, using a 15-ounce can of drained pink salmon. Follow the recipe as written, but add the salmon with the dill and lemon zest in Step 4.

- 12 ounces fettuccine
- 2 teaspoons olive oil
- 4 scallions, thinly sliced
- 2 cloves garlic, minced
- 1 small yellow squash, quartered lengthwise and thinly sliced
- 1 pound salmon fillet, skinned and cut into large chunks
- 1 cup chicken broth
- ¼ teaspoon salt
- ½ cup reduced-fat sour cream
- 1 tablespoon flour
- ¼ cup snipped fresh dill
- 1 teaspoon grated lemon zest

1. In a large pot of boiling water, cook the pasta according to package directions until firm-tender. Drain well.

2. Meanwhile, in a large nonstick skillet, heat the oil over moderate heat. Add the scallions and garlic, and sauté for 3 minutes. Add the squash and cook for 3 minutes or until tender.

3. Add the salmon, broth, ⅔ cup of water, and the salt, and cook for 5 minutes or until the salmon just flakes when tested with a fork.

4. In a small bowl, combine the sour cream and flour. Whisk into the skillet and simmer for 3 minutes or until lightly thickened. Stir in the dill and lemon zest. Toss the salmon and sauce with the hot fettuccine. Serves 4.

Per serving: Calories 573; Fiber 3g; Protein 37g; Total Fat 15g; Saturated Fat 4g; Cholesterol 72mg; Sodium 481mg

Parchment-Baked Salmon with Baby Peas

PREP: 10 MINUTES / COOK: 15 MINUTES

- 2 cups frozen baby peas, thawed
- 2 scallions, thinly sliced
- ¼ cup chopped fresh mint
- 2 tablespoons lemon juice
- 2 teaspoons olive oil
- ¾ teaspoon salt
- 4 salmon fillets, skinned (6 ounces each)

1. Preheat the oven to 450°F. In a medium bowl, toss together the peas, scallions, mint, lemon juice, oil, and ¼ teaspoon of the salt.

2. Spray four 15-inch lengths of parchment paper or foil with nonstick

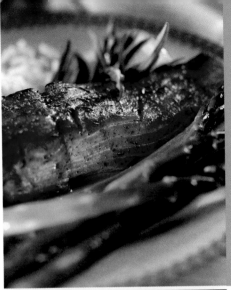

cooking spray. Place the salmon fillets, rounded-side up, on one half of each piece of parchment paper. Sprinkle the salmon with the remaining ½ teaspoon salt and top with the pea mixture. Fold the other half of the paper over the salmon and fold the edges over once or twice to seal the packets.

3. Place the packets on a baking sheet and bake for 12 to 15 minutes or until the packets are puffed and the salmon is medium-rare to medium. Serves 4.

Per serving: Calories 336; Fiber 6g; Protein 39g; Total Fat 14g; Saturated Fat 2g; Cholesterol 94mg; Sodium 641mg

Salmon with Salsa Verde

PREP: 15 MINUTES / COOK: 20 MINUTES

- 1   green bell pepper, cut lengthwise into flat panels
- ½   cup cilantro or parsley, finely chopped
- 3   tablespoons chicken broth or water
- 2   tablespoons lime juice
- 1   tablespoon olive oil
- 1   pickled jalapeño, finely chopped
- 4   salmon steaks (8 ounces each)
- ½   teaspoon each crumbled dried rosemary and salt
- ¼   teaspoon sugar

1. Preheat the broiler. Place the bell pepper pieces, skin-side up, on the broiler rack and broil 4 inches from the heat for 12 minutes or until the skin is blackened. (Leave the oven on.) When the peppers are cool enough to handle, peel and finely chop them. Transfer to a medium bowl and stir in the cilantro, broth, lime juice, oil, and jalapeño; set aside.

2. Rub the salmon with the rosemary, salt, and sugar. Broil 6 inches from the heat, turning once, for 6 minutes or until medium-rare to medium. Serve with the salsa spooned on top. Serves 4.

Per serving: Calories 324; Fiber 0g; Protein 40g; Total Fat 16g; Saturated Fat 2g; Cholesterol 110mg; Sodium 484mg

Broiled Herb-Rubbed Salmon In small bowl, combine ¾ tsp. salt, ½ tsp. sugar, ½ tsp. crumbled dried rosemary, ¼ tsp. dried tarragon, and a pinch ground allspice. Rub into four 6-oz. salmon fillets. Broil 6 inches from heat, without turning, for 5 minutes or until medium-rare. Serves 4. *[Cal 244; Fat 11g; Sod 511mg]*

Salmon Salad Sandwiches Stir together ¼ cup light mayonnaise, 2 tbsp. reduced-fat sour cream, 1 tsp. mustard, and 1 tbsp. each capers, chopped gherkin pickles, chopped fresh dill, and lemon juice. Add 15-oz. can pink salmon and stir to combine. Make 4 sandwiches with 8 slices whole-grain bread, 4 tomato slices, and 8 lettuce leaves. Serves 4. *[Cal 354; Fat 15g; Sod 1103mg]*

Teriyaki Salmon In shallow pie plate, combine 3 tbsp. soy sauce and 2 tsp. each brown sugar, oil, ketchup, and rice vinegar. Add four 8-oz. salmon steaks and marinate 1 hour. Place salmon on baking sheet, spoon marinade over, and bake at 500°F. for 10 minutes or until medium-rare. Serves 4. *[Cal 321; Fat 15g; Sod 890mg]*

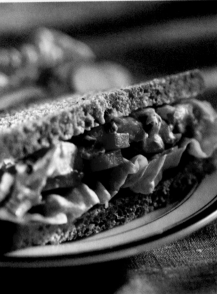
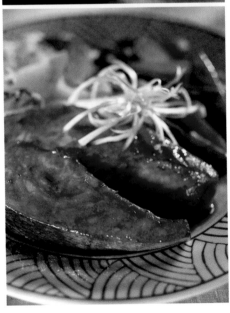

Tuna

Nutritional power
Remarkably lean for so flavorful a fish, tuna provides good amounts of healthful omega-3 fatty acids. It is also an excellent source of B vitamins.

Healthy Highlights

Fresh Tuna
PER 4 OUNCES COOKED

Calories	157
Fiber	0g
Protein	34g
Total Fat	1.4g
Saturated Fat	0.3g
Cholesterol	66mg
Sodium	53mg

NUTRIENTS

	% Daily Value
Niacin	68%
Vitamin B6	59%
Thiamin	38%
Potassium	22%
Magnesium	18%
Vitamin B12	12%

Canned Tuna*
PER 4 OUNCES

Calories	145
Fiber	0g
Protein	27g
Total Fat	3.4g
Saturated Fat	0.9g
Cholesterol	48mg
Sodium	427mg

NUTRIENTS

	% Daily Value
Niacin	33%
Vitamin B12	22%
Vitamin B6	13%

*water-packed white

Tuna with Roasted Red Onion Relish

PREP: 10 MINUTES / COOK: 50 MINUTES

- 2½ teaspoons sugar
- 1 teaspoon salt
- 1¼ teaspoons dried oregano
- ½ teaspoon pepper
- ⅛ teaspoon allspice
- 1½ pounds large red onions, cut into ½-inch cubes
- 4 teaspoons olive oil
- 1 tomato, diced
- 2 tablespoons red wine vinegar
- 4 tuna steaks (6 ounces each)

1. Preheat the oven to 350°F. In a medium bowl, combine the sugar, ½ teaspoon of the salt, the oregano, pepper, and allspice. Add the onions and 2 teaspoons of the oil, tossing well to coat. Transfer to a 9 x 13-inch baking dish, cover with foil, and bake for 30 minutes, stirring occasionally. Uncover and bake for 10 minutes. Transfer to a bowl, stir in the tomato and vinegar, and cool to room temperature.

2. On a grill pan or in a large nonstick skillet, heat the remaining 2 teaspoons oil over moderately high heat. Sprinkle the remaining ½ teaspoon salt over the tuna and cook, turning the fish over midway, for 5 minutes or until medium-rare. Serve with the relish spooned on top. Serves 4.

Per serving: Calories 347; Fiber 3g; Protein 38g; Total Fat 12g; Saturated Fat 3g; Cholesterol 58mg; Sodium 663mg

Chili-Garlic Grilled Tuna

PREP: 10 MINUTES / COOK: 10 MINUTES

Fresh tuna is so dense, meaty, and flavorful that it makes a welcome alternative to beef steaks at a barbecue. If you can't find green jalapeño pepper sauce at your local supermarket, use the regular red-colored hot pepper sauce.

- 2 cloves garlic, minced
- ½ teaspoon each crushed red pepper flakes and salt
- 4 tuna steaks, 1 inch thick (8 ounces each)
- 1 tablespoon jalapeño pepper sauce
- 4 teaspoons olive oil

1. Prepare the grill or preheat the broiler. In a small bowl, combine the garlic, pepper flakes, and salt. With a sharp, thin knife, make several horizontal slits into the sides of each tuna steak. Insert the garlic-pepper flake mixture into the slits.

2. Rub each tuna steak all over with the jalapeño pepper sauce and oil. Grill or broil the tuna steaks 6 inches from the heat for 3 minutes per side or until the tuna is cooked to medium-rare. Serves 4.

Per serving: Calories 333; Fiber 0g; Protein 47g; Total Fat 14g; Saturated Fat 3g; Cholesterol 77mg; Sodium 421mg

Tuna Salad Niçoise

PREP: 15 MINUTES / COOK: 20 MINUTES

Canned tuna is the traditional choice for this summery salad from Provence.

- **3 cloves garlic, peeled**
- **½ pound green beans, cut into 1-inch lengths**
- **¾ pound small red potatoes (about 6), halved**
- **¼ cup balsamic or red wine vinegar**
- **2 tablespoons light mayonnaise**
- **1 tablespoon olive oil**
- **½ teaspoon salt**
- **¼ cup packed fresh basil leaves**
- **1 pound tomatoes, cut into ½-inch-thick wedges**
- **2 cans (6½ ounces each) water-packed tuna, drained**
- **3 cups packed torn romaine lettuce**
- **¼ cup Niçoise olives**

1. In a large pot of boiling water, cook the garlic for 3 minutes to blanch. With a slotted spoon, transfer the garlic to a food processor or blender; set aside. Add the green beans to the boiling water and cook for 4 minutes or until crisp-tender. Remove the beans with a slotted spoon, rinse under cold water, and drain. Add the potatoes to the pot and cook for 12 minutes or until tender; drain.

2. Add the vinegar, mayonnaise, oil, and salt to the garlic in the food processor, and purée. Add the basil and 2 tablespoons of water, and purée.

3. Transfer the dressing to a large bowl. Add the tomatoes, green beans, potatoes, and tuna, tossing to coat. Add the lettuce and toss again. Sprinkle the olives on top. Serves 4.

Per serving: Calories 304; Fiber 6g; Protein 30g; Total Fat 8g; Saturated Fat 1g; Cholesterol 37mg; Sodium 741mg

At the market
Yellowfin is the type of tuna most often available fresh; boneless steaks are the most common form sold. Canned tuna comes in white (albacore) and light versions; white tuna is packed "solid" (usually a single piece of tuna), while light tuna comes in chunks or flakes.

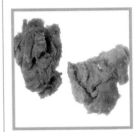

Chunk light tuna (left) and solid white tuna.

Look for Fresh tuna looks more like meat than fish: Yellowfin is deep red. The steaks should have a pleasant saltwater smell; they should look moist and dense, and feel springy to the touch. When selecting canned tuna, do not assume that all water-packed is lower in fat than oil-packed: Since the fat content of tuna can vary with when and where it is caught, always check the fat grams on the label.

Basic cooking Grill or broil tuna steaks for 3 minutes per side, or until medium-rare; or bake for 7 to 10 minutes in a 400° oven.

Tuna Salad Niçoise This light but satisfying salad features a heady basil dressing.

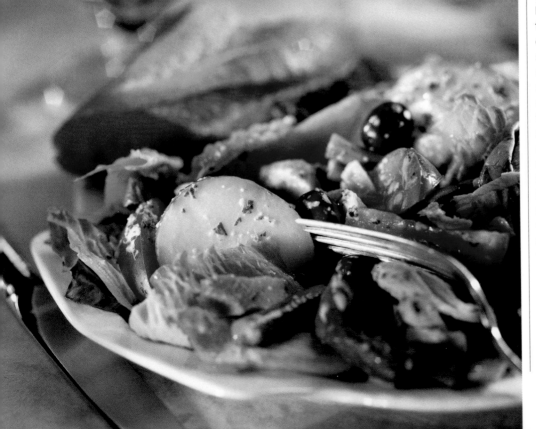

Meaty fish

Nutritional power
Along with plenty of high-quality protein, these lean, satisfying fish supply B vitamins, potassium, and moderate amounts of omega-3 fatty acids.

Healthy Highlights

Swordfish
PER 4 OUNCES COOKED

Calories	176
Fiber	0g
Protein	29g
Total Fat	5.8g
Saturated Fat	1.6g
Cholesterol	57mg
Sodium	130mg

NUTRIENTS

	% Daily Value
Niacin	67%
Vitamin B12	38%
Vitamin B6	22%
Potassium	14%
Magnesium	10%

Monkfish
PER 4 OUNCES COOKED

Calories	110
Fiber	0g
Protein	21g
Total Fat	2.2g
Saturated Fat	0g
Cholesterol	36mg
Sodium	26mg

NUTRIENTS

	% Daily Value
Vitamin B12	20%
Potassium	19%
Vitamin B6	16%
Niacin	15%

Grilled Marinated Swordfish Steaks

PREP: 10 MINUTES / MARINATE: 1 HOUR / COOK: 10 MINUTES

If you want to persuade someone to start eating fish, try this recipe for swordfish in a spicy marinade. Its flavor and texture are much like those of grilled chicken or steak.

- ¼ cup ketchup
- 2 tablespoons balsamic vinegar
- 2 teaspoons light brown sugar
- 2 teaspoons olive oil
- 1 teaspoon red hot pepper sauce
- ½ teaspoon each dried oregano and ground ginger
- ¼ teaspoon salt
- 4 swordfish steaks (6 ounces each)

1. In a shallow bowl, combine the ketchup, vinegar, brown sugar, oil, hot pepper sauce, oregano, ginger, and salt. Add the swordfish and rub the ketchup mixture into both sides. Cover and refrigerate for at least 1 hour.

2. Preheat the grill to medium (or preheat the broiler). Reserving the marinade, grill the swordfish 8 inches from the heat (or broil 6 inches from the heat) for 4 minutes. Turn the fish over, spoon on the reserved marinade, and grill for 4 minutes or until the fish is just cooked through. Serves 4.

Per serving: Calories 230; Fiber 0g; Protein 30g; Total Fat 8g; Saturated Fat 2g; Cholesterol 59mg; Sodium 491mg

Swordfish Kebabs with Lemon-Garlic Sauce

PREP: 20 MINUTES / COOK: 10 MINUTES

Sturdy swordfish is perfect for kebabs—it won't fall apart on the skewer. If using wooden skewers, soak them in cold water for 30 minutes to keep them from scorching.

- 3 cloves garlic, peeled
- ¼ cup lemon juice
- 4 teaspoons olive oil
- 1 tablespoon chopped parsley
- ¼ cup chicken broth
- ½ teaspoon each sugar and salt
- ¼ teaspoon pepper
- 1½ pounds swordfish steaks, skinned and cut into 24 chunks
- 16 cherry tomatoes
- 1 red onion, cut into 8 chunks

1. In a small pot of boiling water, cook the garlic for 2 minutes to blanch. Finely chop the garlic and transfer it to a small bowl along with the lemon juice, 3 teaspoons of the oil, and the parsley. Set the sauce aside.

2. Preheat the broiler. In a medium bowl, combine the broth, sugar, salt, and pepper. Add the fish, tomatoes, and onion, tossing gently to coat. Reserving the broth, alternately thread the fish, tomatoes, and onions onto eight 8-inch skewers.

3. Add the remaining 1 teaspoon oil to the reserved broth mixture. Brush the broth-oil mixture on the skewered fish

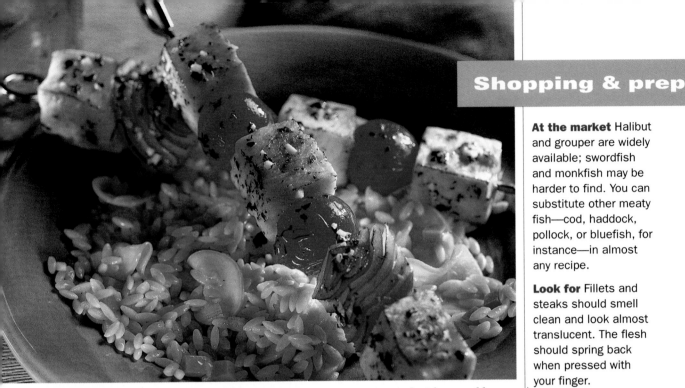

Swordfish Kebabs with Lemon-Garlic Sauce *Serve over orzo tossed with vegetables.*

and vegetables. Broil 6 inches from the heat for 6 minutes, turning the skewers over once, or until the fish is just cooked through and the onion is lightly browned. Spoon the lemon-garlic sauce over the kebabs. Serves 4.

Per serving: Calories 260; Fiber 1g; Protein 31g; Total Fat 11g; Saturated Fat 2g; Cholesterol 59mg; Sodium 504mg

Sautéed Parmesan-Crusted Monkfish

PREP: 20 MINUTES / COOK: 15 MINUTES

Relatively new to the American table, monkfish is so meaty and delicately sweet that it is sometimes called "poor man's lobster." Monkfish fillets are sheathed in a tough membrane, which should be removed before cooking (see how-to photo at right).

- 1½ **pounds monkfish fillets (1 inch thick), membrane removed, thinly sliced into 16 slices**
- ½ **cup grated Parmesan cheese**
- 4 **egg whites**
- ¾ **cup plain dry bread crumbs**
- ½ **teaspoon salt**
- 4 **teaspoons vegetable oil**
- 4 **lemon wedges**

1. Preheat the oven to 400°F. Spray a baking sheet with nonstick cooking spray; set aside. Place the monkfish slices between 2 sheets of wax paper and with the flat side of a small skillet or meat pounder, pound the fish to a ¼-inch thickness.

2. Spread the Parmesan on a sheet of wax paper. In a shallow dish, lightly beat the egg whites with 3 tablespoons of water. In another shallow dish or pie plate, combine the bread crumbs and salt. Dip the fish slices first in the Parmesan, then into the egg whites, then into the bread-crumb mixture, patting the bread crumbs into the fish.

3. In a large nonstick skillet, heat 1 teaspoon of the oil over moderately high heat. Sauté 4 slices of the fish for 1 minute per side or until golden brown and crispy. Transfer to the prepared baking sheet. Repeat with the remaining oil and fish. Bake the fish for 5 minutes or until just cooked through. Serve with the lemon wedges for squeezing. Serves 4.

Per serving: Calories 316; Fiber 1g; Protein 35g; Total Fat 12g; Saturated Fat 3g; Cholesterol 51mg; Sodium 736mg

At the market Halibut and grouper are widely available; swordfish and monkfish may be harder to find. You can substitute other meaty fish—cod, haddock, pollock, or bluefish, for instance—in almost any recipe.

Look for Fillets and steaks should smell clean and look almost translucent. The flesh should spring back when pressed with your finger.

Prep Steaks and fillets come ready to cook, except for monkfish fillets, which have a tough membrane on one side (on monkfish steaks, the membrane runs along the edge). Peel off the membrane before cooking.

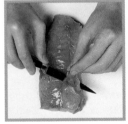

Slide a knife between the monkfish fillet and the membrane, and pull the membrane off.

Basic cooking Follow the Canadian Rule for cooking any fish: Measure the thickness of the fish with a ruler, and cook it about 10 minutes per inch of thickness.

Halibut
PER 4 OUNCES COOKED

Calories	159
Fiber	0g
Protein	30g
Total Fat	3.3g
Saturated Fat	0.5g
Cholesterol	46mg
Sodium	78mg

NUTRIENTS

	% Daily Value
Niacin	41%
Magnesium	30%
Vitamin B12	25%
Vitamin B6	23%
Potassium	22%

Grouper
PER 4 OUNCES COOKED

Calories	133
Fiber	0g
Protein	28g
Total Fat	1.5g
Saturated Fat	0.3g
Cholesterol	53mg
Sodium	60mg

NUTRIENTS

	% Daily Value
Vitamin B6	20%
Potassium	18%
Vitamin B12	13%
Magnesium	10%

Did you know? . . .
Several studies have now indicated that eating fish reduces the risk of heart disease, and many health authorities now advise eating fish at least once or twice each week.

Mushroom-Smothered Baked Halibut

PREP: 20 MINUTES / COOK: 40 MINUTES

The dried mushrooms called porcini (or cèpes, in French) have especially good flavor and aroma, but less expensive dried mushrooms will do just fine for this recipe.

- ¼ ounce dried porcini or other imported dried mushrooms
- 1 cup boiling water
- 4 teaspoons olive oil
- 1 pound button mushrooms, coarsely chopped
- 3 cloves garlic, minced
- ¼ cup chopped parsley
- ¾ teaspoon salt
- 1½ pounds halibut fillet, skinned and cut into 4 pieces
- 2 tablespoons lemon juice
- ¼ teaspoon pepper
- 2 tablespoons plain dry bread crumbs

1. In a small heatproof bowl, combine the dried mushrooms and boiling water, and let stand for 10 minutes or until softened. Reserving the soaking liquid, scoop out the porcini and coarsely chop. Strain the soaking liquid through a coffee filter or a paper towel-lined sieve.

2. In a large nonstick skillet, heat 2 teaspoons of the oil over moderate heat. Add the chopped porcini, the button mushrooms, and garlic, and sauté for 4 minutes or until the fresh mushrooms are tender. Add the mushroom soaking liquid, increase the heat to high, and cook for 5 minutes or until the liquid has evaporated. Stir in the parsley and ¼ teaspoon of the salt.

3. Preheat the oven to 350°F. Spray a 9-inch square glass baking dish with nonstick cooking spray and arrange the fish pieces in a single layer. Sprinkle with the remaining ½ teaspoon salt, the

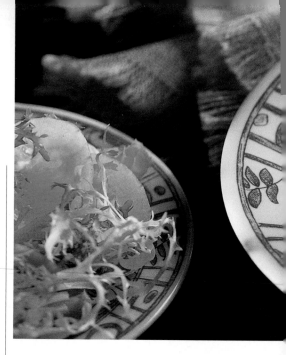

lemon juice, and pepper. Spoon the mushroom mixture on top. Sprinkle on the bread crumbs; drizzle the remaining 2 teaspoons oil over the crumbs. Bake for 30 minutes or until the fish is just cooked through. Serves 4.

Per serving: Calories 284; Fiber 2g; Protein 39g; Total Fat 9g; Saturated Fat 1g; Cholesterol 55mg; Sodium 565mg

Provençal Fish Stew

PREP: 25 MINUTES / COOK: 20 MINUTES

- 1 tablespoon olive oil
- 1 onion, finely chopped
- 4 cloves garlic, minced
- 1 red bell pepper, cut into ½-inch squares
- 1 can (14½ ounces) no-salt-added stewed tomatoes, chopped with their juice
- ⅓ cup chicken broth
- ½ teaspoon each fennel seeds and salt
- ¼ teaspoon cayenne pepper
- ¼ cup Calamata, Gaeta, or other brine-cured olives, pitted and coarsely chopped
- ¾ pound skinned and boned halibut or grouper, cut into 1-inch chunks
- ¾ pound skinned and boned cod or haddock, cut into 1-inch chunks
- ⅓ cup chopped fresh basil

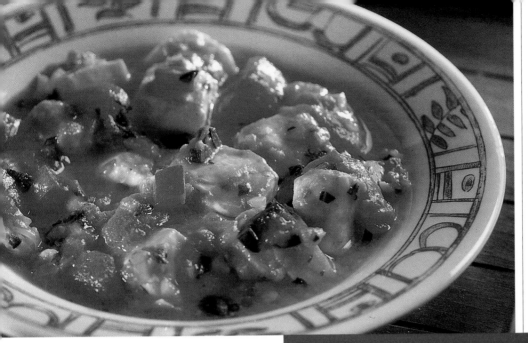

Provençal Fish Stew
Tomatoes, garlic, fennel seeds, olives, and fresh herbs give this stew a true French flavor.

Did you know? . . .
Halibut, grouper, and monkfish all have less than half the fat of an equivalent serving of beef round, one of the leanest cuts of beef.

1. In a large nonstick skillet, heat the oil over moderate heat. Add the onion and garlic, and sauté for 5 minutes or until the onion is soft. Add the bell pepper and cook for 4 minutes or until crisp-tender.

2. Add the tomatoes and their juice, the broth, fennel seeds, salt, cayenne, and olives, and bring to a boil. Reduce to a simmer, add the halibut and cod, cover, and cook for 7 minutes or until the fish is cooked through. Stir in the basil. Serves 4.

Per serving: Calories 276; Fiber 4g; Protein 35g; Total Fat 9g; Saturated Fat 1g; Cholesterol 64mg; Sodium 641mg

Orange-Braised Grouper

PREP: 10 MINUTES / COOK: 25 MINUTES
Grouper is a firm but delicate-tasting fish that is related to sea bass. It's delicious in this citrusy wine sauce.

- 1 tablespoon olive oil
- 4 scallions, thinly sliced
- 2 cloves garlic, minced
- ½ cup dry white wine or chicken broth
- ½ teaspoon grated orange zest
- 1 cup orange juice
- ⅓ cup chicken broth
- ½ teaspoon salt
- ¼ teaspoon pepper

In Japan, where fish forms part of the daily diet, heart disease is remarkably rare.

- 4 grouper fillets (6 ounces each), skinned
- 2 tablespoons chopped parsley

1. In a large skillet, heat 1 teaspoon of the oil over low heat. Add the scallions and garlic, and sauté for 2 minutes or until the scallions are soft. Add the wine, increase the heat to high, and cook for 3 minutes or until the wine is evaporated by half.

2. Add the orange zest, orange juice, broth, salt, and pepper. Bring to a boil and cook for 2 minutes. Reduce to a simmer, add the fish, cover, and cook for 10 minutes or until the fish is just cooked through.

3. Remove the fish from the poaching liquid and transfer to a platter or serving plates. Increase the heat under the skillet to high, add the remaining 2 teaspoons oil, and cook for 5 minutes or until the sauce is lightly thickened and syrupy. Stir in the parsley and spoon the sauce over the fish. Serves 4.

Per serving: Calories 226; Fiber 1g; Protein 34g; Total Fat 5g; Saturated Fat 1g; Cholesterol 63mg; Sodium 472mg

According to one study, the Japanese—who consume perhaps five times as much fish as Americans do—have about one-sixth the incidence of heart disease.

Ocean fish, including swordfish, monkfish, halibut, and grouper, are the best dietary source of iodine, a mineral required for proper thyroid function.

Despite the fact that they live in salt water, marine fish are naturally low in sodium.

Seafood is a good source of fluorine, which, in addition to its well-known role in keeping teeth healthy, also helps prevent calcium loss from bones.

Mild fish

Nutritional power
Snapper, striped bass, and rainbow trout are rich in omega-3 fatty acids; flounder has less of these but is a good source of heart-healthy vitamin E.

Healthy Highlights

Flounder
PER 4 OUNCES COOKED

Calories	133
Fiber	0g
Protein	27g
Total Fat	1.7g
Saturated Fat	0.4g
Cholesterol	77mg
Sodium	119mg

NUTRIENTS

	% Daily Value
Vitamin B12	47%
Magnesium	16%
Vitamin B6	14%
Niacin	13%
Potassium	13%
Vitamin E	11%

Red Snapper
PER 4 OUNCES COOKED

Calories	145
Fiber	0g
Protein	30g
Total Fat	1.9g
Saturated Fat	0.4g
Cholesterol	53mg
Sodium	65mg

NUTRIENTS

	% Daily Value
Vitamin B12	67%
Vitamin B6	26%
Potassium	20%
Magnesium	10%

Broiled Flounder with Herb Butter

PREP: 15 MINUTES / COOK: 5 MINUTES

Fillets of flounder and other thin flatfish fillets are a health-conscious cook's answer to fast food. Remove the fish from the pan as soon as it is done, or it may overcook from the heat of the pan.

- 2 tablespoons unsalted butter, softened
- 2 teaspoons reduced-fat cream cheese (Neufchâtel)
- 1 tablespoon snipped fresh dill
- 1 teaspoon snipped fresh chives or scallion greens
- 1 teaspoon drained horseradish
- ½ teaspoon grated lemon zest
- 4 flounder fillets (6 ounces each)
- 2 tablespoons lemon juice
- ¼ teaspoon salt

1. Preheat the broiler. In a medium bowl, beat together the butter and cream cheese until well combined. Stir in the dill, chives, horseradish, and lemon zest.

2. Sprinkle the flounder with the lemon juice and salt. Broil 6 inches from the heat, without turning the fish over, for 5 minutes or until the flounder is cooked through. Serve the fish topped with the herb butter. Serves 4.

Per serving: Calories 214; Fiber 0g; Protein 32g; Total Fat 8g; Saturated Fat 4g; Cholesterol 99mg; Sodium 295mg

Asian-Style Red Snapper

PREP: 10 MINUTES / COOK: 20 MINUTES

This Chinese-restaurant-style presentation of a whole snapper is a real dinner-party showstopper. Serve with white or brown rice.

- 1 whole red snapper (1¾ pounds)
- 2 tablespoons lower-sodium soy sauce
- 1 tablespoon sherry
- 1 teaspoon light brown sugar
- ¼ teaspoon salt
- 2 scallions, thinly sliced
- 1 tablespoon minced fresh ginger
- 1 tablespoon sesame oil

1. Preheat the oven to 400°F. With a large knife, make several slashes on both sides of the fish. Line a 9 x 13-inch metal baking pan (or small roasting pan) with foil, leaving a 2-inch overhang on both short ends. Fill the pan with water to come up ¼ inch. Place the fish in the pan, cover the pan with foil, and bake for 17 minutes or until the fish is just cooked through.

2. Meanwhile, in a small bowl, combine the soy sauce, sherry, brown sugar, and salt.

3. Using the overhang, lift the fish from the pan and pour off the liquid. Transfer the fish to a serving platter. Spoon the soy mixture over the fish. Sprinkle with the scallions and ginger.

4. In a small saucepan, heat the sesame oil. Pour the hot oil over the fish. Serves 4.

Per serving: Calories 152; Fiber 0g; Protein 22g; Total Fat 5g; Saturated Fat 1g; Cholesterol 38mg; Sodium 511mg

Baked Rolled Sole with Lemon & Oregano

PREP: 15 MINUTES / COOK: 10 MINUTES

Despite its elegant appearance, this is an easy, surefire recipe. Just be sure to lay the fillets smooth-side up (see how-to photo at right) so they will roll easily.

- ¼ **cup plain dry bread crumbs**
- ¼ **cup grated Parmesan cheese**
- 2 **tablespoons chopped parsley**
- 2 **tablespoons raisins or currants**
- ½ **teaspoon dried oregano**
- ½ **teaspoon grated lemon zest**
- ¼ **teaspoon each salt and pepper**
- 4 **sole or flounder fillets (6 ounces each)**
- 2 **teaspoons lemon juice**
- 2 **teaspoons olive oil**

1. Preheat the oven to 400°F. In a small bowl, combine the bread crumbs, Parmesan, parsley, raisins, oregano, lemon zest, salt, and pepper.

2. Place the fish, smooth-side up, on a work surface. Sprinkle the mixture over the fish and roll up from one short end. Place the rolls seam-side down in a 9-inch square glass baking dish. Drizzle the lemon juice and oil over the fish.

3. Bake, uncovered, for 10 minutes or until the fish is just cooked through and the filling is piping hot. Serves 4.

Per serving: Calories 240; Fiber 1g; Protein 35g; Total Fat 6g; Saturated Fat 2g; Cholesterol 86mg; Sodium 434mg

At the market Flounder is one of the most popular fish on the American market, and there are many kinds, such as gray sole, yellowtail flounder, plaice, and petrale. Farm-raised rainbow trout is also widely available. Striped bass and red snapper are less common; substitute yellowtail or silk snapper, or members of the rockfish family, such as ocean perch and Pacific snapper.

Look for Fillets should appear translucent and glistening fresh. Gutted whole fish should have bright, clear, bulging eyes; the gills should be bright red or pink.

Basic cooking Follow the Canadian Rule for cooking any fish: Measure the thickness of the fish with a ruler, and cook it about 10 minutes per inch of thickness.

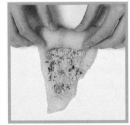

When rolling fillets, place the fish on the work surface with the smooth side up and the muscled (ribbed) side down, and the rolling will go more easily.

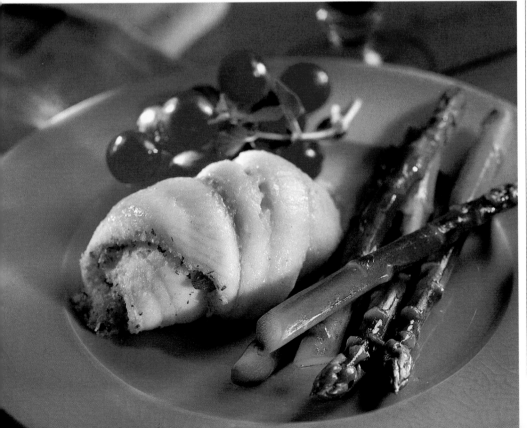

Baked Rolled Sole with Lemon & Oregano *Perfect with asparagus for a spring dinner.*

Healthy Highlights

Rainbow Trout
PER 4 OUNCES COOKED

Calories	191
Fiber	0g
Protein	28g
Total Fat	8.2g
Saturated Fat	2.4g
Cholesterol	77mg
Sodium	48mg

NUTRIENTS

	% Daily Value
Vitamin B12	93%
Niacin	50%
Vitamin B6	23%
Thiamin	18%
Potassium	17%
Calcium	10%

Striped Bass
PER 4 OUNCES COOKED

Calories	140
Fiber	0g
Protein	26g
Total Fat	3.4g
Saturated Fat	0.7g
Cholesterol	117mg
Sodium	100mg

NUTRIENTS

	% Daily Value
Vitamin B12	83%
Vitamin B6	20%
Niacin	15%
Magnesium	14%
Potassium	12%

Did you know? . . .
In a study of two African tribes—one totally vegetarian and the other heavy fish-eaters—the fish-eaters had lower levels of LDL, or "bad," cholesterol.

Sesame-Coated Striped Bass with Spicy Tomato Sauce

PREP: 25 MINUTES / COOK: 25 MINUTES

A thin coating of flour and sesame seeds gives the fish fillets a delicately crunchy crust.

- 5 tablespoons sesame seeds
- ¼ cup flour
- ½ teaspoon each salt and paprika
- 2 egg whites
- 1½ pounds striped bass or red snapper fillets, skinned and cut crosswise into 1-inch-wide strips
- 2 teaspoons olive oil
- 3 cloves garlic, minced
- 1 cup no-salt-added canned tomatoes, finely chopped with their juice
- ½ teaspoon grated orange zest
- ¼ teaspoon each ground ginger and crushed red pepper flakes
- 2 tablespoons orange juice

1. Preheat the oven to 400°F. Spray a large baking sheet with nonstick cooking spray. On a plate or a sheet of wax paper, combine the sesame seeds, flour, ¼ teaspoon of the salt, and the paprika. In a shallow bowl, lightly beat the egg whites with 1 tablespoon of water. Dip the fish first in the egg whites, then in the sesame mixture, pressing the sesame mixture into the fish. Place the fish on the prepared baking sheet.

2. In a large nonstick skillet, heat the oil over low heat. Add the garlic and sauté for 2 minutes or until soft. Add the tomatoes and their juice, orange zest, ginger, red pepper flakes, and the remaining ¼ teaspoon salt. Bring to a boil, reduce to a simmer, cover, and cook for 10 minutes or until the flavors have developed. Add the orange juice and cook for 1 minute.

3. Meanwhile, place the baking sheet in the oven and bake the fish, turning the pieces over once, for 10 minutes or until cooked through and crispy. Spoon the sauce alongside the fish. Serves 4.

Per serving: Calories 309; Fiber 2g; Protein 36g; Total Fat 12g; Saturated Fat 2g; Cholesterol 136mg; Sodium 444mg

Broiled "Buffalo" Fish

PREP: 15 MINUTES / COOK: 5 MINUTES

This unusual fish dish picks up on the idea of Buffalo wings (spicy chicken wings served with a rich blue cheese sauce and celery sticks). For this variation, spice-rubbed fish fillets are accompanied with a relish made with celery, carrot, and parsley tossed with a light blue cheese sauce.

- ½ teaspoon sugar
- ¼ teaspoon each dried oregano, thyme, and salt
- ⅛ teaspoon each cayenne and black pepper
- 4 red snapper or striped bass fillets, skinned (6 ounces each)
- 1¼ ounces Roquefort or other blue cheese, crumbled
- 1 tablespoon red wine vinegar
- 1 tablespoon reduced-fat sour cream
- 2 tablespoons plain nonfat yogurt
- 1 stalk celery, quartered lengthwise and thinly sliced (1 cup)
- 1 small carrot, quartered lengthwise and thinly sliced (¼ cup)
- 1 tablespoon chopped parsley

1. Preheat the broiler. In a small bowl, combine the sugar, oregano, thyme, salt, cayenne, and black pepper. Rub the mixture into one side of the fish; set the fillets aside.

2. In a medium bowl, whisk together the Roquefort, vinegar, and sour cream until well combined. Stir in the yogurt. Stir in the celery, carrot, and parsley.

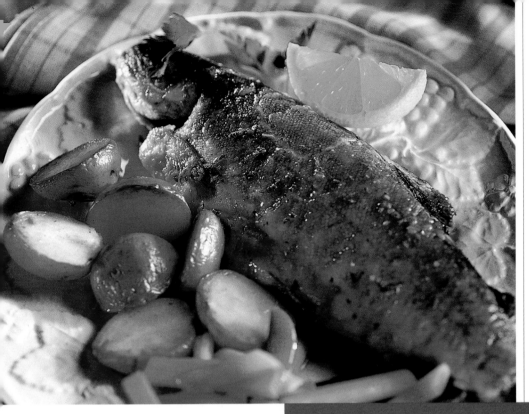

Rainbow Trout à la Meunière *A whole trout with a crusty-brown "coat" is a delectable country-style dish.*

Did you know? . . .
The American Heart Association recommends a well-rounded diet that includes fish (rather than fish-oil supplements) as a means of preventing heart disease.

3. Broil the fish, coated-side up, 6 inches from the heat for 4 to 5 minutes or until just cooked through. Serve the celery relish on the side. Serves 4.

Per serving: Calories 225; Fiber 1g; Protein 38g; Total Fat 6g; Saturated Fat 3g; Cholesterol 72mg; Sodium 449mg

Rainbow Trout à la Meunière

PREP: 20 MINUTES / COOK: 20 MINUTES
Meunière means "miller's wife" and describes foods sautéed with a light coating of flour.

- **4   whole rainbow trout (about 10 ounces each)**
- **½   cup low-fat (1%) milk**
- **¼   cup flour**
- **2   teaspoons vegetable oil**
- **⅓   cup lemon juice**
- **½   cup chicken broth**
- **¾   teaspoon cornstarch**
- **¼   teaspoon salt**
- **4   teaspoons unsalted butter**
- **1   tablespoon chopped parsley**

1. Preheat the oven to 400°F. Dip the trout in the milk and then in the flour, shaking off the excess.

The American Heart Association recommends fish as part of a heart-healthy diet.

2. In a large nonstick skillet, heat 1 teaspoon of the oil over moderately high heat. Add two trout to the pan and sauté, turning once, for 4 minutes or until lightly browned. Transfer to a baking sheet. Repeat with the remaining 1 teaspoon oil and two trout. Bake the trout for 10 minutes or until golden brown and cooked through.

3. Meanwhile, wipe the skillet dry. Pour in the lemon juice and cook for 1 minute. Whisk the broth into the cornstarch, add it to the skillet, and bring to a boil over moderate heat. Stir in the salt. Cook, stirring, for 1 minute or until lightly thickened.

4. Remove the sauce from the heat and swirl in the butter and parsley. Spoon the lemon sauce over the fish. Serves 4.

Per serving: Calories 328; Fiber 0g; Protein 41g; Total Fat 13g; Saturated Fat 4g; Cholesterol 121mg; Sodium 342mg

A health study begun in 1957 included a survey of the dietary habits of its 2,107 male subjects. A follow-up 30 years later revealed that the men who ate the most fish had the lowest risk of heart disease—nearly 40 percent lower than those who ate no fish at all.

A compound called DHA—one of the omega-3 fatty acids found in fish—is vital to brain development in early childhood, especially before the age of two. Researchers suspect that a deficit of DHA in adulthood may be a factor in depression.

Sardines

Nutritional power

In your quest for healthful foods, don't overlook the humble sardine, a rich source of protein, calcium (from the bones), and omega-3 fatty acids.

Healthy Highlights

PER 3¾-OUNCE CAN	
Calories	191
Fiber	0g
Protein	23g
Total Fat	10.5g
Saturated Fat	1.4g
Cholesterol	131mg
Sodium	465mg

NUTRIENTS	
	% Daily Value
Vitamin B12	137%
Calcium	35%
Niacin	24%
Iron	17%
Potassium	12%
Riboflavin	12%

Did you know? . . .
Nutrition experts at the Center for Science in the Public Interest include sardines on their list of five "super foods for seniors."

Rinsing canned sardines (handle them gently to avoid breaking them) will reduce their sodium content, which is often fairly high.

Potato & Sardine Salad

PREP: 20 MINUTES / COOK: 15 MINUTES

The addition of sardines turns this German-style potato salad into a satisfying main dish. Drained canned tuna may be substituted for the sardines.

- 1¼ pounds red potatoes, cut into ½-inch chunks
- ⅓ cup cider vinegar
- 2 teaspoons sugar
- 1 tablespoon grainy mustard
- ½ teaspoon salt
- ¾ cup plain nonfat yogurt
- 1 Granny Smith apple, cut into ½-inch chunks
- 1 red bell pepper, cut into ¼-inch dice
- 1 stalk celery, halved lengthwise and thinly sliced
- ¼ cup finely chopped red onion
- ¼ cup snipped fresh dill
- 2 cans (3¾ ounces each) sardines packed in oil, drained

1. In a large pot of boiling water, cook the potatoes for 12 minutes or until tender; drain.

2. Meanwhile, in a small saucepan, combine the vinegar and sugar, and heat for 1 minute to dissolve the sugar. Transfer the vinegar mixture to a large bowl and whisk in the mustard and salt. Add the hot potatoes to the dressing, tossing to combine. Let stand for 10 minutes to absorb the dressing.

3. Stir in the yogurt, apple, bell pepper, celery, onion, and dill, tossing to combine. Add the sardines, gently toss. Serve at room temperature or chilled. Serves 4.

Per serving: Calories 280; Fiber 4g; Protein 17g; Total Fat 6g; Saturated Fat 1g; Cholesterol 66mg; Sodium 621mg

Fish Cakes with Chutney Mayonnaise

PREP: 15 MINUTES / COOK: 10 MINUTES

Spicy sardine cakes are a tasty new idea (tuna would work in this recipe, too). Their gentle curry flavor is complemented by a creamy mango-chutney sauce.

- 1 slice firm white sandwich bread, crumbled
- 2 tablespoons low-fat (1%) milk
- 4 cans (3¾ ounces each) sardines packed in oil, drained
- 1 teaspoon curry powder
- ½ teaspoon ground ginger
- ¼ teaspoon each salt and pepper
- 2 teaspoons vegetable oil
- 2 tablespoons light mayonnaise
- 2 tablespoons plain nonfat yogurt
- 1 tablespoon mango chutney, finely chopped
- 1 teaspoon Dijon mustard
- 1 teaspoon lemon juice
- ⅛ teaspoon cayenne pepper

1. Preheat the oven to 400°F. In a medium bowl, combine the bread and milk until completely moistened. Add the sardines, curry powder, ginger, salt, and pepper, stirring to combine. Shape into 4 patties.

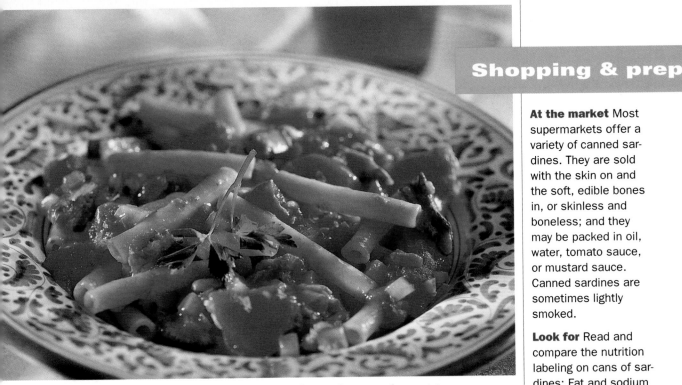

Sicilian Pasta features an interplay of sweet and spicy flavors and appetizing aromas.

At the market Most supermarkets offer a variety of canned sardines. They are sold with the skin on and the soft, edible bones in, or skinless and boneless; and they may be packed in oil, water, tomato sauce, or mustard sauce. Canned sardines are sometimes lightly smoked.

Look for Read and compare the nutrition labeling on cans of sardines: Fat and sodium content varies considerably among the different types.

Basic cooking Although they're not the most common of market fish in the United States, fresh sardines are sometimes available. After cooking the boned fish (sauté them briefly on both sides), you can use them in any of the recipes here.

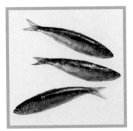

Fresh sardines are milder in flavor than the canned fish, but they boast the same nutritional assets.

---

2. In a large nonstick skillet, heat the oil over moderate heat. Add the fish cakes and cook for 2 minutes per side or until golden brown. Transfer to a baking sheet and bake for 5 minutes or until heated through.

3. Meanwhile, in a small bowl, combine the mayonnaise, yogurt, chutney, mustard, lemon juice, and cayenne. Serve the fish cakes with the chutney mayonnaise. Serves 4.

Per serving: Calories 282; Fiber 0g; Protein 24g; Total Fat 16g; Saturated Fat 2g; Cholesterol 134mg; Sodium 786mg

---

Sicilian Pasta

PREP: 20 MINUTES / COOK: 30 MINUTES

The quintessentially Sicilian combination of fennel and raisins brings a lovely, subtle sweetness to this pasta toss. If you can't get fennel, substitute 3 stalks of celery, diced, and 1 teaspoon crushed fennel seeds.

- **2** teaspoons olive oil
- **1** small onion, finely chopped
- **3** cloves garlic, minced
- **1** small bulb fennel (1 pound), stalks and fronds removed, cut into ¼-inch dice
- **2** cans (14½ ounces each) no-salt-added canned tomatoes, chopped with their juice
- **2** cans (3¾ ounces each) sardines packed in oil, drained
- **½** cup golden raisins
- **½** teaspoon salt
- **⅛** teaspoon cayenne pepper
- **10** ounces ziti
- **1** tablespoon pine nuts, toasted

1. In a large nonstick skillet, heat the oil over moderate heat. Add the onion and garlic, and sauté for 5 minutes or until soft. Add the fennel and sauté for 5 minutes or until soft. Add the tomatoes, sardines, raisins, salt, and cayenne, and bring to a boil. Reduce to a simmer, cover, and cook for 15 minutes or until the sauce is highly flavored.

2. Meanwhile, in a large pot of boiling water, cook the pasta according to package directions until firm-tender. Drain. Toss the hot pasta with the sauce and pine nuts. Serves 4.

Per serving: Calories 515; Fiber 6g; Protein 25g; Total Fat 11g; Saturated Fat 1g; Cholesterol 65mg; Sodium 648mg

Clams

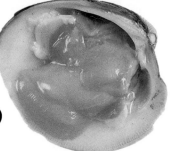

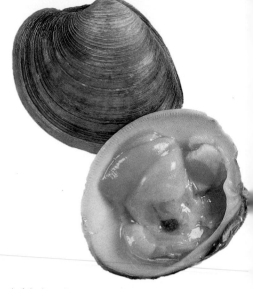

Nutritional power
Clams are a surpris-
ing source of vitamin
C, and an outstand-
ing source of vitamin
B12. They also sup-
ply an impressive
amount of iron and
plenty of copper.

Healthy Highlights

PER ¼ CUP SHUCKED

Calories	42
Fiber	0g
Protein	7g
Total Fat	0.6g
Saturated Fat	0.1g
Cholesterol	19mg
Sodium	32mg

NUTRIENTS

	% Daily Value
Vitamin B12	468%
Iron	44%
Manganese	14%
Vitamin C	12%
Copper	10%

Did you know? . . .
Most people don't
think much about
their intake of cop-
per, but this element
is required for the
body to convert iron
into hemoglobin.
Copper also sup-
ports immune sys-
tem function.

Clams used to be
considered high in
cholesterol, but new
research shows
them to be very low.

Spaghetti with Red Clam Sauce

PREP: 20 MINUTES / COOK: 20 MINUTES

You can make this dish with two 6½-ounce
cans of minced clams, drained. Omit Step 1
and the wine; in Step 2, substitute ⅔ cup
bottled clam juice or chicken broth for the
cooking liquid. Add the clams in Step 4.

- ¾ cup dry white wine
- 2 dozen littleneck or other small hardshell clams
- 1 teaspoon olive oil
- 1 small onion, finely chopped
- 5 cloves garlic, minced
- 2 cups canned no-salt-added tomatoes, chopped with their juice
- ⅓ cup chopped parsley
- ¼ teaspoon pepper
- 12 ounces spaghetti
- ¼ cup grated Parmesan cheese
- 2 teaspoons unsalted butter

1. In a large nonaluminum skillet,
heat the wine over moderate heat. Add
the clams, cover, and cook for 4 minutes
or until the clams open. (Start checking
after 2 minutes and remove the clams as
they open; discard any that do not.)
Strain the cooking liquid through a
fine-meshed sieve lined with paper towels or cheesecloth; measure out ⅔ cup
and set aside. Remove the clams from
their shells and coarsely chop.

2. In a large nonstick skillet, heat the
oil over moderate heat. Add the onion
and garlic, and sauté for 5 minutes or
until soft. Add the tomatoes, parsley,
pepper, and the reserved ⅔ cup cooking
liquid. Bring to a boil, reduce to a simmer, cover, and cook for 10 minutes to
develop the flavors.

3. Meanwhile, in a large pot of boiling
water, cook the pasta according to
package directions until firm-tender.
Drain and transfer to a large bowl.

4. Add the clams to the sauce and
cook for 1 minute to reheat. Pour the
sauce over the pasta and add the
Parmesan and butter, tossing to combine. Serves 4.

Per serving: Calories 478; Fiber 4g;
Protein 22g; Total Fat 7g; Saturated Fat 3g;
Cholesterol 28mg; Sodium 151mg

Baked Spinach-Stuffed Clams

PREP: 15 MINUTES / COOK: 25 MINUTES

Fresh bread crumbs are easy to make; a half-
slice of firm-textured white bread will
yield the ⅓ cup crumbs you'll need for this
recipe. Tear the bread into largish pieces, then
chop it in a mini-food processor, using on/off
pulses, until it's coarsely crumbled.

- 1 dozen cherrystone or other medium-size hardshell clams
- 4 teaspoons olive oil
- ¼ cup finely chopped onion
- 2 cloves garlic, minced
- 4 teaspoons flour
- ⅔ cup low-fat (1%) milk
- ½ teaspoon salt
- ⅛ teaspoon cayenne pepper
- ⅓ cup frozen chopped spinach
- ⅓ cup fresh bread crumbs
- 2 tablespoons grated Parmesan cheese

1. Place the clams in a large skillet
with ½ inch of water. Bring to a boil,
cover, and cook for 4 minutes or until
the clams open. (Start checking after 2
minutes and remove the clams as they

open; discard any that do not.) Transfer the clams to a bowl; when cool enough to handle, remove the top shell halves and discard. Place the shell halves with clams attached on a baking sheet.

2. Preheat the oven to 450°F. In a small saucepan, heat 2 teaspoons of the oil over low heat. Add the onion and garlic, and sauté for 5 minutes or until soft. Whisk in the flour and cook for 1 minute. Whisk in the milk, salt, and cayenne, and cook for 3 minutes or until lightly thickened. Stir in the spinach.

3. In a small bowl, stir together the bread crumbs and Parmesan. Spoon the spinach mixture over the clams. Top with the bread-crumb mixture and drizzle with the remaining 2 teaspoons oil. Bake for 10 minutes or until the clams are piping hot and the crumbs are lightly crisped. Serves 4.

Per serving: Calories 132; Fiber 1g; Protein 9g; Total Fat 6g; Saturated Fat 1g; Cholesterol 19mg; Sodium 414mg

Baked Spinach-Stuffed Clams *get a dinner party off to a deliciously spicy start.*

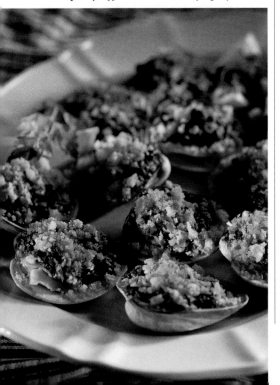

New England Clam Chowder with Corn

PREP: 15 MINUTES / COOK: 25 MINUTES

Crisp corn kernels and a touch of rosemary set this chowder apart. If you can't find in-shell or freshly shucked clams, use two 6½-ounce cans minced clams, drained. Add them in Step 3, cooking for just a minute or so, or until heated through.

- 2 **ounces bacon, finely chopped**
- 1 **small onion, finely chopped**
- 1 **red bell pepper, cut into ½-inch squares**
- ¾ **pound all-purpose potatoes, peeled and cut into ½-inch chunks**
- 1 **cup bottled clam juice or chicken broth**
- ½ **teaspoon each black pepper and salt**
- ¼ **teaspoon dried rosemary, crumbled**
- 1 **cup low-fat (1%) milk**
- 2 **tablespoons flour**
- 1 **cup frozen corn kernels**
- 1 **cup shucked clams (from 2 dozen littlenecks), coarsely chopped**

1. In a large saucepan, cook the bacon with 2 tablespoons of water over low heat for 3 minutes or until the bacon has rendered its fat and is lightly crisped. Add the onion and bell pepper, and cook, stirring frequently, for 5 minutes or until the onion is soft. Add the potatoes, tossing to coat.

2. Stir in the clam juice, 1¼ cups of water, the black pepper, salt, and rosemary, and bring to a boil. Reduce to a simmer, cover, and cook for 10 minutes or until the potatoes are tender.

3. In a small bowl, whisk the milk into the flour until well combined. Stir into the saucepan along with the corn and clams, and cook, stirring frequently, for 5 minutes or until the soup is lightly thickened and the clams are cooked through. Serves 4.

Per serving: Calories 265; Fiber 3g; Protein 14g; Total Fat 10g; Saturated Fat 4g; Cholesterol 31mg; Sodium 584mg

At the market Fresh hardshell clams are available all year round. Atlantic clams, such as littlenecks and cherrystones, are usually found in the East, while Pacific clams such as manilas and littlenecks (different from the East Coast littlenecks) are found in the West.

Look for Clams must be alive when you buy them: If the shells are tightly closed (or if they close when tapped), the clams are alive. Shucked clams should be plump, surrounded by a clear liquid.

Prep Scrub the shells under running water, then shuck them, if necessary, using a clam knife or other knife with a short, sturdy blade: Hold the clam in your palm, hinge toward your thumb, and wedge the knife blade between the shells. Work the blade all around the edge, then cut the muscle at the hinge.

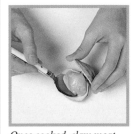

Once cooked, clam meat can be easily scooped from the shell: Use the edge of a spoon to sever the muscle.

Crab

Nutritional power
Crabmeat is a delectable, very low-fat protein source and an excellent source of copper and zinc. Crab also supplies B vitamins, calcium, and potassium.

Healthy Highlights

PER 4 OUNCES COOKED	
Calories	115
Fiber	0g
Protein	23g
Total Fat	2.0g
Saturated Fat	0.3g
Cholesterol	113mg
Sodium	315mg

NUTRIENTS	
	% Daily Value
Vitamin B12	138%
Copper	37%
Zinc	32%
Niacin	19%
Folate	14%
Calcium	12%
Potassium	12%
Vitamin B6	10%

Did you know? . . .
A Dutch study suggests that high zinc levels are associated with a reduced risk of cancer. A serving of crabmeat provides about one-third of your daily zinc requirement.

California Crab Roll

PREP: 15 MINUTES / COOK: 20 MINUTES

A popular sushi-bar selection, the California roll is a tidy assemblage of rice, crabmeat, cucumber, and avocado. Traditionally, the filling would be wrapped in a sheet of nori (dried seaweed); these heartier California rolls are made with flour tortillas.

- ⅓ cup rice
- ¼ teaspoon salt
- 3 tablespoons rice vinegar
- 1½ teaspoons sugar
- 8 flour tortillas (7 inch diameter)
- 8 large Boston lettuce leaves
- 1 pound lump crabmeat, picked over to remove any cartilage
- 1 cucumber, peeled, halved lengthwise, seeded, and cut into 2 x ¼-inch strips
- ½ avocado, cut lengthwise into eighths
- ½ cup jarred roasted red peppers, cut into 8 strips
- 2 tablespoons plus 2 teaspoons lemon juice

1. In a small saucepan, bring ⅔ cup of water to a boil. Add the rice and salt, cover, and simmer for 17 minutes or until tender. Sprinkle the vinegar and sugar over the rice and stir to combine. Let cool to room temperature.

2. Top each tortilla with a lettuce leaf. Spread the rice over the lettuce. Sprinkle the crabmeat on top, then place a cucumber strip, an avocado slice, and a roasted pepper strip on top. Sprinkle each with 1 teaspoon of the lemon juice. Roll up. Serves 4.

Per serving: Calories 418; Fiber 3g; Protein 30g; Total Fat 10g; Saturated Fat 2g; Cholesterol 114mg; Sodium 770mg

Curried Crab Salad

PREP: 15 MINUTES

- 1 teaspoon curry powder
- ½ teaspoon ground coriander
- ¼ teaspoon ground ginger
- ¼ cup light mayonnaise
- 2 tablespoons reduced-fat sour cream
- 1 tablespoon lemon juice
- ¼ teaspoon salt
- ¼ teaspoon red hot pepper sauce
- 1 pound lump crabmeat, picked over to remove any cartilage
- 1 red apple, cut into ¼-inch dice
- 4 cups torn Boston lettuce
- ¼ cup chopped cilantro or parsley

1. In a small skillet, combine the curry powder, coriander, and ginger, and heat over low heat, shaking the pan occasionally, for 1 minute or until lightly toasted. Transfer to a medium bowl and stir in the mayonnaise, sour cream, lemon juice, salt, and hot pepper sauce. Add the crabmeat and apple, tossing to coat.

2. Line plates with the lettuce, top with the crab mixture, and sprinkle with the cilantro. Serves 4.

Per serving: Calories 212; Fiber 2g; Protein 24g; Total Fat 8g; Saturated Fat 2g; Cholesterol 121mg; Sodium 593mg

Maryland Crab Cakes with Tomato-Avocado Relish

PREP: 25 MINUTES / COOK: 10 MINUTES

Crab-cake lovers look for the maximum proportion of crabmeat to bread crumbs; this recipe is designed to please the most finicky fan. The piquant "salsa" served alongside is the perfect complement to the crab cakes.

- 1   large tomato, cut into ¼-inch dice
- ⅓   cup diced avocado
- 2   tablespoons chopped cilantro or parsley
- 2   tablespoons minced red onion
- 1   tablespoon lime juice
- ½   teaspoon salt
- ¼   teaspoon red hot pepper sauce
- 1   slice firm white sandwich bread, crumbled
- ¼   cup low-fat (1%) milk

- 1   pound lump crabmeat, picked over to remove any cartilage
- 2   tablespoons light mayonnaise
- ⅓   cup plain dry bread crumbs
- 4   teaspoons vegetable oil

1. In a medium bowl, combine the tomato, avocado, cilantro, onion, lime juice, ¼ teaspoon of the salt, and the hot pepper sauce. Cover and refrigerate while you prepare the crab cakes.

2. In a medium bowl, thoroughly combine the crumbled bread and milk. Add the crabmeat, mayonnaise, and remaining ¼ teaspoon salt, stirring to combine. Shape into 8 crab cakes and dredge in the dry bread crumbs.

3. Preheat the oven to 400°F. In a large nonstick skillet, heat the oil over moderate heat. Sauté the crab cakes for 2 minutes per side or until golden brown. Transfer the cakes to a baking sheet and bake for 5 minutes or until heated through. Serve the cakes with the tomato-avocado relish. Serves 4.

Per serving: Calories 277; Fiber 2g; Protein 26g; Total Fat 12g; Saturated Fat 2g; Cholesterol 117mg; Sodium 802mg

At the market You're most likely to find live crabs in markets near the coast; cooked crabmeat is widely available fresh, frozen, or canned. Pasteurized crabmeat is a good choice; it keeps longer than other forms.

Look for For big chunks of crab, choose "lump" crabmeat, which is expensive but worth the price. "Backfin" meat comes in smaller pieces, while "flake" crabmeat consists of still smaller bits. The meat should be white and freshsmelling.

Prep Crabmeat is ready to eat as it comes, but you should pick it over: Spread the crabmeat out on a plate and remove any bits of cartilage you find. Handle lump crabmeat gently so that the chunks don't break up.

Curried Crab Salad embellishes luxurious lump crabmeat with a well-seasoned sauce.

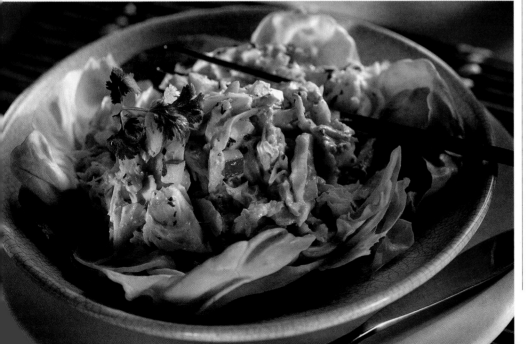

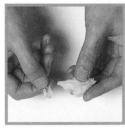

Small pieces of cartilage are sometimes left behind when crabmeat is cleaned. Pick over the meat and remove them.

Mussels & Oysters

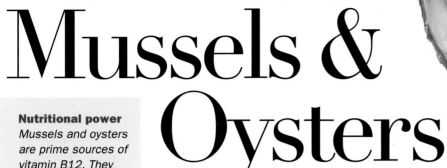

Nutritional power
Mussels and oysters are prime sources of vitamin B12. They are also rich in minerals, including manganese, which is a component of antioxidant enzymes.

Healthy Highlights

Mussels

PER ¼ CUP SHUCKED

Calories	32
Fiber	0g
Protein	5g
Total Fat	0.8g
Saturated Fat	0.2g
Cholesterol	11mg
Sodium	107mg

NUTRIENTS

	% Daily Value
Vitamin B12	75%
Manganese	64%

Oysters

PER ¼ CUP SHUCKED

Calories	42
Fiber	0g
Protein	4g
Total Fat	1.5g
Saturated Fat	0.5g
Cholesterol	33mg
Sodium	131mg

NUTRIENTS

	% Daily Value
Zinc	375%
Vitamin B12	202%
Copper	138%
Iron	22%
Manganese	11%

Pasta with Mussels in Marinara Sauce

PREP: 15 MINUTES / COOK: 20 MINUTES

Mussels in the shell top tomato-sauced linguine for an attractive but simple meal.

- 12 ounces linguine
- 4 teaspoons unsalted butter
- 2 teaspoons olive oil
- 1 small onion, finely chopped
- 5 cloves garlic, minced
- 2 cans (14½ ounces each) no-salt-added tomatoes, chopped with their juice
- 1½ pounds mussels, well scrubbed and debearded
- ⅓ cup chopped fresh basil
- ¼ cup chopped parsley
- ¼ teaspoon each salt and pepper

1. In a large pot of boiling water, cook the pasta according to package directions until firm-tender. Drain, transfer to a large bowl, add the butter, and toss to coat.

2. Meanwhile, in a large skillet, heat the oil over low heat. Add the onion and garlic, and sauté for 5 minutes or until soft. Add the tomatoes and cook, stirring occasionally, for 5 minutes or until the sauce is richly flavored.

3. Add the mussels, cover, and cook for 5 minutes or until the mussels have opened. (Start checking after 2 minutes and remove the mussels as they open; discard any that do not.)

4. When all the mussels have opened, return them to the pan. Add the basil, parsley, salt, and pepper, and cook for 1 minute. Add to the pasta, tossing gently to combine. Serves 4.

Per serving: Calories 473; Fiber 5g; Protein 20g; Total Fat 9g; Saturated Fat 3g; Cholesterol 24mg; Sodium 322mg

Pan-Fried Oysters with Spicy Mustard Sauce

PREP: 10 MINUTES / COOK: 5 MINUTES

Browned in just 2 teaspoons of oil, these delicate crusty oysters barely fit the definition of "fried."

- 4 teaspoons Dijon mustard
- 1 tablespoon chili sauce
- 1 teaspoon lemon juice
- ⅛ teaspoon red hot pepper sauce
- 1½ teaspoons honey
- ¼ teaspoon ground ginger
- ¼ cup flour
- 2 tablespoons yellow cornmeal
- ¼ teaspoon each baking powder and salt
- 1 egg white
- 1 dozen oysters, shucked
- 2 teaspoons olive oil

1. In a small bowl, combine the mustard, chili sauce, lemon juice, red pepper sauce, honey, and ginger; set aside.

2. On a sheet of wax paper, combine the flour, cornmeal, baking powder, and salt. In a small bowl, beat the egg white with 1 tablespoon of water. Dip the oysters first in the egg white, then in the flour mixture.

3. In a large nonstick skillet, heat the oil over moderately high heat. Cook the oysters for 2 minutes per side or until golden brown and crisp. Serve with the mustard sauce spooned alongside. Serves 4.

Per serving: Calories 145; Fiber 0g; Protein 8g; Total Fat 5g; Saturated Fat 1g; Cholesterol 47mg; Sodium 464mg

Creamy Oyster Stew

PREP: 10 MINUTES / COOK: 10 MINUTES

When you shuck the oysters, work over a bowl to catch the liquid: You'll need ½ cup of this so-called "liquor" for the stew. If you are using shucked oysters with too little liquid, fill it out with clam juice or chicken broth.

4   **large slices (2 ounces) Italian bread, without seeds**
2   **teaspoons unsalted butter**
3   **cups low-fat (1%) milk**
¼   **cup flour**
¾   **teaspoon salt**
¼   **teaspoon cayenne pepper**
2   **dozen oysters, shucked, liquor reserved**
¼   **cup chopped parsley**

1. Toast the bread and spread with the butter; set aside.

2. In a large saucepan, whisk the milk into the flour. Stir over low heat until smooth. Add the salt and cayenne, and cook, stirring frequently, for 3 minutes or until lightly thickened and no floury taste remains.

3. Stir in ½ cup of the reserved oyster liquor. Bring the mixture to a simmer, add the oysters, cover, and cook for 3 minutes or just until the edges of the oysters begin to curl. Stir in the parsley.

4. Spoon the stew into individual soup bowls and serve with the buttered toast. Serves 4.

Per serving: Calories 221; Fiber 1g; Protein 14g; Total Fat 7g; Saturated Fat 3g; Cholesterol 59mg; Sodium 708mg

At the market Most mussels sold in the U.S. are "farmed" in safe waters and are available year-round, though scarcer in the summer. Oysters are also farmed; although they are available at other times of the year, they're best in the fall and winter.

Look for Mussels are usually sold live in the shell; oysters are sold live or shucked. The shells should be tightly closed. Shucked oysters are packed in their "liquor," which should be clear, not milky.

Prep To clean mussels, pull out the "beards" (see below) and then scrub under running water. To shuck oysters, use an oyster knife, which has a short, sturdy blade. Protect your hands with a potholder or kitchen towel. Insert the knife at the hinge and twist to break the hinge; work the knife around to sever the muscle, then cut the meat from the shell.

Creamy Oyster Stew One of the fastest, tastiest ways to serve oysters.

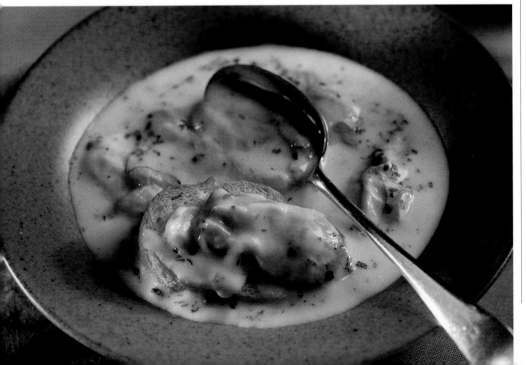

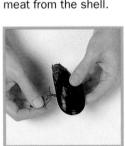

To clean a mussel, grab the "beard" and pull out with a quick, firm tug.

225

Scallops

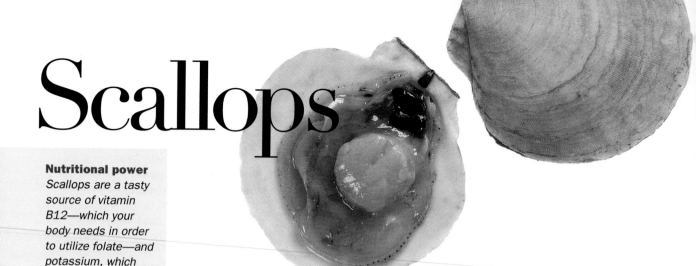

Nutritional power

Scallops are a tasty source of vitamin B12—which your body needs in order to utilize folate—and potassium, which helps control blood pressure.

Healthy Highlights

PER 4 OUNCES RAW	
Calories	99
Fiber	0g
Protein	19g
Total Fat	0.9g
Saturated Fat	0.1g
Cholesterol	37mg
Sodium	182mg

NUTRIENTS	
	% Daily Value
Vitamin B12	28%
Magnesium	16%
Potassium	12%

Did you know? . . .
Scallops contain about twice as much omega-3 fatty acids as does water-packed light tuna.

The cholesterol content of most shellfish is fairly low—lower than that of lean turkey breast. Among shellfish, scallops are the second lowest in cholesterol content—only mussels contain less.

Seviche-Style Scallop Salad

PREP: 25 MINUTES / COOK: 15 MINUTES

True seviche is not cooked, but it's safer to simmer the scallops for a few minutes.

- 1 tablespoon olive oil
- 2 scallions, thinly sliced
- 2 cloves garlic, minced
- 1 teaspoon chili powder
- 1 cup orange juice
- 1 tablespoon no-salt-added tomato paste
- 1 pound sea scallops, halved crosswise
- ¼ cup chopped cilantro
- 2 tablespoons lime juice
- 1 large tomato, cut into ¼-inch dice
- 1 mango, cut into ½-inch chunks
- ½ teaspoon salt

1. In a large nonstick skillet, heat 1 teaspoon of the oil over low heat. Add the scallions, garlic, and chili powder, and cook for 2 minutes or until softened. Add the orange juice and tomato paste, bring to a boil, and cook for 3 minutes or until reduced by one-third.

2. Reduce to a simmer, add the scallops, and cook for 3 minutes or until just cooked through. With a slotted spoon, transfer the scallops to a large bowl.

3. Increase the heat to high and boil the liquid in the skillet for 5 minutes or until reduced to ½ cup. Let the reduced liquid cool slightly, then add to the scallops. Stir in the remaining 2 teaspoons

oil, the cilantro, and lime juice until well combined. Add the tomato, mango, and salt. Serve at room temperature or chilled. Serves 4.

Per serving: Calories 215; Fiber 2g; Protein 21g; Total Fat 5g; Saturated Fat 1g; Cholesterol 38mg; Sodium 491mg

Pasta & Scallops Provençal

PREP: 20 MINUTES / COOK: 20 MINUTES

- 12 ounces ziti
- 1 tablespoon olive oil
- 2 small leeks, white and tender green parts only, halved lengthwise, cut crosswise into ½-inch slices, and well washed
- 4 cloves garlic, minced
- 1 red bell pepper, cut into ½-inch squares
- ½ teaspoon each fennel seeds and dried tarragon
- ⅓ cup chicken broth
- 1½ cups canned no-salt-added tomatoes, chopped with their juice
- 3 tablespoons no-salt-added tomato paste
- ¾ teaspoon salt
- ½ teaspoon grated orange zest
- 1 pound sea scallops, halved crosswise
- ¼ cup grated Parmesan cheese

1. In a large pot of boiling water, cook the pasta according to package directions until firm-tender; drain.

2. Meanwhile, in a large nonstick skillet, heat 2 teaspoons of the oil over low heat. Add the leeks and garlic, and sauté for 4 minutes or until the leeks are tender. Add the remaining 1 teaspoon oil, the bell pepper, fennel seeds, and tarragon, and sauté for 5 minutes or until the pepper is tender.

3. Add the broth, increase the heat to high, and cook for 2 minutes or until the liquid has evaporated. Add the tomatoes, tomato paste, salt, and orange zest; reduce the heat to low and cook for 5 minutes.

4. Add the scallops, cover, and cook for 4 minutes or just until the scallops are cooked through. Transfer to a large bowl, add the pasta and Parmesan, and toss to combine. Serves 4.

Per serving: Calories 536; Fiber 4g; Protein 34g; Total Fat 8g; Saturated Fat 2g; Cholesterol 41mg; Sodium 834mg

Spicy Scallops with Shredded Vegetables *Tender bay scallops keep company with a colorful selection of vegetables in this saucy stir-fry.*

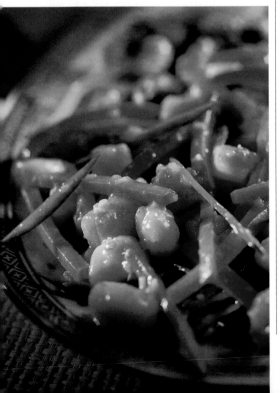

Spicy Scallops with Shredded Vegetables

PREP: 20 MINUTES / COOK: 5 MINUTES

Scallops are an ideal stir-fry component because they cook in a flash. Keep them in mind for other quick meals, too—they require little or no preparation, and there's no waste.

- 1 **pound bay scallops or quartered sea scallops**
- 2 **tablespoons plus 1 teaspoon cornstarch**
- 4 **teaspoons vegetable oil**
- 2 **carrots, cut into 2 x ¼-inch matchsticks**
- 8 **ounces snow peas, strings removed, cut lengthwise into ¼-inch-wide strips**
- 1 **red bell pepper, cut into ¼-inch-wide strips**
- 3 **scallions, cut into 2-inch lengths**
- 1 **tablespoon minced fresh ginger**
- 3 **cloves garlic, minced**
- ¾ **cup chicken broth**
- ½ **teaspoon crushed red pepper flakes**
- ¼ **teaspoon salt**

1. Dredge the scallops in 2 tablespoons of the cornstarch, shaking off the excess. In a large nonstick skillet, heat 2 teaspoons of the oil over moderately high heat. Add the scallops and stir-fry for 2 minutes or until lightly golden. With a slotted spoon, transfer the scallops to a plate.

2. Add the remaining 2 teaspoons oil to the skillet along with the carrots, snow peas, bell pepper, scallions, ginger, and garlic, and stir-fry for 2 minutes or until crisp-tender. In a small bowl, whisk the broth, red pepper flakes, and salt into the remaining 1 teaspoon cornstarch. Pour into the skillet, bring to a boil, and boil for 1 minute. Reduce to a simmer, return the scallops to the pan, and cook for 30 seconds or just until heated through. Serves 4.

Per serving: Calories 213; Fiber 3g; Protein 22g; Total Fat 6g; Saturated Fat 1g; Cholesterol 38mg; Sodium 540mg

At the market Sea scallops, which are about 1½ inches across, are widely available. Bay scallops, about ½ inch across, are sweeter; harvested mainly on the East Coast, they are less common than sea scallops.

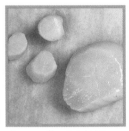

A sea scallop (right) is considerably larger than a bay scallop (left).

Look for Scallops, which are almost always sold shucked, should be plump and shiny; they should smell sweetly fresh, not fishy.

Prep Scallops sometimes have a small piece of tough connective tissue along one side. Pull this off and discard. To substitute sea scallops in a recipe that calls for bay scallops, quarter the sea scallops.

Basic cooking Cook scallops until just opaque throughout; this should be done quickly so that they do not toughen. Sautéing and stir-frying are two good choices for cooking scallops.

Shrimp

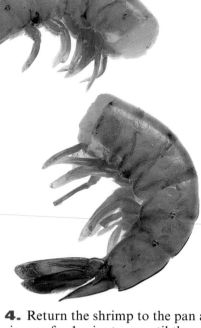

Nutritional power

A low-fat protein source, shrimp provide a good amount of two B vitamins—B12 and niacin. They're also mineral-rich, supplying iron, zinc, and copper.

Healthy Highlights

PER 4 OUNCES COOKED	
Calories	112
Fiber	0g
Protein	24g
Total Fat	1.2g
Saturated Fat	0.3g
Cholesterol	221mg
Sodium	254mg

NUTRIENTS	
	% Daily Value
Vitamin B12	28%
Iron	22%
Niacin	15%
Zinc	12%
Copper	11%

Did you know? . . .

Shrimp are rich in both iron and zinc. Many adults, especially women and the elderly, consume less of both these minerals than their bodies require. Eating more shrimp is a tasty way to get adequate amounts of iron and zinc.

Shrimp Bisque with Croutons

PREP: 20 MINUTES / COOK: 20 MINUTES

A bisque usually derives its richness from heavy cream. This version is rendered "creamy" with low-fat milk and flour.

- 4 slices (½ inch thick) French or Italian bread
- 1 clove garlic, halved
- 1 cup bottled clam juice or chicken broth
- 1 pound medium shrimp, peeled and deveined
- 1 can (8 ounces) no-salt-added tomato sauce
- 2 cups low-fat (1%) milk
- 2 tablespoons flour
- ½ teaspoon each dried tarragon, salt, and pepper
- ¼ cup chopped parsley

1. Preheat the oven to 400°F. Rub the bread with the cut sides of the halved garlic, then cut the bread into ½-inch cubes. Place on a baking sheet and bake for 5 minutes or until lightly toasted. Remove and set aside.

2. In a medium saucepan, bring the clam juice and ¼ cup of water to a simmer. Add the shrimp and cook for 3 minutes or until just done. With a slotted spoon, transfer the shrimp to a bowl. Stir the tomato sauce into the saucepan.

3. In a medium bowl, whisk the milk into the flour, then whisk the mixture into the saucepan. Cook over moderate heat, stirring constantly, for 5 minutes or until the mixture is lightly thickened and no floury taste remains. Stir in the tarragon, salt, pepper, and parsley.

4. Return the shrimp to the pan and simmer for 1 minute or until they are just heated through. Serve topped with the croutons. Serves 4.

Per serving: Calories 256; Fiber 2g; Protein 26g; Total Fat 4g; Saturated Fat 1g; Cholesterol 145mg; Sodium 782mg

Cajun-Style Grilled Shrimp

PREP: 25 MINUTES / MARINATE: 30 MINUTES / COOK: 5 MINUTES

- 1½ teaspoons dried oregano
- 1 teaspoon granulated sugar
- ¾ teaspoon each dried thyme and salt
- ½ teaspoon black pepper
- ¼ teaspoon cayenne pepper
- 1½ pounds large shrimp, peeled and deveined
- 1½ teaspoons vegetable oil
- ⅓ cup ketchup
- 2 tablespoons plus 2 teaspoons red wine vinegar
- ¾ teaspoon light brown sugar
- ½ teaspoon ground ginger
- 2 cups frozen corn kernels, thawed
- 2 scallions, thinly sliced

1. In a medium bowl, combine the oregano, granulated sugar, thyme, salt, black pepper, and cayenne. Add the shrimp and oil, tossing to coat. Cover and refrigerate for 30 minutes.

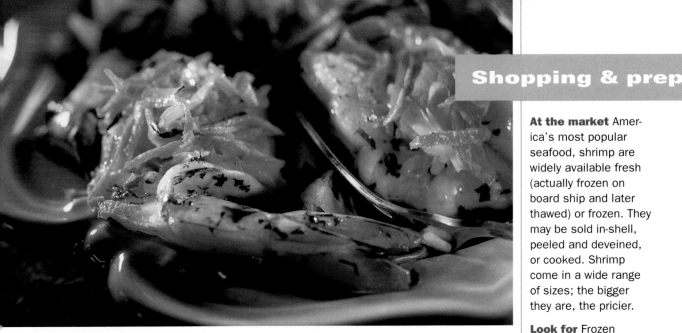

Asian Stuffed Shrimp Butterflied shrimp are crowned with a gingery vegetable topping.

At the market America's most popular seafood, shrimp are widely available fresh (actually frozen on board ship and later thawed) or frozen. They may be sold in-shell, peeled and deveined, or cooked. Shrimp come in a wide range of sizes; the bigger they are, the pricier.

Look for Frozen shrimp should be solidly frozen; thawed shrimp should smell fresh and have firm, glossy shells.

Prep In-shell shrimp need to be peeled and deveined for some recipes (see below).

2. Meanwhile, combine the ketchup, vinegar, brown sugar, and ginger. Stir in the corn and scallions.

3. Preheat the broiler. Broil the shrimp 6 inches from the heat, turning them over once, for 4 minutes or until cooked through. Toss the hot shrimp with the corn mixture. Serves 4.

Per serving: Calories 270; Fiber 2g; Protein 31g; Total Fat 5g; Saturated Fat 1g; Cholesterol 211mg; Sodium 880mg

Asian Stuffed Shrimp

PREP: 30 MINUTES / COOK: 10 MINUTES

- 16   **jumbo shrimp (1½ pounds), peeled and deveined**
- ⅓   **cup chopped cilantro**
- 1   **clove garlic, minced**
- 1   **tablespoon olive oil**
- 2   **carrots, julienned**
- 2   **scallions, cut into 2 x ¼-inch strips**
- 1   **tablespoon minced fresh ginger**
- 2   **tablespoons lower-sodium soy sauce**
- 2   **tablespoons chili sauce**
- 4   **teaspoons lime juice**
- 1   **teaspoon sugar**
- 6   **cups torn romaine lettuce leaves**
- 1   **cucumber, peeled, halved lengthwise, seeded, and sliced**
- 2   **tablespoons chopped fresh mint**

1. With a paring knife, make a cut along the back of the shrimp until you have cut almost, but not quite through, to the other side. In a large bowl, toss together the shrimp, cilantro, garlic, and 1 teaspoon of the oil; set aside.

2. In a large nonstick skillet, heat the remaining 2 teaspoons oil over moderate heat. Add the carrots and scallions, and sauté for 2 minutes. Add the ginger and cook for 2 minutes. Cool the vegetable mixture to room temperature.

3. Preheat the broiler. Place the shrimp, cut-side up, on a broiler pan, pressing them down to flatten slightly. Spoon the vegetable mixture onto the shrimp and broil 6 inches from the heat for 4 minutes or until the shrimp are just cooked through.

4. Meanwhile, in a large bowl, combine the soy sauce, chili sauce, lime juice, and sugar. Add the lettuce, cucumber, and mint, tossing to combine. Serve the shrimp on a bed of the salad mixture. Serves 4.

Per serving: Calories 238; Fiber 3g; Protein 31g; Total Fat 6g; Saturated Fat 1g; Cholesterol 211mg; Sodium 645mg

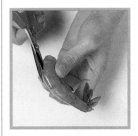

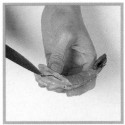

To peel and devein shrimp, make a cut along the center back with kitchen shears or a sharp knife. Remove the shell and legs. Then pick out and remove the black vein that runs down the back. (There are also special gadgets for shelling and deveining; see page 39.)

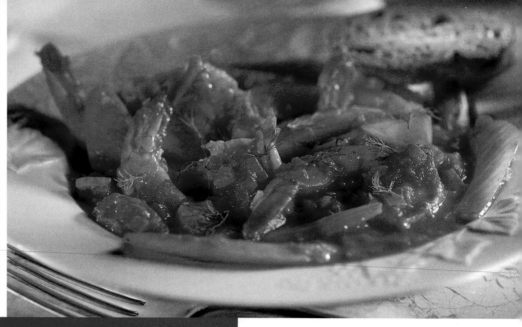

French Shrimp Stew
Save the fennel fronds and use them as a contrasting garnish for this ruby-red stew.

Did you know? . . .
Shrimp are very low in saturated fat. Saturated fat—not dietary cholesterol—is the real villain in elevating blood cholesterol.

Shrimp supply a good amount of omega-3s, which prevent artery-clogging plaques.

Shrimp contain a considerable amount of omega-3 fatty acids— less than fatty fish such as herring, but more than lean fish like cod or haddock. Omega-3s seem to make blood platelets less "sticky," that is, less likely to form artery-clogging plaques.

The results of traditional cholesterol assays—which measured all sterols (a type of fat) as a group—indicated that shrimp were high in cholesterol. But more sophisticated tests show shrimp to have far less cholesterol than previously thought. And, as it turns out, some of the other sterols found in shrimp may have beneficial effects.

French Shrimp Stew
PREP: 30 MINUTES / COOK: 35 MINUTES
Fish and seafood stews from the Mediterranean basin are frequently accented with the licorice-like taste of fennel. Celery may be substituted if necessary.

- 1   red bell pepper, cut lengthwise into flat panels
- ½   teaspoon red hot pepper sauce
- 1   tablespoon olive oil
- 1   small onion, finely chopped
- 2   cloves garlic, minced
- 1   small bulb fennel (trimmed) or 1 large stalk celery, cut into ½-inch pieces
- ⅔   cup canned no-salt-added tomatoes, chopped with their juice
- ½   cup chicken broth
- ¾   teaspoon grated orange zest
- ½   teaspoon salt
- 1   pound medium shrimp, peeled and deveined
- 4   slices French or Italian bread, toasted

1. Preheat the broiler. Place the bell pepper pieces, skin-side up, on the broiler rack and broil 4 inches from the heat for 12 minutes or until the skin is blackened. When the peppers are cool enough to handle, peel them and transfer to a food processor or blender. Add the hot pepper sauce and 1 teaspoon of the oil, and purée.

2. Meanwhile, in a large nonstick skillet, heat the remaining 2 teaspoons oil over moderate heat. Add the onion and garlic, and sauté for 5 minutes or until soft. Add the fennel, and cook for 7 minutes or until tender. Stir in the tomatoes, broth, orange zest, and salt. Bring to a boil, reduce to a simmer, cover, and cook for 5 minutes.

3. Add the shrimp to the skillet and cook for 4 minutes or until just cooked through. Stir the roasted pepper purée into the skillet. Serve the stew with the toast. Serves 4.

Per serving: Calories 228; Fiber 2g; Protein 22g; Total Fat 6g; Saturated Fat 1g; Cholesterol 140mg; Sodium 745mg

Shrimp Scampi
PREP: 20 MINUTES / COOK: 10 MINUTES

- 2   teaspoons olive oil
- 5   cloves garlic, minced
- 1½ pounds large shrimp, peeled and deveined
- ¾   teaspoon salt
- ½   cup dry vermouth or white wine
- ½   teaspoon cornstarch blended with 1 teaspoon water
- ⅓   cup chopped parsley

¾ **teaspoon grated lemon zest**
2 **teaspoons lemon juice**
1 **tablespoon unsalted butter**

1. In a large nonstick skillet, heat the oil over moderate heat. Add the garlic and sauté for 1 minute or until soft. Add the shrimp and salt, and sauté for 3 minutes or until the shrimp are pink. With a slotted spoon, transfer the shrimp to a plate.

2. Add the vermouth to the pan and cook for 1 minute. Stir in the cornstarch mixture and cook, stirring, for 1 minute. Return the shrimp to the pan and stir in the parsley, lemon zest, lemon juice, and butter. Serves 4.

Per serving: Calories 232; Fiber 0g; Protein 29g; Total Fat 8g; Saturated Fat 3g; Cholesterol 218mg; Sodium 646mg

Shrimp Oreganata

PREP: 30 MINUTES / COOK: 5 MINUTES

This zesty appetizer couldn't be easier: You just toss shrimp with a marinade, top with tomato and cheese, and bake.

¼ **cup chopped parsley**
¼ **cup chopped fresh mint**
½ **teaspoon grated lemon zest**
1 **tablespoon lemon juice**
2 **teaspoons olive oil**
1½ **teaspoons dried oregano**
⅛ **teaspoon cayenne pepper**
1 **pound large shrimp, peeled and deveined**
1 **large tomato, finely chopped**
3 **ounces feta cheese, crumbled**

1. In a large bowl, combine the parsley, mint, lemon zest, lemon juice, oil, oregano, and cayenne. Add the shrimp, tossing well to coat.

2. Preheat the oven to 450°. Place the shrimp on a large baking sheet. Top with the tomato and feta. Bake for 4 minutes, without turning, or until the shrimp are cooked through and the feta is melted. Serves 4.

Per serving: Calories 192; Fiber 1g; Protein 23g; Total Fat 9g; Saturated Fat 4g; Cholesterol 159mg; Sodium 383mg

Shrimp Cocktail Stir together ½ cup chili sauce, 1 tbsp. balsamic vinegar, 2 tsp. honey, ½ tsp. mustard, ½ tsp. red hot pepper sauce, ¼ tsp. salt, and 2 tbsp. minced red onion. Serve with ¾ lb. cooked large shrimp. Garnish with lemon wedges and parsley. Serves 4. *[Cal 136; Fat 1g; Sod 816mg]*

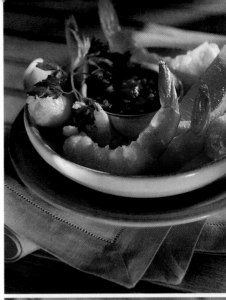

Baby Shrimp Salad Stir together ¼ cup light mayonnaise, 2 tbsp. plain low-fat yogurt, ½ tsp. grated lemon zest, 1 tbsp. lemon juice, and ¼ tsp. salt. Add 1 finely chopped celery stalk and 1½ cups halved seedless red grapes. Stir in 10 oz. cooked baby shrimp. Serve on a bed of lettuce. Serves 4. *[Cal 180; Fat 6g; Sod 438mg]*

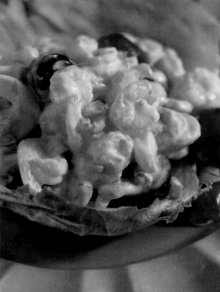

Shrimp Rolls Combine 3 tbsp. light mayonnaise, 1 tbsp. cider vinegar, ¼ tsp. each sugar and pepper. Add 1½ cups coleslaw mix (pre-shredded cabbage and carrots); toss well. Add 12 oz. cooked medium shrimp, chopped; toss. Spoon into 4 sandwich rolls. Serves 4. *[Cal 264; Fat 7g; Sod 530mg]*

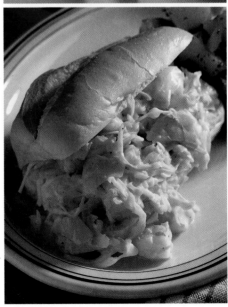

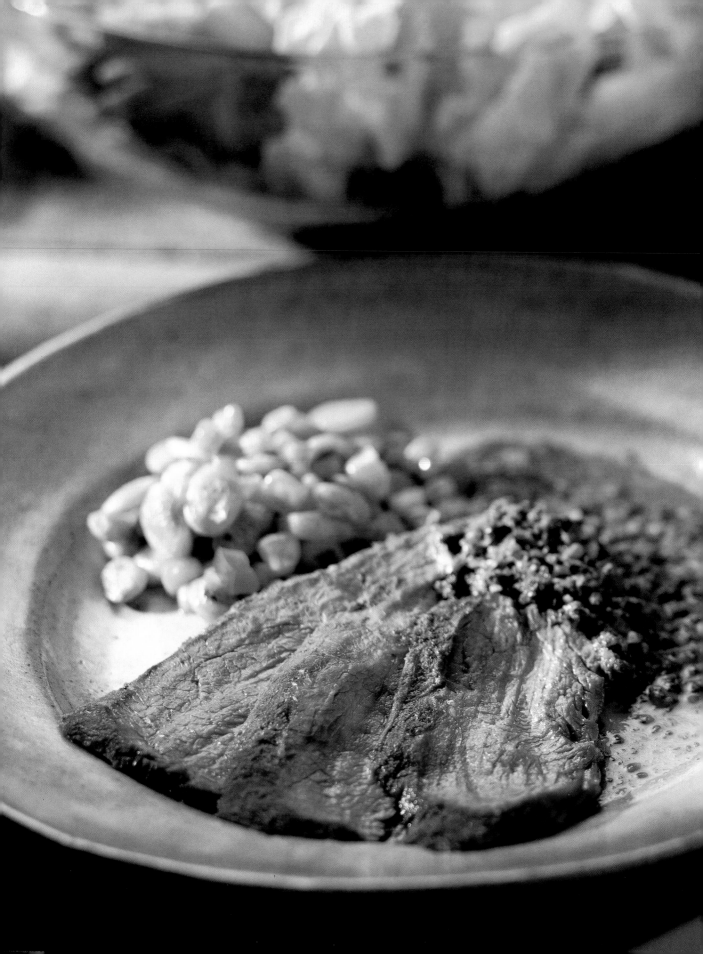

Broiled Flank Steak with Chimichurri Sauce

Beef round

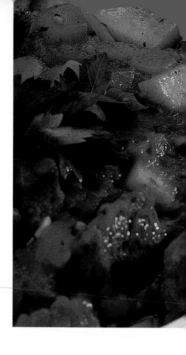

Nutritional power

Portions from the round are the leanest cuts of beef. An excellent protein source, beef round also supplies many of the B vitamins as well as iron and zinc.

Healthy Highlights

PER 3 OUNCES COOKED	
Calories	184
Fiber	0g
Protein	30g
Total Fat	6.0g
Saturated Fat	2.1g
Cholesterol	77mg
Sodium	38mg

NUTRIENTS	
	% Daily Value
Vitamin B12	38%
Zinc	25%
Iron	17%
Niacin	16%
Riboflavin	12%
Vitamin B6	12%

Did you know? . . .
Meat can certainly be part of a healthful diet if it is carefully selected and sensibly prepared. Unfortunately, Americans eat much of their beef in the form of fast-food hamburgers and cheeseburgers, which may have up to 45 grams of fat per serving.

Louisiana Beef Stew

PREP: 25 MINUTES / COOK: 50 MINUTES

The tomatoes that enliven this beef stew are a rich source of lycopene, a disease-fighting carotenoid.

- 1 **pound well-trimmed bottom round of beef, cut into ½-inch chunks**
- 2 **tablespoons flour**
- 1 **tablespoon vegetable oil**
- 1 **small onion, finely chopped**
- 2 **cloves garlic, minced**
- 2 **carrots, thinly sliced**
- 1 **pound all-purpose potatoes, peeled and cut into ½-inch chunks**
- 3 **cups canned no-salt-added tomatoes, chopped with their juice**
- 3 **tablespoons each molasses and red wine vinegar**
- ¾ **teaspoon each ground ginger and salt**

1. Dredge the beef in the flour, shaking off the excess. In a Dutch oven or flameproof casserole, heat the oil over moderately high heat. Cook the beef for 3 minutes or until lightly browned. Transfer the beef to a plate.

2. Reduce the heat to moderate, add the onion and garlic to the pan, and sauté for 5 minutes. Add the carrots and cook for 3 minutes. Add the potatoes, the tomatoes and their juice, the molasses, vinegar, ginger, and salt, and bring to a boil. Reduce to a simmer, cover, and cook for 30 minutes or until the potatoes are tender.

3. Return the beef to the pan, cover, and simmer for 5 minutes or until the beef is cooked through. Serves 4.

Per serving: Calories 383; Fiber 5g; Protein 30g; Total Fat 10g; Saturated Fat 3g; Cholesterol 67mg; Sodium 551mg

Pot Roast with Carrots & Sweet Potatoes

PREP: 15 MINUTES / COOK: 3 HOURS

This pot roast cooks for three hours, but it doesn't need any attention while it cooks.

- 2½ **pounds well-trimmed eye round of beef**
- 2 **cloves garlic, slivered**
- 1 **teaspoon each dried thyme and salt**
- ¼ **teaspoon pepper**
- 1 **large onion, thinly sliced**
- 4 **carrots, thickly sliced**
- 1¼ **pounds sweet potatoes, peeled and cut into ½-inch chunks**
- 1 **can (14½ ounces) no-salt-added stewed tomatoes, chopped with their juice**
- ½ **cup chicken broth**

1. Preheat the oven to 350°F. Cut slits all over the meat and insert the slivers of garlic. Rub the meat with the thyme, salt, and pepper.

2. Place the meat in a Dutch oven or covered casserole small enough to hold the meat and vegetables tightly. Add the onion, carrots, and sweet potatoes. Pour the tomatoes and their liquid, and the broth on top. Cover tightly with foil, place the lid on top, and bake for 3 hours or until the meat is very tender.

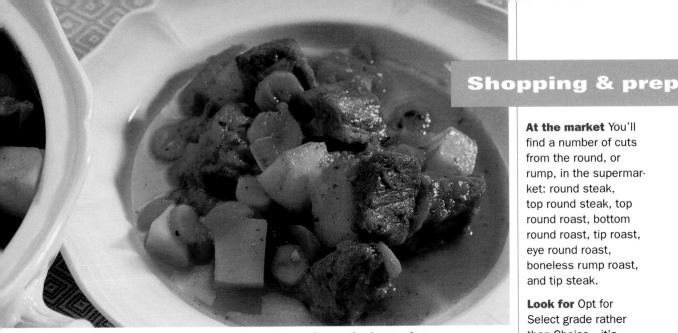

Louisiana Beef Stew is tangy with wine vinegar and a touch of ground ginger.

3. Transfer the meat and vegetables to a platter. Skim fat from the pan juices. Slice the meat and serve with the vegetables; top with pan juices. Serves 6.

Per serving: Calories 379; Fiber 6g; Protein 44g; Total Fat 9g; Saturated Fat 3g; Cholesterol 102mg; Sodium 615mg

Beef Moussaka

PREP: 20 MINUTES / COOK: 1 HOUR

Sweet spices and fresh mint flavor this wonderful Greek casserole.

1½	pounds eggplant, peeled and sliced lengthwise into ½-inch-thick slices
2	teaspoons olive oil
1	large onion, finely chopped
3	cloves garlic, minced
1	pound lean ground round
1	can (15 ounces) no-salt-added tomato sauce
¼	cup chopped fresh mint
½	teaspoon salt
¼	teaspoon cinnamon
⅛	teaspoon allspice
1¾	cups low-fat (1%) milk
2	tablespoons flour
2	ounces feta cheese, crumbled
2	tablespoons grated Parmesan cheese

1. Place the eggplant (in several layers if necessary) on a heatproof plate that will fit in a large skillet without touching the sides of the pan. Place a wire rack in the skillet and fill the skillet with 1 inch of water. (The rack should sit above, not in, the water.) Bring the water to a simmer, place the plate on the rack, cover, and steam for 12 minutes or until tender. Remove from the skillet.

2. Meanwhile, preheat the oven to 375°F. Spray a 7 x 11-inch baking dish with nonstick cooking spray. In a large nonstick skillet, heat the oil over low heat. Add the onion and garlic, and sauté for 5 minutes or until tender. Crumble in the beef and sauté for 5 minutes or until no longer pink. Add the tomato sauce, mint, salt, cinnamon, and allspice, and simmer for 5 minutes.

3. In a medium saucepan, whisk the milk into the flour, stirring until smooth. Cook, stirring constantly, for 5 minutes or until lightly thickened. Spoon half the meat mixture into the bottom of the baking dish. Top with half the eggplant and half the white sauce. Repeat with the remaining meat mixture, eggplant, and white sauce. Sprinkle the feta and Parmesan cheese on top. Bake for 35 minutes or until the top is golden brown. Serves 6.

Per serving: Calories 330; Fiber 3g; Protein 21g; Total Fat 18g; Saturated Fat 8g; Cholesterol 65mg; Sodium 437mg

At the market You'll find a number of cuts from the round, or rump, in the supermarket: round steak, top round steak, top round roast, bottom round roast, tip roast, eye round roast, boneless rump roast, and tip steak.

Look for Opt for Select grade rather than Choice—it's much leaner. Beef round has very little marbling (streaks of fat) and should have little or no exterior fat.

Prep If any exterior fat remains on the meat, trim it off with a sharp knife. For the leanest possible ground beef, cut a piece of top round into cubes or chunks (roughly 1½ inches square) and chop them in a food processor.

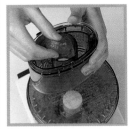

To make ground beef, drop the chunks of top round through the feed tube and chop by pulsing the processor on and off.

Basic cooking Lean-round is best cooked by moist heat—in a braised dish, stew, or casserole.

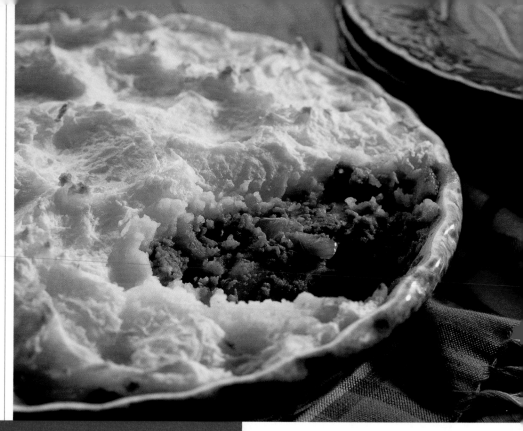

Shepherd's Pie *is a warming, meaty main dish with a garlic-scented potato crust.*

Did you know? . . .
The complete protein in beef helps your body utilize the incomplete protein in vegetables, legumes, and grains when you eat these foods along with beef.

Eating beef along with grains or legumes helps you absorb more of their iron.

Many older people suffer from an insufficient intake of dietary protein, leading to a loss of muscle strength and impairment of immune function. Including even small amounts of beef in their meals would give such people a big protein bonus.

Because beef supplies two kinds of iron (heme and non-heme iron), while plant foods, such as spinach, contain only non-heme iron, eating a little beef with iron-rich vegetables or legumes will help you better absorb the non-heme iron from the plant foods.

Shepherd's Pie

PREP: 20 MINUTES / COOK: 50 MINUTES

Shepherd's pie, as the name suggests, was originally made with lamb. Many cooks, however, prefer to use beef. The sweet Hungarian paprika used in this recipe can be found in the spice section—usually packed in a red and green tin.

1½	**pounds all-purpose potatoes, peeled and thinly sliced**
3	**cloves garlic, peeled and crushed**
¾	**teaspoon salt**
¼	**cup low-fat (1%) milk**
2	**teaspoons vegetable oil**
1	**onion, finely chopped**
2	**carrots, thinly sliced**
1	**teaspoon Hungarian paprika**
1	**teaspoon each ground coriander and cumin**
½	**teaspoon each cinnamon and pepper**
1	**pound lean ground round**
1	**can (8 ounces) no-salt-added tomato sauce**

1. In a medium pot, combine the potatoes, garlic, ¼ teaspoon of the salt, and water to cover. Bring to a boil and cook for 12 minutes or until the potatoes are tender. Drain; transfer the potatoes and garlic to a bowl. Add the milk and mash the potatoes with a potato masher or handheld mixer until smooth; set aside.

2. Preheat the oven to 375°F. In a large nonstick skillet, heat the oil over moderate heat. Add the onion and carrots, and cook for 7 minutes. Add the paprika, coriander, cumin, cinnamon, and pepper, and cook for 1 minute. Remove from the heat and stir in the beef, tomato sauce, and the remaining ½ teaspoon salt.

3. Spoon into a 9-inch pie plate. Spread the potato mixture on top. Place on a baking sheet and bake for 30 minutes or until the potato topping is golden brown. Serves 6.

Per serving: Calories 302; Fiber 3g; Protein 18g; Total Fat 15g; Saturated Fat 5g; Cholesterol 53mg; Sodium 370mg

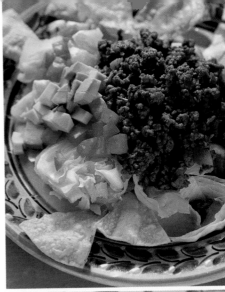

Italian Beef Rolls

PREP: 25 MINUTES / COOK: 15 MINUTES

This Sicilian-style recipe features beef slices wrapped around a piquant filling made with black olives, capers, and raisins. For a dressy occasion, you can slice each roll crosswise into about six pieces and arrange them atop a bed of rice or orzo pasta.

- 1 **pound well-trimmed bottom round of beef, cut into 8 thin slices**
- ⅓ **cup chopped parsley**
- ¼ **cup chopped fresh basil**
- ¼ **cup Gaeta, Calamata, or other brine-cured black olives, pitted and coarsely chopped**
- 3 **tablespoons plain dry bread crumbs**
- 2 **tablespoons capers, rinsed and drained**
- 2 **tablespoons raisins**
- 1 **teaspoon grated lemon zest**
- ¼ **teaspoon pepper**
- 2 **tablespoons flour**
- 2 **teaspoons olive oil**
- 2 **cups canned no-salt-added tomatoes, finely chopped with their juice**

1. One at a time, place the meat slices between 2 layers of wax paper and pound to a ⅛-inch thickness; set aside.

2. In a medium bowl, combine the parsley, basil, olives, bread crumbs, capers, raisins, lemon zest, and pepper. Spread the mixture over the beef slices. Roll the slices up from one short end. Fasten with a toothpick. Dredge the beef rolls in the flour, shaking off the excess.

3. In a large nonstick skillet, heat the oil over moderate heat. Cook the beef rolls, turning them as they brown, for 4 minutes or until browned all over. Add the tomatoes and bring to a boil. Reduce to a simmer, cover, and cook for 10 minutes or until the beef is cooked through. Serve the beef rolls with the sauce. Serves 4.

Per serving: Calories 292; Fiber 2g; Protein 28g; Total Fat 13g; Saturated Fat 3g; Cholesterol 67mg; Sodium 615mg

Taco Salad Brown 1 lb. lean ground round with 1 tbsp. chili powder, ½ tsp. each cumin and coriander in 2 tsp. oil. Stir in ¼ cup salsa. For each serving, top 1 cup shredded lettuce with 1 cup meat mixture, ¼ cup diced tomato, 2 tbsp. diced avocado, and ½ cup baked tortilla chips. Serves 4. *[Cal 375; Fat 25g; Sod 315mg]*

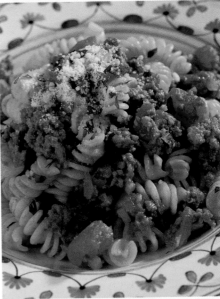

Beef & Tomato Pasta Sauce In large skillet, sauté ¼ cup each minced onion and carrot, and 3 minced garlic cloves in 1 tbsp. oil. Add 2½ cups chopped no-salt-added tomatoes, 1 tbsp. tomato paste, and ½ tsp. salt; simmer 10 minutes. Add 12 oz. lean ground round; simmer 2 minutes. Cook 12 oz. pasta; toss with sauce and ¼ cup Parmesan. Sprinkle with parsley. Serves 4. *[Cal 611; Fat 21g; Sod 500mg]*

Chunky Beef Chili Sauté 3 minced scallions, 2 minced garlic cloves, 1 tbsp. chili powder, 1 tsp. ground cumin, and ½ tsp. oregano in 2 tsp. oil for 1 minute. Add 1 lb. lean ground round, stir to brown. Add 16-oz. can red kidney beans, drained, 14½-oz. can no-salt-added stewed tomatoes, and 1 cup corn kernels; simmer 5 minutes. Serves 4. *[Cal 443; Fat 23g; Sod 257mg]*

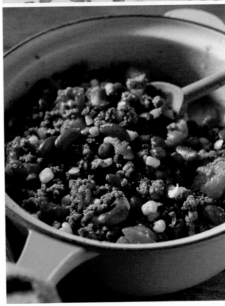

Beef sirloin

Nutritional power

An iron-rich protein source, this lean cut also supplies plenty of vitamin B12 and zinc. Served with vegetables and grains, sirloin makes a healthful meal.

Healthy Highlights

PER 3 OUNCES COOKED

Calories	195
Fiber	0g
Protein	25g
Total Fat	9.8g
Saturated Fat	3.9g
Cholesterol	76mg
Sodium	54mg

NUTRIENTS

	% Daily Value
Vitamin B12	40%
Zinc	35%
Vitamin B6	19%
Niacin	18%
Iron	17%
Riboflavin	14%
Potassium	11%

Did you know? . . .

Through scientifically planned breeding and feeding, beef is now 27 percent leaner than it was 20 years ago. In addition, butchers now trim far more fat from retail cuts of beef, leaving as little as 1/10 inch.

Quick Beef Burgundy
PREP: 25 MINUTES / COOK: 40 MINUTES

- 2 ounces bacon, coarsely chopped
- 1 pound well-trimmed beef sirloin, cut into ½-inch chunks
- 2 tablespoons flour
- 1 cup frozen pearl onions
- 4 cloves garlic, peeled and halved
- 2 carrots, halved lengthwise and cut into 2-inch lengths
- ½ pound small button mushrooms, quartered
- 4 ounces fresh shiitake mushrooms or button mushrooms, trimmed and thickly sliced
- ⅔ cup each dry red wine and chicken broth
- 1 tablespoon tomato paste
- ½ teaspoon each dried thyme and salt

1. In a Dutch oven or flameproof casserole, heat the bacon and ¼ cup of water over moderate heat for 4 minutes or until the bacon has rendered its fat. Leave bacon in pan. Dredge the beef in the flour, shaking off the excess. Sauté the beef for 3 minutes or until lightly browned on both sides. Transfer the beef to a plate.

2. Add the pearl onions and garlic to the pan and sauté for 5 minutes. Add the carrots and sauté for 7 minutes. Add the button and shiitake mushrooms, and cook for 4 minutes.

3. Add the wine, increase the heat to high, and cook for 5 minutes or until reduced by half. Add the broth, tomato paste, thyme, and salt, and simmer for 10 minutes. Return the beef to the pan and simmer for 3 minutes. Serves 4.

Per serving: Calories 309; Fiber 3g; Protein 29g; Total Fat 14g; Saturated Fat 5g; Cholesterol 79mg; Sodium 683mg

Double-Pepper Steak
PREP: 10 MINUTES / COOK: 10 MINUTES

- 2 teaspoons coarsely ground black pepper
- 4 well-trimmed sirloin steaks (4 ounces each)
- 2 teaspoons vegetable oil
- 1 red or yellow bell pepper, cut into 2 x ½-inch strips
- 1 green bell pepper, cut into 2 x ½-inch strips
- 2 tablespoons brandy, bourbon, or Scotch
- 1 cup chicken broth
- ¼ teaspoon salt
- 2 tablespoons reduced-fat sour cream
- ¾ teaspoon flour

1. Pat the black pepper onto both sides of the steaks. In a large nonstick skillet, heat the oil over moderately high heat. Add the beef and cook for 2 minutes per side for medium-rare. Transfer the steaks to a plate.

2. Reduce the heat to moderate, add the bell peppers to the pan, and cook for 3 minutes or until crisp-tender. Off the heat, add the brandy, then cook for 30 seconds. Add the broth and salt, bring to a boil, and cook for 1 minute.

3. In a small bowl, combine the sour cream and flour. Stir the sour cream mixture into the pan and cook, stirring, for 1 minute or until lightly thickened. Reduce to a simmer, return the steaks to the pan, and cook just until reheated. Serve the steaks with the sauce and bell peppers spooned on top. Serves 4.

Per serving: Calories 219; Fiber 1g; Protein 25g; Total Fat 9g; Saturated Fat 3g; Cholesterol 72mg; Sodium 477mg

Beef Stroganoff

PREP: 15 MINUTES / COOK: 10 MINUTES

As elegant as it may sound, beef Stroganoff (named for a Russian diplomat) can be a quick dish to prepare. Reduced-fat sour cream makes it a healthful one, too.

1   tablespoon vegetable oil
1   pound well-trimmed beef sirloin, cut into 3 x 1-inch strips
3   scallions, thinly sliced
½   pound mushrooms, thinly sliced
⅓   cup canned no-salt-added tomatoes, chopped with their juice
1   tablespoon tomato paste
½   teaspoon each dried tarragon and salt
¼   teaspoon black pepper
⅛   teaspoon cayenne pepper
¼   cup reduced-fat sour cream
4   slices Italian or French bread, toasted

Double-Pepper Steak *Coarsely ground black pepper coats the steaks; colorful bell peppers, cooked in broth, brandy, and sour cream, serve as the sauce.*

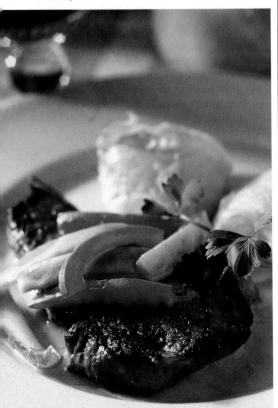

1. In a large nonstick skillet, heat 2 teaspoons of the oil over moderately high heat. Add the beef and sauté for 2 to 3 minutes or until lightly browned and just cooked through. With a slotted spoon, transfer the meat to a plate.

2. Add the remaining 1 teaspoon oil, the scallions, and mushrooms to the pan and cook, stirring frequently, for 3 minutes or until the mushrooms begin to release their juice. Add the tomatoes, tomato paste, tarragon, salt, black pepper, and cayenne, and bring to a boil. Cook for 1 minute. Remove from the heat and stir in the sour cream.

3. Return the meat to the pan, stirring to combine. Serve the stew with the toasted bread. Serves 4.

Per serving: Calories 310; Fiber 2g; Protein 30g; Total Fat 12g; Saturated Fat 4g; Cholesterol 74mg; Sodium 578mg

Grilled Herb-Rubbed Steak

PREP: 5 MINUTES / COOK: 10 MINUTES

1   teaspoon dried rosemary, crumbled
½   teaspoon each dried thyme and salt
¼   teaspoon each sugar and pepper
4   well-trimmed sirloin steaks (4 ounces each)
2   teaspoons olive oil

1. Preheat the grill to medium (or preheat the broiler).

2. In a small bowl, combine the rosemary, thyme, salt, sugar, and pepper. Rub the mixture into the steaks. Rub the oil over the beef.

3. Grill the steaks 8 inches from the heat (or broil 6 inches from the heat) for 3 minutes per side for medium-rare. Serves 4.

Per serving: Calories 189; Fiber 0g; Protein 26g; Total Fat 8g; Saturated Fat 3g; Cholesterol 76mg; Sodium 346mg

At the market Four cuts of sirloin steak are sold at retail: Round bone, flat bone, pinbone, and top sirloin, which may be bone-in or boneless. Any of these cuts can be used in these recipes.

Look for For lean meat, buy Select rather than Choice grade. The beef itself should be bright red, and any fat around the edge of the steak should be white, not yellowish.

Prep Sirloin steak is often sold with a thin layer of fat around the edge. Trim this off before cooking the meat. (For these recipes, weigh the meat after trimming.)

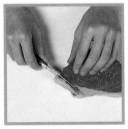

Use a sharp knife with a sawing motion to trim any external fat from steaks.

Basic cooking Though lean, sirloin is tender enough to be broiled or grilled. It's also excellent when briefly braised.

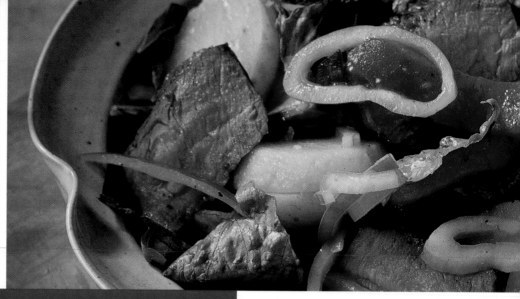

Steak & Potato Salad *To turn a warm potato salad into a hearty, low-fat main dish, add sliced sirloin, extra helpings of vegetables, and a light vinaigrette.*

Did you know? . . .
One ounce of lean beef supplies more protein than two egg whites.

Buy beef labeled "Select" rather than "Choice"—the former is far lower in fat.

Iron-deficiency anemia is the most common nutrient-deficiency problem in the United States. This nutritional shortfall can result in fatigue, irritability, and lowered immunity. Women are especially susceptible to this condition, and should pay particular attention to their intake of iron-rich foods.

A study of iron consumption among women revealed that when equal amounts of iron were consumed, women who included red meat in their meals absorbed more iron than women who ate chicken or fish, or who were vegetarians.

Steak & Potato Salad

PREP: 20 MINUTES / COOK: 20 MINUTES
STANDING TIME: 10 MINUTES

1½	pounds small all-purpose potatoes
2	red bell peppers, cut lengthwise into flat panels
1	clove garlic, peeled and halved
⅓	cup chicken broth
2	tablespoons balsamic vinegar
1	tablespoon Dijon mustard
1	tablespoon honey
½	teaspoon each salt and black pepper
1	large red onion, halved and thinly sliced
2	well-trimmed sirloin steaks (8 ounces each)
6	cups torn romaine or iceberg lettuce

1. In a medium pot of boiling water, cook the potatoes for 20 minutes, until tender. When cool enough to handle, peel and cut into ½-inch-thick slices.

2. Meanwhile, preheat the broiler. Place the bell pepper pieces, skin-side up, on the broiler rack and broil 4 inches from the heat for 12 minutes or until the skin is blackened. When the peppers are cool enough to handle, peel them and cut into ½-inch-wide strips. Leave the broiler on.

3. Rub a salad bowl with the cut garlic; discard the garlic. Add the broth, vinegar, mustard, honey, ¼ teaspoon each of the salt and black pepper, and whisk to combine. Add the bell peppers, potatoes, and onion, tossing to coat.

4. Rub the sirloin with the remaining ¼ teaspoon each salt and black pepper. Broil 4 minutes per side for medium-rare. Let stand for 10 minutes, then thinly slice across the grain and cut the slices into 2-inch lengths. Add to the bowl along with the lettuce and toss well. Serves 4.

Per serving: Calories 371; Fiber 5g; Protein 32g; Total Fat 7g; Saturated Fat 3g; Cholesterol 76mg; Sodium 543mg

Fajitas with Tomato Relish

PREP: 25 MINUTES / MARINATE: 1 HOUR
COOK: 15 MINUTES / STANDING TIME:
10 MINUTES

2	well-trimmed sirloin steaks (8 ounces each)
¼	cup lime juice
½	teaspoon salt
¼	teaspoon black pepper
2	teaspoons vegetable oil
1	pound tomatoes, halved, seeded, and coarsely chopped
⅓	cup chopped cilantro
2	scallions, thinly sliced

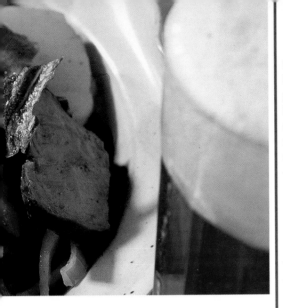

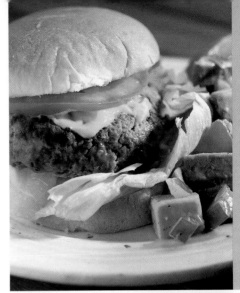

1 pickled jalapeño pepper, minced
⅓ cup diced avocado
2 red bell peppers, cut lengthwise into flat panels
1 large onion, sliced into ¼-inch-thick rounds
½ teaspoon chili powder
4 cups shredded iceberg lettuce
4 flour tortillas (7-inch diameter)

1. Sprinkle the steaks with 2 tablespoons of the lime juice, ¼ teaspoon of the salt, the black pepper, and the oil. Cover and refrigerate for 1 hour, turning the steak once.

2. Meanwhile, to make the relish, combine the tomatoes, cilantro, scallions, jalapeño, 1 tablespoon of the lime juice, and the remaining ¼ teaspoon salt. Fold in the avocado. Refrigerate.

3. Preheat the broiler. Gently toss the bell peppers and onion with the remaining 1 tablespoon lime juice and the chili powder. Broil the onion and peppers, skin-side up, 6 inches from the heat for 8 minutes, turning the onions once. Peel the peppers and cut into strips.

4. Broil the steaks 6 inches from the heat for 3 minutes per side for medium-rare. Let stand for 10 minutes, then thinly slice across the grain. Serve with the relish, peppers, onion, lettuce, and tortillas. Serves 4.

Per serving: Calories 367; Fiber 5g; Protein 31g; Total Fat 13g; Saturated Fat 3g; Cholesterol 76mg; Sodium 557mg

Deviled Hamburger

Combine 1½ lbs. lean ground sirloin, 3 tbsp. ketchup, 1 tbsp. rinsed capers, 1 tbsp. Dijon mustard, and ½ tsp. each salt and pepper. Shape into 4 patties. Broil 6 inches from heat for 3 to 4 minutes per side for medium-rare. Serve on bun with lettuce, mustard, and tomato. Serves 4. *[Cal 467; Fat 23g; Sod 939mg]*

Argentinian Beef & Fruit Kebabs

Toss ¾ lb. well-trimmed sirloin, cut into 1-inch chunks, with 2 minced garlic cloves, 2 tbsp. lime juice, 1 tsp. oregano, and ½ tsp. each salt, pepper, and sugar. Soften 16 dried apricot halves in boiling water; drain. Thread beef and apricots on 8 skewers. Broil 6 inches from heat for 3 minutes per side for medium-rare. Serves 4. *[Cal 165; Fat 5g; Sod 335mg]*

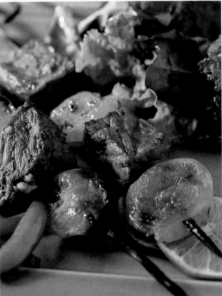

Barbecued Beef Sandwich

Combine ½ cup ketchup, 1 tbsp. red wine vinegar, 2 tsp. brown sugar, ½ tsp. ground ginger, and ½ tsp. yellow mustard. Brush half of mixture over one side of two well-trimmed 8-ounce sirloin steaks. Broil 6 inches from heat for 4 minutes. Turn, brush on remaining mixture, and broil 3 minutes for medium-rare. Thinly slice and place on 4 buns. Serves 4. *[Cal 330; Fat 8g; Sod 662mg]*

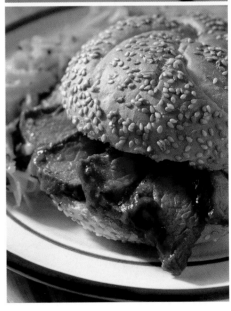

Flank steak

Nutritional power

You don't have to give up steak to eat healthfully: Lean yet richly flavorful, flank steak supplies even more of vitamins B12 and B6 than other lean beef cuts.

Healthy Highlights

PER 3 OUNCES COOKED

Calories	201
Fiber	0g
Protein	24g
Total Fat	11.1g
Saturated Fat	4.7g
Cholesterol	60mg
Sodium	61mg

NUTRIENTS

	% Daily Value
Vitamin B12	48%
Zinc	34%
Niacin	20%
Iron	17%
Vitamin B6	16%
Potassium	10%

Did you know? . . .
Most people think of bananas when they think of potassium sources, but beef is also a very good source of this mineral, which helps maintain the body's fluid balance. A 3-ounce portion of broiled flank steak supplies almost as much potassium as a small banana.

Broiled Flank Steak with Chimichurri Sauce

PREP: 15 MINUTES / COOK: 10 MINUTES
STANDING TIME: 10 MINUTES

Chimichurri is the favorite condiment for meat in Argentina, a nation of meat lovers. It's a thick vinaigrette rounded out with herbs, garlic, and hot chilies.

- ¾ teaspoon salt
- ½ teaspoon each ground coriander, cumin, and dried oregano
- 1 well-trimmed flank steak (1 pound)
- 2 garlic cloves, peeled
- 1 cup packed cilantro leaves
- ½ cup packed parsley leaves
- 1 pickled jalapeño, finely chopped
- ⅓ cup chicken broth
- 2 tablespoons red wine vinegar
- 2 teaspoons olive oil

1. In a small bowl, combine ¼ teaspoon of the salt, the coriander, cumin, and oregano. Rub into both sides of the flank steak; set aside.

2. To make the sauce: In a small pot of boiling water, cook the garlic for 2 minutes to blanch. Transfer to a food processor and add the cilantro, parsley, jalapeño, broth, vinegar, oil, and the remaining ½ teaspoon salt. Process until smooth.

3. Preheat the broiler. Broil the flank steak 6 inches from the heat for 4 minutes per side for medium-rare. Let stand for 10 minutes, then thinly slice across the grain. Serve with the chimichurri sauce spooned on top. Serves 4.

Per serving: Calories 210; Fiber 1g; Protein 24g; Total Fat 11g; Saturated Fat 4g; Cholesterol 57mg; Sodium 657mg

Steak & Pasta Salad

PREP: 15 MINUTES / COOK: 20 MINUTES
STANDING TIME: 10 MINUTES

Narrow strips of broiled steak are perfect for tossing with pasta and a pesto-like sauce.

- 1 well-trimmed flank steak (1 pound)
- 1 teaspoon salt
- ½ teaspoon each pepper and dried thyme
- 4 cloves garlic, peeled
- 10 ounces fusilli
- 1 cup packed fresh basil leaves
- 1 cup evaporated skimmed milk
- 3 tablespoons red wine vinegar
- 2 cups cherry tomatoes, halved
- 2 cups frozen corn kernels, thawed

1. Preheat the broiler. Sprinkle the steak with ¼ teaspoon of the salt, ¼ teaspoon of the pepper, and the thyme. Broil the steak 6 inches from the heat for 4 minutes per side for medium-rare. Let stand for 10 minutes, then thinly slice across the grain. Cut the slices into 1-inch-wide strips.

2. Meanwhile, in a large pot of boiling water, cook the garlic for 2 minutes to blanch. Remove with a slotted spoon and transfer to a food processor. Add the pasta to the boiling water and cook according to package directions until firm-tender. Drain.

3. Add the basil, evaporated milk, vinegar, the remaining ¾ teaspoon salt, and ¼ teaspoon pepper to the garlic and process to a smooth purée. Transfer the sauce to a large bowl. Add the hot pasta to the sauce along with the steak, tomatoes, and corn. Toss well. Serve at room temperature or chilled. Serves 4.

Per serving: Calories 590; Fiber 6g; Protein 41g; Total Fat 11g; Saturated Fat 4g; Cholesterol 60mg; Sodium 741mg

Stir-Fried Steak with Vegetables

PREP: 20 MINUTES / COOK: 10 MINUTES

Just 12 ounces of beef serves four handsomely when combined with plenty of vegetables—which is how meat is most often used in Asia, home of the stir-fry.

- 1 **tablespoon lower-sodium soy sauce**
- 1 **tablespoon dry sherry**
- 1 **tablespoon plus 1 teaspoon cornstarch**
- ⅛ **teaspoon baking soda**
- ¾ **pound well-trimmed flank steak, cut for stir-fry (see how-to photos at right)**
- ½ **cup chicken broth**
- 1 **tablespoon rice vinegar**
- ¾ **teaspoon sugar**
- 1 **tablespoon vegetable oil**
- 1 **tablespoon finely chopped fresh ginger**
- 3 **cloves garlic, minced**
- 1 **red bell pepper, cut into 2 x ¼-inch strips**
- ½ **pound asparagus, trimmed and cut into 2-inch lengths**
- 2 **cups shredded Napa cabbage**
- 3 **scallions, thinly sliced**

1. In a medium bowl, combine the soy sauce, sherry, 1 tablespoon of the cornstarch, and the baking soda. Add the beef, tossing to coat. In a small bowl, whisk together the broth, vinegar, sugar, and the remaining 1 teaspoon cornstarch; set aside.

2. In a large nonstick skillet, heat 2 teaspoons of the oil over moderately high heat. Add the beef and stir-fry for 2 to 3 minutes or until just cooked through. With a slotted spoon, transfer the beef to a plate.

3. Add the remaining 1 teaspoon oil, the ginger, and garlic to the pan and stir-fry for 30 seconds. Add the bell pepper and asparagus, and cook for 2 minutes. Add the Napa cabbage and scallions, and cook for 2 minutes.

4. Stir the broth mixture to recombine, add to the skillet, and bring to a boil. Cook, stirring, for 1 minute. Reduce to a simmer, return the beef to the pan, and cook for 30 seconds or until just heated through. Serves 4.

Per serving: Calories 214; Fiber 2g; Protein 20g; Total Fat 10g; Saturated Fat 3g; Cholesterol 43mg; Sodium 391mg

At the market A popular cut, flank steak is widely available.

Look for Buy Select grade beef rather than Choice, which is much fattier. Flank steak should have virtually no marbling of fat through the lean tissue.

Prep Cut flank steak into thin strips for stir-fries and sautés (see below).

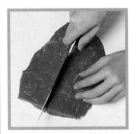

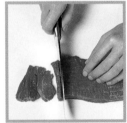

First cut the whole steak in half lengthwise, with the grain. Then cut each piece crosswise (and across the grain) into thin strips.

Basic cooking Cook flank steak only to medium-rare, or it will become tough. Carve broiled steak very thinly across the grain and on a sharp diagonal. This cuts across the meat's fibers and makes it more tender.

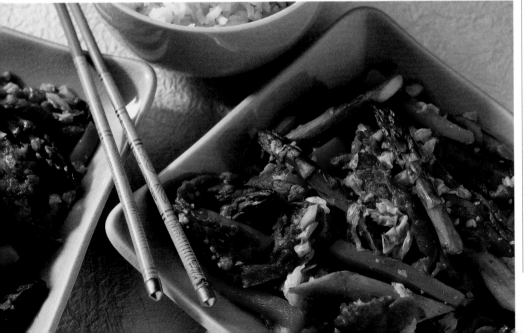

Stir-Fried Steak with Vegetables *Serve with white or brown rice—and chopsticks.*

Veal

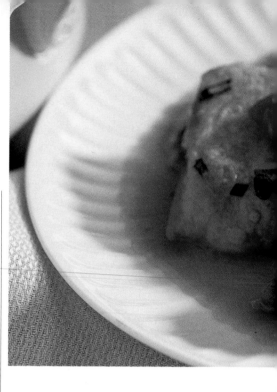

Nutritional power
Lower in fat than all but the very leanest beef cuts, veal is an exceptional source of niacin, which keeps your skin, nerves, and digestive system healthy.

Healthy Highlights

PER 3 OUNCES COOKED	
Calories	192
Fiber	0g
Protein	29g
Total Fat	7.8g
Saturated Fat	2.2g
Cholesterol	106mg
Sodium	71mg

NUTRIENTS	
	% Daily Value
Niacin	43%
Zinc	23%
Vitamin B12	18%
Riboflavin	17%
Vitamin B6	12%

Did you know? . . .
Because veal is so lean, it requires careful cooking to keep it from becoming tough. But you don't have to slather veal with fat to maintain its tenderness: Just use moderate heat, and never overcook it. This will protect the meat's delicate texture.

Saltimbocca

PREP: 15 MINUTES / COOK: 10 MINUTES

So tasty that they seem to jump in your mouth—that's what "saltimbocca" means in Italian—these delectable little rolls of veal, ham, and cheese are worthy of the name.

- 8   slices veal scaloppine (¾ pound), pounded ⅛ inch thick
- ½   teaspoon each dried sage and salt
- 8   very thin slices baked ham (about 2 ounces)
- ½   cup shredded Fontina cheese (2 ounces)
- 2   tablespoons flour
- 2   teaspoons olive oil
- ¼   cup dry white wine
- ½   cup chicken broth
- 1   teaspoon cornstarch blended with 1 tablespoon water
- ¼   cup chopped parsley

1. Sprinkle one side of the veal with the sage and salt. Place a piece of ham on each piece of veal; sprinkle with the Fontina. Roll up from one short end (see how-to photo, opposite page) and secure with toothpicks.

2. Dredge the veal rolls in the flour, shaking off the excess. In a large nonstick skillet, heat the oil over moderate heat. Add the veal rolls and cook for 4 minutes or until lightly browned.

3. Add the wine to the pan, increase the heat to high, and cook for 1 minute, scraping up any browned bits from the pan. Add the broth and simmer for 1 minute. Stir in the cornstarch mixture and cook, stirring constantly, for 1 minute or until lightly thickened. Stir in the parsley. Serve the veal with the sauce spooned on top. Serves 4.

Per serving: Calories 218; Fiber 0g; Protein 25g; Total Fat 9g; Saturated Fat 4g; Cholesterol 90mg; Sodium 762mg

Veal Scaloppine with Mushrooms

PREP: 15 MINUTES / COOK: 10 MINUTES

Scaloppine, or pounded veal cutlets, cook in a matter of minutes.

- 8   slices veal scaloppine (¾ pound), pounded ⅛ inch thick
- 2   tablespoons flour
- 1   tablespoon olive oil
- 2   cloves garlic, minced
- ¾   pound mushrooms, thinly sliced
- ¼   teaspoon each crumbled dried rosemary, salt, and pepper
- ¾   cup chicken broth
- ½   teaspoon grated lemon zest
- 1   tablespoon lemon juice
- 1   teaspoon cornstarch blended with 1 tablespoon water

1. Dredge the veal in the flour, shaking off the excess. In a large nonstick skillet, heat 1 teaspoon of the oil over moderately high heat. Add half of the veal and sauté for 1 minute per side or until golden brown and just cooked through. Transfer to a platter. Repeat with another 1 teaspoon oil and the remaining veal.

2. Add the remaining 1 teaspoon oil and the garlic to the skillet, reduce the heat to moderate, and cook for 30 sec-

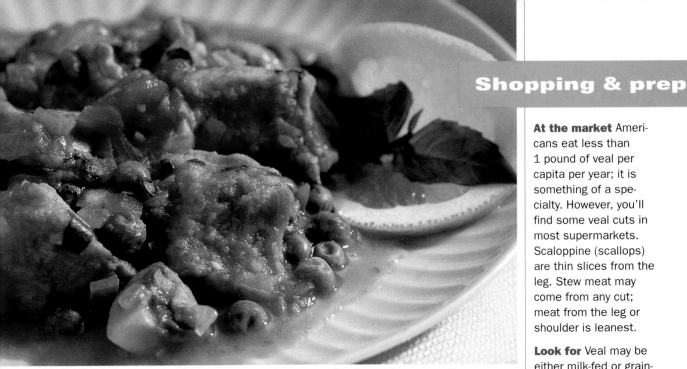

Veal Stew with Orange & Basil A lively jolt of citrus brightens the tomato flavor.

At the market Americans eat less than 1 pound of veal per capita per year; it is something of a specialty. However, you'll find some veal cuts in most supermarkets. Scaloppine (scallops) are thin slices from the leg. Stew meat may come from any cut; meat from the leg or shoulder is leanest.

Look for Veal may be either milk-fed or grain-fed. Milk-fed veal is a pale pink and exceptionally tender. Grain-fed veal is darker in color (though not as red as mature beef) and somewhat less tender than milk-fed.

Basic cooking Cook veal gently. Be extra careful when cooking it by dry heat methods, such as broiling.

onds. Add the mushrooms, rosemary, salt, and pepper to the pan and sauté for 4 minutes or until the mushrooms have released their juice.

3. Stir the broth, lemon zest, and lemon juice into the pan and bring to a boil. Add the cornstarch mixture and cook, stirring constantly, for 1 minute or until lightly thickened. Spoon the sauce over the veal. Serves 4.

Per serving: Calories 167; Fiber 1g; Protein 21g; Total Fat 6g; Saturated Fat 1g; Cholesterol 66mg; Sodium 399mg

---

Veal Stew with Orange & Basil

PREP: 20 MINUTES / COOK: 1 HOUR

You can buy veal for stewing already cut up, or buy 1 pound of boneless veal and cut it into chunks yourself.

- 2 **teaspoons olive oil**
- 1 **pound veal stew meat, cut into ½-inch chunks**
- 2 **tablespoons flour**
- 1 **onion, finely chopped**
- 2 **cloves garlic, minced**
- ½ **pound small mushrooms, quartered**
- 1 **cup canned no-salt-added tomatoes, chopped with their juice**

- 1 **teaspoon grated orange zest**
- ½ **cup orange juice**
- ½ **teaspoon salt**
- 1 **cup frozen peas**
- ¼ **cup chopped fresh basil**

1. Preheat the oven to 350°F. In a nonstick Dutch oven or flameproof casserole, heat the oil over moderate heat. Dredge the veal in the flour, shaking off the excess. Sauté the veal, working in batches if necessary, for 4 minutes or until golden brown. With a slotted spoon, transfer the veal to a plate.

2. Add the onion and garlic to the pan and sauté for 3 minutes or until the onion is crisp-tender. Add the mushrooms and sauté for 5 minutes or until they begin to release their juices.

3. Add the tomatoes and their juice, the orange zest, orange juice, and salt to the pan and bring to a boil. Return the veal to the pan, cover, and bake for 45 minutes or until the veal is tender. Stir in the peas and basil, and cook for 5 minutes or until the peas are heated through. Serves 4.

Per serving: Calories 246; Fiber 4g; Protein 28g; Total Fat 6g; Saturated Fat 1g; Cholesterol 95mg; Sodium 436mg

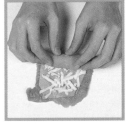

To prepare the Saltimbocca (opposite page), lay a similar-sized piece of ham on each veal scallop. Sprinkle with cheese and roll the scallops tidily but not too tightly.

Pork loin

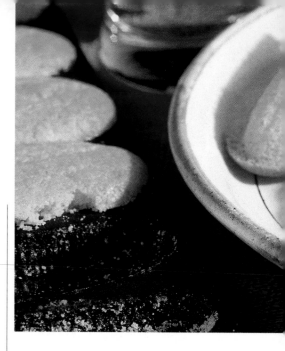

Nutritional power

Pork is the number-one dietary source of thiamin; it offers impressive amounts of other B vitamins as well. And pork is now far leaner than it used to be.

Healthy Highlights

PER 3 OUNCES COOKED	
Calories	173
Fiber	0g
Protein	24g
Total Fat	7.8g
Saturated Fat	2.9g
Cholesterol	67mg
Sodium	43mg

NUTRIENTS	
	% Daily Value
Thiamin	37%
Niacin	20%
Vitamin B6	17%
Riboflavin	14%
Zinc	14%
Potassium	11%

Did you know? . . .
There is a significant difference between cuts of pork loin: A 3-ounce cooked portion from the blade loin has about 13 grams of fat, while the center loin contains less than 7 grams of fat per serving. (The figures in the nutrient lists above are an average of several loin cuts.)

Sweet & Sour Pork
PREP: 10 MINUTES / COOK: 10 MINUTES

- 1 can (8 ounces) juice-packed pineapple chunks, drained, juice reserved
- ¼ cup chili sauce
- 3 tablespoons rice vinegar
- ¼ cup chicken broth
- 1 tablespoon plus ½ teaspoon sugar
- 1 tablespoon cornstarch
- ¼ teaspoon salt
- 1 tablespoon lower-sodium soy sauce
- 1 tablespoon dry sherry
- ¼ teaspoon pepper
- 1 pound well-trimmed boneless center-cut pork loin, cut into 1-inch chunks
- 1 tablespoon vegetable oil
- 1 tablespoon minced fresh ginger
- 1 large carrot, thinly sliced
- 8 ounces sugar snap peas, strings removed

1. In a small bowl, combine the reserved pineapple juice, chili sauce, vinegar, broth, 1 tablespoon of the sugar, 1 teaspoon of the cornstarch, and the salt; set aside.

2. In a medium bowl, combine the soy sauce, sherry, the remaining 2 teaspoons cornstarch, remaining ½ teaspoon sugar, and the pepper. Add the pork and toss well to coat.

3. In a large nonstick skillet, heat the oil over moderately high heat. Add the pork and stir-fry for 4 minutes or until golden brown and just cooked through. With a slotted spoon, transfer the pork to a plate.

4. Add the ginger to the pan and cook for 30 seconds. Add the carrot and sugar snaps, and stir-fry for 3 minutes or until crisp-tender. Stir in the pineap- ple chunks. Pour in the pineapple-chili sauce mixture and bring to a boil. Cook, stirring constantly, for 1 minute or until lightly thickened. Reduce to a simmer, return the pork to the pan, and cook just until heated through. Serves 4.

Per serving: Calories 310; Fiber 3g; Protein 27g; Total Fat 10g; Saturated Fat 3g; Cholesterol 67mg; Sodium 656mg

Stir-Fried Pork with Vermicelli
PREP: 20 MINUTES / COOK: 15 MINUTES

- 10 ounces vermicelli or capellini
- 2 tablespoons cornstarch
- 1 tablespoon lower-sodium soy sauce
- 1 tablespoon sherry
- ¾ teaspoon salt
- ½ teaspoon sugar
- ¾ pound well-trimmed boneless center-cut pork loin, cut into 2 x ¼-inch matchsticks
- 1 tablespoon vegetable oil
- 3 scallions, thinly sliced
- 2 tablespoons minced fresh ginger
- 3 cloves garlic, minced
- 1 yellow summer squash, halved lengthwise and thinly sliced
- 1 red bell pepper, cut into ½-inch squares
- ¾ cup chicken broth

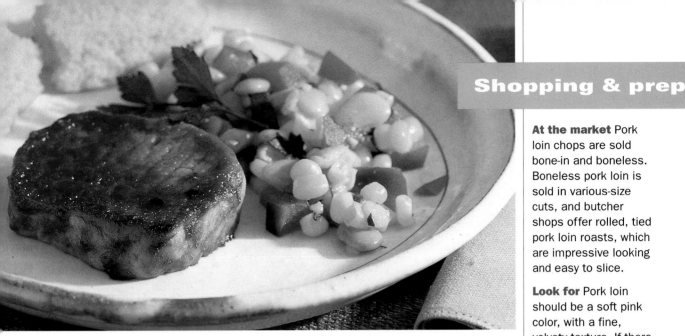

Barbecued Pork is brushed with an herbed tomato-and-vinegar sauce as it broils.

1. In a large pot of boiling water, cook the pasta according to package directions until firm-tender; drain.

2. Meanwhile, in a medium bowl, combine 5 teaspoons of the cornstarch, the soy sauce, sherry, ¼ teaspoon of the salt, and the sugar. Add the pork, tossing well to coat.

3. In a large nonstick skillet, heat 2 teaspoons of the oil over moderate heat. Add the pork, scallions, ginger, and garlic, and stir-fry for 3 minutes or until the pork is just cooked through. Transfer the pork to a plate.

4. Add the remaining 1 teaspoon oil, the squash, and bell pepper to the pan and sauté for 4 minutes or until the squash and pepper are crisp-tender. Add the drained vermicelli and the remaining ½ teaspoon salt, and cook for 1 to 2 minutes, stirring constantly, until the noodles are lightly browned.

5. In a small bowl, combine the broth, ⅓ cup of water, and the remaining 1 teaspoon cornstarch. Pour the broth mixture into the pan and bring to a boil. Return the pork to the pan and cook, stirring, for 1 minute or until the pasta is nicely coated. Serves 4.

Per serving: Calories 467; Fiber 3g; Protein 29g; Total Fat 10g; Saturated Fat 2g; Cholesterol 50mg; Sodium 837mg

Barbecued Pork

PREP: 10 MINUTES / COOK: 15 MINUTES

- ⅓ **cup ketchup**
- 2 **tablespoons red wine vinegar**
- 1 **tablespoon molasses**
- 1 **teaspoon dark brown sugar**
- ½ **teaspoon red hot pepper sauce**
- ¼ **teaspoon each crumbled dried rosemary and sage**
- ⅛ **teaspoon black pepper**
- ⅛ **teaspoon liquid smoke (optional)**
- 1 **pound well-trimmed boneless center-cut pork loin, cut into 4 slices**

1. In a small saucepan, combine the ketchup, vinegar, molasses, brown sugar, hot pepper sauce, rosemary, sage, black pepper, and liquid smoke. Cook over low heat for 5 minutes or until the barbecue sauce is lightly thickened.

2. Preheat the broiler. Brush the pork with half of the barbecue sauce and broil 6 inches from the heat for 4 minutes. Turn the pork over, brush with the remaining sauce, and broil for 4 minutes or until the pork is cooked through but still juicy. Serves 4.

Per serving: Calories 219; Fiber 0g; Protein 25g; Total Fat 8g; Saturated Fat 3g; Cholesterol 67mg; Sodium 308mg

At the market Pork loin chops are sold bone-in and boneless. Boneless pork loin is sold in various-size cuts, and butcher shops offer rolled, tied pork loin roasts, which are impressive looking and easy to slice.

Look for Pork loin should be a soft pink color, with a fine, velvety texture. If there is bone in the meat, it should be reddish rather than white.

Prep Pork requires little preparation except for the removal of any external fat.

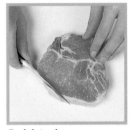

Pork loin chops can come with as much as a ¼-inch layer of fat on the outside. Use a sharp paring knife to trim it before cooking.

Basic cooking Overcooking will toughen pork loin, which is very lean. The meat should reach an internal temperature of 160°, but you can remove a roast from the oven when the thermometer registers 155°. Let stand for 15 minutes before serving; during this time, the temperature will rise to 160°.

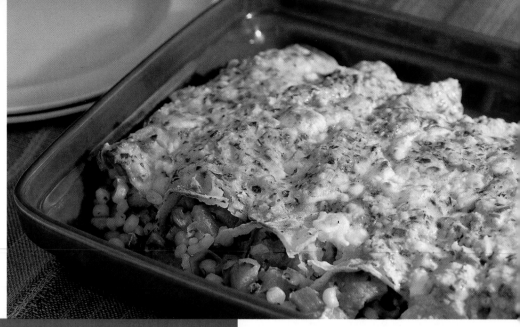

Pork Enchiladas *are baked in a creamy green-chili sauce and topped with melted feta cheese.*

Did you know? . . .
Although pork loin has slightly more total fat than loin cuts of beef, pork has less saturated fat.

The fat content of pork has been markedly lowered through new farming practices.

Advances in the breeding and raising of pigs have resulted in a marked drop in the fat content of the meat. Overall fat and saturated fat have both been cut by about 30 percent. In addition, cholesterol is about 10 percent lower than it was as recently as the early 1980s.

Many people overcook pork because health authorities formerly recommended that it be cooked to 170° to avoid any danger of trichinosis. However, the risk of trichinosis in commercially raised pork is now virtually nil, so it's safe to cook pork to 160° and serve it when it is still deliciously juicy and slightly pink.

Maple Pork Chops

PREP: 10 MINUTES / COOK: 10 MINUTES

4	well-trimmed center-cut loin pork chops (6 ounces each)
2	tablespoons orange juice
½	teaspoon each dried sage and salt
¼	teaspoon pepper
2	tablespoons maple syrup
1	tablespoon orange marmalade
½	teaspoon light brown sugar

1. Preheat the broiler. Sprinkle both sides of the pork chops with the orange juice, sage, salt, and pepper.

2. In a small bowl, combine the maple syrup, marmalade, and brown sugar. Brush the chops with half of the maple-syrup mixture and broil 6 inches from the heat for 3 to 4 minutes or until lightly browned.

3. Turn the chops over and brush with the remaining maple-syrup mixture. Broil for 3 minutes or until browned and cooked through but still juicy. Serves 4.

Per serving: Calories 216; Fiber 0g; Protein 26g; Total Fat 7g; Saturated Fat 3g; Cholesterol 70mg; Sodium 345mg

Pork Enchiladas

PREP: 20 MINUTES / COOK: 30 MINUTES

1	tablespoon vegetable oil
4	scallions, thinly sliced
3	cloves garlic, minced
1	can (4 ounces) chopped mild green chilies, drained
1	pickled jalapeño pepper, finely chopped
⅔	cup chopped cilantro
2	tablespoons lime juice
⅔	cup low-fat (1%) milk
1	tablespoon flour
¾	pound well-trimmed boneless center-cut pork loin, cut into 2 x ¼-inch strips
½	teaspoon salt
1	large tomato, coarsely chopped
½	cup frozen corn kernels, thawed
8	corn tortillas (6 inch diameter)
⅓	cup crumbled feta cheese

1. In a large nonstick skillet, heat 2 teaspoons of the oil over moderate heat. Add the scallions, garlic, mild chilies, and jalapeño, and cook for 2 minutes or until the scallions and garlic are tender. Transfer the mixture to a food processor; add ⅓ cup of the cilantro and the lime juice, and process until smooth. Add the milk and flour and process until well combined.

2. Preheat the oven to 350°F. In the same skillet, heat the remaining 1 teaspoon oil over moderate heat. Add the

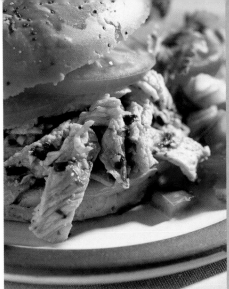

pork, sprinkle with the salt, and sauté for 3 minutes or until just cooked through. Remove the pan from the heat and stir in the tomato, corn, and the remaining ⅓ cup cilantro. Spoon the pork mixture down the center of each tortilla and roll up.

3. Spoon ¼ cup of the sauce into a 7 x 11-inch baking dish. Place the enchiladas, seam-side down, in the dish and spoon the remaining sauce on top. Cover with foil and bake for 15 minutes. Uncover, sprinkle the feta on top, and return to the oven for 5 minutes or until the cheese is just melted. Serves 4.

Per serving: Calories 365; Fiber 5g; Protein 26g; Total Fat 13g; Saturated Fat 4g; Cholesterol 62mg; Sodium 798mg

Mustard & Honey-Glazed Roast Pork

PREP: 10 MINUTES / COOK: 35 MINUTES
STANDING TIME: 10 MINUTES

No fat is added to the meat, but it comes out of the oven juicy and temptingly glossy.

- ½ **teaspoon salt**
- ¼ **teaspoon dried rosemary, crumbled**
- 1 **clove garlic, minced**
- 1 **pound well-trimmed boneless center-cut pork loin**
- 2 **tablespoons honey**
- 4 **teaspoons Dijon mustard**
- 1 **teaspoon lemon juice**

1. Preheat the oven to 425°F. Rub the salt, rosemary, and garlic into the pork. Place the roast in a small roasting pan lined with foil and roast for 20 minutes.

2. Meanwhile, in a small bowl, combine the honey, mustard, and lemon juice. Brush half of the honey-mustard mixture over the top of the roast. Return the pork to the oven and roast, basting twice with the honey-mustard mixture, for 15 minutes or until the pork is just cooked through and nicely glazed. Let stand for 10 minutes before slicing. Serves 4.

Per serving: Calories 208; Fiber 0g; Protein 24g; Total Fat 8g; Saturated Fat 3g; Cholesterol 67mg; Sodium 467mg

Spicy Pork Sandwich In saucepan, heat ⅓ cup cider vinegar, 2 tbsp. water, 3 minced garlic cloves, ¼ cup minced cilantro, ½ tsp. salt, and ¼ tsp. pepper. Add 1 lb. well-trimmed pork loin in 4 pieces. Cook until tender, slice, return to pan; stir in 2 tbsp. ketchup. Serve on buns with tomato slices. Serves 4. *[Cal 304; Fat 9g; Sod 681mg]*

Pork Satay with Curry Sauce Toss 1 lb. well-trimmed pork loin, cut into ½-inch cubes, with 2 tsp. curry powder and ½ tsp. each sugar, salt, and pepper. Thread on 4 skewers. Stir together ¾ cup plain low-fat yogurt, 1 tbsp. chopped mango chutney, and ½ tsp. curry powder. Broil skewers for 5 minutes, turning once. Serve with yogurt mixture. Serves 4. *[Cal 211; Fat 7g; Sod 422mg]*

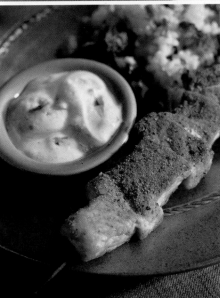

Pork Piccata Dredge 8 thin slices pork loin (1 lb.) in 2 tbsp. flour. Heat 1 tbsp. oil in large nonstick skillet. Add pork, cook until browned on both sides; remove. Stir together 1 tsp. cornstarch, ½ cup chicken broth, 3 tbsp. lemon juice, 3 tbsp. chopped parsley, and ½ tsp. salt. Add to pan, simmer 1 minute. Spoon over pork. Serves 4. *[Cal 216; Fat 10g; Sod 484mg]*

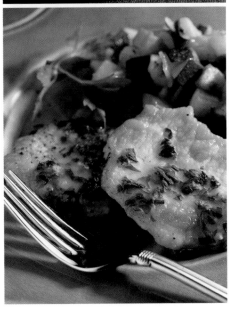

Pork tenderloin

Nutritional power
The choicest cut of pork, tenderloin is also the leanest. A serving has only 1.4 grams of saturated fat—which is even less than skinless chicken legs.

Healthy Highlights

PER 3 OUNCES COOKED

Calories	139
Fiber	0g
Protein	24g
Total Fat	4.1g
Saturated Fat	1.4g
Cholesterol	67mg
Sodium	48mg

NUTRIENTS

	% Daily Value
Thiamin	53%
Niacin	20%
Riboflavin	19%
Vitamin B6	18%
Zinc	15%
Potassium	12%

Did you know? . . .
Fresh pork is a more healthful choice by far than pork sausages, which may have more than 25 grams of fat (and sometimes more than 1000 milligrams of sodium) per serving. This is true of frankfurters, salami, and bologna, as well as fresh pork sausage.

Pork Rolls Stuffed with Apricots

PREP: 25 MINUTES / COOK: 40 MINUTES

For this guest-worthy dish, you first flatten two ½-pound pieces of pork into thin scallops (see how-to photographs, opposite page).

- ½ cup fresh bread crumbs
- ¼ cup plus 2 tablespoons chopped dried apricots
- 3 tablespoons finely chopped red onion
- 3 tablespoons finely chopped fresh basil
- 2 tablespoons grated Parmesan cheese
- 1 pound well-trimmed pork tenderloin
- ½ cup apricot nectar
- ½ cup chicken broth
- 1 tablespoon lemon juice
- 1 teaspoon Worcestershire sauce
- 2 teaspoons cornstarch blended with 1 tablespoon water
- ¼ teaspoon salt

1. Preheat the oven to 350°F. Spray a small baking dish with nonstick cooking spray. In a small bowl, combine the bread crumbs, ¼ cup of the apricots, the onion, basil, and Parmesan.

2. Halve the tenderloin lengthwise. Working with one half at a time, place between 2 sheets of plastic wrap. With the flat side of a small skillet or a meat pounder, pound the pork to a ¼-inch thickness. Halve each piece crosswise for a total of 4 pieces.

3. Spread the apricot mixture over the pork and press to flatten. Roll up each piece of pork from one short end. Place the pork rolls, seam-side down, in the prepared baking dish and bake for 35 to 40 minutes or until the meat is cooked through but still juicy.

4. Meanwhile, in a small saucepan, combine the remaining 2 tablespoons apricots, the apricot nectar, broth, lemon juice, Worcestershire sauce, cornstarch mixture, and salt. Bring to a simmer, stirring, and cook for 1 minute or until lightly thickened. Cut the pork rolls into 4 to 6 slices each and serve with the apricot sauce. Serves 4.

Per serving: Calories 226; Fiber 2g; Protein 26g; Total Fat 5g; Saturated Fat 2g; Cholesterol 76mg; Sodium 423mg

Orange-Glazed Roast Pork

PREP: 10 MINUTES / COOK: 30 MINUTES
STANDING TIME: 10 MINUTES

As roasts go, this one is super-fast, because pork tenderloin is a cut that cooks quickly.

- ¼ cup orange marmalade
- 1 tablespoon ketchup
- 2 teaspoons cider vinegar
- ¼ teaspoon Worcestershire sauce
- ½ teaspoon each ground coriander, cumin, and salt
- ¼ teaspoon ground ginger
- 1 pound well-trimmed pork tenderloin

1. Preheat the oven to 425°F. Press the marmalade through a fine-mesh sieve to remove any solid bits. In a small bowl, combine the strained marmalade, ketchup, vinegar, and Worcestershire sauce. In another small bowl, combine the coriander, cumin, salt, and ginger. Rub the spice mixture into the pork.

2. Line a small roasting pan with foil. Place the pork in the pan and roast for 10 minutes. Brush half of the marmalade mixture over the pork and roast for 10 minutes. Brush with the remaining marmalade mixture and roast for

10 minutes or until the pork is cooked through but still juicy. Let stand for 10 minutes before slicing. Serves 4.

Per serving: Calories 195; Fiber 0g; Protein 24g; Total Fat 4g; Saturated Fat 1g; Cholesterol 67mg; Sodium 397mg

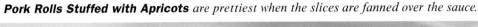

Pork Medallions Milanese

PREP: 10 MINUTES / COOK: 20 MINUTES

This adaptation of a classic veal recipe substitutes a minimal amount of olive oil for the usual copious quantities of butter.

- ¼ **cup grated Parmesan cheese**
- ⅓ **cup plain dry bread crumbs**
- 1 **egg white**
- 1 **pound well-trimmed pork tenderloin, cut crosswise into 4 pieces**
- 1 **tablespoon olive oil**
- 4 **lemon wedges**

1. Preheat the oven to 400°. Place the Parmesan on a sheet of wax paper. Place the bread crumbs on another sheet of wax paper. In a small bowl, beat the egg white with 1 tablespoon of water.

2. Dredge the pork in the Parmesan, pressing it on. Dip the pork in the egg white, then in the bread crumbs, patting the crumbs onto the pork.

3. In a large nonstick skillet, heat the oil over moderate heat. Add the pork and cook for 3 minutes per side or until golden brown and crisp. Transfer to a baking sheet and bake for 10 to 15 minutes, or until cooked through but still juicy. Serve with the lemon wedges. Serves 4.

Per serving: Calories 254; Fiber 0g; Protein 30g; Total Fat 11g; Saturated Fat 3g; Cholesterol 84mg; Sodium 239mg

At the market Pork tenderloin is something of a specialty item; if your supermarket doesn't carry it, try a butcher shop or gourmet shop.

Look for The tenderloin is a long, slender piece of meat, only about 2 inches in diameter. Tenderloin is darker in color than other cuts of pork: The meat should be a clear light red.

Prep To make the Pork Rolls Stuffed with Apricots (opposite page), the tenderloin needs to be pounded thin (see below).

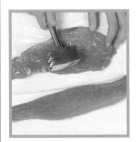

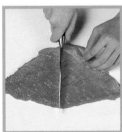

Halve a 1-pound piece of tenderloin lengthwise. Place each piece of pork between sheets of plastic wrap. Working from the center out, use a meat pounder to thin the pork to a ¼-inch thickness (top photo). Then cut each pounded portion crosswise (bottom).

Pork Rolls Stuffed with Apricots *are prettiest when the slices are fanned over the sauce.*

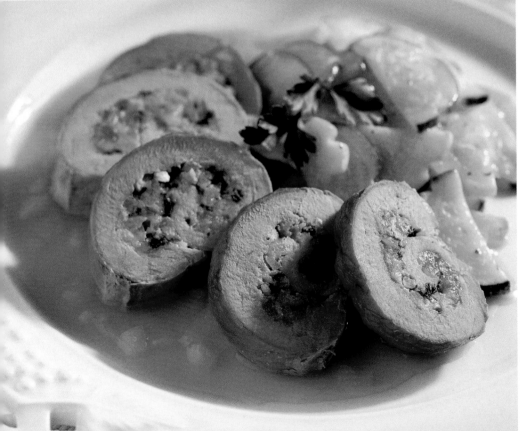

251

Ham

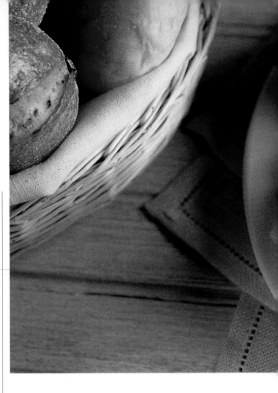

Nutritional power

A rich source of B vit-amins and protein, ham is surprisingly low in fat. The sodium content can be quite high, but reduced-sodium hams are available.

Healthy Highlights

PER 3 OUNCES

Calories	133
Fiber	0g
Protein	21g
Total Fat	4.7g
Saturated Fat	1.6g
Cholesterol	47mg
Sodium	1128mg

NUTRIENTS

	% Daily Value
Thiamin	39%
Niacin	22%
Vitamin B6	20%
Zinc	15%
Riboflavin	13%
Vitamin B12	10%

Did you know? . . .

American country-style hams, such as Virginia's Smithfield hams, are dry-salted, smoked for several weeks, and then aged for a year or longer. The salting and smoking pre-serve the meat, but the ham still must be cooked (after soaking to remove some of the salt) before you eat it.

Peppery Ham & Swiss Strata

PREP: 15 MINUTES / SOAK: 30 MINUTES
COOK: 55 MINUTES

A strata is a layered casserole of bread, beaten eggs, and cheese; ham adds extra protein and a wealth of flavor. Rye bread complements the Swiss cheese and ham.

- 6 slices (5 ounces total) rye bread, cut into 1-inch-wide strips
- 1 large tomato, seeded and coarsely chopped
- 6 ounces thinly sliced ham, slivered
- 4 ounces Swiss cheese, shredded
- 2 cups low-fat (1%) milk
- 1 egg
- 4 egg whites
- 3 tablespoons grated Parmesan cheese
- ½ teaspoon cayenne pepper

1. Using one-third of the bread, make a layer in the bottom of an 8-inch square glass baking dish. Top with half of the tomato, half of the ham, and half of the Swiss cheese. Repeat with another one-third of the bread and the remaining tomato, ham, and Swiss cheese. Top with a final layer of bread.

2. In a medium bowl, whisk together the milk, whole egg, egg whites, Parme-san, and cayenne. Pour the mixture over the bread mixture, cover with foil, and let soak for 30 minutes in the refrigerator.

3. Preheat the oven to 350°F. Bake the strata, covered, for 30 minutes. Uncover and bake for 25 minutes or until the strata is nicely puffed, golden brown, and set. Serves 4.

Per serving: Calories 392; Fiber 3g; Protein 30g; Total Fat 17g; Saturated Fat 9g; Cholesterol 111mg; Sodium 1074mg

Ham & Sweet Potato Salad

PREP: 30 MINUTES / COOK: 15 MINUTES

The sweet potatoes and ginger-lime dressing set this salad apart from the ordinary.

- 1 pound sweet potatoes (2 medium), peeled and cut into ½-inch chunks
- 3 tablespoons grated fresh ginger
- ⅓ cup lime juice
- 2 tablespoons honey
- 1 tablespoon olive oil
- 1 teaspoon Dijon mustard
- ¼ teaspoon black pepper
- 2 pears (about 6 ounces each), peeled, quartered lengthwise, cored, and sliced ¼ inch thick
- ½ pound baked ham, cut into ½-inch chunks
- 1 red bell pepper, cut into 2-inch-long matchsticks
- ½ cup thinly sliced red onion
- 6 cups torn Boston or leaf lettuce

1. In a medium pot of boiling water, cook the sweet potatoes for 12 minutes or until tender.

2. Meanwhile, working over a large bowl, squeeze the ginger with your fin-gers to extract the ginger juice; discard the solids. Whisk in the lime juice, honey, oil, mustard, and black pepper.

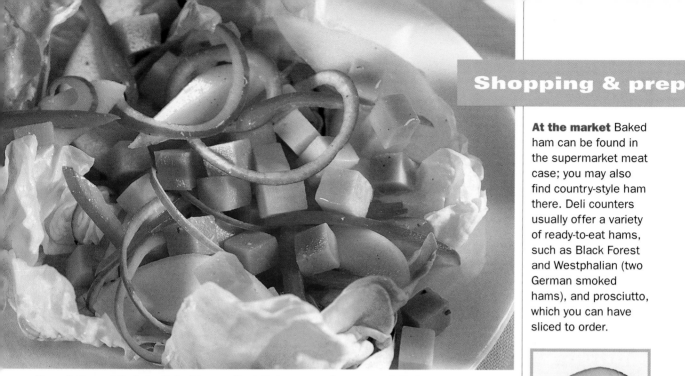

Ham & Sweet Potato Salad is equally delicious served warm or chilled.

3. Drain the sweet potatoes well and add to the bowl with the lime mixture, tossing to coat. Add the pears, ham, bell pepper, and onion, and toss again. Serve the salad on a bed of lettuce. Serves 4.

Per serving: Calories 332; Fiber 6g; Protein 16g; Total Fat 9g; Saturated Fat 2g; Cholesterol 34mg; Sodium 906mg

Bow Ties with Smoked Ham & Asparagus

PREP: 25 MINUTES / COOK: 25 MINUTES

- **10** ounces bow-tie pasta
- **¾** pound asparagus, trimmed and cut into 1-inch lengths
- **2** teaspoons olive oil
- **2** large onions, halved and thinly sliced
- **1** teaspoon sugar
- **½** teaspoon dried oregano
- **¼** teaspoon black pepper
- **1** large red bell pepper, cut into ½-inch squares
- **4** ounces smoked ham, cut into ¼-inch dice
- **⅔** cup chicken broth
- **¾** teaspoon grated lemon zest
- **¼** teaspoon salt
- **1** teaspoon cornstarch blended with 1 tablespoon water
- **⅓** cup chopped fresh basil
- **1** tablespoon lemon juice

1. In a large pot of boiling water, cook the pasta according to package directions until firm-tender. Add the asparagus for the last 2 minutes of cooking time. Drain.

2. Meanwhile, in a large nonstick skillet, heat the oil over moderate heat. Add the onions, sugar, oregano, and black pepper, and sauté for 12 minutes or until the onions are light golden and very tender. Add the bell pepper and ham, and cook for 5 minutes or until the pepper is crisp-tender.

3. Add the drained pasta and asparagus, the broth, lemon zest, and salt, and simmer until the pasta is heated through. Stir in the cornstarch mixture and cook for 1 minute, stirring constantly, until lightly thickened. Remove from the heat and stir in the basil and lemon juice. Serves 4.

Per serving: Calories 399; Fiber 5g; Protein 19g; Total Fat 5g; Saturated Fat 1g; Cholesterol 13mg; Sodium 736mg

At the market Baked ham can be found in the supermarket meat case; you may also find country-style ham there. Deli counters usually offer a variety of ready-to-eat hams, such as Black Forest and Westphalian (two German smoked hams), and prosciutto, which you can have sliced to order.

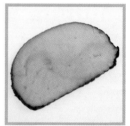

Turkey ham—cooked, cured turkey thigh meat— can be substituted for ham.

Look for Baked hams should be pink and finely grained; country hams range from pink to deep red. Read the label: Reduced-sodium and extra-lean hams are good choices.

Prep Trim any external fat from ham before cooking or serving.

Basic cooking These recipes call for ready-to-eat ham. However, when serving ham that is labeled "cook before eating," you'll need to heat the ham to an internal temperature of 160°. Hams labeled "fully cooked" may be heated to 140° to enhance their flavor.

Lamb

Nutritional power

Exceptionally flavor-ful, lamb is a super source of vitamin B12, niacin, and zinc. Like other types of red meat, it also supplies a good amount of iron.

Healthy Highlights

PER 3 OUNCES COOKED*	
Calories	196
Fiber	0g
Protein	26g
Total Fat	9.5g
Saturated Fat	3.5g
Cholesterol	85mg
Sodium	65mg

NUTRIENTS	
	% Daily Value
Vitamin B12	38%
Zinc	31%
Niacin	27%
Riboflavin	14%
Iron	11%

an average of loin, leg, and shoulder

Did you know? . . .
Lamb is leaner than it used to be, thanks to advances in breeding. And most retail cuts of lamb now carry just ¼ inch of external fat.

Avoid packaged ground lamb; 3 ounces, cooked, may contain as much as 17 grams of fat.

Grilled Lamb Chops with Mint Salsa

PREP: 20 MINUTES / COOK: 10 MINUTES

A pourable vinegar-based mint sauce is traditional with lamb; this update features a chunky mint salsa made with bell peppers, scallions, garlic, and lemon.

- 2 cloves garlic, peeled
- ½ cup chopped fresh mint
- ¼ cup diced red bell pepper
- 1 scallion, thinly sliced
- 1 teaspoon grated lemon zest
- 3 tablespoons rice vinegar
- ½ teaspoon lemon juice
- 2¼ teaspoons sugar
- ½ teaspoon salt
- ½ teaspoon dried oregano
- 4 well-trimmed loin lamb chops (5 ounces each)

1. In a small pot of boiling water, cook the garlic for 2 minutes to blanch. Drain. When cool enough to handle, finely chop and transfer to a medium bowl. Add the mint, bell pepper, scallion, lemon zest, vinegar, lemon juice, 2 teaspoons of the sugar, and ¼ teaspoon of the salt; set aside.

2. In a small bowl, combine the oregano, the remaining ¼ teaspoon each sugar and salt. Rub the mixture onto both sides of the chops and let stand for 10 minutes.

3. Preheat the grill to medium (or preheat the broiler). Grill the chops 8 inches from the heat (or broil 6 inches from the heat) for 3½ minutes per side for medium-rare. Serve the chops with the mint salsa spooned on top. Serves 4.

Per serving: Calories 204; Fiber 1g; Protein 26g; Total Fat 8g; Saturated Fat 3g; Cholesterol 81mg; Sodium 366mg

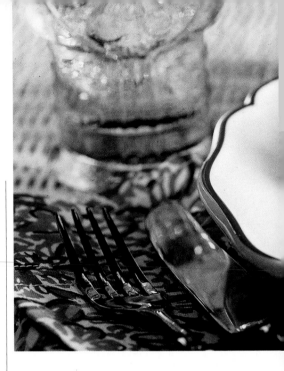

Szechuan Lamb with Scallions

PREP: 20 MINUTES / COOK: 10 MINUTES

- 2 tablespoons lower-sodium soy sauce
- 1 tablespoon dry sherry or white wine
- 1 tablespoon cornstarch
- ¼ teaspoon crushed red pepper flakes
- ¾ pound well-trimmed leg of lamb, thinly sliced and then cut into ½-inch-wide strips
- 1 tablespoon vegetable oil
- 1 yellow bell pepper, cut into 2-inch-long matchsticks
- 1 red bell pepper, cut into 2-inch-long matchsticks
- 1 pickled jalapeño pepper, finely chopped
- 3 cloves garlic, minced
- 1 tablespoon minced fresh ginger
- 10 scallions, cut into 2-inch lengths
- ¼ teaspoon each salt and sugar

1. In a medium bowl, combine the soy sauce, sherry, cornstarch, and red pepper flakes. Add the lamb, tossing to coat. In a large nonstick skillet, heat 2 teaspoons of the oil over moderately high heat. Add the lamb to the pan and stir-fry for 2 minutes or until just cooked through. With a slotted spoon, transfer the lamb to a plate.

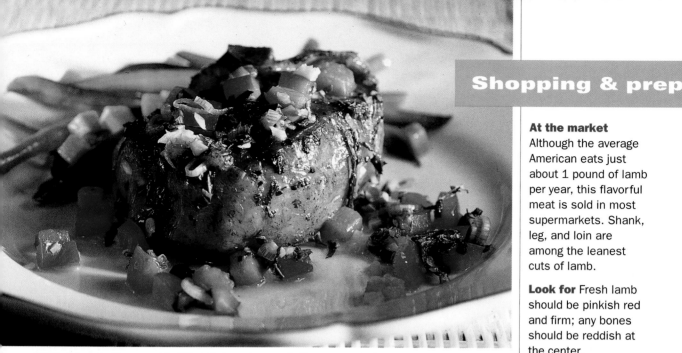

Grilled Lamb Chops with Mint Salsa *A tangy bell-pepper relish accompanies the chops.*

2. Add the remaining 1 teaspoon oil to the skillet along with the bell peppers, jalapeño, garlic, and ginger, and stir-fry for 2 minutes or until the bell peppers are crisp-tender. Add the scallions, salt, and sugar, and cook for 1 minute. Return the lamb to the skillet and cook for 1 minute or just until heated through. Serves 4.

Per serving: Calories 185; Fiber 2g; Protein 19g; Total Fat 7g; Saturated Fat 2g; Cholesterol 55mg; Sodium 559mg

Lamb Curry

PREP: 15 MINUTES / COOK: 1 HOUR

This unusual curry cooks in a coconut-almond sauce flavored with curry spices.

- 2 teaspoons vegetable oil
- 1 pound well-trimmed boneless lamb shoulder, cut into ½-inch chunks
- 1 large onion, finely chopped
- 1 red bell pepper, diced
- 1 teaspoon turmeric
- ¾ teaspoon each ground cumin and coriander
- ½ teaspoon ground ginger
- ¼ teaspoon each ground cardamom and sugar
- ¼ cup flaked coconut
- ¼ cup sliced natural almonds
- 1¼ cups plain low-fat yogurt
- ½ cup no-salt-added tomato sauce
- ¾ teaspoon salt
- ¾ cup frozen peas
- ½ cup chopped cilantro or parsley

1. In a large nonstick skillet, heat the oil over moderately high heat. Working in batches, add the lamb and sauté for 4 minutes or until browned. Transfer the lamb to a plate.

2. Reduce the heat to moderate, add the onion and bell pepper, and sauté for 7 minutes or until the onion is golden brown. Add the turmeric, cumin, coriander, ginger, cardamom, and sugar, and cook for 2 minutes or until the spices are fragrant. Transfer the mixture to a blender; add the coconut, almonds, and ⅔ cup of water, and process until smooth. Return to the pan, stir in ¼ cup of the yogurt, the tomato sauce, and salt, and bring to a simmer.

3. Return the lamb to the pan, cover, and cook for 35 minutes. Stir in the peas, cover, and cook for 10 minutes or until the lamb is tender. Stir in the cilantro and the remaining 1 cup yogurt. Serves 4.

Per serving: Calories 348; Fiber 3g; Protein 30g; Total Fat 16g; Saturated Fat 5g; Cholesterol 79mg; Sodium 618mg

At the market
Although the average American eats just about 1 pound of lamb per year, this flavorful meat is sold in most supermarkets. Shank, leg, and loin are among the leanest cuts of lamb.

Look for Fresh lamb should be pinkish red and firm; any bones should be reddish at the center.

Prep There shouldn't be much external fat on lamb, but do trim off any that you see.

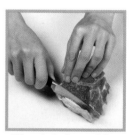

Although the layer of fat on most chops these days is minimal, it's more healthful to trim it to nothing before cooking.

Basic cooking When broiling, roasting, or grilling lamb, don't cook it beyond medium-rare or it will lose its rich flavor. Lamb cooked by moist-heat methods, such as stewing or braising, can be cooked longer.

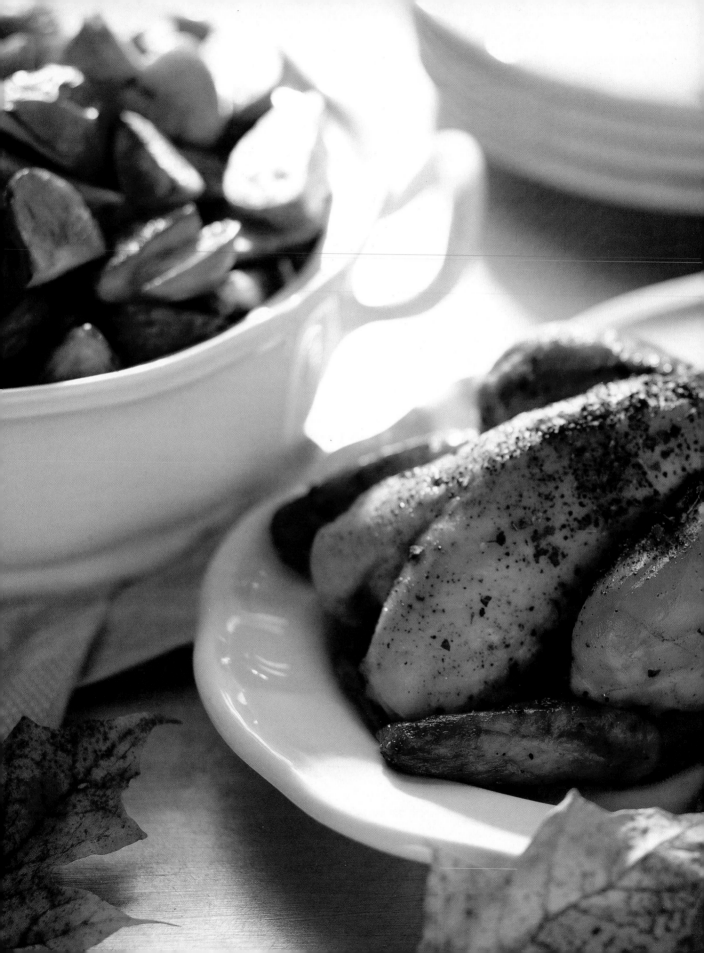

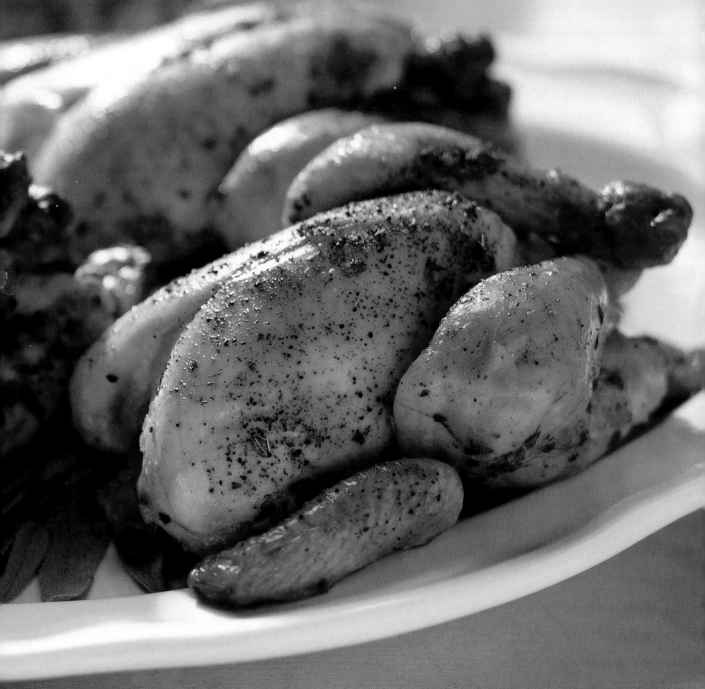

Chicken & Turkey

Roasted Game Hens with Garlic Potatoes

Whole chicken & game hens

Nutritional power
Always an impressive dish, a whole bird (eaten without the skin) provides plenty of protein, little saturated fat, and good amounts of B vitamins and zinc.

Healthy Highlights

Whole Chicken*
PER 3 OUNCES COOKED

Calories	162
Fiber	0g
Protein	25g
Total Fat	6.3g
Saturated Fat	1.7g
Cholesterol	76mg
Sodium	73mg

NUTRIENTS

	% Daily Value
Niacin	39%
Vitamin B6	20%
Zinc	12%

*meat only, no skin

Did you know? . . .
A University of Minnesota study found that no significant fat is transferred from the skin to the meat when chicken is cooked. So when roasting, broiling, or grilling chicken (or game hens), it's okay to leave the skin on during cooking as long as you remove it before eating.

Roasted Game Hens with Garlic Potatoes

PREP: 15 MINUTES / COOK: 1 HOUR

Potatoes roasted with game hens absorb lots of fat—unless the birds are skinned first.

- 1 **pound small red potatoes (about 8), quartered**
- 1 **pound small Yukon Gold potatoes (about 8), quartered**
- 1 **tablespoon olive oil**
- 8 **cloves garlic, peeled**
- ¾ **teaspoon salt**
- 1 **teaspoon each dried oregano and chili powder**
- ¼ **teaspoon pepper**
- 2 **Cornish game hens (1¼ pounds each), skinned**

1. Preheat the oven to 425°F. In a large pot of boiling water, cook the potatoes 5 minutes to blanch. Drain.

2. Meanwhile, place the oil and garlic in a large roasting pan and bake for 5 minutes. Add the drained potatoes to the pan, sprinkle with ¼ teaspoon of the salt, and bake for 15 minutes, shaking the pan occasionally and turning the potatoes as they brown.

3. In a small bowl, combine the oregano, chili powder, pepper, and the remaining ½ teaspoon salt. Rub the hens with the spice mixture. Place, breast-side up, on the potatoes and cook for 30 to 35 minutes or until the hens are cooked through. Halve the hens to serve. Serves 4.

Per serving: Calories 414; Fiber 4g; Protein 37g; Total Fat 9g; Saturated Fat 2g; Cholesterol 148mg; Sodium 571mg

Braised Lemon Chicken

PREP: 20 MINUTES / COOK: 35 MINUTES

- 1 **broiler-fryer chicken (3 to 3½ pounds)**
- 3 **tablespoons flour**
- 1 **tablespoon vegetable oil**
- 4 **cloves garlic, minced**
- 3 **scallions, thinly sliced**
- ¾ **cup chicken broth**
- 1 **teaspoon grated lemon zest**
- ⅓ **cup lemon juice**
- 2 **tablespoons sugar**
- ½ **teaspoon salt**
- 1 **teaspoon cornstarch blended with 1 tablespoon water**
- ¼ **cup chopped cilantro**

1. Cut the chicken into 8 pieces (2 thighs, 2 drumsticks, and 2 breasts cut in half; discard the wings and back or save for stock). Skin the chicken and dredge in the flour, shaking off the excess. In a large nonstick skillet, heat the oil over moderate heat. Sauté the chicken for 3 minutes per side or until golden. Transfer the chicken to a plate.

2. Add the garlic and scallions to the pan and sauté for 1 minute or until the scallions are tender. Add the broth, ½ cup of water, the lemon zest, lemon juice, sugar, and salt, and bring to a boil. Return the drumsticks and thighs to the pan; reduce to a simmer, cover, and cook for 10 minutes. Return the chicken breasts to the pan, re-cover, and cook for 15 minutes or until the chicken is tender. Transfer the chicken to a platter.

3. Return the liquid in the pan to a boil, stir in the cornstarch mixture, and cook, stirring constantly, for 1 minute or until lightly thickened. Stir in the cilantro and spoon the sauce over the chicken. Serves 4.

Per serving: Calories 306; Fiber 1g; Protein 39g; Total Fat 9g; Saturated Fat 2g; Cholesterol 124mg; Sodium 630 mg

Herb-Roasted Chicken

PREP: 10 MINUTES
COOK: 1 HOUR 5 MINUTES

1   **broiler-fryer chicken (3 to 3½ pounds), trimmed of excess fat**
¾   **teaspoon dried rosemary**
1   **teaspoon salt**
½   **teaspoon each dried marjoram and sage**
6   **large cloves garlic, unpeeled**
½   **cup chicken broth**
2   **teaspoons lemon juice**
1   **tablespoon flour**

1. Preheat the oven to 425°F. Sprinkle the cavity of the chicken with ½ tea- spoon of the rosemary and ¼ teaspoon each of the salt, marjoram, and sage. Place the garlic in the cavity.

2. In a small bowl, combine the remaining ¾ teaspoon salt and remaining ¼ teaspoon each rosemary, marjoram, and sage. Carefully lift the skin of the breast and thighs and rub the herb mixture underneath.

3. Place the chicken, breast-side down, on a rack in a roasting pan, and roast for 30 minutes. Turn breast-side up and roast for 30 minutes or until cooked through. Transfer to a platter.

4. Add the broth, lemon juice, and ¼ cup of water to the roasting pan and stir, scraping up the browned bits. Pour the drippings into a gravy separator, then pour the defatted juices into a small saucepan. Blend the flour with ¼ cup of water, add to the pan, and cook over medium heat, stirring, until the gravy is thickened. Serve the gravy alongside the chicken. Remove the skin before eating. Serves 4.

Per serving: Calories 232; Fiber 0g; Protein 39g; Total Fat 6g; Saturated Fat 2g; Cholesterol 124mg; Sodium 852mg

At the market Whole chickens come in several sizes. Young, tender broiler-fryers range from 2½ to 5 pounds. Roasters are larger—from 3½ to 6 pounds. Rock Cornish hens range from ¾ to 2 pounds.

Look for Choose a chicken with a meaty breast. The skin color will depend on the chicken's breed and diet, and does not affect nutritional value.

Prep Rinse the chicken under cold running water. Remove any visible fat. To reduce the risk of food poisoning, wash utensils, work surface, and hands with hot, soapy water after preparing raw chicken.

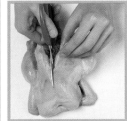

To halve a game hen, cut through the breastbone, then along the backbone.

Basic cooking To avoid salmonella risk, cook a whole chicken until a thermometer inserted in the thigh reads 180° (the meat will be white, and juices will run clear— not pink—when the meat is pierced).

Herb-Roasted Chicken *is redolent with rosemary, marjoram, sage, and garlic.*

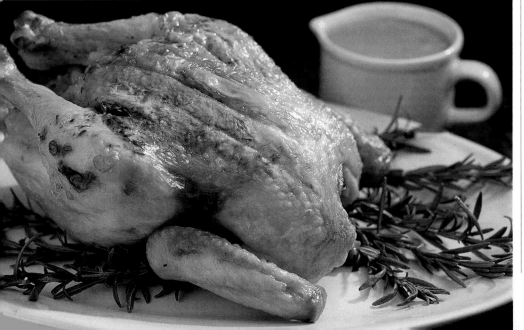

Cornish Game Hens*

PER 3 OUNCES COOKED

Calories	114
Fiber	0g
Protein	20g
Total Fat	3.3g
Saturated Fat	0.8g
Cholesterol	90mg
Sodium	54mg

NUTRIENTS

	% Daily Value
Niacin	27%
Vitamin B6	16%
Riboflavin	11%

meat only, no skin

Did you know? . . .
Chicken is almost always a good menu choice, but beware of what fast-food restaurants do to it: Those breaded chicken nuggets have more than 17 grams of fat per serving; oversized specialty chicken sandwiches with special sauces may have as much as 40 grams of fat.

It's safer not to cook poultry with stuffing in the cavity; however, "stuffing" a bird under the skin with a flavoring mixture is perfectly safe.

Coq au Vin Blanc

PREP: 25 MINUTES / COOK: 1 HOUR

Our white-wine version of this French country stew is much lower in fat than the original.

2	slices bacon, chopped
1	broiler-fryer chicken (3 to 3½ pounds)
3	tablespoons flour
2	cups frozen pearl onions, thawed
2	carrots, halved lengthwise and cut into 1-inch lengths
½	pound small mushrooms, halved
¾	cup dry white wine
¾	cup chicken broth
¾	teaspoon salt
½	teaspoon dried rosemary, crumbled
¼	teaspoon each dried sage and pepper
1½	teaspoons cornstarch blended with 1 tablespoon water
¼	cup chopped parsley

1. In a Dutch oven or flameproof casserole, combine the bacon and ¼ cup of water over moderate heat. Cook for 4 minutes or until the bacon has rendered its fat and is lightly crisped. Cut the chicken into 8 pieces (2 thighs, 2 drumsticks, and 2 breasts cut in half; discard the wings and back or save for stock). Skin the chicken and dredge in the flour, shaking off the excess. Sauté the chicken in the bacon drippings for 3 minutes per side or until golden brown. Transfer the chicken to a plate.

2. Add the pearl onions and carrots to the pan and cook for 10 minutes or until the onions are golden. Add the mushrooms and cook for 4 minutes or until they begin to release their juices.

3. Add the wine to the pan, increase the heat to high, and cook for 3 minutes, scraping up any browned bits that cling to the bottom of the pan. Add the broth, salt, rosemary, sage, and pepper, and bring to a boil. Return the chicken thighs and drumsticks to the pan; reduce to a simmer, cover, and cook for 15 minutes. Add the breasts, re-cover, and cook for 15 minutes or until the chicken is cooked through.

4. Transfer the chicken to a serving platter. Bring the sauce to a boil, stir in the cornstarch mixture, and cook, stirring constantly, for 1 minute or until lightly thickened. Stir in the parsley and spoon over the chicken. Serves 4.

Per serving: Calories 386; Fiber 2g; Protein 42g; Total Fat 14g; Saturated Fat 5g; Cholesterol 133mg; Sodium 894mg

Grilled Game Hens Diablo

PREP: 15 MINUTES / MARINATE: 1 HOUR
COOK: 15 MINUTES

The "devilish" touch here is the marinade, made with chili sauce and hot pepper sauce.

5	tablespoons chili sauce
2	teaspoons olive oil
1	teaspoon red hot pepper sauce
½	teaspoon each salt and black pepper
½	teaspoon grated lemon zest
3	cloves garlic, minced
2	Cornish game hens (about 1¼ pounds each), halved (see how-to photo, page 259) and skinned
2	tablespoons red wine vinegar
1	red bell pepper, diced
1	stalk celery, cut into ¼-inch dice

1. In a shallow pan, combine 2 tablespoons of the chili sauce, the oil, hot pepper sauce, salt, black pepper, lemon zest, and garlic. Add the hens, turn to coat, cover, and refrigerate for 1 hour.

2. Meanwhile, in a medium bowl, combine the remaining 3 tablespoons chili sauce, the vinegar, bell pepper, and celery. Set aside.

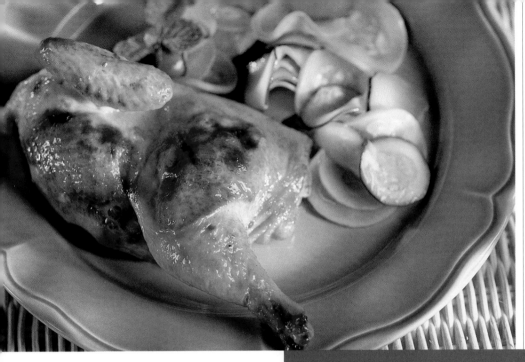

Greek-Style Roasted Game Hens A "stuffing" made with Greek olives, sun-dried tomatoes, garlic, and mint is rubbed under the skin before roasting.

Did you know? . . .

Skinless light-meat chicken may be as much as 80 percent leaner than trimmed beef (the difference depends on the cut and grade of the beef).

Remove the skin and you subtract nearly half the fat from roast chicken.

3. Preheat the grill to medium (or preheat the broiler). Reserving the marinade, grill the hens, breast-side down, 8 inches from the heat (or broil 6 inches from the heat) for 8 minutes; brush with the reserved marinade as they cook. Turn the hens over and brush with the marinade. Grill or broil for 6 minutes or until the hens are just cooked through. Serve with the pepper-celery relish. Serves 4.

Per serving: Calories 242; Fiber 1g; Protein 33g; Total Fat 8g; Saturated Fat 2g; Cholesterol 148mg; Sodium 728mg

Greek-Style Roasted Game Hens

PREP: 20 MINUTES / COOK: 30 MINUTES
The hens have a savory tomato-olive mixture stuffed under the skin.

- ¼ **cup sun-dried tomato halves (not oil-packed)**
- ⅓ **cup chopped fresh mint**
- ¼ **cup Calamata or other brine-cured black olives, pitted and chopped**
- ¼ **cup golden raisins**
- 2 **cloves garlic, finely chopped**
- ½ **teaspoon grated lemon zest**
- ¼ **teaspoon salt**
- 2 **Cornish game hens (1¼ pounds each), halved (see how-to photo, page 259)**

1. Preheat the oven to 425°F. In a small saucepan, bring 1 cup of water to a boil. Add the sun-dried tomatoes and cook for 5 minutes to blanch. Reserving 2 tablespoons of the cooking liquid, drain the tomatoes. Place the reserved cooking liquid in a medium bowl. When cool enough to handle, coarsely chop the sun-dried tomatoes and add them to the bowl.

2. Add the mint, olives, raisins, garlic, lemon zest, and salt to the sun-dried tomatoes, stirring to combine. Using your fingers, carefully lift the game hens' breast skin and as much of the thigh skin as you can without tearing it. Place one-fourth of the sun-dried tomato stuffing mixture under the skin of each hen half.

3. Place the hens, skin-side up, on a rack in a roasting pan, and roast for 25 minutes or until they are cooked through. Remove the skin before eating. Serves 4.

Per serving: Calories 223; Fiber 2g; Protein 28g; Total Fat 7g; Saturated Fat 1g; Cholesterol 120mg; Sodium 374mg

Chicken is rich in niacin (vitamin B3), which may play a role in cancer protection. Laboratory experiments at the University of Kentucky suggest that niacin may help prevent certain precancerous changes at the cellular level.

It's best to roast a whole chicken on a rack, which allows the fat to drip off as the bird cooks.

Chickens sold in stores are inspected by the USDA or by state systems with equivalent standards. Grading, however, is voluntary; Grade A chickens are, naturally, of the highest quality.

Chicken breasts

Nutritional power

One of the leanest of all meats, skinless chicken breast is a superlative protein source for the health-conscious. B vitamins are a healthy bonus.

Healthy Highlights

PER 3 OUNCES COOKED

Calories	128
Fiber	0g
Protein	25g
Total Fat	2.6g
Saturated Fat	0.7g
Cholesterol	65mg
Sodium	54mg

NUTRIENTS

	% Daily Value
Niacin	36%
Vitamin B6	14%

Did you know? . . .

A three-ounce portion of cooked skinless chicken breast supplies about half of your daily protein requirement.

The fat in chicken is mostly monounsaturated, which some researchers believe lowers blood cholesterol.

Chicken breast is a fairly good source of some minerals, including iron, potassium, and zinc.

Baked Moroccan Chicken & Couscous

PREP: 20 MINUTES / COOK: 35 MINUTES

This dish offers a satisfying and healthful balance of carbohydrate and protein.

- 1 teaspoon each ground cumin and coriander
- ¾ teaspoon salt
- ½ teaspoon each ground ginger, cinnamon, and pepper
- 4 skinless, bone-in chicken breast halves (8 ounces each)
- 2 teaspoons olive oil
- 1 small onion, finely chopped
- 3 cloves garlic, minced
- 1 cup couscous
- 1½ cups boiling water
- ¼ cup chopped cilantro or parsley
- ¼ cup chopped dates or raisins
- 2 tablespoons lemon juice

1. In a small bowl, combine the cumin, coriander, ½ teaspoon of the salt, the ginger, cinnamon, and pepper. Rub the spice mixture onto the chicken.

2. Preheat the oven to 375°F. In a large nonstick skillet, heat the oil over moderate heat. Add the chicken and cook for 3 minutes per side. Transfer the chicken to a plate.

3. Add the onion and garlic to the pan and sauté for 5 minutes. Add the couscous, boiling water, and the remaining ¼ teaspoon salt; stir, cover, remove from the heat, and let stand for 5 minutes. With a fork, gently stir in the cilantro and dates.

4. Make 4 mounds of the couscous mixture in a 9 x 13-inch baking dish and place a chicken breast half on each mound. Sprinkle the chicken with lemon juice, cover with foil, and bake for 10 minutes. Uncover and bake for 10 minutes or until the chicken is cooked through. Serve each person a mound of couscous topped with a chicken breast half. Serves 4.

Per serving: Calories 435; Fiber 3g; Protein 47g; Total Fat 5g; Saturated Fat 1g; Cholesterol 101mg; Sodium 558mg

Chicken Strips with Two Sauces

PREP: 15 MINUTES / COOK: 15 MINUTES

- ½ cup plain dry bread crumbs
- ¼ teaspoon salt
- 2 egg whites
- 1¼ pounds skinless, boneless chicken breasts, cut into 1-inch-wide strips
- 4 teaspoons vegetable oil
- ⅓ cup ketchup
- 2 tablespoons mango chutney, finely chopped
- 5 teaspoons lime juice
- ½ teaspoon ground ginger
- ⅓ cup plain low-fat yogurt
- 2 tablespoons light mayonnaise
- 2 scallions, thinly sliced
- ½ teaspoon dried tarragon

1. Preheat the oven to 350°F. On a sheet of wax paper, combine the bread crumbs and salt. In a shallow bowl, beat the egg whites with 2 tablespoons of water. Dip the chicken first into the egg whites, then into the bread crumbs.

2. In a large nonstick skillet, heat 2 teaspoons of the oil over moderate heat. Add half the chicken and cook for 2 minutes on one side, then transfer to a large baking sheet, browned-side up. Repeat with the remaining 2 teaspoons oil and chicken. Bake the chicken for 10 minutes or until cooked through.

3. Meanwhile, in a bowl, combine the ketchup, chutney, 1 tablespoon of the lime juice, and the ginger. In another bowl, combine the yogurt, mayonnaise, scallions, the remaining 2 teaspoons lime juice, and the tarragon. Serve the chicken with the two sauces. Serves 4.

Per serving: Calories 350; Fiber 1g; Protein 38g; Total Fat 10g; Saturated Fat 2g; Cholesterol 86mg; Sodium 772mg

Grilled Chicken with Parsley Sauce

PREP: 10 MINUTES / COOK: 10 MINUTES

- 4 skinless, boneless chicken breast halves (5 ounces each)
- ½ teaspoon each salt, paprika, and ground coriander
- ¼ teaspoon sugar
- 1 cup packed parsley leaves, preferably flat-leaf
- ¼ cup chicken broth
- 1 tablespoon lemon juice
- 2 teaspoons olive oil

1. Preheat the grill to medium (or preheat the broiler). Rub the chicken with ¼ teaspoon of the salt, and all of the paprika, coriander, and sugar. Grill the

Southern "Fried" Chicken is briefly sautéed, then oven-baked.

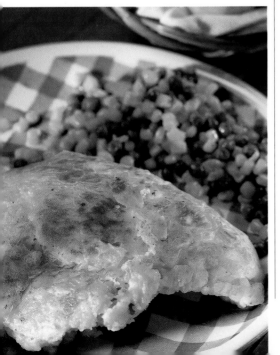

chicken 8 inches from the heat (or broil 6 inches from the heat) for 6 to 8 minutes per side, until cooked through.

2. Meanwhile, in a food processor, purée the parsley, broth, lemon juice, oil, and the remaining ¼ teaspoon salt. Spoon the sauce over the chicken. Serves 4.

Per serving: Calories 190; Fiber 1g; Protein 34g; Total Fat 4g; Saturated Fat 1g; Cholesterol 82mg; Sodium 460mg

Southern "Fried" Chicken

PREP: 10 MINUTES / MARINATE: 30 MINUTES / COOK: 30 MINUTES

- 1 cup low-fat (1.5%) buttermilk
- 1 tablespoon honey
- ½ teaspoon each cayenne pepper and salt
- ¼ teaspoon black pepper
- 4 skinless, bone-in chicken breasts (8 ounces each)
- ½ cup flour
- 1 tablespoon vegetable oil

1. In a large bowl, whisk together the buttermilk, honey, cayenne, ¼ teaspoon of the salt, and the black pepper. Add the chicken, turning to coat. Cover and marinate in the refrigerator for at least 30 minutes.

2. Preheat the oven to 400°F. Lift the chicken from its marinade and dredge in the flour, shaking off the excess. In a large nonstick skillet, heat the oil over moderate heat. Sauté the chicken, bone-side up, for 4 minutes or until golden brown. Turn the chicken over and cook for 3 minutes. Transfer to a baking sheet lined with foil and bake, bone-side down, for 20 minutes or until the chicken is cooked through. Sprinkle with the remaining ¼ teaspoon salt. Serves 4.

Per serving: Calories 326; Fiber 1g; Protein 44g; Total Fat 7g; Saturated Fat 2g; Cholesterol 105mg; Sodium 435mg

At the market Perennially popular chicken breasts are sold whole or halved and in several forms: bone-in with skin, boneless with skin, and boneless, skinless. You can even buy skinless chicken breasts cut into bite-size nuggets—though at a premium price.

Look for Chicken should look plump and smell fresh.

Prep For some recipes, you'll need to pound boneless chicken breasts to flatten them to a uniform thickness.

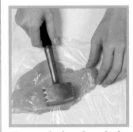

To pound a boneless chicken breast, place it between two sheets of plastic wrap and pound it gently with the flat side of a meat pounder or a small, heavy skillet.

Basic cooking To preserve the juiciness of chicken breasts, cook them quickly (especially when broiling or baking), but long enough that the meat is fully tender and the juices run clear when the meat is pierced.

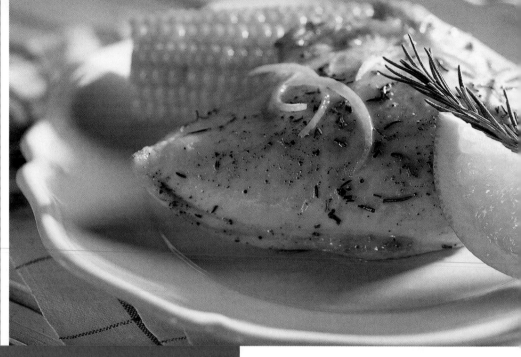

Grilled Wine-Marinated Chicken Breasts calls for just seven ingredients, but they add up to bold, sophisticated flavor.

Did you know? . . . According to the National Broiler Council, when buying chicken parts, one-fourth of consumers buy only white meat (i.e., breasts).

Chicken is a good source of selenium, an antioxidant mineral.

When meat or poultry is grilled, carcinogenic substances can form as fat drips onto the fire; these substances are deposited back on the food in the form of smoke. But a study funded by the National Cancer Institute demonstrated that when chicken is marinated (the researchers used a marinade based on oil, vinegar, lemon juice, and mustard), the amount of these substances formed is greatly reduced.

Chicken Parmigiana
PREP: 10 MINUTES / COOK: 20 MINUTES

- ½ cup grated Parmesan cheese
- ½ cup plain dry bread crumbs
- 2 egg whites
- 4 skinless, boneless chicken breast halves (5 ounces each)
- 1 tablespoon olive oil
- ¼ cup shredded part-skim mozzarella
- 2 tablespoons tomato sauce

1. Preheat the oven to 400°F. Place the Parmesan on one sheet of wax paper and the bread crumbs on another. In a shallow bowl, beat the egg whites with 2 tablespoons of water. Dip the chicken into the Parmesan, then into the egg whites, and then the bread crumbs.

2. In a large nonstick skillet, heat the oil over moderate heat. Sauté the chicken for 3 minutes per side. Transfer the chicken to a baking sheet, sprinkle with the mozzarella; spoon the tomato sauce on top. Bake for 10 minutes or until the chicken is cooked through. Serves 4.

Per serving: Calories 313; Fiber 1g; Protein 42g; Total Fat 10g; Saturated Fat 4g; Cholesterol 94mg; Sodium 501mg

Grilled Wine-Marinated Chicken Breasts
PREP: 10 MINUTES / MARINATE: 3 HOURS / COOK: 15 MINUTES

- ½ cup dry white wine
- 1 tablespoon olive oil
- 4 cloves garlic, peeled and lightly crushed
- ¾ teaspoon each crumbled dried rosemary and salt
- ½ teaspoon pepper
- 3 strips orange zest (3 x ½ inch)
- 4 skinless, bone-in chicken breast halves (8 ounces each)

1. In a shallow nonreactive pan, combine the wine, oil, garlic, rosemary, salt, pepper, and orange zest. Add the chicken, turning to coat. Cover and marinate in the refrigerator for at least 3 hours, turning the chicken several times.

2. Preheat the grill to medium (or preheat the broiler). Reserving the marinade, grill the chicken, bone-side up, 8 inches from the heat (or broil 6 inches from the heat) for 8 minutes. Turn the chicken over, brush with the marinade, and grill or broil for 7 minutes or until the chicken is cooked through. Serves 4.

Per serving: Calories 317; Fiber 0g; Protein 54g; Total Fat 8g; Saturated Fat 2g; Cholesterol 148mg; Sodium 350mg

Parchment-Baked Chicken Forestière

PREP: 30 MINUTES / COOK: 40 MINUTES

Dishes described as "à la forestière" are prepared with mushrooms, potatoes, and ham or bacon—simple ingredients that a hunter might have on hand.

- 1½ **pounds red potatoes (about 6 medium), cut into ½-inch cubes**
- ¾ **teaspoon salt**
- ½ **teaspoon pepper**
- 2 **teaspoons olive oil**
- 3 **cloves garlic, minced**
- ½ **pound mushrooms, thinly sliced**
- 2 **ounces smoked ham, chopped**
- ½ **teaspoon dried sage**
- 4 **skinless, boneless chicken breast halves (5 ounces each)**
- 8 **parsley sprigs**
- 4 **thin lemon slices, seeded**

1. In a medium pot of boiling water, cook the potatoes for 5 minutes to blanch. Drain; toss with ½ teaspoon of the salt and ¼ teaspoon of the pepper.

2. Meanwhile, preheat the oven to 400°F. In a large nonstick skillet, heat the oil over moderate heat. Add the garlic and sauté for 1 minute. Add the mushrooms and sauté for 5 minutes. Add the potatoes, ham, and sage, tossing to coat.

3. Cut four 18-inch lengths of parchment paper or foil. Make a mound of mushroom-potato mixture on one half of each sheet. Place the chicken on top and sprinkle with the remaining ¼ teaspoon each salt and pepper. Top each breast with 2 parsley sprigs and a lemon slice. Fold the parchment or foil over the chicken and make several folds to seal the packets.

4. Place the packets on a baking sheet and bake for 20 to 25 minutes or until the chicken and potatoes are cooked through. Serves 4.

Per serving: Calories 356; Fiber 4g; Protein 40g; Total Fat 5g; Saturated Fat 1g; Cholesterol 89mg; Sodium 748mg

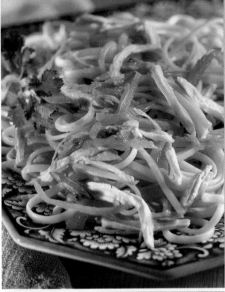

Chinese Chicken Salad Cook 8 oz. linguine. Combine 3 tbsp. light soy sauce, 2 tbsp. rice vinegar, 1 tbsp. sesame oil, ¾ tsp. each sugar and ginger, and ¼ tsp. salt. Toss with ¾ lb. cooked shredded chicken breast, 2 shredded carrots, 1 slivered red bell pepper, 2 sliced scallions, and the pasta. Serves 4. *[Cal 415; Fat 8g; Sod 674mg]*

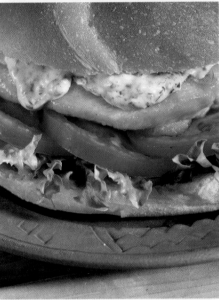

Chicken Sandwich with Lemon-Basil Mayo In food processor, combine ½ cup fresh basil, ¼ cup light mayonnaise, 2 tbsp. lemon juice, and ¼ tsp. salt; purée. Dredge 4 chicken cutlets (4 oz. each) in 2 tbsp. flour. Sauté in 1 tbsp. oil for 3 minutes per side or until done. Place 4 lettuce leaves on 4 hard rolls. Top each with tomato slices, cutlet, and basil mixture. Serves 4. *[Cal 394; Fat 12g; Sod 646mg]*

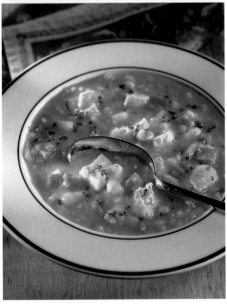

Chicken & White Bean Soup In saucepan, combine 15-oz. can rinsed white beans, mashed with 2½ cups chicken broth, 2 tbsp. tomato paste, 2 tsp. red wine vinegar, 1 diced red bell pepper, ⅓ cup minced onion, 3 cloves minced garlic, ¼ tsp. each salt and red pepper flakes, and ¾ lb. skinless, boneless chicken breasts, cut into chunks. Simmer until chicken is cooked. Serves 4. *[Cal 189; Fat 3g; Sod 1093mg]*

Did you know? . . .
A hamburger made from regular ground beef contains more than 8 times as much saturated fat as the equivalent portion of skinless chicken breast.

Chicken should always be marinated in the refrigerator—not on the counter. The same is true of thawing frozen chicken. You can also thaw frozen chicken safely in the microwave.

Chicken can be marinated (in a covered dish in the refrigerator) for up to two days.

Chicken & Egg Noodle Stir-Fry

PREP: 20 MINUTES / COOK: 15 MINUTES

Sliced chicken and vegetables are served over a crisp Asian-style noodle "pancake."

- **8 ounces thin egg noodles**
- **1 tablespoon vegetable oil**
- **1 large onion, thinly sliced**
- **2 cloves garlic, minced**
- **1 large carrot, thinly sliced**
- **1 red bell pepper, cut into ½-inch-wide strips**
- **10 ounces skinless, boneless chicken breasts, thinly sliced crosswise**
- **2 cups chicken broth**
- **2 tablespoons dry sherry**
- **1 tablespoon cornstarch**
- **1 teaspoon sugar**
- **¾ teaspoon ground ginger**
- **½ teaspoon salt**

1. In a large pot of boiling water, cook the noodles according to package directions until firm-tender. Drain.

2. Meanwhile, in a large nonstick skillet, heat 2 teaspoons of the oil over moderately high heat. Add the onion and garlic, and sauté for 3 minutes or until crisp-tender. Add the carrot and bell pepper, and sauté for 3 minutes. Add the chicken and cook for 3 minutes or until just done.

3. In a small bowl, whisk together the broth, ½ cup of water, the sherry, cornstarch, sugar, ginger, and salt. Add to the skillet and bring to a boil. Cook, stirring constantly, for 1 minute or until lightly thickened. Transfer the chicken and vegetable mixture to a bowl.

4. Add the remaining 1 teaspoon oil to the pan along with the noodles. Cook without stirring for 3 minutes or until the noodles begin to brown on the bottom. Turn the noodles over and continue cooking, pressing down, until they are golden brown and have formed a flat cake. Slide the cake onto a serving platter. Return the chicken mixture to the skillet and cook just until heated through. Pour over the noodle cake and cut into wedges to serve. Serves 4.

Per serving: Calories 398; Fiber 4g; Protein 26g; Total Fat 8g; Saturated Fat 1g; Cholesterol 95mg; Sodium 885mg

Chicken wings have about three times as much fat as chicken breasts.

Chicken is a good source of selenium, a mineral that is a component of the antioxidant enzyme glutathione peroxidase. This enzyme plays a major role in detoxifying free radicals.

Creole-Style Chicken
Chicken in a spicy tomato sauce, cooked with bell peppers and served with rice, is Louisiana's answer to comfort food.

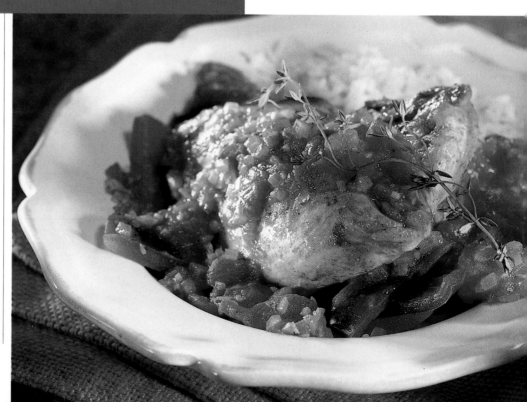

Creole-Style Chicken

PREP: 15 MINUTES / COOK: 40 MINUTES

Cooked tomatoes are a rich source of lycopene, a phytochemical that is a promising cancer-fighter.

1 cup rice
¾ teaspoon salt
4 teaspoons olive oil
1 teaspoon paprika
4 skinless, bone-in chicken breast halves (8 ounces each)
1 small onion, finely chopped
4 cloves garlic, minced
1 red bell pepper, cut into 2 x ½-inch strips
1 green bell pepper, cut into 2 x ½-inch strips
¼ teaspoon each dried thyme and black pepper
⅛ teaspoon cayenne pepper
1 can (14½ ounces) no-salt-added stewed tomatoes, chopped with their juice
½ cup chicken broth

1. In a medium saucepan, bring 2¼ cups of water to a boil. Add the rice and ¼ teaspoon of the salt, reduce to a simmer, cover, and cook for 17 minutes or until the rice is tender.

2. Meanwhile, in a large nonstick skillet, heat 2 teaspoons of the oil over moderate heat. Add the paprika and stir for 10 seconds. Add the chicken and cook for 2 minutes per side or until richly browned. Transfer the chicken to a plate. Add the remaining 2 teaspoons oil, the onion, and garlic to the pan and sauté for 3 minutes or until the onion is lightly browned.

3. Add the bell peppers, thyme, black pepper, cayenne, and the remaining ½ teaspoon salt to the pan and cook, stirring, for 5 minutes or until the bell peppers are crisp-tender. Add the tomatoes and broth, and bring to a boil. Reduce to a simmer, return the chicken to the pan, cover, and cook for 20 minutes or until the chicken is just cooked through. Serve over the rice. Serves 4.

Per serving: Calories 459; Fiber 4g; Protein 46g; Total Fat 8g; Saturated Fat 1g; Cholesterol 101mg; Sodium 703mg

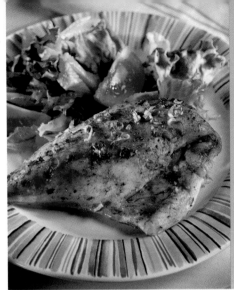

Jerk Chicken Combine 6 sliced scallions, 2 tbsp. red wine vinegar, 2 tsp. brown sugar, ¾ tsp. each black pepper and salt, and ½ tsp. each allspice and cayenne. Rub onto 4 skinless, bone-in chicken breast halves (8 oz. each). Broil 7 minutes per side or until done. Serves 4. *[Cal 292; Fat 6g; Sod 563mg]*

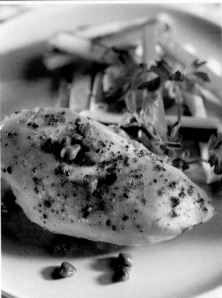

Grilled Chicken with Caper Dressing Combine ½ tsp. each salt and oregano, ¼ tsp. each sugar and pepper. Rub mixture onto 4 skinless, boneless chicken breast halves (5 oz. each). Grill or broil 6 inches from heat for 4 minutes per side or until done. Combine 3 tbsp. lemon juice, 1 tbsp. olive oil, and 1 tbsp. rinsed capers. Spoon on top. Serves 4. *[Cal 191; Fat 5g; Sod 479mg]*

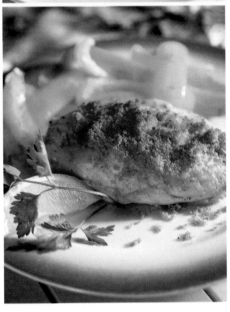

Mustard Crumb Chicken Combine 2 tbsp. Dijon mustard with ½ tsp. each honey and lemon juice. Sprinkle ½ tsp. each salt and pepper over 4 skinless, boneless chicken breast halves (5 oz. each). Brush with mustard mixture. Broil, mustard-side up, for 7 minutes. Sprinkle ¼ cup dry bread crumbs over, gently pressing. Drizzle with 1 tbsp. oil; broil until cooked through. Serves 4. *[Cal 224; Fat 6g; Sod 620mg]*

Chicken legs

Nutritional power
Although higher in fat than white meat, chicken legs (thighs and drumsticks) are a more concentrated source of minerals, including zinc and some iron.

Healthy Highlights

Chicken Thighs*

PER 3 OUNCES COOKED

Calories	166
Fiber	0g
Protein	21g
Total Fat	8.3g
Saturated Fat	2.3g
Cholesterol	76mg
Sodium	64mg

NUTRIENTS

	% Daily Value
Niacin	22%
Zinc	15%
Riboflavin	11%

meat only, no skin

Did you know? . . .
Chicken drumsticks and thighs offer richly flavored meat similar to that of goose. However, chicken is considerably lower in fat than goose.

Mushroom-Stuffed Chicken Thighs

PREP: 20 MINUTES / COOK: 40 MINUTES

- 2 slices bacon, chopped
- 1 small onion, finely chopped
- 2 cloves garlic, minced
- 4 ounces mushrooms, chopped
- ½ teaspoon dried rosemary, crumbled
- ¼ teaspoon each salt and pepper
- 2 slices firm white sandwich bread, toasted and crumbled
- ¼ cup chopped parsley
- 4 skinless, boneless chicken thighs (4 ounces each)
- 2 teaspoons olive oil
- ½ cup dry white wine
- ⅔ cup chicken broth
- 1 teaspoon cornstarch blended with 1 tablespoon water

1. In a large nonstick skillet, cook the bacon over low heat for 2 minutes or until it begins to render its fat. Add the onion and garlic, and sauté for 5 minutes. Add the mushrooms, ¼ teaspoon of the rosemary, the salt, and pepper, and sauté for 4 minutes. Transfer to a bowl and stir in the bread and parsley. Cool to room temperature.

2. Place a chicken thigh between 2 sheets of plastic wrap and pound to a ⅛-inch thickness. Repeat for all the thighs. Spoon the stuffing over them, and roll up from one short end to form packages. Secure with toothpicks.

3. In a large nonstick skillet, heat the oil over moderate heat. Add the chicken rolls and cook for 5 minutes or until golden. Add the wine, increase the heat to high, and cook for 3 minutes. Add the broth and the remaining ¼ teaspoon rosemary. Cover and simmer for 15 minutes or until the chicken is cooked through.

4. Transfer the chicken to plates. Bring the liquid to a boil, add the cornstarch mixture, and cook, stirring, for 1 minute or until lightly thickened. Spoon the sauce over the chicken. Serves 4.

Per serving: Calories 282; Fiber 1g; Protein 26g; Total Fat 14g; Saturated Fat 4g; Cholesterol 101mg; Sodium 571mg

Chicken with Plum Barbecue Sauce

PREP: 10 MINUTES / COOK: 35 MINUTES

- 1 can (8 ounces) no-salt-added tomato sauce
- ⅓ cup plum jam
- 1 tablespoon cider vinegar
- 2 cloves garlic, minced
- ½ teaspoon red hot pepper sauce
- ½ teaspoon each ground ginger and salt
- 1 teaspoon each chili powder, ground cumin, and coriander
- 8 chicken drumsticks (2 pounds total), skinned

1. In a medium saucepan, combine the tomato sauce, jam, vinegar, garlic, hot pepper sauce, ginger, and salt, and bring to a boil. Reduce to a simmer, cover, and cook for 10 minutes. Uncover and cook for 5 minutes or until the plum sauce is thick enough to coat a spoon and the flavors have blended. Cool to room temperature. Measure out ½ cup of the plum sauce and set aside; use the rest as a baste.

2. Preheat the broiler. In a small bowl, stir together the chili powder, cumin, and coriander. Rub the chicken with the spice mixture. Broil the chicken 6 inches from the heat for 3 minutes per side. Brush with half of the basting mixture and broil for 5 minutes longer. Turn the

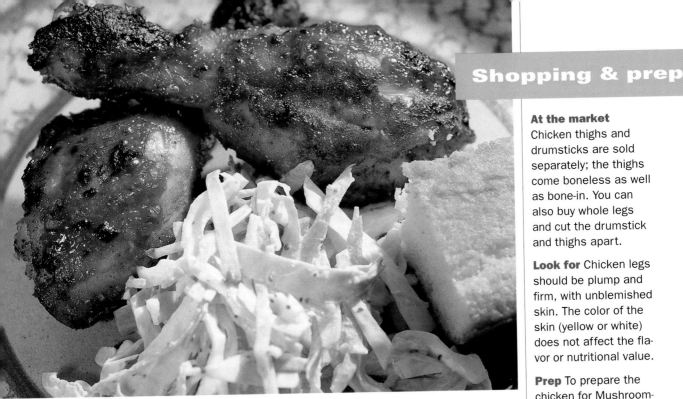

Chicken with Plum Barbecue Sauce *Spicy chicken is brushed with a tangy-sweet sauce.*

At the market
Chicken thighs and drumsticks are sold separately; the thighs come boneless as well as bone-in. You can also buy whole legs and cut the drumstick and thighs apart.

Look for Chicken legs should be plump and firm, with unblemished skin. The color of the skin (yellow or white) does not affect the flavor or nutritional value.

Prep To prepare the chicken for Mushroom-Stuffed Chicken Thighs (opposite page), the boneless thighs are first pounded thin and then stuffed and rolled (see below).

chicken over, brush with the remaining baste, and broil for 7 minutes or until cooked through. Serve the chicken with the reserved sauce. Serves 4.

Per serving: Calories 248; Fiber 2g; Protein 27g; Total Fat 6g; Saturated Fat 1g; Cholesterol 84mg; Sodium 423mg

Risotto with Chicken & Wild Mushrooms

PREP: 15 MINUTES / COOK: 55 MINUTES

Arborio is an Italian rice that makes the creamiest risotto. If you can't get Arborio, regular rice can be used instead.

2　teaspoons olive oil
1　pound skinless, boneless chicken thighs, cut into 1-inch pieces
1　small onion, finely chopped
½　pound fresh shiitake mushrooms, trimmed and thinly sliced
½　pound button mushrooms, sliced
1¼　cups Arborio rice
⅔　cup dry white wine
1½　cups chicken broth
¼　teaspoon salt
3　tablespoons Parmesan cheese
½　teaspoon pepper

1. In a large nonstick saucepan, heat the oil over moderate heat. Add the chicken and cook for 5 minutes. Transfer the chicken to a plate.

2. Add the onion to the pan and sauté for 5 minutes. Add the shiitakes and cook for 5 minutes. Add the button mushrooms and sauté for 4 minutes.

3. Add the rice, stir to coat, and add the wine. Cook until the wine has been absorbed, about 4 minutes. Combine the broth with 2 cups of water. Add 1½ cups of broth mixture to the rice along with the salt and cook, stirring occasionally, for 12 minutes or until the liquid has been absorbed. Add 1 cup of the broth mixture and cook, stirring occasionally, for 10 minutes or until the liquid has been absorbed.

4. Add the remaining 1 cup broth mixture, return the chicken to the pan, and cook for 7 minutes or until the rice is creamy but not mushy. Stir in the Parmesan and pepper. Serves 4.

Per serving: Calories 409; Fiber 6g; Protein 31g; Total Fat 9g; Saturated Fat 2g; Cholesterol 97mg; Sodium 710mg

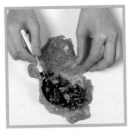

After pounding boneless chicken thighs to a uniform thickness, spoon the stuffing over them, leaving a border. Then roll up from one short side; secure with toothpicks.

Basic cooking
Chicken thighs and legs can stand up to fairly long braising. After cooking, even though the meat is dark, the juices should run clear when the meat is pierced with a sharp knife or skewer.

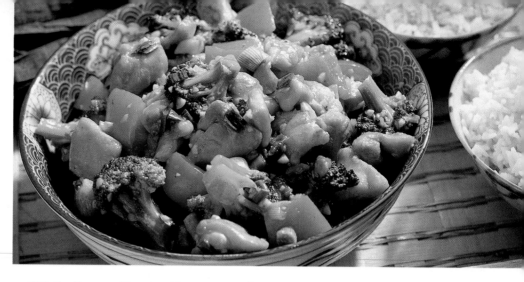

Chicken-Cashew Stir-Fry This boldly flavorful Chinese-style dish includes broccoli and red bell pepper.

Healthy Highlights

Drumsticks*

PER 3 OUNCES COOKED

Calories	143
Fiber	0g
Protein	23g
Total Fat	4.8g
Saturated Fat	1.3g
Cholesterol	75mg
Sodium	68mg

NUTRIENTS

	% Daily Value
Niacin	18%
Zinc	17%
Riboflavin	11%
Vitamin B6	10%

*meat only, no skin

Did you know? . . .

Chicken legs and thighs supply more zinc than do chicken breasts. Zinc plays a key role in cell growth and division. In this capacity, zinc helps your body heal itself when you are injured.

The dark meat (legs and thighs) of chicken contains only slightly more cholesterol than the white meat.

Chicken Paprikash

PREP: 20 MINUTES / COOK: 35 MINUTES

- 2 teaspoons vegetable oil
- 4 chicken legs, split and skinned (12 ounces each)
- 2 tablespoons plus 2 teaspoons flour
- 1 onion, finely chopped
- 4 cloves garlic, minced
- 1 tablespoon paprika
- 1 green bell pepper, coarsely chopped
- ½ cup dry white wine
- ½ cup chicken broth
- 2 tablespoons tomato paste
- ½ teaspoon salt
- ¼ teaspoon caraway seeds (optional)
- 1 jarred roasted red pepper, rinsed and drained
- ¼ cup reduced-fat sour cream

1. In a large nonstick skillet, heat the oil over moderate heat. Dredge the chicken in 2 tablespoons of the flour. Sauté for 3 minutes per side or until golden; transfer the chicken to a plate.

2. Add the onion and garlic to the pan and sauté for 5 minutes. Stir in the paprika. Add the bell pepper and ¼ cup of water, and cook, stirring, for 5 minutes. Add the wine, increase the heat to high, and cook for 2 minutes.

3. Add the broth, tomato paste, salt, and caraway seeds, and bring to a boil. Return the chicken to the pan, cover, and simmer for 15 minutes or until chicken is cooked through.

4. Meanwhile, in a food processor, combine the roasted pepper, sour cream, and the remaining 2 teaspoons flour, and purée. Stir the mixture into the pan and cook for 3 minutes or until lightly thickened. Serves 4.

Per serving: Calories 287; Fiber 2g; Protein 29g; Total Fat 10g; Saturated Fat 3g; Cholesterol 109mg; Sodium 649mg

Chicken-Cashew Stir-Fry

PREP: 20 MINUTES / COOK: 15 MINUTES

- 3 cups broccoli florets
- 1 tablespoon lower-sodium soy sauce
- 1 tablespoon dry sherry
- 4 teaspoons cornstarch
- ¾ pound skinless, boneless chicken thighs, cut into ½-inch chunks
- 2 teaspoons vegetable oil
- 1 tablespoon minced fresh ginger
- 3 cloves garlic, minced
- 1 red bell pepper, coarsely diced
- ½ cup chicken broth
- 3 tablespoons chili sauce
- ¼ teaspoon salt
- 2 scallions, thinly sliced
- ¼ cup cashews, coarsely chopped

1. In a steamer, cook the broccoli for 3 minutes or until crisp-tender; set aside. In a medium bowl, combine the soy sauce, sherry, and 3 teaspoons of the cornstarch. Add the chicken and toss.

2. In a large nonstick skillet, heat the oil. Add the chicken and stir-fry for 3 minutes. Transfer to a plate. Add the ginger and garlic, and stir-fry for 30 seconds. Add the broccoli and bell pepper, and stir-fry for 2 minutes.

3. Add the broth, chili sauce, and salt, and bring to a boil. In a small bowl, combine the remaining 1 teaspoon cornstarch with 1 tablespoon water; add to the pan and stir for 1 minute or until lightly thickened. Return the chicken to the pan; add the scallions and cook for 1 minute. Stir in the cashews. Serves 4.

Per serving: Calories 252; Fiber 4g; Protein 23g; Total Fat 10g; Saturated Fat 2g; Cholesterol 71mg; Sodium 715mg

---

Thai-Style Chicken

PREP: 25 MINUTES / COOK: 20 MINUTES

- 2 teaspoons vegetable oil
- 4 skinless, boneless chicken thighs (4 ounces each)
- 3 cloves garlic, minced
- 2 tablespoons minced fresh ginger
- ⅔ cup chicken broth
- 2 tablespoons ketchup
- 1 pickled jalapeño pepper, minced
- ½ teaspoon salt
- 2 tablespoons lime juice
- ¼ cup each chopped basil and mint
- 6 ounces vermicelli, broken in thirds
- 2 cups finely shredded Napa cabbage or iceberg lettuce
- 2 scallions, thinly sliced

1. In a large nonstick skillet, heat the oil over moderate heat. Add the chicken and cook for 3 minutes per side or until golden brown. Transfer to a plate.

2. Add the garlic and ginger to the pan and cook for 1 minute. Add the broth, ketchup, jalapeño, and salt. Return the chicken to the pan, cover, and simmer for 12 minutes or until the chicken is cooked through. Stir in the lime juice, basil, and mint.

3. Meanwhile, in a large pot of boiling water, cook the pasta according to package directions until firm-tender; drain. Divide the vermicelli among 4 plates. Top with the cabbage, spoon the chicken and sauce on top, and sprinkle with the scallions. Serves 4.

Per serving: Calories 345; Fiber 2g; Protein 29g; Total Fat 8g; Saturated Fat 2g; Cholesterol 94mg; Sodium 718mg

Baked Walnut Chicken In food processor, grind ⅓ cup walnuts, ¼ cup dry bread crumbs, and ½ tsp. each grated lemon zest and salt. Dip 4 split, skinned chicken legs (2½ lbs.) in 2 egg whites, then in walnut mixture, patting it on. Bake at 400° F for 25 to 30 minutes or until done. Serves 4. *[Cal 330; Fat 14g; Sod 542mg]*

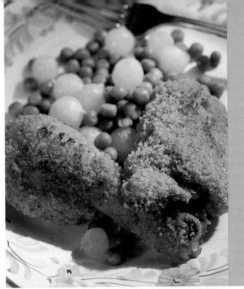

Mom's Chicken-Noodle Soup In medium saucepan, combine 2 cups water, 1 cup chicken broth, 1 sliced celery stalk, 1 sliced carrot, 1 minced garlic clove, and ¼ tsp. salt. Bring to boil. Add ⅓ cup ditalini (or other small pasta) and 1 lb. skinless, boneless chicken thighs, cut into ½-inch chunks. Cover and simmer 10 minutes or until pasta and chicken are done. Serves 4. *[Cal 181; Fat 5g; Sod 519mg]*

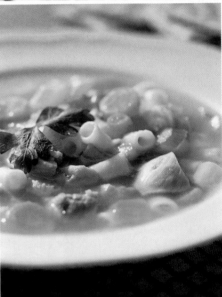

Spiced Yogurt Chicken In shallow pan, combine 2 cups plain low-fat yogurt, ½ cup chopped cilantro, 1 tsp. each cumin, coriander, ginger, salt, and pepper. Set half of mixture aside. To remaining mixture, add 4 split, skinned chicken legs (2½ lbs.); marinate 1 hour. Discard marinade; broil chicken for 7 minutes per side or until done. Serve with reserved yogurt mixture, if desired. Serves 4. *[Cal 289; Fat 9g; Sod 663mg]*

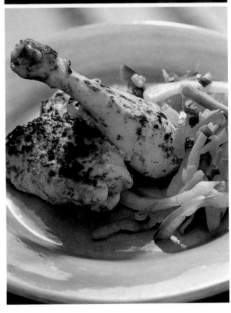

Whole turkey

Nutritional power

A roast turkey is the definitive holiday bird. Eaten without the skin, and accompanied with a low-fat stuffing, turkey makes a healthfully balanced meal.

Healthy Highlights

PER 3 OUNCES COOKED*

Calories	145
Fiber	0g
Protein	25g
Total Fat	4.2g
Saturated Fat	1.4g
Cholesterol	65mg
Sodium	60mg

NUTRIENTS

	% Daily Value
Niacin	23%
Vitamin B6	20%
Zinc	17%
Iron	11%

*meat only, no skin

Did you know? . . .

From a food-safety standpoint, it's best to cook the stuffing as "un-stuffing"— that is, outside the turkey. Cooking the stuffing separately also means that it will not absorb fat from the turkey— and the unstuffed turkey will cook in far less time.

Cajun-Spiced Turkey

PREP: 15 MINUTES / COOK: 3 HOURS

- 2 tablespoons green hot pepper sauce
- 2 tablespoons vegetable oil
- 1 teaspoon salt
- 2 teaspoons each dried oregano, dried thyme, and sugar
- ½ teaspoon each black pepper and cayenne pepper
- 1 turkey (13 pounds)
- 1 lemon, pricked with a fork
- 2 tablespoons flour
- 2 cups chicken or turkey broth

1. In a small bowl, combine the hot pepper sauce, oil, salt, oregano, thyme, sugar, black pepper, and cayenne. Rub the spice mixture under the skin of the turkey's breast meat and drumsticks. Place the lemon in the cavity of the turkey.

2. Roast according to the roasting instructions in "Basic cooking," opposite page.

3. Transfer the turkey to a cutting board; discard the lemon. Pour the pan juices into a gravy separator and then pour the defatted juices into a small saucepan. Whisk together the flour and broth, and add to the pan juices. Cook, stirring, for 4 minutes or until the gravy is lightly thickened. Remove turkey skin before eating. Serves 12.

Per serving: Calories 431; Fiber 0g; Protein 71g; Total Fat 13g; Saturated Fat 4g; Cholesterol 186mg; Sodium 584mg

Apricot-Cornbread Stuffing

PREP: 15 MINUTES / COOK: 40 MINUTES

- 1 cup dried apricot halves
- 1 cup boiling water
- 6 ounces sweet Italian sausage, casings removed
- 1 onion, finely chopped
- 2 cloves garlic, minced
- ½ teaspoon dried sage
- ¼ teaspoon salt
- 7 cups crumbled cornbread (1½ pounds)
- 1 can (10 ounces) water-packed chestnuts, drained and chopped
- 2 cups chicken broth
- 1 tablespoon unsalted butter, melted

1. Preheat the oven to 450°F. In a small heatproof bowl, combine the apricots and boiling water; set aside. Meanwhile, crumble the sausage into a large nonstick skillet and cook over moderate heat for 5 minutes or until it has browned and rendered its fat. Add the onion, garlic, sage, and salt, and sauté for 5 minutes or until the onion is soft. Transfer to a large bowl.

2. Drain the apricots and coarsely chop. Add the apricots, cornbread, and chestnuts to the bowl. Drizzle with the broth and butter, tossing to coat. Spoon into a 9 x 13-inch pan, cover with foil, and bake for 20 minutes. Uncover and bake for 10 minutes. Serves 12.

Per serving: Calories 280; Fiber 3g; Protein 7g; Total Fat 11g; Saturated Fat 4g; Cholesterol 48mg; Sodium 781mg

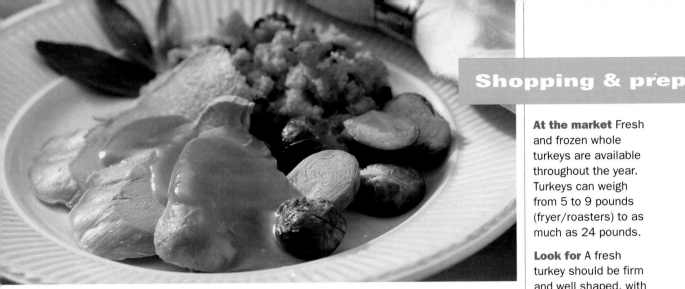

Teriyaki Turkey with Apricot-Cornbread Stuffing A mixed-cuisine combo that works.

At the market Fresh and frozen whole turkeys are available throughout the year. Turkeys can weigh from 5 to 9 pounds (fryer/roasters) to as much as 24 pounds.

Look for A fresh turkey should be firm and well shaped, with creamy white skin. Frozen turkeys should be solidly frozen.

Prep Remove the giblets and neck from the cavity. Rinse the turkey under cold running water and remove any pinfeathers.

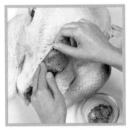

To season the turkey, carefully lift the skin over the breast and drumsticks, and rub the seasoning mixture underneath.

Basic cooking Have the turkey at room temperature. Place on a rack in a roasting pan and pour 2 cups of water into the pan. Roast, covered, in a preheated 350°F oven for 12 minutes per pound, or until the thigh meat registers 170°F. Uncover for the last 40 minutes of roasting.

Teriyaki Turkey

PREP: 15 MINUTES / COOK: 3 HOURS

- ⅓ cup lower-sodium soy sauce
- 2 tablespoons honey
- 2 tablespoons sesame oil
- 1 teaspoon grated orange zest
- ¼ teaspoon ground cinnamon
- 1 turkey (13 pounds)
- 1 head of garlic, unpeeled
- 2 tablespoons flour
- ¼ teaspoon salt
- 2 cups chicken or turkey broth

1. In a small bowl, combine the soy sauce, honey, sesame oil, orange zest, and cinnamon. Rub the mixture under the skin of the turkey's breast and drumsticks. Place the garlic in the cavity of the turkey.

2. Roast according to the roasting instructions in "Basic cooking," at right.

3. Transfer the turkey to a cutting board; discard the garlic. Pour the pan juices into a gravy separator and then pour the defatted juices into a small saucepan. Whisk together the flour, salt, and broth, and add to the pan juices. Cook, stirring, for 4 minutes or until the gravy is lightly thickened. Remove turkey skin before eating. Serves 12.

Per serving: Calories 457; Fiber 0g; Protein 72g; Total Fat 14g; Saturated Fat 4g; Cholesterol 186mg; Sodium 667mg

Two-Mushroom Stuffing

PREP: 25 MINUTES / COOK: 55 MINUTES

- 10 ounces whole-wheat sourdough bread, cut into 1-inch chunks (8 cups)
- 2 tablespoons olive oil
- 1 large onion, finely chopped
- 3 cloves garlic, minced
- 1 pound button mushrooms, sliced
- 12 ounces fresh shiitake mushrooms, trimmed and sliced
- ¾ teaspoon salt
- ½ teaspoon each crumbled dried rosemary and pepper
- 2 cups chicken broth

1. Preheat the oven to 450°F. Place the bread on a baking sheet and bake for 10 minutes or until crusty and partially dry. Transfer to a large bowl.

2. In a Dutch oven, heat 1 tablespoon of the oil over moderate heat. Add the onion and garlic, and sauté for 5 minutes. Add the button and shiitake mushrooms, salt, rosemary, and pepper, and cook, stirring, for 7 minutes.

3. Add the mushroom mixture to the bread, tossing to combine. Add the broth and the remaining 1 tablespoon oil and toss again. Transfer to a 9 x 13-inch pan, cover with foil, and bake for 30 minutes. Serves 12.

Per serving: Calories 114; Fiber 2g; Protein 4g; Total Fat 3g; Saturated Fat 1g; Cholesterol 0mg; Sodium 467mg

Turkey breast

Nutritional power

The leanest of all meats, turkey breast has a mild flavor that makes it a versatile cooking ingredient. It supplies a lot of high-quality protein and B vitamins.

Healthy Highlights

PER 3 OUNCES COOKED*

Calories	115
Fiber	0g
Protein	26g
Total Fat	0.6g
Saturated Fat	0.2g
Cholesterol	71mg
Sodium	44mg

NUTRIENTS

	% Daily Value
Niacin	32%
Vitamin B6	24%
Zinc	10%

*meat only, no skin

Did you know? . . .
If you've been advised to watch your intake of saturated fat (everyone should, but it's especially important for people with high cholesterol), skinless turkey breast should be on your table frequently. It contains less saturated fat than any other meat.

Turkey Enchiladas

PREP: 20 MINUTES / COOK: 35 MINUTES

The tortillas, filled with turkey and salsa, are baked in a creamy tomato-chili sauce.

- 1 tablespoon olive oil
- 1 pound skinless, boneless turkey breast, cut into 2 x ½-inch strips
- 1 red bell pepper, cut into ½-inch pieces
- 4 scallions, thinly sliced
- 3 cloves garlic, minced
- 1 teaspoon chili powder
- ⅓ cup reduced-sodium salsa
- 8 corn tortillas (6-inch diameter)
- 1 can (4 ounces) mild green chilies, drained
- 3 tablespoons no-salt-added tomato paste
- 1 pickled jalapeño pepper
- 2 tablespoons flour
- 2 cups low-fat (1%) milk
- 6 tablespoons shredded Cheddar cheese (1½ ounces)

1. Preheat the oven to 375°F. In a large nonstick skillet, heat 2 teaspoons of the oil over moderate heat. Add the turkey and cook for 3 minutes or until just cooked through. With a slotted spoon, transfer the turkey to a bowl.

2. Add the remaining 1 teaspoon oil, the bell pepper, scallions, and garlic to the pan and cook for 4 minutes or until crisp-tender. Stir in the chili powder. Transfer to the bowl with the turkey. Stir in the salsa. Spoon the mixture down the center of the tortillas, roll them up, and place, seam-side down, in a 7 x 11-inch glass baking dish.

3. In a food processor, combine the green chilies, tomato paste, and jalapeño, and process until smooth. Add the flour and milk, and blend. Pour the mixture over the enchiladas.

Bake for 25 minutes or until the enchiladas are piping hot. Sprinkle with the Cheddar. Serves 4.

Per serving: Calories 412; Fiber 4g; Protein 39g; Total Fat 11g; Saturated Fat 4g; Cholesterol 86mg; Sodium 510mg

Ricotta-Stuffed Turkey Breast

PREP: 25 MINUTES
COOK: 1 HOUR 5 MINUTES

The turkey is pounded so that it can be rolled (see how-to photos, opposite page) around a spinach and ricotta filling.

- 4 teaspoons olive oil
- 4 cloves garlic, minced
- ½ package (10 ounces) frozen chopped spinach
- ⅔ cup part-skim ricotta cheese
- 1 egg white
- ½ teaspoon grated orange zest
- ¼ teaspoon pepper
- 1 skinless, boneless turkey breast half (3¾ pounds)
- ¾ teaspoon salt
- ½ teaspoon dried rosemary, crumbled

1. Preheat the oven to 375°F. In a large nonstick skillet, heat 2 teaspoons of the oil over low heat. Add the garlic and sauté for 1 minute. Add the spinach and cook, stirring occasionally, for 4 minutes or until tender. Let cool.

2. In a small bowl, combine the ricotta, egg white, orange zest, and pepper. Stir in the spinach mixture. Place the turkey between 2 sheets of wax paper or foil and pound to a ¾-inch thickness. Sprinkle with ¼ teaspoon of the salt. Spread the ricotta mixture on the turkey and roll up from one long side. Tie the roast to secure it, then place seam-side down in a small roasting pan.

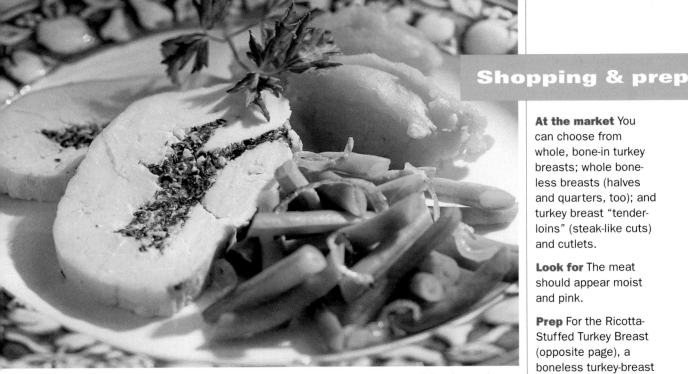

Ricotta-Stuffed Turkey Breast makes elegant holiday fare or a special family meal.

At the market You can choose from whole, bone-in turkey breasts; whole bone-less breasts (halves and quarters, too); and turkey breast "tender-loins" (steak-like cuts) and cutlets.

Look for The meat should appear moist and pink.

Prep For the Ricotta-Stuffed Turkey Breast (opposite page), a boneless turkey-breast half is pounded to an even thickness so that it can be stuffed and rolled (see below).

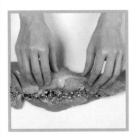

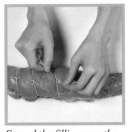

Spread the filling over the pounded turkey breast, leaving a little space at the edges. Roll from one long side and tie in a few places with kitchen string.

Basic cooking Whole turkey breast should be cooked to an internal temperature of 170°. Don't overcook, or the meat will be dry.

3. Brush with the remaining 2 teaspoons oil and sprinkle with the remaining ½ teaspoon salt and the rosemary. Roast for 1 hour or until browned and cooked through. Serves 8.

Per serving: Calories 294; Fiber 0g; Protein 56g; Total Fat 5g; Saturated Fat 2g; Cholesterol 138mg; Sodium 368mg

Turkey Chow Mein
PREP: 20 MINUTES / COOK: 15 MINUTES

This Chinese-American stir-fry is usually served over fried noodles. This lower-fat interpretation calls for linguine instead.

- 8 **ounces linguine, broken in half**
- 2 **tablespoons lower-sodium soy sauce**
- 1 **tablespoon plus 1½ teaspoons cornstarch**
- ½ **teaspoon red hot pepper sauce**
- 1 **pound skinless, boneless turkey breast, cut into thin strips**
- 1 **tablespoon vegetable oil**
- 1 **red bell pepper, cut into ½-inch squares**
- 1 **carrot, thinly sliced**
- 1 **tablespoon minced fresh ginger**
- 2 **cloves garlic, minced**
- 4 **ounces mushrooms, sliced**
- ⅔ **cup chicken broth**
- ¼ **teaspoon salt**

1. In a large pot of boiling water, cook the pasta according to package directions until firm-tender. Drain. Meanwhile, in a medium bowl, whisk together the soy sauce, 1 tablespoon of the cornstarch, and the hot pepper sauce. Add the turkey, tossing to coat.

2. In a large nonstick skillet, heat 2 teaspoons of the oil over moderately high heat. Add the turkey and stir-fry for 4 minutes or until lightly golden and just cooked through. With a slotted spoon, transfer the turkey to a plate.

3. Add the remaining 1 teaspoon oil, the bell pepper, carrot, ginger, and garlic, and stir-fry until crisp-tender. Add the mushrooms and stir-fry until softened. Whisk together the broth, salt, and the remaining 1½ teaspoons cornstarch. Add to the skillet and cook, stirring constantly, for 1 minute or until lightly thickened. Add the turkey and pasta, and cook until the pasta and turkey are heated through. Serves 4.

Per serving: Calories 410; Fiber 3g; Protein 37g; Total Fat 6g; Saturated Fat 1g; Cholesterol 70mg; Sodium 703mg

Turkey Stroganoff

A lightened sour cream sauce lets the flavors and colors of the fresh ingredients shine through.

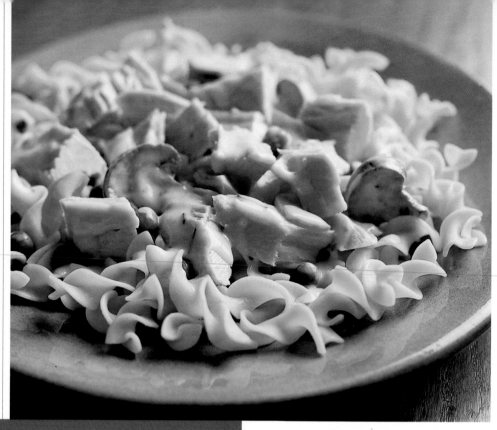

Did you know? . . .
Skinless turkey breast has about the same amount of protein, vitamin B6, and niacin as beef top round, but only about one-sixth the fat.

With barely 1 gram of fat per serving, skinless turkey breast is the leanest meat of all.

When buying cooked turkey breast at the deli counter, try to get fresh roasted turkey rather than packaged turkey products, which may have added broth or water, starch, sugar, oil, and preservatives.

Turkey breast can be substituted for veal in many recipes.

Americans have a proprietary feeling about our traditional holiday bird, but per capita, more turkey is eaten in Israel than in the United States. France takes third place, after the U.S.

Turkey Stroganoff

PREP: 10 MINUTES / COOK: 20 MINUTES

The carrots and green peas in this updated classic add nutritional value (notably beta carotene, fiber, and potassium) as well as a touch of color. The turkey and vegetables are delicious served over egg noodles, though you could also try the yolk-free noodles now available.

8	ounces medium egg noodles
2	tablespoons olive oil
1	pound skinless, boneless turkey breast, cut into 2 x ½-inch strips
2	carrots, thinly sliced
½	pound small mushrooms, halved
¾	cup lower-sodium chicken broth
1	cup frozen peas
½	teaspoon each salt and pepper
¼	teaspoon dried rosemary, crumbled
½	cup reduced-fat sour cream
1	tablespoon flour

1. In a large pot of boiling water, cook the noodles according to package directions until firm-tender. Drain.

2. Meanwhile, in a large skillet, heat 1 tablespoon of the oil over moderate heat. Add the turkey and sauté for 3 minutes or until just cooked through. With a slotted spoon, transfer the turkey to a plate.

3. Add the remaining 1 tablespoon oil to the skillet. Add the carrots and mushrooms and sauté for 3 minutes or until the mushrooms begin to give up their liquid.

4. Add the broth, ½ cup of water, the peas, salt, pepper, and rosemary, and bring to a boil. Reduce to a simmer and cook, uncovered, for 2 minutes or until the carrots are tender.

5. In a small bowl, combine the sour cream and flour. Whisk the sour cream mixture into the skillet. Return the turkey (and any juices that have accumulated on the plate) to the skillet and cook for 2 minutes or until the sauce is thickened. Serve over the hot egg noodles. Serves 4.

Per serving: Calories 522; Fiber 5g; Protein 42g; Total Fat 15g; Saturated Fat 4g; Cholesterol 134mg; Sodium 609mg

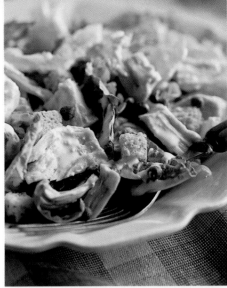

Turkey Cutlets with Mole Sauce

PREP: 15 MINUTES / COOK: 45 MINUTES

This intriguing list of ingredients hints at the complexity of flavors in this variation on a mole poblano—a classic Mexican sauce that always contains a hint of chocolate.

- 1 tablespoon olive oil
- 1 small onion, thinly sliced
- 2 cloves garlic, minced
- 1½ teaspoons chili powder
- ½ cup canned no-salt-added tomatoes, chopped with their juice
- 1 pickled jalapeño pepper, chopped
- ¼ cup each sliced banana and prunes
- 1 tablespoon sesame seeds, toasted
- 1 teaspoon unsweetened cocoa
- 1 teaspoon reduced-fat peanut butter
- 1 corn tortilla, torn into pieces
- 1½ teaspoons red wine vinegar
- ¼ teaspoon each ground cumin, coriander, cinnamon, and salt
- ½ cup chicken broth
- 1 pound skinless, boneless turkey breast, cut into 4 thick slices

1. In a large nonstick saucepan, heat 1 teaspoon of the oil over moderate heat. Add the onion and garlic, and sauté for 5 minutes or until the onion is tender. Add the chili powder, stir to coat, and cook for 1 minute.

2. Add the tomatoes, jalapeño, banana, prunes, sesame seeds, cocoa, peanut butter, tortilla, vinegar, cumin, coriander, cinnamon, and salt. Add the broth and ¼ cup of water and bring to a boil. Transfer the mixture to a food processor and process until smooth. Return the mole sauce to the saucepan, bring to a boil, reduce to a simmer, cover, and cook for 30 minutes or until the sauce is richly flavored and thick.

3. Meanwhile, in a nonstick skillet, heat the remaining 2 teaspoons oil over moderately high heat. Add the turkey and cook for 2 minutes per side or until lightly browned. Add the sauce and cook for 3 minutes or until the turkey is cooked through. Serves 4.

Per serving: Calories 251; Fiber 3g; Protein 30g; Total Fat 7g; Saturated Fat 1g; Cholesterol 70mg; Sodium 416mg

Turkey Caesar

Combine ¼ cup light mayonnaise, 2 tbsp. lemon juice, and 3 tbsp. Parmesan. Toss with 6 cups torn romaine lettuce, ½ pound diced cooked turkey breast, ¼ cup seasoned croutons, and 1 tbsp. capers. Serves 4. *[Cal 162; Fat 6g; Sod 315mg]*

Turkey-Cheddar Sandwich

Combine ¼ cup spicy brown mustard and 4 tsp. honey. Spread the mixture on 4 slices of whole-grain bread. Top each with 3 oz. roast turkey, 4 slices of apple, 1 oz. sliced Cheddar cheese, curly leaf lettuce, and a second slice of bread. Serves 4. *[Cal 459; Fat 16g; Sod 673mg]*

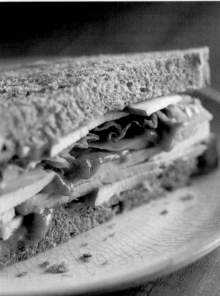

Turkey Minestrone

In saucepan, combine one 13¾-oz. can chicken broth, one 14½-oz. can no-salt-added stewed tomatoes, 1 cup water, 1 cup cooked small pasta shells, 1 cup frozen peas, and 2 cups cubed cooked turkey breast. Bring to a boil and cook for 5 minutes to heat through. Sprinkle each serving with 2 tbsp. Parmesan. Serves 4. *[Cal 270; Fat 7g; Sod 749mg]*

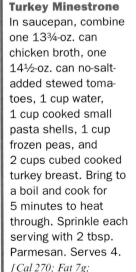

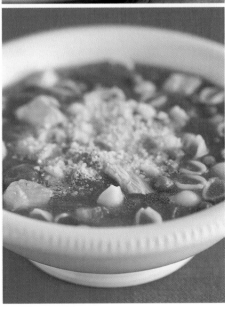

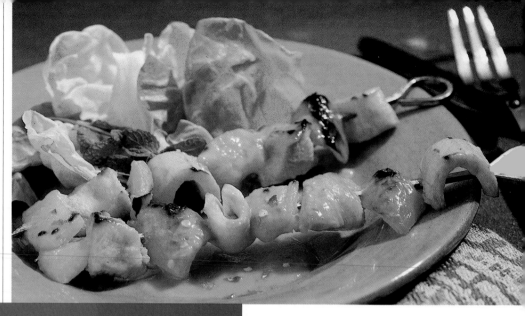

Turkey Satay *These skewers of turkey, peppers, cucumber, and pineapple can be broiled in the oven or grilled outdoors.*

Did you know? . . .
A serving of skinless turkey breast supplies more iron than the equivalent portion of pork tenderloin.

Skinless turkey breast is a better source of iron than pork tenderloin.

American turkey consumption increased by more than 100 percent between 1970 and 1990. In 1996, annual consumption of turkey rose by more than half a pound per person—to a total of more than 14 pounds.

Do you nod off after Thanksgiving dinner? Credit the combination of turkey (which is rich in the amino acid tryptophan) and lots of carbohydrates. Tryptophan makes you feel relaxed and sleepy; the carbohydrate enhances the brain's uptake of this amino acid.

With just over half a gram of total fat and just a trace of saturated fat, turkey breast is even leaner than many types of fish.

Turkey Gumbo

PREP: 15 MINUTES / COOK: 50 MINUTES

When cut-up okra is cooked, a substance in the vegetable thickens its cooking liquid much as cornstarch would.

- 2 teaspoons olive oil
- 1 pound skinless, boneless turkey breast, cut into 1-inch chunks
- 2 ounces smoked ham, chopped
- 1 onion, finely chopped
- 2 scallions, thinly sliced
- 1 red bell pepper, coarsely chopped
- 1 tablespoon flour
- ½ package (10 ounces) frozen sliced okra, minced
- 1 cup chicken broth
- 4 cups kale or spinach, shredded
- ½ teaspoon each dried thyme and marjoram
- ¼ teaspoon salt
- ⅛ teaspoon cayenne pepper

1. In a nonstick Dutch oven or flameproof casserole, heat the oil over moderately high heat. Add the turkey and ham, and cook for 5 minutes or until the turkey is lightly browned. Transfer the turkey and ham to a plate.

2. Add the onion and scallions to the pan and sauté for 5 minutes. Add the bell pepper and sauté for 4 minutes. Stir in the flour until well coated. Add the okra and stir until the okra has broken up and is well combined. Gradually add the broth and ⅔ cup of water, stirring constantly, until the sauce is smooth.

3. Add the kale, thyme, marjoram, salt, and cayenne. Bring to a boil, reduce to a simmer, cover, and cook, stirring occasionally, for 30 minutes or until the gumbo is lightly thickened. Return the turkey and ham to the pan and cook for 2 minutes or until the turkey is cooked through. Serves 4.

Per serving: Calories 247; Fiber 7g; Protein 35g; Total Fat 5g; Saturated Fat 1g; Cholesterol 77mg; Sodium 697mg

Turkey Satay

PREP: 15 MINUTES / MARINATE: 1 HOUR
COOK: 10 MINUTES

- ½ cup lime juice
- 2 tablespoons honey
- 2 tablespoons peanut butter
- ½ teaspoon each crushed red pepper flakes and salt
- 1 pound skinless, boneless turkey breast, cut into ½-inch chunks
- 1 large cucumber, peeled, halved, seeded and cut into 16 pieces
- 1 red bell pepper, cut into 16 pieces
- 2 tablespoons finely chopped fresh basil or mint
- 16 fresh or canned pineapple chunks

1. In a medium bowl, whisk together the lime juice, honey, peanut butter, red pepper flakes and salt. Set aside ¼ cup of the mixture. Add the turkey, cucumber, bell pepper, and basil to the mixture remaining in the bowl, tossing well. Cover and refrigerate for 1 hour.

2. Preheat the broiler. Thread the turkey, vegetables, and pineapple onto eight 10-inch skewers. Broil 6 inches from the heat for 6 minutes, turning once. To serve, spoon the reserved sauce over the skewers. Serves 4.

Per serving: Calories 249; Fiber 2g; Protein 31g; Total Fat 5g; Saturated Fat 1g; Cholesterol 70mg; Sodium 393mg

Turkey Scaloppine

PREP: 15 MINUTES / COOK: 10 MINUTES

This update of a recipe usually made from veal is a light main dish suitable for company.

- **2 tablespoons lemon juice**
- **½ teaspoon salt**
- **2 teaspoons plus 1 tablespoon olive oil**
- **6 cups shredded romaine lettuce**
- **1 scallion, thinly sliced**
- **1 pound skinless, boneless turkey breast, cut into 8 thin slices**
- **2 tablespoons flour**
- **1 large tomato, diced**

1. In a large bowl, whisk together the lemon juice, ¼ teaspoon of the salt, and 2 teaspoons of the oil. Add the lettuce and scallion; toss well.

2. In a large nonstick skillet, heat the remaining 1 tablespoon oil over moderately high heat. Dredge the turkey in the flour, shaking off the excess. Working in batches, sauté the turkey for 2 minutes per side or until golden brown and cooked through.

3. Place the turkey on 4 plates, top with the tomato. Sprinkle with the remaining ¼ teaspoon salt. Top with the salad. Serves 4.

Per serving: Calories 216; Fiber 2g; Protein 30g; Total Fat 7g; Saturated Fat 1g; Cholesterol 70mg; Sodium 358mg

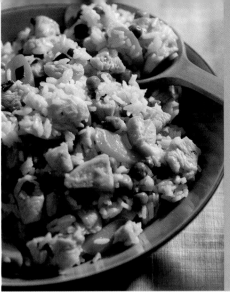

Turkey Fried Rice
In large nonstick skillet, heat 1 tbsp. oil. Sauté 1 sliced carrot, 3 sliced scallions, and 2 minced garlic cloves. Add 3 cups cooked rice, ¾ lb. diced cooked turkey breast, 1 cup frozen peas, 1 tbsp. soy sauce, ½ tsp. each ground ginger and salt. Heat through. Serves 4. *[Cal 344; Fat 5g; Sod 641mg]*

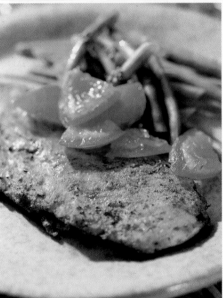

Tandoori Turkey In bowl, combine 1½ tsp. each ground cumin, coriander, turmeric, and chili powder; 1 tsp. each ground cardamom and pepper; ½ tsp. salt; and ⅓ cup plain low-fat yogurt. Rub mixture onto four 4-oz. slices of skinless, boneless turkey breast. Marinate 2 hours. Broil for 5 minutes per side or until cooked through. Top with 1 tomato, sliced. Serves 4. *[Cal 162; Fat 2g; Sod 375mg]*

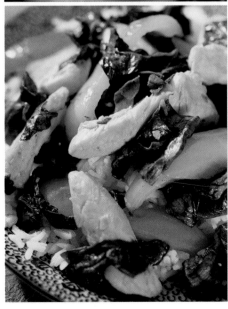

Turkey-Garlic Stir-Fry
In large nonstick skillet, heat 1 tbsp. oil over moderate heat. Add 1 each sliced red and yellow bell pepper and 3 cloves minced garlic, and cook until tender. Add 1 lb. skinless, boneless turkey breast, cut into thin strips; cook 2 minutes. Add 10-oz. package fresh spinach and ½ tsp. salt, and cook until spinach is wilted and turkey is cooked through. Serves 4. *[Cal 185; Fat 4g; Sod 402mg]*

Ground turkey

Nutritional power

The perfect lower-fat substitute for ground beef or pork, ground turkey breast makes any burger, meat loaf, pasta sauce, or chili a far more healthful dish.

Healthy Highlights

PER 3 OUNCES COOKED*	
Calories	115
Fiber	0g
Protein	26g
Total Fat	0.6g
Saturated Fat	0.2g
Cholesterol	71mg
Sodium	44mg

NUTRIENTS	
	% Daily Value
Niacin	32%
Vitamin B6	24%
Zinc	10%

*turkey breast

Did you know? . . .

A 3-ounce turkey burger made with ground turkey breast is a lean, mean, protein machine with less than 1 gram of fat. Served on a whole-wheat bun with lettuce and tomato, it's a nutritious main dish. Compare this to a fast-food hamburger: Even the "lean" version has 12 grams of fat.

Tomato-Glazed Turkey Meat Loaf

PREP: 10 MINUTES / COOK: 55 MINUTES

- 2 teaspoons olive oil
- 1 onion, chopped
- 2 cloves garlic, minced
- 1 large carrot, minced
- 1½ pounds lean ground turkey breast
- 3 slices (2 ounces total) firm-textured white sandwich bread, crumbled
- ¼ cup low-fat (1%) milk
- 1 egg
- 1 teaspoon dried sage
- ¾ teaspoon each salt and pepper
- ⅓ cup ketchup

1. Preheat the oven to 350°F. Spray a 5 x 8½ x 3-inch loaf pan with nonstick cooking spray.

2. In a large nonstick skillet, heat the oil over moderate heat. Add the onion and garlic, and cook, stirring, for 5 minutes or until the onion is softened. Add the carrot and cook, stirring, for 4 minutes or until the carrot is crisp-tender. Set aside to cool slightly.

3. In a large bowl, combine the bread and milk. Add the ground turkey, the sautéed vegetable mixture, the egg, ¾ teaspoon of the sage, ½ teaspoon of the salt, and all of the pepper, and mix well. Transfer the meat loaf mixture to the prepared pan.

4. In a small bowl, combine the ketchup with the remaining ¼ teaspoon each sage and salt. Spread the ketchup mixture evenly over the top of the meat loaf and bake for 45 minutes or until cooked through and firm. Serves 6.

Per serving: Calories 217; Fiber 2g; Protein 31g; Total Fat 4g; Saturated Fat 1g; Cholesterol 106mg; Sodium 576mg

Turkey Meatballs & Spaghetti

PREP: 30 MINUTES / COOK: 20 MINUTES

Because ground turkey breast is so lean, you need a trick or two to keep it moist. Mixing the meat with milk-soaked bread works well.

- 4 teaspoons olive oil
- 1 small onion, finely chopped
- 3 cloves garlic, minced
- 1 slice firm-textured white sandwich bread, crumbled
- ¼ cup low-fat (1%) milk
- 1 pound lean ground turkey breast
- 3 tablespoons grated Parmesan cheese
- ¾ teaspoon salt
- ¼ teaspoon each dried sage and pepper
- 3 tablespoons flour
- 2 cans (14½ ounces each) canned no-salt-added tomatoes, chopped with their juice
- 1 can (8 ounces) no-salt-added tomato sauce
- 12 ounces spaghetti

1. In a small nonstick skillet, heat 1 teaspoon of the oil over low heat. Add the onion and garlic, and sauté for 5 minutes or until the onion is tender. Transfer to a large bowl, add the bread and milk, and stir to moisten. Add the turkey, Parmesan, ½ teaspoon of the salt, the sage, and pepper. Mix well to combine, then shape into 20 meatballs.

2. Dredge the meatballs in the flour, shaking off the excess. In a large nonstick skillet, heat the remaining 3 teaspoons oil over moderate heat. Add the meatballs and cook, turning, for 4 minutes or until lightly browned all over.

3. Add the tomatoes and their juice, the tomato sauce, and the remaining ¼ teaspoon salt, and bring to a boil.

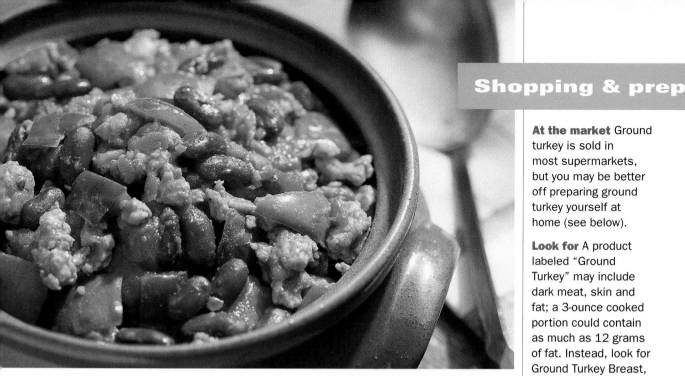

Turkey Chili is a quick and easy main dish with robust, well-rounded seasonings.

Reduce to a simmer and cook for 10 minutes or until the meatballs are cooked through and the sauce is flavorful.

4. Meanwhile, in a large pot of boiling water, cook the pasta according to package directions until firm-tender. Drain and transfer to a large bowl. Add the meatballs and sauce, tossing to combine. Serves 4.

Per serving: Calories 621; Fiber 5g; Protein 45g; Total Fat 9g; Saturated Fat 2g; Cholesterol 74mg; Sodium 654mg

Turkey Chili

PREP: 15 MINUTES / COOK: 20 MINUTES

For a party, you can double or triple this crowd-pleasing recipe. Serve the chili with warm cornbread or tortillas.

1   tablespoon vegetable oil
1   onion, finely chopped
3   cloves garlic, minced
1   green bell pepper, cut into ½-inch squares
1   red bell pepper, cut into ½-inch squares
2   teaspoons chili powder
¾   teaspoon each oregano, ground cumin, and coriander

1   pound lean ground turkey breast
1   can (14½ ounces) no-salt-added stewed tomatoes, chopped with their juice
1   can (8 ounces) no-salt-added tomato sauce
2   tablespoons no-salt-added tomato paste
½   teaspoon salt
¼   teaspoon black pepper
1   can (15 ounces) red kidney beans, rinsed and drained

1. In a Dutch oven or flameproof casserole, heat the oil over moderate heat. Add the onion and garlic, and sauté for 5 minutes or until the onion is soft. Add the bell peppers and sauté for 5 minutes or until soft.

2. Stir in the chili powder, oregano, cumin, and coriander, and cook for 1 minute. Add the ground turkey and sauté for 3 minutes or until no longer pink. Add the stewed tomatoes, tomato sauce, tomato paste, salt, and black pepper, and bring to a simmer. Add the beans and cook for 3 minutes or until heated through. Serves 4.

Per serving: Calories 321; Fiber 10g; Protein 37g; Total Fat 6g; Saturated Fat 1g; Cholesterol 70mg; Sodium 529mg

At the market Ground turkey is sold in most supermarkets, but you may be better off preparing ground turkey yourself at home (see below).

Look for A product labeled "Ground Turkey" may include dark meat, skin and fat; a 3-ounce cooked portion could contain as much as 12 grams of fat. Instead, look for Ground Turkey Breast, which is made from skinless white meat.

Prep For the leanest possible ground turkey, buy a skinless turkey breast portion and chop it in a food processor (see below).

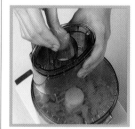

Cut skinless turkey breast into 1-inch chunks. Coarsely grind the turkey in a food processor with on-and-off pulses, taking care not to turn it into a paste.

Basic cooking To help keep ground turkey moist, handle it lightly: Don't compact it when shaping burgers, meatballs or meat loaf.

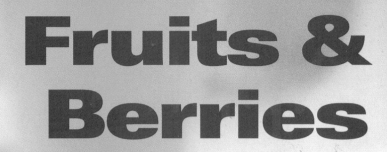

Fruits & Berries

Honeydew-Lime Tart

Apples & Pears

Nutritional power
One of America's most popular snack fruits, the apple supplies some vitamin C as well as potassium. Eat the peel to get the full measure of fiber.

Healthy Highlights

Apples*
PER 1 MEDIUM

Calories	81
Fiber	3.7g
Protein	0g
Total Fat	0.5g
Saturated Fat	0.1g
Cholesterol	0mg
Sodium	0mg

NUTRIENTS	
	% Daily Value
Vitamin C	13%

*with skin

Did you know? . . .
Some of the fiber in apples is pectin, which may help lower blood cholesterol.

Apples should be stored in the refrigerator. At room temperature they quickly begin to decline in quality: Their flesh becomes mushy, and they lose some of their vitamin content.

Squash & Apple Soup

PREP: 25 MINUTES / COOK: 40 MINUTES
Garnish this autumnal purée with very thin, unpeeled apple slices.

- 1 tablespoon olive oil
- 1 small onion, halved and thinly sliced
- 3 cloves garlic, crushed and peeled
- 1 tablespoon minced fresh ginger
- 1 pickled jalapeño, finely chopped
- 1½ pounds butternut squash, peeled, seeded, and thinly sliced
- 2 teaspoons sugar
- 1 pound McIntosh apples, peeled and thinly sliced
- 1 pound Granny Smith apples, peeled and thinly sliced
- 1½ teaspoons chili powder
- ½ teaspoon salt
- ¼ teaspoon dried thyme
- 1½ cups chicken broth

1. In a Dutch oven, heat the oil over moderate heat. Add the onion, garlic, ginger, and jalapeño, and sauté for 5 minutes or until the onion is soft. Add the squash, sprinkle with the sugar, and sauté for 5 minutes or until the squash is crisp-tender.

2. Add the apples, chili powder, salt, and thyme, stirring to coat. Add the broth and 1½ cups of water, and bring to a boil. Reduce to a simmer, partially cover, and cook for 30 minutes or until the squash is very tender. Transfer to a food processor and purée. If necessary, gently reheat. Serves 4.

Per serving: Calories 241; Fiber 7g; Protein 3g; Total Fat 5g; Saturated Fat 1g; Cholesterol 0mg; Sodium 755mg

Pork Chops with Fresh Pear Salsa

PREP: 20 MINUTES / COOK: 10 MINUTES
Try this tangy salsa with roast chicken or turkey, or on a roast-beef sandwich.

- ¾ pound Bosc or Bartlett pears
- 1 red bell pepper, cut into ½-inch squares
- ⅓ cup finely chopped red onion
- 3 tablespoons honey
- 2 tablespoons apple cider vinegar
- ½ teaspoon red hot pepper sauce
- ¾ teaspoon each salt and dried sage
- ½ teaspoon black pepper
- ¼ teaspoon ground ginger
- 2 cloves garlic, minced
- 4 well-trimmed center-cut pork chops (6 ounces each)

1. Peel the pears and cut them into ½-inch chunks. Transfer to a large bowl. Add the bell pepper, onion, honey, vinegar, hot pepper sauce, and ¼ teaspoon of the salt. Toss to combine. Refrigerate until serving time.

2. Preheat the broiler. In a small bowl, combine the sage, black pepper, ginger, garlic, and the remaining ½ teaspoon salt. Rub the mixture into both sides of the chops. Broil 6 inches from the heat for 3 to 4 minutes per side or until cooked through but still juicy. Serve with the pear salsa. Serves 4.

Per serving: Calories 339; Fiber 3g; Protein 35g; Total Fat 10g; Saturated Fat 3g; Cholesterol 93mg; Sodium 523mg

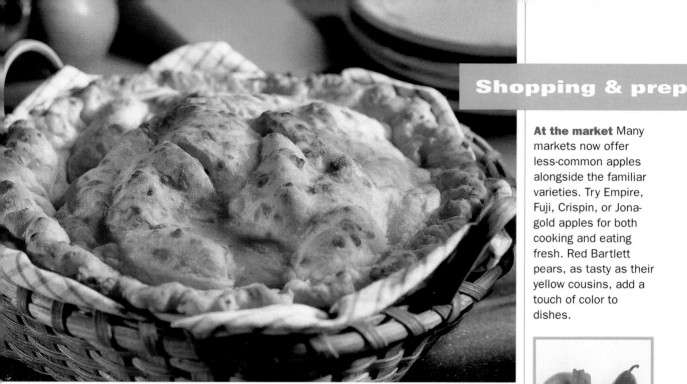

Apple Pie with Cheddar Crust Tart apples are concealed beneath a savory crust.

Apple Pie with Cheddar Crust

PREP: 30 MINUTES / CHILL: 1 HOUR
COOK: 40 MINUTES

A slice of double-crust pie topped with a slab of Cheddar is very high in fat. Try this single-crust pie with Cheddar mixed into the dough.

CRUST:
- 1   cup flour
- 1   tablespoon sugar
- ½   teaspoon baking powder
- ¼   teaspoon salt
- ⅛   teaspoon cayenne pepper
- 3   tablespoons cold unsalted butter, cut up
- 2   tablespoons solid vegetable shortening
- 1   cup shredded sharp Cheddar cheese (4 ounces)
- ⅓   cup ice water

FILLING:
- 2½ pounds Granny Smith apples, peeled and thinly sliced
- ½   cup sugar
- 2   tablespoons flour
- 1   tablespoon lemon juice
- ½   teaspoon cinnamon

1. For the crust: In a medium bowl, combine the flour, sugar, baking powder, salt, and cayenne. With a pastry blender or two knives, cut in the butter and shortening until the mixture resembles coarse meal. Stir in the cheese until well combined. Sprinkle on the ice water and stir just until the dough leaves the sides of the bowl. Shape into a flat disk, wrap in plastic wrap, and refrigerate for at least 1 hour.

2. Preheat the oven to 450°F. For the filling: In a large bowl, toss together the apples, sugar, flour, lemon juice, and cinnamon. Spoon into a 9-inch glass pie plate.

3. On a lightly floured surface, roll the dough out to a 13-inch round and drape over the apples. Crimp the edges to seal. Make 2 slashes in the dough for steam vents. Place on a baking sheet with sides and bake for 20 minutes. Reduce the heat to 350°F and bake for 20 minutes or until the crust is golden brown and the apples are tender. If the crust begins to brown too much before the apples are tender, tent with foil. Serves 8.

Per serving: Calories 315; Fiber 3g; Protein 6g; Total Fat 13g; Saturated Fat 7g; Cholesterol 27mg; Sodium 191mg

At the market Many markets now offer less-common apples alongside the familiar varieties. Try Empire, Fuji, Crispin, or Jonagold apples for both cooking and eating fresh. Red Bartlett pears, as tasty as their yellow cousins, add a touch of color to dishes.

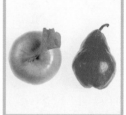

The spicy Crispin apple (formerly called Mutsu) is new to American markets. It's a cross between Golden Delicious and a Japanese apple, Indo. Sweet, juicy Red Bartlett pears are a treat for the eye as well as the palate: They turn a brilliant crimson when ripe.

Look for Choose hard apples with unbruised skin. Buy firm, unblemished pears a few days before you'll eat them; pears are sold underripe and need time to ripen at room temperature.

Prep When you need apple or pear wedges, use a disk-shaped corer-slicer on peeled or unpeeled fruit. To just core apples, use an apple corer—basically a metal tube with a pointed tip, set into a handle.

Chicken Normandy
Apples, sage, and a touch of apple brandy in a cream sauce are lovely complements to sautéed chicken.

Healthy Highlights

Pears*

PER 1 MEDIUM	
Calories	98
Fiber	4.0g
Protein	1g
Total Fat	0.7g
Saturated Fat	0g
Cholesterol	0mg
Sodium	0mg

NUTRIENTS	
	% **Daily Value**
Vitamin C	12%

*with skin

Did you know? . . .
Most of the vitamin C in pears is found in the skin.

Asian pears, which you'll find in some gourmet shops and in Asian markets, are apple-shaped but taste like pears. Juicy and very crisp, Asian pears contain about one-third more fiber than regular pears.

Most of the fiber in pears is insoluble—the kind that helps prevent diverticulosis and colon cancer.

Canned pears packed in juice or water may be substituted for fresh in many recipes. They do contain considerably less vitamin C than fresh pears.

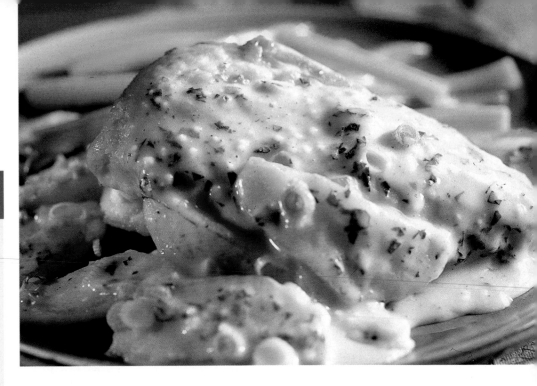

Chicken Normandy

PREP: 10 MINUTES / COOK: 30 MINUTES

Normandy is home to bountiful orchards and lush pastures for dairy cows. Dishes from this French region often include apples and cream.

- 2 **teaspoons vegetable oil**
- 4 **skinless, boneless chicken breast halves (1 pound total)**
- 2 **tablespoons plus 1 teaspoon flour**
- 3 **scallions, thinly sliced**
- ¾ **pound McIntosh, Cortland, or Empire apples, peeled, halved, and thinly sliced**
- ¾ **pound Granny Smith or Crispin apples, peeled, halved, and thinly sliced**
- 3 **tablespoons applejack, Calvados, or brandy**
- ¾ **cup chicken broth**
- ½ **teaspoon each salt and pepper**
- ¼ **teaspoon dried sage**
- 3 **tablespoons reduced-fat sour cream**
- 2 **tablespoons chopped parsley**

1. In a large nonstick skillet, heat the oil over moderate heat. Dredge the chicken in 2 tablespoons of the flour, shaking off the excess. Sauté the chicken for 3 minutes per side or until golden brown. Transfer the chicken to a plate.

2. Add the scallions to the pan and cook for 1 minute or until tender. Add the apples and sauté for 5 minutes or until lightly browned. Remove the pan from the heat and add the applejack. Return the pan to the heat and cook for 30 seconds or until the liquid has evaporated. Add ¼ cup of the broth and ¼ teaspoon each of the salt and pepper to the pan and simmer gently for 4 minutes or until the apples are tender but not falling apart. Remove with a slotted spoon; set aside.

3. Add the remaining ½ cup broth to the pan along with the sage and the remaining ¼ teaspoon each salt and pepper. Bring to a boil. Reduce to a simmer, return the chicken to the pan, cover, and cook for 5 to 7 minutes or until the chicken is cooked through. Return the apples to the pan and simmer gently for 1 minute or until heated through.

4. In a small bowl, whisk together the sour cream and the remaining 1 teaspoon flour. Stir it into the pan and simmer, stirring constantly, for 2 minutes or until lightly thickened. Stir in the parsley. Serves 4.

Per serving: Calories 300; Fiber 3g; Protein 28g; Total Fat 6g; Saturated Fat 2g; Cholesterol 70mg; Sodium 569mg

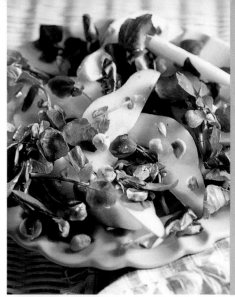

Pear Strudel

PREP: 20 MINUTES / COOK: 50 MINUTES

You could also make this strudel with apples. Use Cortland, Northern Spy, or another cooking variety that will hold its shape.

- ⅓ **cup frozen apple juice concentrate**
- 1 **tablespoon lemon juice**
- ¼ **teaspoon each salt and pepper**
- 2 **pounds firm-ripe pears, such as Bartlett or Bosc, peeled and coarsely chopped**
- ⅓ **cup dried sweetened cranberries or currants**
- 6 **sheets phyllo dough**
- 2 **tablespoons plus 1 teaspoon unsalted butter, melted**
- 2 **tablespoons plus 1 teaspoon sugar**

1. In a large skillet, bring the apple juice concentrate, lemon juice, salt, and pepper to a boil over moderate heat. Add the pears, reduce to a simmer, and cook, uncovered, for 10 minutes or until the pears are crisp-tender and the liquid has evaporated. Stir in the cranberries. Cool to room temperature.

2. Preheat the oven to 400°F. On a work surface, lay 2 sheets of phyllo dough on top of one another with the long side facing you. Brush with 2 teaspoons of the butter and sprinkle with 2 teaspoons of the sugar. Repeat two more times, using 2 sheets of phyllo, 2 teaspoons of butter, and 2 teaspoons of sugar for each layer.

3. Spoon the pear mixture along the lower third of the phyllo, leaving a 2-inch border at each end. Fold the short ends in over the filling, then roll up from the long side jelly-roll fashion. Brush the roll with the remaining 1 teaspoon butter and sprinkle with the remaining 1 teaspoon sugar.

4. Place the roll on an ungreased baking sheet; make several diagonal slashes on the top of the roll. Bake for 40 minutes or until crisp and golden brown. Cool for 10 minutes before serving. Serves 6.

Per serving: Calories 243; Fiber 4g; Protein 2g; Total Fat 6g; Saturated Fat 3g; Cholesterol 12mg; Sodium 192mg

Pear & Hazelnut Salad In large bowl, whisk ¼ cup lime juice, 2 tbsp. honey, and 1 tsp. olive oil. Add 4 Bartlett pears, cut into thin wedges. Add 4 cups watercress; toss. Sprinkle salad with ¼ cup coarsely chopped toasted hazelnuts. Serves 4. *[Cal 193; Fat 6g; Sod 17mg]*

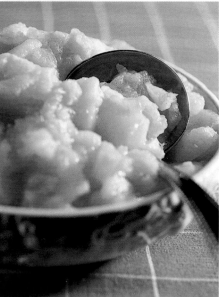

Chunky Apple & Pear Sauce In medium saucepan, combine 2 large apples and 2 large pears, peeled and diced. Add 2 tbsp. sugar (or more to taste), 2 tbsp. lemon juice, and ¼ tsp. each cinnamon and ginger. Cook over low heat, stirring often, for 10 minutes or until tender. Lightly mash with a potato masher or immersion blender. Serve warm or chilled. Serves 4. *[Cal 139; Fat 1g; Sod 2mg]*

Apple-Pear Crisp Preheat oven to 375°F. In 8-in. square baking pan, toss 1½ lbs. each peeled, sliced pears and peeled, sliced apples with 3 tbsp. lemon juice, 2 tbsp. sugar, ½ tsp. ginger, and ¼ tsp. salt. In small bowl, mix 3 tbsp. each white and brown sugars, ½ tsp. cinnamon, and ¼ tsp. salt. Cut in 2 tbsp. unsalted butter. Sprinkle over fruit. Bake 40 minutes. Serves 4. *[Cal 351; Fat 7g; Sod 294mg]*

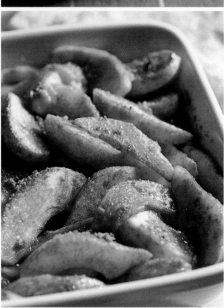

Apricots

Nutritional power

These golden fruits are "good as gold" nutritionally. An outstanding source of beta carotene, apricots also supply considerable vitamin C and potassium.

Healthy Highlights

Fresh Apricots
PER 1 CUP

Calories	79
Fiber	4.0g
Protein	2g
Total Fat	0.6g
Saturated Fat	0g
Cholesterol	0mg
Sodium	2mg

NUTRIENTS

	% Daily Value
Vitamin A	86%
Vitamin C	28%
Potassium	16%

Dried Apricots
PER ¼ CUP

Calories	77
Fiber	2.9g
Protein	1g
Total Fat	0.1g
Saturated Fat	0g
Cholesterol	0mg
Sodium	3mg

NUTRIENTS

	% Daily Value
Vitamin A	47%
Potassium	15%
Iron	11%

Grilled Chicken with Fresh Apricot Sauce

**PREP: 20 MINUTES / MARINATE: 1 HOUR
COOK: 15 MINUTES**

You can make the sauce with drained canned apricots when fresh apricots aren't available. Use one 16-ounce can and rinse the fruit if it's packed in syrup.

- ¾ cup apricot nectar
- 2 tablespoons balsamic vinegar
- 1 tablespoon sesame oil
- 2 scallions, chopped
- 2 teaspoons grated fresh ginger
- 2 cloves garlic, chopped
- 4 skinless, boneless chicken breast halves (1 pound total)
- 1 teaspoon cornstarch blended with 1 tablespoon water
- ½ teaspoon salt
- 10 ounces fresh apricots, sliced
- 2 scallions, sliced (optional)

1. In a medium bowl, whisk together the apricot nectar, vinegar, sesame oil, scallions, ginger, and garlic. Measure out ½ cup, transfer to a medium saucepan, and set aside. Add the chicken to the mixture remaining in the bowl, tossing to coat. Marinate at room temperature for 1 hour or in the refrigerator for up to 4 hours.

2. Preheat the broiler. Broil the chicken 6 inches from the heat, turning halfway through, for 12 minutes or until cooked through.

3. Meanwhile, add the cornstarch mixture and salt to the saucepan of reserved apricot nectar mixture. Bring to a simmer over moderate heat, stir-ring. Add the apricots and cook for 2 minutes or until the sauce is slightly thickened and the apricots are fork-tender. Serve the chicken with the sauce spooned on top, garnished with the scallions. Serves 4.

Per serving: Calories 222; Fiber 1g; Protein 28g; Total Fat 5g; Saturated Fat 1g; Cholesterol 66mg; Sodium 351mg

Apricot Bavarian

PREP: 20 MINUTES / CHILL: 4 HOURS

Fresh apricots have a short season; canned fruit can stand in, if necessary. You'll need about four 16-ounce cans, well drained.

- 1 can (12 ounces) low-fat evaporated milk
- 2 envelopes unflavored gelatin
- ¼ cup boiling water
- 4 cups sliced fresh apricots (1¼ pounds)
- 5 tablespoons light brown sugar
- 5 tablespoons honey
- ¼ cup heavy cream
- 1 tablespoon lemon juice
- ⅛ teaspoon cinnamon
- 1 pinch of nutmeg

1. Place the evaporated milk in a large metal bowl and place in the freezer for 1 hour or until semi-frozen (slushy).

2. Meanwhile, in a small bowl, sprinkle the gelatin over ¼ cup of cold water and let stand for 5 minutes. Transfer the gelatin to a blender or food processor, add the boiling water, and process for 30 seconds or until dissolved. Add 3 cups of the sliced apricots, 4 tablespoons each of the brown sugar and honey, the heavy cream, 2 teaspoons of the lemon juice, the cinnamon, and nutmeg, and process until smooth. Refrigerate the apricot purée for 1 to 1½ hours or until the texture of raw egg whites. (Or quick-chill in a bowl set in a larger bowl of ice water.)

3. When the evaporated milk is slushy, beat with an electric mixer at high speed until soft peaks form. Fold the beaten milk into the chilled apricot mixture. Pour into an 8-cup serving bowl or 8 individual 1-cup dishes. Chill for at least 3 hours or until set.

4. Coarsely dice the remaining 1 cup apricots and combine with the remaining 1 tablespoon each brown sugar and honey, and 1 teaspoon lemon juice. Serve the sweetened diced apricots with the bavarian. Serves 8.

Per serving: Calories 180; Fiber 1g; Protein 6g; Total Fat 4g; Saturated Fat 2g; Cholesterol 18mg; Sodium 64mg

Grilled Chicken with Fresh Apricot Sauce *is tangy with balsamic vinegar; ginger and garlic flavor the sauce, too.*

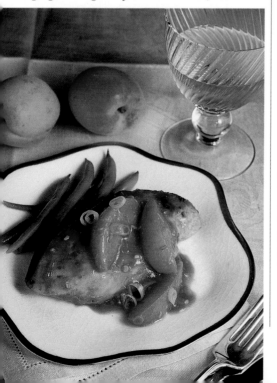

Apricot "Poundcake"

PREP: 20 MINUTES / COOK: 45 MINUTES
With just 2 tablespoons of butter, it's not a real poundcake, but it's a delicious one.

1⅔	**cups dried apricots, chopped**
¾	**cup unsweetened applesauce**
2	**tablespoons unsalted butter**
2	**tablespoons light olive oil**
¼	**cup low-fat (1.5%) buttermilk**
3	**eggs**
2	**teaspoons vanilla extract**
2	**teaspoons grated orange zest**
1½	**cups sugar**
3½	**cups cake flour**
1	**teaspoon each baking powder and salt**
½	**teaspoon baking soda**

1. Preheat the oven to 350°F. Spray a 10-inch tube pan with a removable bottom with nonstick cooking spray.

2. In a medium saucepan, combine ⅓ cup of the apricots, the applesauce, and ½ cup of water. Simmer for 5 minutes or until the apricots are softened. Transfer to a food processor or blender. Add the butter, oil, and buttermilk, and process until smooth. Set the apricot mixture aside to cool slightly, then beat in the eggs, vanilla, and orange zest, blending just until smooth. Transfer to a large bowl. Stir in the sugar.

3. In a medium bowl, stir together the cake flour, baking powder, salt, and baking soda. Fold the flour mixture into the apricot mixture in 3 additions. Fold in the remaining 1⅓ cups apricots and scrape into the prepared pan.

4. Bake for 40 minutes or until a cake tester inserted halfway between the sides and the center comes out clean. Cool in the pan on a wire rack for 10 minutes. Loosen the cake from the pan, remove the sides, and set the cake on the rack to cool completely. Serves 16.

Per serving: Calories 242; Fiber 1g; Protein 4g; Total Fat 5g; Saturated Fat 2g; Cholesterol 44mg; Sodium 223mg

At the market Most apricots sold in the U.S. are grown in California; they're available from May through summer's end. You can also sometimes buy locally-grown apricots in the summer. Imported apricots are sold in December and January.

Look for Apricots are highly perishable, so they're usually picked underripe to help them withstand shipping. Buy fruits that are firm but not rock-hard; the skin should be orangy-gold, with no greenish tinge. Ripen apricots at home in a paper bag at room temperature; when they're ripe, eat them immediately or refrigerate for a few days.

Prep Apricots are easy to peel if you drop them in boiling water for about 20 seconds; cool in cold water.

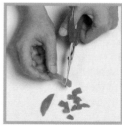

It's easiest to chop or dice dried apricots with kitchen scissors if you spray the blades with nonstick cooking spray. Cut the apricots into strips, then cut the strips into bits.

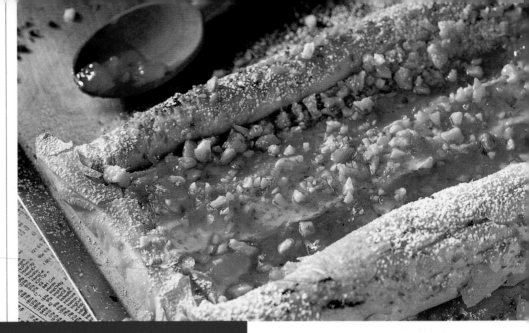

Apricot Danish
Layers of flaky phyllo pastry frame a cream-cheese filling topped with apricot purée and chopped nuts.

Did you know? . . .
It's a good idea to substitute chopped dried apricots for raisins in your favorite recipes: The apricots contain nearly 1000 percent more beta carotene.

When buying canned apricots, opt for juice- or water-packed rather than syrup-packed.

Canned apricots may be substituted for fresh in most recipes; juice- or water-packed fruit is the best choice. Apricots packed in heavy or extra-heavy syrup have three to four times as many calories as water-packed. The extra calories are "empty" calories that come from sugar.

Drying concentrates the apricot's impressive nutrient value. Dried apricots make a good cereal topping as well as a healthful substitute for raisins in breads, cakes, and cookies.

Dried apricots are often treated with sulfur dioxide to keep their color bright. Those allergic to sulfites should look for unsulfured apricots in health-food stores.

Apricot-Pecan Stuffing

PREP: 20 MINUTES / COOK: 1 HOUR

- 8   cups white and whole-wheat bread cubes (¾ inch)
- 1   tablespoon olive oil
- 2   stalks celery, chopped
- 1   large red onion, finely chopped
- ½   teaspoon each dried thyme and sage
- 1¼   cups lower-sodium chicken broth
- 1½   cups chopped dried apricots
- 1   egg
- ¼   cup chopped parsley
- ¼   cup chopped toasted pecans
- ¼   teaspoon each salt and pepper

1. Preheat the oven to 375°F. Spread the bread on a baking sheet and bake for 8 to 10 minutes, or until dried out. Remove the bread from the oven and lower the temperature to 350°F.

2. In a large skillet, heat the oil over moderate heat. Add the celery, onion, thyme, and sage, and cook for 8 minutes. Add 1 cup of the broth and the apricots. Bring to a simmer and cook for 5 minutes or until the apricots are softened. Transfer the apricot mixture to a large bowl and set aside to cool.

3. In a small bowl, whisk together the egg and the remaining ¼ cup broth. Stir the egg mixture into the cooled apricot mixture along with the parsley, pecans, salt, and pepper. Add the bread cubes, tossing until well combined.

4. Spray a 9 x 13-inch baking dish with nonstick cooking spray. Spoon the stuffing mixture in and cover with foil. Bake for 25 minutes. Remove the foil and bake for 10 minutes or until crisp and heated through. Serves 10.

Per serving: Calories 171; Fiber 4g; Protein 5g; Total Fat 5g; Saturated Fat 1g; Cholesterol 21mg; Sodium 302mg

Apricot Danish

PREP: 25 MINUTES / COOK: 45 MINUTES

- ¾   cup dried apricots, chopped
- ½   cup plus 2 tablespoons packed light brown sugar
- 2   teaspoons vanilla extract
- ½   teaspoon ground ginger
- 4   ounces nonfat cream cheese
- 6   gingersnaps (1 ounce), crushed
- 2   tablespoons unsalted butter, melted
- 2   tablespoons vegetable oil
- 12   sheets frozen phyllo dough, thawed
- 3   tablespoons chopped hazelnuts or walnuts
- ⅓   cup apricot preserves
- 1   tablespoon confectioners sugar

1. In a small saucepan, combine the apricots, ¼ cup of the brown sugar, and ½ cup of water. Bring to a simmer over medium heat and cook for 10 minutes or until softened. Transfer the apricot mixture to a blender or food processor, add 1 teaspoon of the vanilla, and process to a smooth purée.

2. In a medium bowl, with an electric mixer, cream ¼ cup of the brown sugar, the ground ginger, the remaining 1 teaspoon vanilla, and the cream cheese. In a small bowl, combine the gingersnap crumbs and the remaining 2 tablespoons brown sugar.

3. In a small dish, combine the butter and oil. Place the phyllo on a work surface and cover with a towel. Spray a baking sheet with nonstick cooking spray. Lay 2 sheets of phyllo on the baking sheet and brush lightly with some of the butter mixture. Sprinkle with 1 tablespoon of the gingersnap crumbs. Repeat the layering with more butter mixture (save some for the top of the pastry), and the remaining phyllo and crumbs.

4. Preheat the oven to 375°F. Spoon the cream cheese mixture down the center of the dough in a 1½-inch-wide strip; stop 1 inch short of the short ends. Spoon the apricot purée in two 1½-inch-wide strips, one on either side of the cheese. Roll the long sides of the pastry in toward the center until they just begin to cover the apricot. Roll the short sides in and press firmly to seal (if not firmly sealed, the phyllo may start to unfold as it bakes). The finished size should be 13 x 6½ inches.

5. Brush the crust lightly with the remaining butter mixture. Sprinkle the nuts over the filling and bake for 30 to 35 minutes or until golden and crisped. Meanwhile, in a small saucepan, melt the apricot preserves with 1 tablespoon of water over low heat. Brush the preserves over the warm pastry. Sprinkle with the confectioners sugar. Serves 8.

Per serving: Calories 318; Fiber 1g; Protein 5g; Total Fat 10g; Saturated Fat 3g; Cholesterol 9mg; Sodium 242mg

Chocolate-Dipped Apricots In double boiler, melt 2 oz. semi-sweet chocolate with ½ tsp. solid vegetable shortening. Cool to room temperature. Dip 24 dried apricots into chocolate mixture, coating one half of each apricot. Dry on a wire rack before serving. Serves 6. *[Cal 115; Fat 3g; Sod 4mg]*

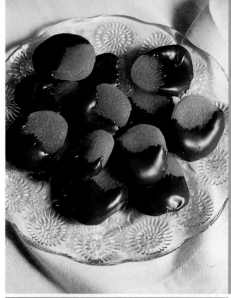

Fresh Apricots Poached in Syrup In medium saucepan, bring 1 cup water, ½ cup sugar, and ½ tsp. ground ginger to a boil. Boil for 3 minutes. Add 8 fresh apricots, cover, and cook for 10 minutes or until tender. Remove from heat and stir in 1 tsp. vanilla. Cool apricots in syrup. Chill to serve. Serves 4. *[Cal 134; Fat 0g; Sod 1mg]*

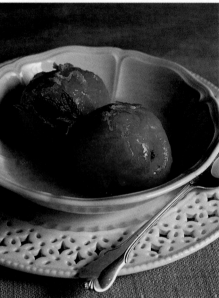

Warm Apricot Compote In medium saucepan, bring ½ cup apricot nectar, ½ cup orange juice, ¼ cup sugar, 2 tbsp. lemon juice, and ¼ tsp. cardamom to a boil. Add ¾ pound dried apricots. Simmer 20 minutes or until tender. Serve warm, at room temperature, or chilled. Serves 4. *[Cal 285; Fat 1g; Sod 12mg]*

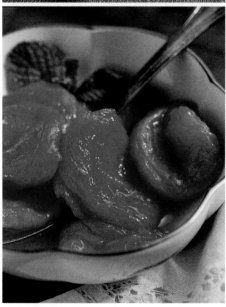

Avocado

Nutritional power
Their texture tells you that avocados are high in fat—but it's mostly monoun- saturated fat, the type that has a posi- tive effect on blood cholesterol levels.

Healthy Highlights

PER ½ CUP*	
Calories	118
Fiber	3.7g
Protein	1g
Total Fat	11g
Saturated Fat	1.8g
Cholesterol	0mg
Sodium	7mg

NUTRIENTS	
	% Daily Value
Potassium	15%
Folate	11%
Copper	10%
Vitamin B6	10%
Vitamin C	10%

⅓ medium avocado

Did you know? . . .
The avocado is a source of lutein, a carotenoid that seems to help pre- vent age-related macular degenera- tion, an eye disease that affects the elderly.

A medium avocado supplies 20 percent of the daily adult requirement of vita- min E, which is a potent antioxidant.

Avocado & Ham Antipasto with Guacamole Dressing

PREP: 20 MINUTES

The favorite Mexican dip is used as a sauce in this inventive first-course dish. Cucumber provides a crunchy contrast to the velvety avocado.

- 1 avocado, cut lengthwise into thin wedges
- 1 tomato, diced
- ¼ cup finely chopped red onion
- ¼ cup chopped cilantro or parsley
- 2 tablespoons red wine vinegar
- ½ teaspoon ground cumin
- ¼ teaspoon salt
- 1 cucumber, peeled and thinly sliced
- 2 ounces smoked ham, cut into matchsticks

1. Measure out ¼ cup of the avocado and coarsely chop. Transfer to a bowl and stir in the tomato, onion, cilantro, vinegar, cumin, and salt. Set the dress- ing aside.

2. Divide the remaining avocado and the cucumber and ham among 4 serving plates. Spoon the guacamole dressing on top. Serves 4.

Per serving: Calories 120; Fiber 2g; Protein 5g; Total Fat 9g; Saturated Fat 2g; Cholesterol 7mg; Sodium 358mg

Avocado "Sushi" Salad

PREP: 20 MINUTES / COOK: 20 MINUTES

Authentic sushi rolls are tricky to make, but you can enjoy similar flavors in this appetizer, a simple presentation of rice on greens. Use soft lettuce in place of spinach if you prefer.

- 1 cup rice
- ¼ teaspoon salt
- ¼ cup rice vinegar
- 2 tablespoons each lower-sodium soy sauce and lime juice
- 4 teaspoons sugar
- 1 carrot, cut into ¼-inch dice
- 2 small avocados, cut into ¼-inch dice
- 24 small spinach leaves

1. In a medium saucepan, bring 2 cups of water to a boil. Add the rice and salt, cover, and simmer for 17 minutes or until tender.

2. Meanwhile, in a small saucepan, bring the vinegar, soy sauce, lime juice, and sugar to a boil. Remove from the heat. Stir into the cooked rice. Transfer the seasoned rice to a bowl and let cool to room temperature.

3. Stir the carrot and avocado into the rice. Dividing evenly, spoon the mixture into four 8-ounce ramekins or bowls

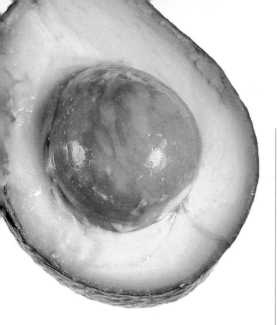

Mixed Greens with Creamy Avocado Dressing

PREP: 15 MINUTES

1   avocado, cut into chunks
¼   cup plain low-fat yogurt
½   teaspoon grated lemon zest
1   tablespoon lemon juice
½   teaspoon salt
4   cups sliced romaine lettuce
4   cups watercress or curly endive
2   scallions, thinly sliced

1. In a food processor or blender, combine the avocado, yogurt, lemon zest, lemon juice, salt, and 1 tablespoon of water, and process until smooth.

2. Transfer the dressing to a large bowl. Add the lettuce, watercress, and scallions, tossing to coat. Serves 4.

Per serving: Calories 106; Fiber 3g; Protein 4g; Total Fat 8g; Saturated Fat 1g; Cholesterol 1mg; Sodium 325mg

At the market There are two types of avocado most often seen in markets: the Hass, which has a pebbly, almost black skin (pictured on opposite page), and the Fuerte, which is larger, with smoother, greener skin.

Look for Choose a heavy avocado with unbroken skin. The fruit should yield to gentle pressure. If necessary, leave it at room temperature for a few days to soften.

Prep Peel and slice avocados close to serving time; their flesh darkens when exposed to air. To halve the fruit, run a knife lengthwise around the avocado, sliding it around the pit, then twist the halves. Remove the pit by twisting it out with a knife blade (see below).

and gently but firmly press down. Arrange the spinach on serving plates and invert the molded rice salads onto the spinach. Serves 4.

Per serving: Calories 322; Fiber 3g; Protein 6g; Total Fat 12g; Saturated Fat 2g; Cholesterol 0mg; Sodium 473mg

*Avocado **"Sushi" Salad** features Japanese flavors in a sophisticated side dish.*

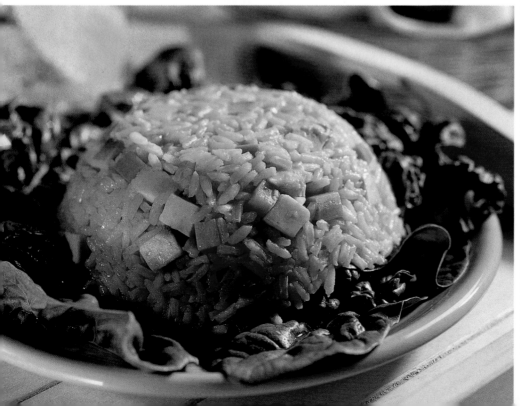

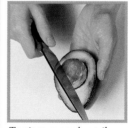

To pit an avocado, strike the pit lightly but sharply with the blade of a chef's knife. Then twist the blade to "unscrew" the pit and lift it out (attached to the blade).

Bananas

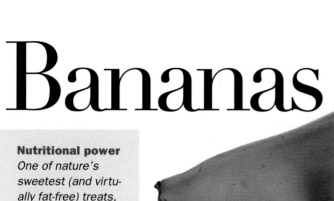

Nutritional power

One of nature's sweetest (and virtually fat-free) treats, the banana offers a healthy helping of potassium along with vitamin C and B vitamins.

Healthy Highlights

PER 1 MEDIUM	
Calories	109
Fiber	2.8g
Protein	1g
Total Fat	0.6g
Saturated Fat	0.2g
Cholesterol	0mg
Sodium	1mg

NUTRIENTS	
	% Daily Value
Vitamin B6	34%
Vitamin C	18%
Potassium	16%

Did you know? . . .
Your body's supply of vitamin B6 must be replenished each day, and eating bananas is a good way to do it. Vitamin B6 plays a role in antibody production, so an adequate supply of this nutrient strengthens immunity. A USDA study revealed that many Americans—particularly the elderly—don't get enough vitamin B6.

Banana Raita

PREP: 10 MINUTES / COOK: 10 MINUTES
CHILL: 2 HOURS

A raita is a yogurt-based Indian condiment meant to be served as a cooling contrast to highly spiced dishes.

- 2 teaspoons vegetable oil
- 1 small onion, finely chopped
- ½ teaspoon each ground coriander and cumin
- ¼ teaspoon ground cardamom
- ⅛ teaspoon ground ginger
- 1 pound bananas (2 to 3), mashed
- ½ teaspoon salt
- ⅛ teaspoon cayenne pepper
- 2 cups plain low-fat yogurt

1. In a small skillet, heat the oil over moderate heat. Add the onion and sauté for 5 minutes or until golden. Stir in the coriander, cumin, cardamom, and ginger, and cook for 1 minute or until fragrant.

2. Add the bananas and stir to incorporate the spices. Transfer the banana mixture to a bowl and stir in the salt, cayenne, and yogurt. Cover and refrigerate for 2 hours or until well chilled. Makes 3½ cups.

Per ½ cup: Calories 98; Fiber 1g; Protein 4g; Total Fat 3g; Saturated Fat 1g; Cholesterol 4mg; Sodium 212mg

Banana-Pecan Bread

PREP: 15 MINUTES
COOK: 1 HOUR 25 MINUTES

If your banana-bread recipe calls for a stick (or two) of butter, try this one instead—it's made with just 3 tablespoons of oil.

- 1 cup old-fashioned rolled oats
- ⅓ cup pecans
- 3 very ripe bananas (1 pound)
- 1 cup low-fat (1.5%) buttermilk
- 3 tablespoons vegetable oil
- 2 egg whites
- 1 teaspoon vanilla extract
- ½ cup each granulated sugar and packed dark brown sugar
- 2 cups flour
- 2½ teaspoons baking powder
- ½ teaspoon baking soda
- ¼ teaspoon salt

1. Preheat the oven to 350°F. Spray a 9 x 5-inch loaf pan with nonstick cooking spray. In a small baking pan, toast the oats, stirring them occasionally, for 10 minutes or until lightly browned. At the same time, in another small baking pan, toast the pecans for 7 minutes or until fragrant and lightly browned. When the pecans are cool enough to handle, coarsely chop them.

2. In a large bowl, with a potato masher or fork, mash the bananas until

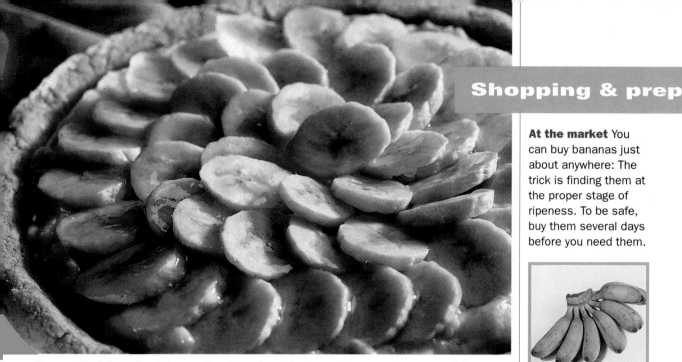

Banana Pudding Pie A layer of apricot-glazed bananas sits atop a banana pudding.

At the market You can buy bananas just about anywhere: The trick is finding them at the proper stage of ripeness. To be safe, buy them several days before you need them.

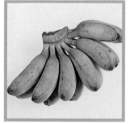

Sweet and petite Lady bananas (also called finger bananas) have a firmer, drier flesh than regular bananas, and a hint of strawberry in their flavor.

Look for Buy firm, unblemished bananas, either green-tipped or fully yellow. Beware of grayish bananas: They've probably been stored at too cool a temperature, and will never ripen.

Prep Store bananas in a paper bag at room temperature if they need ripening. Sliced bananas will darken when exposed to air; to keep them from turning brown, toss the slices with a little citrus juice. To prevent bananas from getting overripe, store them in the refrigerator. The skin will turn an alarming black, but the bananas themselves will be fine.

not quite smooth. Add the buttermilk, oil, egg whites, vanilla, and granulated and brown sugars, and mix until well blended; set aside.

3. In a small bowl, combine the flour, baking powder, baking soda, and salt. Fold the dry ingredients into the banana mixture along with the oats and pecans until just combined. Do not overmix. Spoon the batter into the prepared pan, smoothing the top. Bake for 1 hour and 25 minutes or until a cake tester inserted in the center comes out clean. Cool in the pan on a rack for 10 minutes. Turn out of the pan onto the rack to cool completely. Serves 8.

Per serving: Calories 384; Fiber 3g; Protein 8g; Total Fat 10g; Saturated Fat 1g; Cholesterol 2mg; Sodium 339mg

Banana Pudding Pie

PREP: 15 MINUTES / COOK: 10 MINUTES
This impressive single-crust pie is crowned with a layer of jam-glazed banana slices.

- **8** ounces vanilla wafers (about 48)
- **1** tablespoon plus ½ cup sugar
- **1** tablespoon vegetable oil
- **¼** cup cornstarch
- **⅛** teaspoon each salt and nutmeg
- **3** cups low-fat (1%) milk
- **1** teaspoon vanilla extract
- **2** teaspoons unsalted butter
- **4** large bananas (1½ pounds), thinly sliced
- **¼** cup apricot jam, melted

1. Preheat the oven to 350°F. In a food processor, combine the vanilla wafers and 1 tablespoon of the sugar, and process to crumbs. Add the oil and ¼ cup of water, and process until well combined. Press the mixture into a 9-inch pie plate to form a pie shell. Bake for 10 minutes or until set.

2. Meanwhile, in a medium saucepan, combine the remaining ½ cup sugar, the cornstarch, salt, and nutmeg. Whisk in the milk until well combined. Cook over moderate heat, stirring, for 7 minutes or until the mixture has come to a boil and is thickened. Remove from the heat and stir in the vanilla and butter. Let cool slightly.

3. Fold 1 cup of the bananas into the cooled pudding. Spoon the pudding mixture into the pie shell and arrange the remaining bananas in a circular pattern on top. Brush the jam over the bananas. Serves 8.

Per serving: Calories 334; Fiber 1g; Protein 5g; Total Fat 8g; Saturated Fat 3g; Cholesterol 6mg; Sodium 176m

Blueberries

Nutritional power
Blueberries are packed with pectin (a form of soluble fiber) as well as vitamin C, and are rich in antioxidants.

Healthy Highlights

PER 1 CUP	
Calories	81
Fiber	3.9g
Protein	1g
Total Fat	0.6g
Saturated Fat	0g
Cholesterol	0mg
Sodium	9mg

NUTRIENTS	
	% Daily Value
Vitamin C	32%
Manganese	21%

Did you know? . . .
In a USDA analysis of the antioxidant capacities of fruits and vegetables, blueberries ranked first among fruits. A 3½-ounce portion of blueberries was found to have the same antioxidant power (in the test tube) as 1270 milligrams of vitamin C.

The blueberry's color comes from pigments called anthocyanosides, which are antioxidants.

Blueberry Semifreddo

PREP: 10 MINUTES / COOK: 10 MINUTES
FREEZE: 4 HOURS / STAND: 30 MINUTES

This molded frozen dessert is meltingly creamy. Semifreddo means "half-frozen."

- 4 cups blueberries
- ½ cup sugar
- ⅛ teaspoon allspice
- 1 cup low-fat (1%) milk
- 1 tablespoon flour
- 1 container (15 ounces) part-skim ricotta cheese
- ⅓ cup reduced-fat sour cream
- ¼ cup honey
- ¾ teaspoon vanilla extract

1. In a medium saucepan, combine the blueberries, sugar, and allspice, and simmer over moderate heat for 5 minutes or until lightly thickened. Cool to room temperature.

2. Meanwhile, in a small saucepan, whisk the milk into the flour. Cook, stirring, for 5 minutes or until the mixture is lightly thickened. Cool to room temperature, then transfer to a food processor. Add the ricotta, sour cream, honey, and vanilla, and process until smooth. Transfer to a bowl and fold in 2 cups of the blueberry sauce. (Refrigerate the remaining sauce until serving time.)

3. Line a 9 x 5-inch glass loaf pan with plastic wrap, leaving a 2-inch overhang. Spoon the blueberry-ricotta mixture into the pan, smoothing the top. Cover with plastic wrap and freeze for 4 hours.

4. To serve, let stand for 30 minutes at room temperature, then unmold onto a serving platter. Cut into slices and serve with the reserved blueberry sauce. Serves 8.

Per serving: Calories 229; Fiber 2g; Protein 8g; Total Fat 6g; Saturated Fat 4g; Cholesterol 21mg; Sodium 92mg

Fresh Blueberry Jam

PREP: 10 MINUTES / COOK: 20 MINUTES

It's fun to make this jam with fruit you've picked yourself at a berry farm. Jam put up by this method is not meant for long storage; refrigerate it and use it within about a week.

- 3 cups blueberries
- 1 cup sugar
- 2 tablespoons lemon juice
- 4 strips (3 x ½ inch) orange zest
- ½ teaspoon ground cinnamon
- ¼ teaspoon salt
- 1 teaspoon vanilla extract

1. In a large pot of boiling water, sterilize 2 half-pint canning jars and lids.

2. In a medium saucepan, combine the blueberries, sugar, lemon juice, orange zest, cinnamon, and salt, and cook over

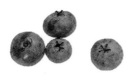

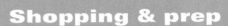

moderate heat, stirring frequently, for 20 minutes or until thick. Remove from the heat. Discard the zest and stir in the vanilla. Spoon the jam into the sterilized jars. Makes 1½ cups.

Per tablespoon: Calories 44; Fiber 0g; Protein 0g; Total Fat 0g; Saturated Fat 0g; Cholesterol 0mg; Sodium 25mg

Blueberry Scones

PREP: 15 MINUTES / COOK: 25 MINUTES

We've made our "cream scones" with low-fat buttermilk instead of heavy cream. Scones are tastiest when served warm.

- ⅓ **cup low-fat (1.5%) buttermilk**
- 1 **egg, separated**
- 1½ **cups flour**
- 2 **tablespoons plus 2 teaspoons sugar**
- 1½ **teaspoons baking powder**
- ¼ **teaspoon each baking soda and salt**
- 3 **tablespoons cold unsalted butter**
- 1½ **cups blueberries**
- 1 **teaspoon grated lemon zest**

1. Preheat the oven to 375°F. In a small bowl, combine the buttermilk and egg yolk; set aside.

2. In a large bowl, combine the flour, 2 tablespoons of the sugar, the baking powder, baking soda, and salt. With a pastry blender or two knives, cut in the butter until the mixture resembles coarse crumbs. Add the blueberries and lemon zest, stirring until well mixed.

3. Make a well in the center of the dry ingredients, add the buttermilk mixture, and, with a fork, combine until a soft dough is formed. (If the mixture is too dry, add up to 2 tablespoons more buttermilk.)

4. Transfer the dough to a lightly floured surface and knead 4 or 5 times until well mixed. Transfer to an ungreased baking sheet and shape into a 7-inch round disk. Lightly beat the egg white and brush over the dough. Sprinkle with the remaining 2 teaspoons sugar. Cut the round into 6 wedges. Bake for 25 minutes or until a cake tester inserted in the center comes out clean. Cool on a wire rack. Serves 6.

Per serving: Calories 231; Fiber 2g; Protein 5g; Total Fat 7g; Saturated Fat 4g; Cholesterol 52mg; Sodium 290mg

At the market You'll find blueberries at the supermarket for much of the year, but they're tastiest (and cheapest) when locally grown berries are in season. Because out-of-season berries are imported, the price is far higher —and their flavor doesn't compare to that of local berries.

Look for Choose plump berries; those with a waxy "bloom" on the surface are freshest. If the box is stained with juice, the berries at the bottom may be spoiled or crushed.

Prep Pick over the berries, removing any green, withered, or squashed ones. Pull off the berry stems with your fingers.

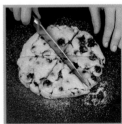

Pat the dough for the Blueberry Scones (at left) into a 7-inch round disk, then cut the round into six wedges.

Blueberry Scones *A British institution, scones are delightful for afternoon tea or brunch.*

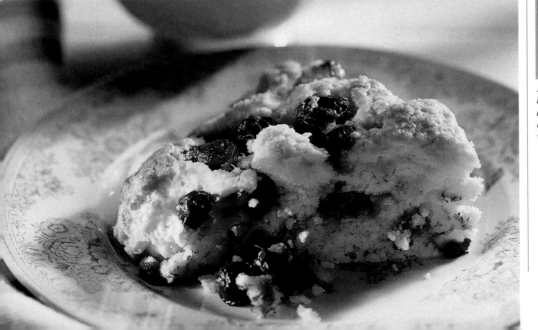

Cherries

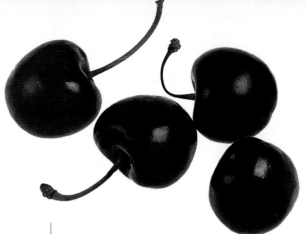

Nutritional power

The irresistible cherry is notable for its vitamin C; sour cherries have even more vitamin C than sweet ones. Both kinds supply beta carotene, as well.

Healthy Highlights

Sweet Cherries
PER 1 CUP PITTED

Calories	104
Fiber	3.3g
Protein	2g
Total Fat	1.4g
Saturated Fat	0.3g
Cholesterol	0mg
Sodium	0mg

NUTRIENTS

	% Daily Value
Vitamin C	17%
Potassium	11%

Sour Cherries
PER 1 CUP PITTED

Calories	78
Fiber	2.5g
Protein	2g
Total Fat	0.5g
Saturated Fat	0.1g
Cholesterol	0mg
Sodium	5mg

NUTRIENTS

	% Daily Value
Vitamin A	40%
Vitamin C	27%

Did you know?
Studies show that cherry juice may neutralize the enzymes that cause tooth decay.

Chocolate & Cherry Pudding

PREP: 25 MINUTES / COOK: 10 MINUTES
CHILL: 30 MINUTES

The cherries are not cooked—just layered in—so they retain all of their vitamin C.

- 3 tablespoons flour
- 3 tablespoons cornstarch
- ½ cup sugar
- ¼ teaspoon salt
- 3 cups low-fat (1%) milk
- 1 egg
- 2 teaspoons vanilla extract
- 2 ounces semisweet chocolate, finely chopped
- 2 cups fresh or thawed frozen cherries, halved and pitted
- 12 chocolate wafer cookies, coarsely chopped

1. In a medium saucepan, whisk together the flour, cornstarch, sugar, and salt. Whisk in the milk. Bring to a simmer over moderate heat, stirring frequently. Simmer for 2 minutes or until the pudding has thickened slightly.

2. In a small bowl, lightly beat the egg. Gradually beat ¾ cup of the hot pudding into the egg, then whisk the warmed egg mixture back into the pan and cook until the pudding starts to simmer. Remove from the heat and stir in the vanilla. Scrape the pudding into a bowl and place plastic wrap directly on the surface to prevent a skin from forming. Cool to room temperature and refrigerate for 30 minutes or until chilled, then whisk until smooth. Stir in all but 2 tablespoons of the chopped chocolate.

3. Dividing the ingredients evenly among six 6-ounce dessert dishes, make

layers as follows: cherries (use half of the total), pudding (use half), all of the wafer cookies, the remaining cherries and pudding. Sprinkle with the reserved chopped chocolate. Serves 6.

Per serving: Calories 293; Fiber 1g; Protein 7g; Total Fat 7g; Saturated Fat 3g; Cholesterol 41mg; Sodium 233mg

Fresh Cherry Sundaes

PREP: 1 HOUR / COOK: 5 MINUTES
FREEZE: 1 HOUR 30 MINUTES

Unsweetened frozen cherries work perfectly well in this tempting treat.

- 1 pint vanilla low-fat frozen yogurt
- ¾ cup chopped pitted cherries plus 1 cup halved pitted cherries (from 1¼ pounds unpitted)
- ¼ cup chopped toasted almonds (½ ounce)
- ½ cup cherry or raspberry jam
- 2 teaspoons cornstarch mixed with 1 tablespoon water
- 1 teaspoon vanilla extract
- ⅛ teaspoon almond extract

1. Let the frozen yogurt stand in the refrigerator for 30 minutes or until softened. Scoop the softened frozen yogurt into a medium bowl and stir in the chopped cherries and 2 tablespoons of the almonds. Return the bowl to the freezer and freeze for 1½ hours or until refrozen.

2. Meanwhile, in a medium saucepan, combine the halved cherries, jam, and cornstarch mixture. Bring to a simmer

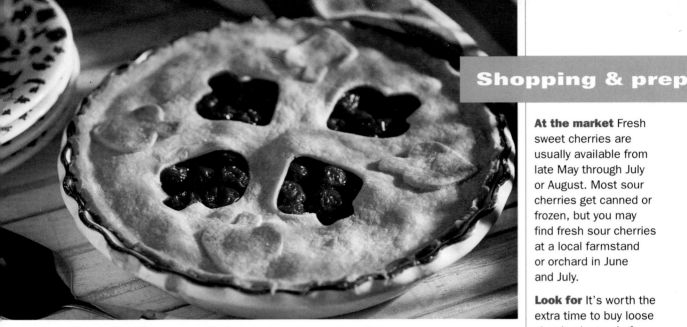

Sour Cherry Pie This gently spiced pie is dressed up with cookie-cutter cut-outs.

At the market Fresh sweet cherries are usually available from late May through July or August. Most sour cherries get canned or frozen, but you may find fresh sour cherries at a local farmstand or orchard in June and July.

Look for It's worth the extra time to buy loose cherries instead of prepackaged. Fresh cherries should be plump, firm, and shiny, with flexible green stems still attached. If the fruit is sticky, it's been damaged and is leaking juice.

Prep If you need to pit cherries for a recipe, a cherry pitter (see below) is the best tool. However, an old-fashioned hairpin (not a bobby pin) or a paper clip can also be used for the job.

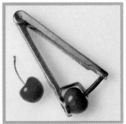

This handy little tool quickly pops the pits out of cherries. (It works nicely on olives, too.)

over moderate heat, stirring, and cook for 1 minute or until thickened. Stir in the vanilla and almond extracts.

3. Serve the frozen yogurt with warm or room-temperature cherry sauce. Sprinkle with the remaining 2 tablespoons almonds. Serves 4.

Per serving: Calories 262; Fiber 2g; Protein 5g; Total Fat 4g; Saturated Fat 1g; Cholesterol 5mg; Sodium 77mg

Sour Cherry Pie

PREP: 30 MINUTES / CHILL: 1 HOUR
COOK: 45 MINUTES

This British-style pie has a top crust only. You can either cut simple steam vents in the pie top, or dress it up a bit with cut-outs as shown above. To make cut-outs, use 2-inch cookie cutters to cut out shapes from the dough round before you put it over the pie. After placing the dough on the pie, position the cut-out pieces decoratively on top.

- 1 **cup all-purpose flour**
- 4 **teaspoons plus ⅔ cup sugar**
- ½ **teaspoon salt**
- 3 **tablespoons unsalted butter**
- 1 **tablespoon solid vegetable shortening**
- 5 **cups jarred sour cherries (packed in light syrup), drained**
- 2 **tablespoons honey**
- 1 **tablespoon lemon juice**
- ¼ **cup cornstarch**
- ⅛ **teaspoon ground allspice (optional)**
- 1 **tablespoon low-fat (1%) milk**

1. In a medium bowl, combine the flour, 3 teaspoons of the sugar, and the salt. With a pastry blender or 2 knives, cut in the butter and shortening until the mixture resembles coarse meal. Stir 2½ to 3 tablespoons ice water into the flour mixture until just combined. Flatten the dough into a disk, wrap in plastic wrap, and refrigerate for at least 1 hour.

2. Preheat the oven to 375°F. In a large bowl, stir together the cherries, honey, lemon juice, ⅔ cup of the sugar, the cornstarch, and allspice. Transfer to a 9-inch pie plate.

3. On a lightly floured surface, roll the dough out to a 12-inch round. Place the dough on top of the pie, crimping the edges to seal to the rim of the pie plate. Brush the crust with the milk and sprinkle with the remaining 1 teaspoon sugar. With a sharp knife, cut 3 or 4 slits in the crust to act as steam vents.

4. Place the pie on a baking sheet with sides and bake for 45 to 50 minutes or until bubbly and hot in the center. Serve warm or at room temperature. Serves 6.

Per serving: Calories 448; Fiber 1g; Protein 4g; Total Fat 8g; Saturated Fat 4g; Cholesterol 16mg; Sodium 201mg

Cranberries

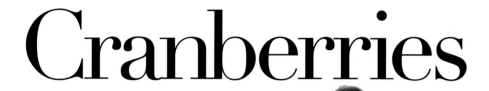

Nutritional power
Now available all year round, fresh, frozen, or dried cranberries bring their cheerful color—and a good bit of vitamin C—to condiments and desserts.

Healthy Highlights

PER 1 CUP RAW	
Calories	47
Fiber	4.0g
Protein	0g
Total Fat	0.2g
Saturated Fat	0g
Cholesterol	0mg
Sodium	1mg

NUTRIENTS	
	% Daily Value
Vitamin C	22%

Did you know? . . .
Cranberries contain ellagic acid, an antioxidant nutrient with significant cancer-fighting properties. Combined with their rich supply of vitamin C, that makes cranberries a potent "health food."

Whether it's the vitamin C or some as-yet-unidentified compound in the berries, cranberry juice seems to have a protective effect against urinary tract infections.

Cranberry-Cherry Relish

PREP: 10 MINUTES / COOK: 15 MINUTES

It's not easy to alter entrenched preferences in the cranberry-sauce department, but this spicy, fragrant three-fruit rendition may just do the trick.

- 1 bag (12 ounces) fresh or frozen (unthawed) cranberries
- 2 cups jarred water-packed sour cherries, drained
- 1 navel orange, unpeeled, coarsely chopped
- ¾ cup granulated sugar
- ½ cup packed light brown sugar
- ½ teaspoon cinnamon
- ¼ teaspoon each crushed red pepper flakes and salt
- ½ teaspoon vanilla extract

1. In a medium saucepan, combine the cranberries, cherries, orange, granulated sugar, brown sugar, cinnamon, red pepper flakes, and salt.

2. Cook over moderately low heat, stirring frequently, for 15 minutes or until the berries pop and the sauce is very thick. Cool to room temperature. Stir in the vanilla. Makes 5½ cups.

Per ¼ cup: Calories 64; Fiber 1g; Protein 0g; Total Fat 0g; Saturated Fat 0g; Cholesterol 0mg; Sodium 30mg

Cranberry Tart

PREP: 25 MINUTES / COOK: 45 MINUTES
CHILL: 1 HOUR

A slender layer of semisweet chocolate lines the tart shell, adding unexpected flavor.

- 1 cup flour
- 3 tablespoons plus 1 cup granulated sugar
- ¼ teaspoon salt
- 4 tablespoons unsalted butter, cut up
- 2 tablespoons reduced-fat cream cheese (Neufchâtel)
- ¼ cup ice water
- 1 ounce semisweet chocolate, melted
- 1 pound cranberries, fresh or frozen (unthawed)
- ¼ cup seedless raspberry jam, melted
- ¾ cup plain nonfat yogurt

1. In a large bowl, combine the flour, 1 tablespoon of the granulated sugar, and the salt. With a pastry blender or two knives, cut in the butter and cream cheese until the mixture resembles coarse meal. Stir in the ice water until just combined. Flatten into a disk, wrap in plastic wrap, and refrigerate for at least 1 hour.

2. Preheat the oven to 400°F. On a lightly floured surface, roll the dough out to a 13-inch round. Fit into a 9-inch tart pan with a removable bottom. Line the shell with foil and fill with dried beans or pie weights. Bake for 10 minutes or until just set. Remove the foil and beans, and bake for 12 minutes or until golden brown. Let cool slightly. Brush the bottom of the tart shell with the melted chocolate and let stand for 5 minutes or until set.

3. In a medium saucepan, combine the cranberries, ¼ cup of water, and 1 cup of the sugar, and bring to a boil. Cook for 8 minutes or until the berries have popped and the sauce is thick. Cool to room temperature. Spoon into the prepared shell and brush with the melted jam. In a small bowl, combine the yogurt and remaining 2 tablespoons sugar. Serve with the tart. Serves 6.

Per serving: Calories 421; Fiber 4g; Protein 5g; Total Fat 11g; Saturated Fat 6g; Cholesterol 25mg; Sodium 145mg

Cranberry Fool *is one of the best things ever to happen to berries. Replacing the heavy cream with milk is a great idea, too.*

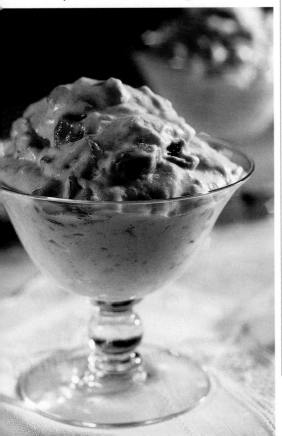

Cranberry Fool

PREP: 20 MINUTES / COOK: 20 MINUTES
CHILL: 45 MINUTES

The name of this fluffy, frivolous dessert may come from the French word "fou," which means crazy or extravagant. Or, perhaps, from the verb "fouetter," meaning to whip.

- **1 cup evaporated whole milk**
- **1 bag (12 ounces) fresh or frozen cranberries, unthawed**
- **½ cup plus 3 tablespoons sugar**
- **¼ teaspoon cinnamon**
- **⅛ teaspoon allspice**
- **½ teaspoon vanilla extract**
- **1 envelope unflavored gelatin**
- **¼ cup reduced-fat sour cream**

1. Pour the evaporated milk into a large mixing bowl, and place it in the freezer for 30 minutes.

2. Meanwhile, in a medium saucepan, combine the cranberries, ½ cup of the sugar, the cinnamon, and allspice, and cook over moderate heat for 15 minutes or until the berries have popped and the sauce is thick. Cool to room temperature, then stir in the vanilla.

3. In a measuring cup, soften the gelatin for 5 minutes in ¼ cup cold water. Place the cup in a pan of simmering water and heat for 2 minutes or until the gelatin has dissolved. Cool to room temperature.

4. Stir the sour cream into the superchilled evaporated milk. With an electric mixer, beat until soft peaks form. Beat in the remaining 3 tablespoons sugar, and beat until stiff peaks form. Beat in the gelatin mixture. Place in the refrigerator for 15 minutes to chill, whisking occasionally until the mixture begins to mound. Fold in the cranberry mixture. Return to the refrigerator and chill for 30 minutes or until set. Serves 4.

Per serving: Calories 292; Fiber 3g; Protein 7g; Total Fat 7g; Saturated Fat 4g; Cholesterol 23mg; Sodium 80mg

At the market
Cranberries are sold in plastic bags. In the fall, you'll find them in the produce section. After the holidays, try the frozen-food case if they're no longer displayed with the fresh fruit.

Look for Bagged berries are usually in fine condition, but squeeze the bag to make sure they're nice and firm.

Prep Rinse the cranberries and remove any stems or damaged berries. Cranberries that have been frozen should not be thawed before using.

Basic cooking Many recipes call for cranberries to be cooked "until they pop." This stage is reached when the skins split; you'll hear a faint spluttering noise as it happens.

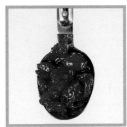

After a few minutes of cooking, cranberries will "pop" and deflate.

Dried Figs

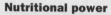

Nutritional power
The tiny seeds that give figs their unique texture also supply a lot of dietary fiber. Potassium, manganese, iron, and calcium are among figs' other benefits.

Healthy Highlights

PER ¼ CUP*	
Calories	127
Fiber	4.6g
Protein	2g
Total Fat	0.6g
Saturated Fat	0.1g
Cholesterol	0mg
Sodium	5mg

NUTRIENTS	
	% Daily Value
Potassium	12%
Manganese	10%

about 3 small figs

Did you know? . . .
Although you may occasionally find them at a fancy fruit shop, fresh figs are very perishable: Most figs that are grown are sold dried. But dried figs are just as nutritious as fresh.

The medicinal use of figs goes back to ancient times. More recently, researchers in Tokyo have had some success using a chemical from figs to treat cancer.

Pasta with Bacon, Figs & "Cream" Sauce

PREP: 20 MINUTES / COOK: 20 MINUTES
Figs, like raisins and prunes, are a delicious— and healthful—addition to savory dishes.

- ½ **pound dried figs, cut into ¼-inch chunks**
- 2 **cups boiling water**
- 1 **teaspoon olive oil**
- 2 **slices bacon, cut crosswise into ¼-inch-wide strips**
- 1 **onion, finely chopped**
- 4 **teaspoons flour**
- 1 **can (12 ounces) low-fat (1%) evaporated milk**
- 12 **ounces penne pasta**
- 2 **tablespoons reduced-fat cream cheese (Neufchâtel)**
- ¾ **teaspoon salt**
- ½ **teaspoon pepper**
- ⅓ **cup grated Parmesan cheese**
- ¼ **cup chopped parsley**

1. In a heatproof bowl, combine the figs and boiling water and let stand for 10 minutes or until softened. Drain, reserving ½ cup of the soaking liquid.

2. In a large nonstick skillet, heat the oil over moderate heat. Add the bacon and cook for 4 minutes or until lightly crisped. Add the onion and sauté for 7 minutes or until lightly golden. Whisk in the flour until coated. Gradually add the evaporated milk, and cook, stirring, for 3 minutes or until lightly thickened.

3. Meanwhile, in a large pot of boiling water, cook the penne according to package directions until firm-tender. Drain and transfer to a large bowl.

4. Whisk the cream cheese, the reserved fig soaking water, the salt, and pepper into the skillet and cook for 1 minute or until the cream cheese has melted. Add the sauce, drained figs, Parmesan, and parsley to the hot pasta, tossing well to combine. Serves 4.

Per serving: Calories 683; Fiber 8g; Protein 24g; Total Fat 15g; Saturated Fat 5g; Cholesterol 33mg; Sodium 787mg

Fig & Almond Cookies

PREP: 25 MINUTES / CHILL: 1 HOUR
COOK: 1 HOUR 5 MINUTES

- 2¼ **cups flour**
- ½ **teaspoon each baking soda and salt**
- 4 **tablespoons unsalted butter**
- 2 **tablespoons solid vegetable shortening**
- ⅔ **cup sugar**
- 1 **egg**
- 3 **tablespoons low-fat (1%) milk**
- 1 **teaspoon grated lemon zest**
- 1 **pound dried figs, cut into ¼-inch bits**
- ¼ **cup whole almonds**
- 2 **tablespoons honey**
- 2 **teaspoons lemon juice**
- ¼ **teaspoon ground ginger**

1. In a small bowl, combine the flour, baking soda, and salt. In a medium bowl with an electric mixer, beat the butter and shortening until creamy. Beat in the sugar until light and fluffy. Beat in the egg and milk until well combined. Beat in the lemon zest. Stir in the dry ingredients just until combined. Divide the dough in half, pat each half into a rectangle, wrap in plastic wrap, and refrigerate for at least 1 hour.

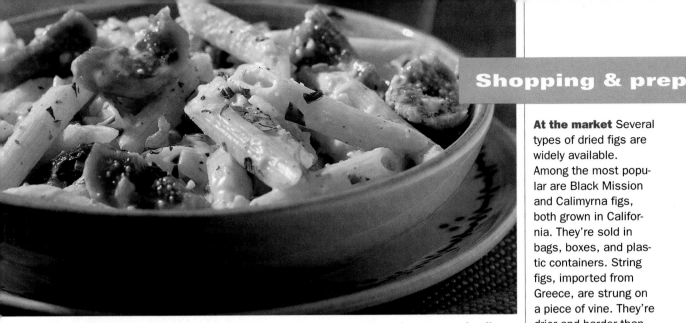

Pasta with Bacon, Figs & "Cream" Sauce The sauce is made with evaporated milk.

At the market Several types of dried figs are widely available. Among the most popular are Black Mission and Calimyrna figs, both grown in California. They're sold in bags, boxes, and plastic containers. String figs, imported from Greece, are strung on a piece of vine. They're drier and harder than other types of figs.

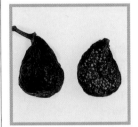

These are Calfornia Black Mission figs. The figs shown on the opposite page are Calimyrnas.

Look for They may be dried, but figs should be plump and soft. Squeeze the package to make sure.

Prep To make chopping sticky figs easier, first spray the knife (or the blades of kitchen shears) with nonstick cooking spray, or coat lightly with vegetable oil.

2. In a medium saucepan, combine the figs and 1½ cups of water. Bring to a boil, reduce to a simmer, cover, and cook for 30 minutes or until the figs are soft. Uncover and cook for 5 minutes or until no liquid remains. Transfer the figs to a food processor along with the almonds. Process to a smooth purée. Stir in the honey, lemon juice, and ginger. Cool to room temperature.

3. Preheat the oven to 350°F. Spray a baking sheet with nonstick cooking spray. On a lightly floured surface, roll each dough half to a 5 x 9-inch rectangle. Spoon half of the filling down the center of one rectangle, leaving a 2-inch border on the long sides and a ½-inch border at each end. Fold the ends in over the filling, then starting on a long side, roll the dough over the filling, jelly-roll fashion. Repeat with the second dough half and remaining filling.

4. Place the rolls, seam-side down, and 4 inches apart on the prepared baking sheet. Bake for 30 minutes or until golden brown and firm to the touch. Cool for 10 minutes on the pan, then carefully transfer to a wire rack to cool completely. Cut each roll into 12 slices. Makes 2 dozen.

Per cookie: Calories 157; Fiber 2g; Protein 2g; Total Fat 4g; Saturated Fat 2g; Cholesterol 14mg; Sodium 81mg

Dried Figs Poached in Red Wine

PREP: 5 MINUTES / COOK: 40 MINUTES

For a stylish dinner-party dessert, serve the figs in goblets accompanied with delicate wafer cookies. For a more casual meal, partner the poached fruit with gingersnaps.

2	cups dry red wine
½	cup sugar
6	whole black peppercorns
1	bay leaf
16	dried figs (10½ ounces)
¼	cup reduced-fat sour cream

1. In a medium saucepan, combine the wine, sugar, peppercorns, and bay leaf. Bring to a boil over moderate heat. Add the figs, reduce to a simmer, cover, and cook for 35 minutes or until tender. With a slotted spoon, transfer the figs to a bowl and set aside.

2. Increase the heat to high and boil the liquid for 5 minutes or until reduced to a medium syrup (about ½ cup). Remove from the heat, discard the bay leaf, and pour over the figs. Cool to room temperature and refrigerate.

3. Serve the figs topped with some of the syrup and a dollop of sour cream. Serves 4.

Per serving: Calories 321; Fiber 7g; Protein 4g; Total Fat 3g; Saturated Fat 1g; Cholesterol 5mg; Sodium 22mg

Grapefruit

Nutritional power

In addition to its rich supply of vitamin C, grapefruit provides potassium, dietary fiber, and, if it's red or pink grapefruit, some beta carotene as well.

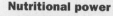

Healthy Highlights

PER 1 MEDIUM	
Calories	78
Fiber	2.6g
Protein	2g
Total Fat	0.2g
Saturated Fat	0g
Cholesterol	0mg
Sodium	0mg

NUTRIENTS	
	% Daily Value
Vitamin C	132%
Potassium	12%

Did you know? . . .

Grapefruit is rich in pectin, a type of dietary fiber that seems to reduce LDL cholesterol.

Researchers have discovered chemical compounds in grapefruit that cause the body to absorb more of certain medications. If you take your medication with grapefruit juice, check with your doctor to be sure this does not pose a problem.

Grapefruit with Spiced Red-Currant Sauce

PREP: 15 MINUTES / COOK: 5 MINUTES
CHILL: 1 HOUR

Delicious as a dessert, this ruby-hued fruit cup also makes a pleasing addition to a brunch menu. You can prepare it a day or two ahead of time and keep it in a covered bowl in the refrigerator.

- 2 pink grapefruits
- 1 white grapefruit
- ⅓ cup red currant jelly
- ½ teaspoon ground ginger
- ¼ teaspoon white pepper
- ⅛ teaspoon allspice
- 1 tablespoon lemon juice

1. With a small paring knife, peel the grapefruits. Working over a bowl to catch the juice, separate the grapefruit sections from the membranes; reserve any juice that collects in the bowl.

2. In a small skillet, combine the jelly, ginger, pepper, and allspice. Bring to a simmer and cook for 1 minute.

3. Pour the jelly mixture into a medium bowl and stir in the lemon juice and 1 tablespoon of the reserved grapefruit juice. Add the grapefruit and toss to combine. Serve chilled. Serves 4.

Per serving: Calories 126; Fiber 1g; Protein 1g; Total Fat 0g; Saturated Fat 0g; Cholesterol 0mg; Sodium 10mg

Grapefruit-Broiled Salmon

PREP: 20 MINUTES / COOK: 10 MINUTES

Tart citrus is the perfect counterpoint to rich fish, and lemon isn't the only fruit that fills the bill. Here, a lively grapefruit salad complements broiled salmon.

- 3 grapefruits
- 1 red bell pepper, diced
- 1 celery stalk, cut into ¼-inch dice
- ¼ cup finely chopped red onion
- 2 teaspoons olive oil
- 1 teaspoon Dijon mustard
- ½ teaspoon salt
- 4 boneless salmon fillets, with skin (6 ounces each)
- ½ teaspoon dried oregano
- ¼ teaspoon black pepper

1. With a small paring knife, peel the grapefruits. Working over a bowl to catch the juice, separate the grapefruit sections from the membranes; reserve any juice that collects in the bowl. Halve the grapefruit sections crosswise and transfer to a salad bowl. Add the bell pepper, celery, onion, oil, mustard, and ¼ teaspoon of the salt. Toss to combine and refrigerate until serving time.

2. Preheat the broiler. Place the salmon, skin-side down, on a broiler rack. Sprinkle 3 tablespoons of the reserved grapefruit juice, the oregano, black pepper, and the remaining ¼ teaspoon salt over the salmon. Broil 6 inches from the heat for 8 minutes or until just cooked through. Serve the salmon with the grapefruit salad. Serves 4.

Per serving: Calories 402; Fiber 2g; Protein 35g; Total Fat 21g; Saturated Fat 4g; Cholesterol 100mg; Sodium 430mg

Crab & Grapefruit Salad

PREP: 25 MINUTES

Crabmeat is the classic choice for this refreshing salad, but you could also opt for shrimp or good-sized cubes of poached chicken breast.

- 4 grapefruits
- 2 tablespoons light mayonnaise
- 1 tablespoon finely chopped mango chutney
- 2 teaspoons Dijon mustard
- 1 teaspoon sesame oil
- ¼ teaspoon each salt and pepper
- ¾ pound lump crabmeat, picked over to remove any cartilage
- 2 cups watercress, tough stems trimmed
- 1 Belgian endive, cut crosswise into ½-inch-wide strips
- 1 head Bibb lettuce, separated into leaves

1. With a small paring knife, peel the grapefruits. Working over a bowl to catch the juice, separate the grapefruit sections from the membranes; reserve any juice that collects in the bowl.

2. In a medium bowl, whisk together the mayonnaise, chutney, mustard, sesame oil, salt, pepper, and 3 tablespoons of reserved grapefruit juice.

3. Add the crabmeat, tossing to combine. Add the watercress, endive, and grapefruit sections, and toss. Serve the salad on a bed of Bibb lettuce. Serves 4.

Per serving: Calories 220; Fiber 2g; Protein 19g; Total Fat 5g; Saturated Fat 1g; Cholesterol 88mg; Sodium 549mg

At the market You'll find grapefruit in the supermarket all year round.

Look for Choose nice round grapefruits that feel heavy in your hand (that means they'll be juicy). The skin should be glossy, but a few dull or brown patches are not a bad sign.

Prep To cut neat segments from a grapefruit, first peel the fruit, using a sharp knife to remove all the white pith, which is unpleasantly bitter. Also remove the outer layer of membrane that surrounds the fruit. Working over a bowl to catch the juice, free the segments from the membranes (see below).

Crab & Grapefruit Salad Tart grapefruit and greens serve as foils for sweet crab.

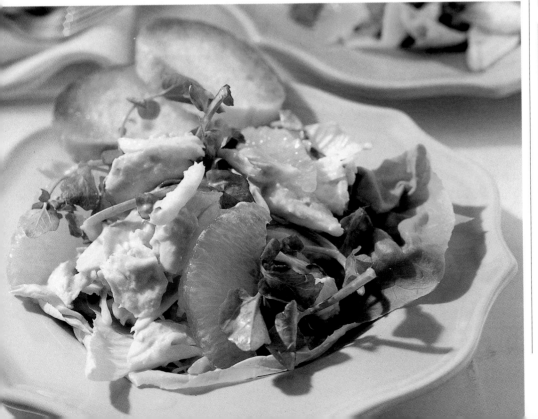

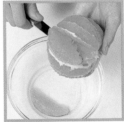

Carefully slice between each dividing membrane and the grapefruit pulp to release the segments.

Grapes & Raisins

Nutritional power
First found in wine, a cholesterol-lowering phytochemical called resveratrol is also present in red grapes. Grapes and raisins also supply potassium and fiber.

Healthy Highlights

Grapes
PER 1 CUP

Calories	114
Fiber	1.6g
Protein	1g
Total Fat	0.9g
Saturated Fat	0.3g
Cholesterol	0mg
Sodium	3mg

NUTRIENTS

	% Daily Value
Vitamin C	28%
Potassium	10%
Thiamin	10%

Raisins
PER ¼ CUP

Calories	124
Fiber	1.7g
Protein	1g
Total Fat	0.2g
Saturated Fat	0.1g
Cholesterol	0mg
Sodium	5mg

NUTRIENTS

	% Daily Value
Potassium	10%

Did you know? . . .
Grapes are a good source of boron, which helps keep bones strong.

Grape & Raisin Coffeecake

PREP: 15 MINUTES / COOK: 55 MINUTES

- 1⅓ cups flour
- 1¼ teaspoons baking powder
- ½ teaspoon baking soda
- ¼ teaspoon salt
- 4 tablespoons unsalted butter, at room temperature
- ⅔ cup plus ¼ cup sugar
- 1 egg
- 2 egg whites
- ¾ cup low-fat (1.5%) buttermilk
- 1 teaspoon vanilla extract
- ½ cup raisins
- ¼ cup pecans or walnuts
- ¾ teaspoon cinnamon
- 2 cups seedless red and/or green grapes

1. Preheat the oven to 350°F. Spray a 9-inch square baking pan with nonstick cooking spray; set aside. In a small bowl, combine the flour, baking powder, baking soda, and salt.

2. In a large bowl with an electric mixer, cream the butter and ⅔ cup of the sugar until light and fluffy. Add the whole egg and egg whites, one at a time, beating until well combined. Beat in the buttermilk and vanilla. Fold the dry ingredients into the butter mixture. Fold in the raisins.

3. In a food processor, combine the remaining ¼ cup sugar, the pecans, and cinnamon, pulsing until the nuts are coarsely ground. Spoon half of the batter into the pan and sprinkle with half of the nut mixture. Top with the remaining batter, the grapes, and the remaining nut mixture. Bake for 55 minutes or until a cake tester inserted in the center comes out clean. Serves 8.

Per serving: Calories 329; Fiber 2g; Protein 6g; Total Fat 10g; Saturated Fat 5g; Cholesterol 45mg; Sodium 263mg

Chicken Véronique

PREP: 15 MINUTES / COOK: 20 MINUTES

This is a variation on the classic Sole Véronique. A combination of red and green grapes makes the prettiest dish.

- 2 teaspoons olive oil
- 4 skinless, boneless chicken breast halves (5 ounces each)
- 2 tablespoons flour
- ½ cup dry white wine
- ¾ cup chicken broth
- ½ teaspoon salt
- ¼ teaspoon each crumbled dried rosemary and pepper
- 2 cups seedless red and/or green grapes, halved
- 3 tablespoons reduced-fat sour cream
- ¼ cup chopped parsley

1. In a large nonstick skillet, heat the oil over moderate heat. Dredge the chicken in the flour, shaking off and reserving the excess. Sauté the chicken

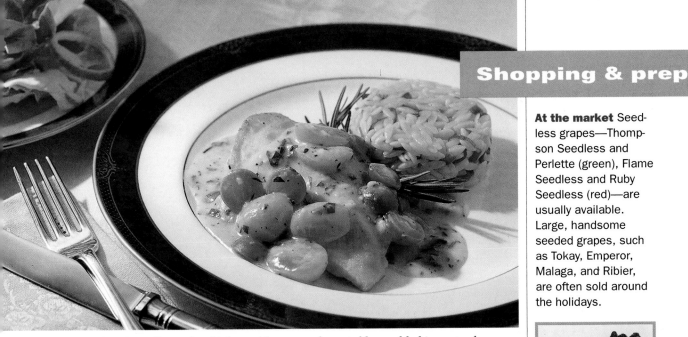

Chicken Véronique Serve the chicken with orzo and vegetables molded in custard cups.

At the market Seedless grapes—Thompson Seedless and Perlette (green), Flame Seedless and Ruby Seedless (red)—are usually available. Large, handsome seeded grapes, such as Tokay, Emperor, Malaga, and Ribier, are often sold around the holidays.

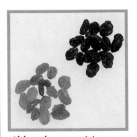

Although most raisins are made from Thompson Seedless grapes, raisins come in two colors: Brown raisins are sun-dried and left as is after drying, while golden raisins are oven-dried and treated with sulfur dioxide to keep them from darkening.

for 2 minutes per side or until golden brown. Add the wine, increase the heat to high, and cook for 2 minutes.

2. Add the broth, salt, rosemary, and pepper, and bring to a boil. Reduce to a simmer, cover, and cook for 5 minutes or until the chicken is cooked through. Add the grapes, cover, and cook for 5 minutes or until tender.

3. In a small bowl, whisk together the sour cream and the reserved flour. Stir the mixture into the pan and cook, stirring constantly, for 2 minutes or until lightly thickened. Transfer the chicken to serving plates. Stir the parsley into the sauce and spoon over the chicken. Serves 4.

Per serving: Calories 292; Fiber 2g; Protein 35g; Total Fat 6g; Saturated Fat 2g; Cholesterol 86mg; Sodium 589mg

Raisin Bars

PREP: 10 MINUTES / COOK: 25 MINUTES

- 2 **cups raisins**
- 2 **cups boiling water**
- 1¼ **cups flour**
- ½ **teaspoon baking powder**
- ¼ **teaspoon baking soda**
- ½ **teaspoon cinnamon**
- ¼ **teaspoon ground nutmeg**
- ⅛ **teaspoon ground cloves**
- 4 **tablespoons unsalted butter, at room temperature**
- ½ **cup packed dark brown sugar**
- 2 **tablespoons molasses**
- 1 **egg**
- 1 **egg white**

1. Preheat the oven to 350°F. Spray a 9-inch square metal baking pan with nonstick cooking spray. Dust with flour; set aside. In a small heatproof bowl, combine the raisins with the boiling water. Let sit for 5 minutes; drain.

2. In a small bowl, combine the flour, baking powder, baking soda, cinnamon, nutmeg, and cloves. In a large bowl, with an electric mixer, beat the butter, brown sugar, and molasses until creamy. Add the whole egg and egg white, one at a time, beating well after each addition. Stir in the dry ingredients.

3. Fold the raisins into the batter. Spread the batter in the prepared pan. Bake for 25 minutes or until the top is springy to the touch and lightly golden. Cool the cake in the pan on a rack, then cut into 24 bars. Makes 24 cookies.

Per cookie: Calories 103; Fiber 1g; Protein 2g; Total Fat 2g; Saturated Fat 1g; Cholesterol 14mg; Sodium 32mg

Look for Choose a well-shaped bunch of plump grapes, avoiding bunches with withered, shriveled, or crushed fruit. Check the color: Green grapes that are yellow-green are sweetest; the tastiest red grapes are a warm crimson color. The grapes should not be pale around the stems, and the stems should be pliable.

Prep Don't rinse grapes until shortly before serving.

Kiwifruit

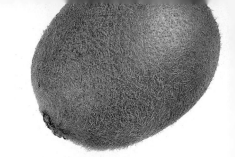

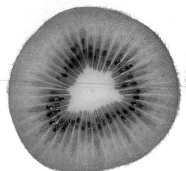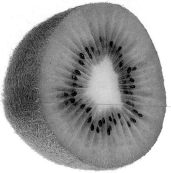

Nutritional power
Following its debut as the darling of upscale chefs, the kiwi, a great source of vitamin C, fiber, and potassium, has become a popular snack fruit.

Healthy Highlights

PER 1 MEDIUM	
Calories	46
Fiber	2.6g
Protein	1g
Total Fat	0.3g
Saturated Fat	0g
Cholesterol	0mg
Sodium	4mg

NUTRIENTS	
	% Daily Value
Vitamin C	123%

Did you know? . . .
Two kiwifruits—a healthy snack—supply more potassium than a medium banana.

Kiwifruit contains an enzyme called actinidin, which breaks down protein. So mashed or puréed kiwifruit can serve as a tenderizing marinade. Leave it on the meat for at least 15 minutes.

A kiwifruit contains almost as much vitamin C as a small orange.

Chicken Salad with Kiwi & Lime-Ginger Dressing

PREP: 25 MINUTES / COOK: 10 MINUTES

You might call this an updated Waldorf salad: In place of apples, walnuts, and mayonnaise, this California-style salad is made with kiwifruit and water chestnuts, and tossed with a tangy chili vinaigrette. Slices of broiled chicken make the salad a meal.

½	teaspoon each dried tarragon, salt, and pepper
4	skinless, boneless chicken breast halves (5 ounces each)
½	teaspoon grated lime zest
3	tablespoons lime juice
3	tablespoons chili sauce
1	tablespoon honey
1	teaspoon olive oil
¾	teaspoon ground ginger
4	cups sliced romaine lettuce
4	kiwifruit, peeled and cut into ½-inch cubes
½	cup canned sliced water chestnuts, rinsed and cut into strips

1. Preheat the broiler. Rub the tarragon, ¼ teaspoon of the salt, and the pepper into the chicken. Broil 6 inches from the heat for 4 minutes per side or until cooked through. Cool to room temperature and slice crosswise into ½-inch slices.

2. Meanwhile, in a large bowl, whisk together the lime zest, lime juice, chili sauce, honey, oil, ginger, and the remaining ¼ teaspoon salt.

3. Add the romaine, kiwi, and water chestnuts, tossing to combine. Add the chicken and toss again. Serves 4.

Per serving: Calories 268; Fiber 4g; Protein 35g; Total Fat 3g; Saturated Fat 1g; Cholesterol 82mg; Sodium 564mg

Kiwi with Ricotta Cream

PREP: 15 MINUTES

Macerating kiwifruit in a mixture of sugar and lime juice produces a tasty syrup that forms the sauce for this dessert. The creamy topping is surprisingly low in fat.

¼	cup plus 2 tablespoons sugar
¼	cup lime juice
8	kiwifruit, peeled and cut into ½-inch cubes
½	teaspoon grated lime zest
½	cup part-skim ricotta cheese
2	tablespoons reduced-fat sour cream

1. In a medium bowl, combine ¼ cup of the sugar and the lime juice. Add the kiwi, tossing to combine. Cover and refrigerate until serving time.

2. In a small bowl, combine the lime zest, ricotta, sour cream, and the remaining 2 tablespoons sugar. Serve the kiwi with its syrup, topped with the ricotta cream. Serves 4.

Per serving: Calories 224; Fiber 5g; Protein 6g; Total Fat 4g; Saturated Fat 2g; Cholesterol 12mg; Sodium 53mg

Red Snapper with Kiwi Relish

PREP: 10 MINUTES / COOK: 10 MINUTES

You don't need a thick, heavy sauce to turn basic fish fillets into a dressy dinner. This colorful uncooked relish, made with kiwifruit, cucumber, red bell pepper, and scallions, fancies up—and flavors up—simple broiled snapper fillets.

- 4 **kiwifruit, peeled and cut into ½-inch cubes**
- 1 **red bell pepper, diced**
- 1 **small cucumber, peeled and cut into ¼-inch dice (½ cup)**
- 1 **scallion, thinly sliced**

- 2 **tablespoons honey**
- ¾ **teaspoon each salt, ground coriander, and cumin**
- ⅛ **teaspoon crushed red pepper flakes**
- 4 **red snapper fillets, with skin (6 ounces each)**
- 2 **tablespoons lime juice**

1. In a medium bowl, combine the kiwi, bell pepper, cucumber, scallion, honey, ¼ teaspoon each salt, coriander, and cumin, and the red pepper flakes. Cover and refrigerate.

2. Preheat the broiler. Place the fish on a broiler pan, skin-side down. Sprinkle the fillets with the lime juice, and the remaining ½ teaspoon each salt, coriander, and cumin. Broil 6 inches from the heat for 7 minutes or until the fish is lightly browned and starts to flake. Serve the fish topped with the kiwi relish. Serves 4.

Per serving: Calories 264; Fiber 3g; Protein 36g; Total Fat 3g; Saturated Fat 1g; Cholesterol 63mg; Sodium 555mg

Red Snapper with Kiwi Relish *The fruit-and-vegetable relish is sweet and slightly hot.*

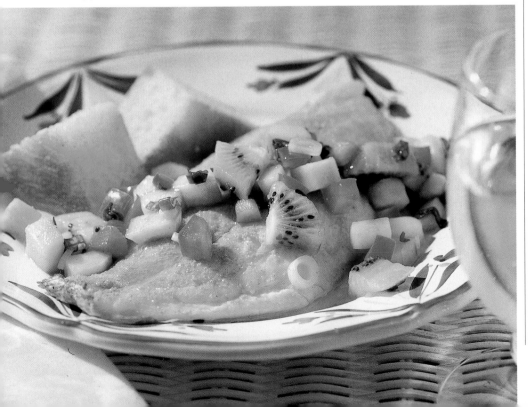

At the market
Kiwifruit are grown in both California (November through May) and New Zealand (June through October), so they're always available. As they've become more popular, their price has dropped markedly.

Look for Kiwis are usually firm when sold, but they readily ripen at room temperature. (When ready to eat, a kiwi is about as yielding as a ripe peach.) Choose plump, unbruised fruits; avoid any with shriveled skin.

Prep You can eat a kiwifruit skin and all; though it's a bit furry, the skin is good for you. Or peel it and then slice it. Instead of using a peeler to peel a kiwi, use a spoon (see below).

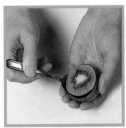

Cut the kiwi in half, then use a spoon to scoop out the flesh in one piece.

Basic cooking
Kiwifruit, like pineapple, contains an enzyme that keeps gelatin from setting, so it should not be used in gelatin desserts.

Lemons & Limes

Nutritional power
Bursting with vitamin C, these tart fruits serve as fat-free, virtually sodium-free seasonings for all sorts of foods and beverages.

Healthy Highlights

Lemon
PER 1 MEDIUM

Calories	17
Fiber	1.6g
Protein	1g
Total Fat	0.2g
Saturated Fat	0g
Cholesterol	0mg
Sodium	1mg

NUTRIENTS

	% Daily Value
Vitamin C	52%

Lime
PER 1 MEDIUM

Calories	20
Fiber	1.9g
Protein	1g
Total Fat	0.1g
Saturated Fat	0g
Cholesterol	0mg
Sodium	1mg

NUTRIENTS

	% Daily Value
Vitamin C	32%

Did you know? . . .
Add fresh lemon or lime juice to frozen or canned to boost the vitamin C content while brightening the flavor.

Key Lime Parfait
PREP: 1 HOUR 40 MINUTES
COOK: 5 MINUTES / CHILL: 2 HOURS

Key limes (originally grown in the Florida Keys) are golf-ball-size, yellow-skinned fruits. Key limes are sold in some gourmet shops; their bottled juice is widely available.

- 1 can (12 ounces) evaporated milk
- 1 envelope unflavored gelatin
- ½ cup confectioners sugar
- ½ cup reduced-fat sour cream
- ½ teaspoon grated lime zest
- ½ cup bottled Key lime juice or fresh lime juice

1. Pour the evaporated milk into a large mixing bowl and place in the freezer until ice crystals begin to form, about 1 hour.

2. In a glass measuring cup, sprinkle the gelatin over ¼ cup cold water and let stand for 5 minutes or until softened. Place the cup in a pan of simmering water and heat for 4 minutes or until the gelatin has dissolved. Cool to room temperature.

3. Beat the partially frozen evaporated milk until soft peaks form. Gradually beat in the confectioners sugar and continue whipping until stiff peaks form. Beat in the sour cream. Beat in the lime zest and cooled gelatin mixture until well combined. Place the bowl in the refrigerator and chill for 30 minutes or until the mixture begins to mound.

4. Fold the lime juice into the milk mixture. Transfer to 8 parfait glasses and chill for 2 hours. Serves 8.

Per serving: Calories 125; Fiber 0g; Protein 5g; Total Fat 6g; Saturated Fat 3g; Cholesterol 19mg; Sodium 60mg

Lemon-Limeade
PREP: 15 MINUTES / COOK: 10 MINUTES

"Simple syrup"—a boiled sugar syrup—is the secret to the best lemonade. This recipe has the extra advantage of lively lime juice.

- 1½ cups sugar
- 6 strips (3 x ½ inch) lemon zest
- 6 strips (3 x ½ inch) lime zest
- ¾ cup fresh lemon juice
- ¾ cup fresh lime juice

1. In a small saucepan, combine the sugar, 1 cup of water, and the lemon and lime zests. Bring to a boil over moderate heat and boil for 5 minutes. Let the syrup cool to room temperature; discard the zest. Transfer to a large jar or juice container, add the lemon and lime juices, and shake to combine.

2. To serve: Spoon ¼ cup of the lemon-lime mixture into an 8-ounce glass. Add ⅓ cup of water or seltzer and stir to combine. Add 2 ice cubes and serve. Serves 12.

Per serving: Calories 105; Fiber 0g; Protein 0g; Total Fat 0g; Saturated Fat 0g; Cholesterol 0mg; Sodium 1mg

Tomato-Vegetable Salad with Lemon Vinaigrette

PREP: 20 MINUTES / COOK: 10 MINUTES

When you dice the lemons, pour the juice from the cutting board into a measuring cup and save it to use in the dressing. Have a third lemon on hand in case you need more juice.

- 1 yellow or red bell pepper, cut lengthwise into flat panels
- 2 lemons
- ¼ cup lemon juice
- 1 tablespoon olive oil
- ½ teaspoon salt
- ¼ teaspoon black pepper
- ¼ teaspoon sugar
- 3 large tomatoes, cut into 1-inch chunks
- 1 stalk celery, thinly sliced
- ¼ cup chopped fresh basil

1. Preheat the broiler. Place the pepper pieces, skin-sides up, on the broiler pan and broil for 12 minutes or until the skin is charred. When cool enough to handle, peel and thinly slice.

2. With a paring knife, peel the lemons. Cut into ¼-inch dice, discarding the seeds. In a large bowl, whisk together the lemon juice, oil, salt, black pepper, and sugar.

3. Add the lemon pieces to the bowl along with the tomatoes, celery, basil, and roasted pepper. Toss well to combine. Serves 4.

Per serving: Calories 87; Fiber 3g; Protein 2g; Total Fat 4g; Saturated Fat 1g; Cholesterol 0mg; Sodium 318mg

At the market Both lemons and limes are available throughout the year.

Look for Pick firm, heavy, bright-colored lemons and limes that have fine-grained, glossy skins. Large-pored skin can be an indication of very thick pith and less juice.

Prep If a recipe calls for the zest as well as the juice or pulp of the lemon or lime, be sure to remove the zest first. Rolling the fruit under the palm of your hand (or warming it under hot water) will make it easier to squeeze the juice.

Tomato-Vegetable Salad with Lemon Vinaigrette *Like oranges or grapefruit, lemons are delicious in salads. The slightly sweet dressing balances their tartness.*

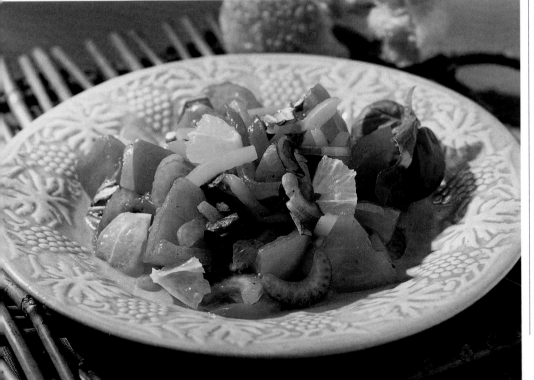

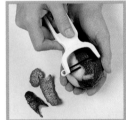

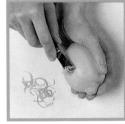

Here are two ways to peel off the zest (the outermost, colored part of the peel) from a lemon or lime. You can use a vegetable peeler and then sliver the zest with a knife. Or, you can use a special zesting tool, which pulls the zest off in thin strands.

Mangoes

Nutritional power
Its golden-orange flesh tips you off to the mango's stellar beta-carotene content. This tropical delight also supplies lots of vitamin C and even some vitamin E.

Healthy Highlights

PER 1 CUP

Calories	107
Fiber	3.0g
Protein	1g
Total Fat	0.4g
Saturated Fat	0.1g
Cholesterol	0mg
Sodium	3mg

NUTRIENTS

	% Daily Value
Vitamin A	129%
Vitamin C	77%
Vitamin B6	11%

Did you know? . . .
Much of the dietary fiber in mangoes is pectin, a form of soluble fiber that has been shown to reduce blood cholesterol.

Ripe mangos usually have a red "blush," but Evergreen, a new variety, is green-skinned when ripe. But its flesh is deep orange, and, like any other mango, the Evergreen is rich in vitamins C and A.

Mango & Shrimp Salad

PREP: 20 MINUTES / COOK: 5 MINUTES

- ⅓ cup lemon juice
- 1 bay leaf
- ¼ teaspoon crushed red pepper flakes
- ¼ teaspoon salt
- 1 pound medium shrimp, peeled and deveined
- ¼ cup chili sauce
- 1 tablespoon olive oil
- 1 red bell pepper, slivered
- 1 cup cherry tomatoes, halved
- 1 cucumber, halved lengthwise, seeded, and cut into half-rounds
- 2 mangoes (2¼ pounds total), peeled and cut into ½-inch cubes
- 8 lettuce leaves
  Cilantro sprigs, for garnish

1. In a large skillet, combine 2 cups of water, 1 tablespoon of the lemon juice, the bay leaf, red pepper flakes, and salt. Bring to a boil over moderate heat. Add the shrimp, reduce to a simmer, cover, and cook for 4 minutes or until pink and firm. Drain the shrimp and set aside to cool to room temperature.

2. In a large bowl, whisk together the chili sauce, oil, and the remaining lemon juice. Add the shrimp, bell pepper, tomatoes, cucumber, and mangoes, tossing to combine. Line plates with the lettuce and top with the shrimp mixture. Garnish with cilantro. Serves 4.

Per serving: Calories 286; Fiber 3g; Protein 21g; Total Fat 6g; Saturated Fat 1g; Cholesterol 140mg; Sodium 513mg

Grilled Pork Chops with Mango Barbecue Sauce

PREP: 15 MINUTES / COOK: 10 MINUTES

- 1 mango (1 pound), peeled and cut into large chunks
- 1 small onion, finely chopped
- ¼ cup balsamic vinegar
- 3 tablespoons packed dark brown sugar
- 2 tablespoons no-salt-added tomato paste
- ½ teaspoon salt
- ¼ teaspoon crushed red pepper flakes
- 4 well-trimmed center-cut pork chops (8 ounces each)

1. In a medium saucepan, combine the mango, onion, vinegar, brown sugar, tomato paste, salt, and red pepper flakes. Bring to a boil over moderate heat. Reduce to a simmer, cover, and cook for 10 minutes or until the sauce is thickened and the mango is very soft. Mash the mango with a spoon and set aside to cool to room temperature.

2. Preheat the broiler. Set aside half of the mango sauce to be served with the pork chops. Brush one side of the chops with half of the remaining sauce and broil 6 inches from the heat for 4 minutes. Turn the chops over, brush with the remaining sauce, and broil for 4 minutes or until cooked through but still juicy. Serve with the reserved sauce. Serves 4.

Per serving: Calories 316; Fiber 2g; Protein 34g; Total Fat 8g; Saturated Fat 3g; Cholesterol 93mg; Sodium 383mg

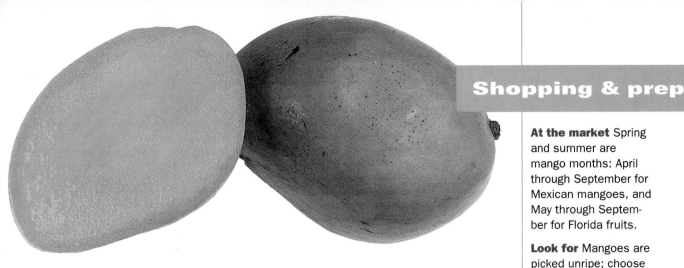

Mango Mousse

PREP: 20 MINUTES / CHILL: 2 HOURS

This pretty, refreshing dessert is most welcome after a rich meal. And there's a nutritional bonus: Mango plus lime juice equals lots of vitamin C.

- **2 mangoes (2¼ pounds total), peeled and sliced**
- **¼ cup lime juice**
- **½ teaspoon ground ginger**
- **1 envelope unflavored gelatin**
- **3 tablespoons sugar**
- **½ cup reduced-fat sour cream**

1. In a food processor, purée the mangoes with the lime juice and ginger.

2. In a small bowl, sprinkle the gelatin over ¼ cup of water. Let stand for 5 minutes or until softened. Meanwhile, in a small saucepan, combine the sugar and ¼ cup of water, and bring to a boil. Stir the gelatin into the sugar mixture and cook, stirring, for 1 minute or just until the gelatin is dissolved.

3. Add the sugar-gelatin mixture to the mango purée and process until well combined. Add the sour cream and process briefly just to blend.

4. Spoon into dessert bowls or glasses, cover, and refrigerate for 2 hours or until chilled and set. Serves 4.

Per serving: Calories 211; Fiber 2g; Protein 4g; Total Fat 5g; Saturated Fat 2g; Cholesterol 10mg; Sodium 26mg

At the market Spring and summer are mango months: April through September for Mexican mangoes, and May through September for Florida fruits.

Look for Mangoes are picked unripe; choose a smooth, unbruised fruit with a reddish or orange tint to its skin.

Prep Ripen mangoes at room temperature until fragrant; black freckles are also a sign of ripeness. To cut, hold the mango stem-end up and make two vertical cuts, one on either side of the large, flat pit. Remove these two side pieces, then cut off the band of flesh that remains around the edges of the pit. Peel the flesh or cube (see below).

Mango & Shrimp Salad The lush sweetness of mango is the perfect complement to the meaty texture and flavors of shrimp in this main course salad.

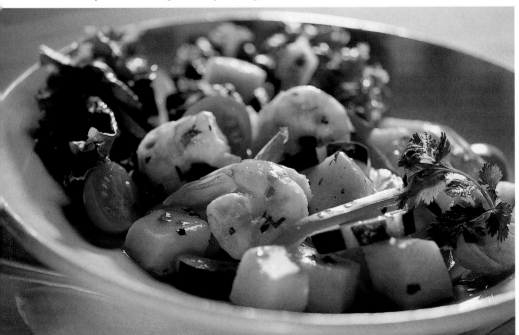

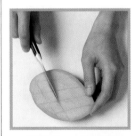

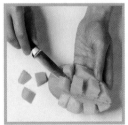

To cube a mango, make criss-cross cuts down to, but not through, the skin of one the side pieces (top photo). Pop the piece inside out and slice off the cubes.

Melons

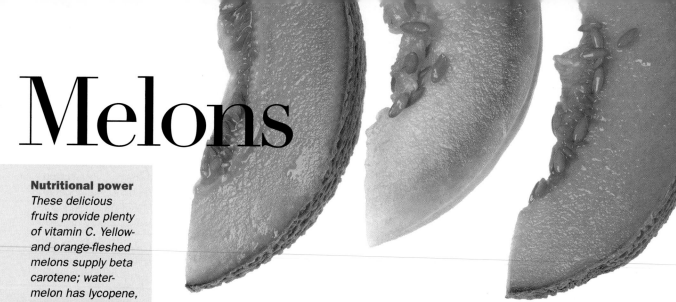

Nutritional power
These delicious fruits provide plenty of vitamin C. Yellow- and orange-fleshed melons supply beta carotene; watermelon has lycopene, another carotenoid.

Healthy Highlights

Cantaloupe
PER 1 CUP

Calories	55
Fiber	1.2g
Protein	1g
Total Fat	0.4g
Saturated Fat	0.1g
Cholesterol	0mg
Sodium	14mg

NUTRIENTS

	% Daily Value
Vitamin C	110%
Vitamin A	101%
Potassium	16%

Honeydew
PER 1 CUP

Calories	60
Fiber	1.0g
Protein	1g
Total Fat	0.2g
Saturated Fat	0g
Cholesterol	0mg
Sodium	17mg

NUTRIENTS

	% Daily Value
Vitamin C	70%
Potassium	15%

Festive Melon Bowl

PREP: 40 MINUTES

Use a small cookie cutter or a melon baller to cut the holes in the watermelon "bowl."

- ½ small watermelon (7 pounds)
- 1 cantaloupe, cut into balls (4 cups)
- ½ honeydew melon (2½ pounds), cut into balls (3 cups)
- 2 cups seedless red or green grapes
- 2 cups fresh or canned pineapple cubes
- 3 tablespoons sugar
- 2 cups plain low-fat yogurt
- ¼ cup reduced-fat sour cream
- ¼ cup honey
- 2 teaspoons lime juice
- 1 pinch of allspice

1. With a melon baller, cut the watermelon into balls, remove the seeds, and transfer to a large bowl (reserve the shell). Add the melons, grapes, and pineapple; sprinkle the fruit with 1 tablespoon of the sugar. Chill the fruit and watermelon shell until serving time.

2. In a small bowl, combine the yogurt, sour cream, honey, remaining 2 tablespoons sugar, the lime juice, and allspice. Chill until serving time.

3. Spoon as much of the fruit mixture as will fit in the watermelon "bowl," reserving the rest for refills. Serve the yogurt sauce on the side. Serves 16.

Per serving: Calories 132; Fiber 2g; Protein 3g; Total Fat 2g; Saturated Fat 1g; Cholesterol 3mg; Sodium 32mg

Honeydew-Lime Tart

PREP: 35 MINUTES / COOK: 15 MINUTES
CHILL: 3 HOURS

CRUST:
- 1½ cups flour
- 1½ tablespoons sugar
- ¾ teaspoon salt
- 4½ tablespoons unsalted butter
- 1½ tablespoons solid vegetable shortening

FILLING & TOPPING:
- 7 tablespoons sugar
- 3 tablespoons flour
- 2 tablespoons cornstarch
- ¼ teaspoon salt
- ¼ teaspoon ground ginger (optional)
- 2½ cups low-fat (1%) milk
- 1 egg
- 2 teaspoons grated lime zest
- 1 teaspoon vanilla extract
- ¾ pound peeled, seeded honeydew melon, cut into thin slices
- 8 lime wedges

1. For the crust: In a medium bowl, combine the flour, sugar, and salt. With a pastry blender or 2 knives, cut in the butter and shortening until the mixture resembles coarse meal. Stir 2½ to 3 tablespoons ice water into the flour mixture until just combined. Flatten the dough into a disk, wrap in plastic wrap, and refrigerate for at least 1 hour.

2. Preheat the oven to 400°F. Spray an 11-inch tart pan with a removable bottom with nonstick cooking spray. On a lightly floured surface, roll out the dough to a 13½-inch circle and fit into the pan. Prick the dough in several places with a fork and bake for 8 to 10 minutes or until crisped and golden. Cool on a rack for at least 10 minutes.

3. Meanwhile, for the filling: In a medium saucepan, whisk together the sugar, flour, cornstarch, salt, and ginger. Whisk in the milk. Bring to a simmer over medium heat, whisking constantly, and cook for 1 minute. In a small bowl, lightly beat the egg. Whisk in some of the hot milk mixture, then whisk the warmed egg back into the pan along with the lime zest and vanilla. Bring just to a simmer, remove from the heat, and pour into the cooled tart shell. Place plastic wrap directly on the surface of the custard to keep a skin from forming. Refrigerate for 2 hours or until chilled.

4. Arrange the honeydew slices on top of the custard. Serve the tart with the lime wedges for squeezing. Serves 8.

Per serving: Calories 297; Fiber 1g; Protein 6g; Total Fat 11g; Saturated Fat 5g; Cholesterol 47mg; Sodium 326mg

Orange-Cantaloupe Sherbet

PREP: 15 MINUTES
FREEZE: 2 TO 3 HOURS

4   cups cantaloupe cubes (¾ inch)
¾   cup low-fat (1.5%) buttermilk
⅓   cup corn syrup
¼   cup orange juice
⅓   cup sugar
1   teaspoon grated orange zest

1. In a food processor, purée the cantaloupe. Transfer to a bowl and stir in the buttermilk, corn syrup, orange juice, sugar, and orange zest.

2. Freeze in an ice cream machine, or, to still-freeze, place in a 9 x 13 x 2-inch pan and freeze for 2 to 3 hours or until almost frozen. Cut into chunks and process in a food processor until smooth. If not serving right away, refreeze, but let soften in the refrigerator for 30 minutes before serving. Serves 4.

Per serving: Calories 226; Fiber 1g; Protein 3g; Total Fat 1g; Saturated Fat 1g; Cholesterol 3mg; Sodium 71mg

In the market Summer is peak season for domestically grown melons, but imported cantaloupes and honeydews are nearly always available.

Look for Cantaloupes and honeydews should have a smooth indentation at the stem end (this indicates that the melon was picked ripe). Their skin color should tend toward yellow-gold rather than green. A honeydew should have a velvety skin; the "netting" on a cantaloupe should cover the whole surface, with no breaks. A watermelon's rind should look somewhat dull and waxy, rather than shiny; the pale underside should be yellowish, not greenish. Once a melon is picked, it won't get any sweeter; but if you leave a melon at room temperature for a day or two, it will get softer and juicier.

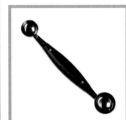

A melon baller makes it easy to prepare attractive fruit salads and desserts. This inexpensive gadget has a different-size scoop at each end.

Festive Melon Bowl *is a simply carved watermelon shell filled with a rainbow of fruit.*

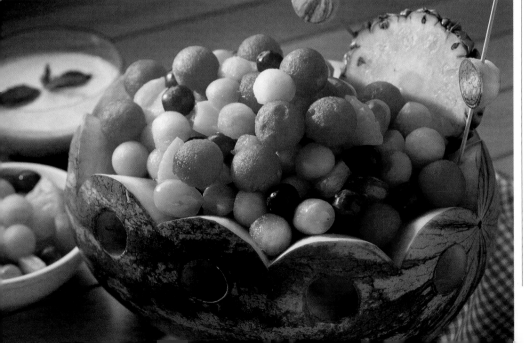

Smoked Turkey & Melon Salad This summertime salad is sparked with a honey-mustard dressing and fresh basil.

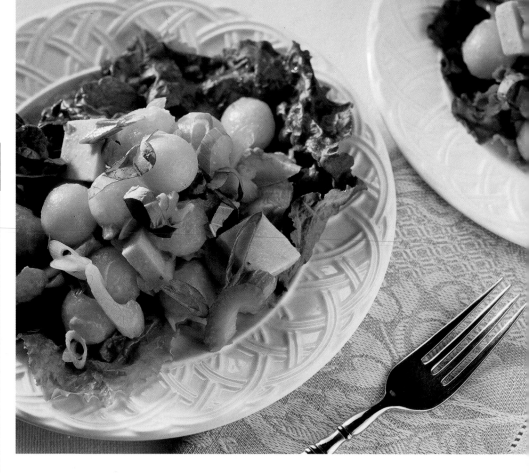

Healthy Highlights

Watermelon

PER 1 CUP

Calories	49
Fiber	0.8g
Protein	1g
Total Fat	0.7g
Saturated Fat	0.1g
Cholesterol	0mg
Sodium	3mg

NUTRIENTS

	% Daily Value
Vitamin C	25%
Vitamin A	11%
Vitamin B6	11%

Did you know? . . .
Watermelon is rich in lycopene, a carotenoid that seems to offer protection against prostate cancer. One large study showed that men who ate 10 or more servings per week of lycopene-rich foods had a 45 percent reduction in prostate cancer risk.

Cut watermelons are a tempting choice because you can more easily judge their ripeness, but keep in mind that melons lose vitamin C when they are cut. If you do buy a half or quarter melon, choose one that's been tightly wrapped in plastic and kept chilled.

Watermelon Ice with Chocolate "Seeds"

PREP: 15 MINUTES
FREEZE: 3 HOURS

This fool-the-eye frozen dessert looks like it's dotted with watermelon seeds, but they're actually chocolate chips. Soften the ice in the refrigerator for 30 minutes before serving.

5	cups cubed watermelon (1½ pounds)
¼	cup corn syrup
¼	cup honey
1	tablespoon lemon juice
¼	cup mini chocolate chips

1. Remove as many seeds as possible from the watermelon cubes. In a food processor or blender, purée the watermelon and push through a strainer if there appear to be any seeds left. In a medium bowl, combine the watermelon purée, ½ cup of water, the corn syrup, honey, and lemon juice.

2. Freeze in an ice cream machine, or, to still-freeze: place in a 9 x 13 x 2-inch pan and freeze for 2 to 3 hours or until almost frozen. Cut into chunks and process in a food processor until smooth. Fold in the chocolate chips, pack into a plastic container, and re-freeze until firm. Serves 6.

Per serving: Calories 158; Fiber 1g; Protein 1g; Total Fat 3g; Saturated Fat 1g; Cholesterol 0mg; Sodium 20mg

Spicy Cantaloupe Antipasto

PREP: 20 MINUTES

Serve this salad soon after you make it; if you leave the cantaloupe in the vinaigrette for too long, the melon juice will dilute the dressing.

¼	cup orange juice
2	tablespoons red wine vinegar
1	tablespoon olive oil
1	tablespoon chopped fresh mint
1	teaspoon honey
½	teaspoon hot red pepper sauce
¼	teaspoon salt

1 cantaloupe, cut into ¾-inch cubes
   (4 cups)
6 ounces part-skim mozzarella
   cheese, cut into ½-inch cubes
   (1½ cups)
3 cups thinly sliced romaine lettuce
1 cup thinly sliced radicchio or red
   cabbage

1. In a large bowl, whisk together
the orange juice, vinegar, oil, mint,
honey, hot pepper sauce, and salt.
Add the cantaloupe and mozzarella,
tossing well to coat.

2. Toss the romaine and radicchio
together and line 4 salad plates with
the mixture. With a slotted spoon, top
the lettuce with the melon-cheese
mixture. Serve the remaining dressing
on the side. Serves 4.

*Per serving: Calories 217; Fiber 2g;
Protein 13g; Total Fat 11g; Saturated Fat 5g;
Cholesterol 25mg; Sodium 370mg*

Smoked Turkey & Melon Salad

PREP: 20 MINUTES

3 cups honeydew and/or cantaloupe
   balls
¾ pound smoked turkey breast, cut
   into ½-inch cubes
½ cup thinly sliced celery
2 scallions, sliced
2 tablespoons slivered fresh basil
2 tablespoons chopped toasted
   walnuts or pecans
2 tablespoons honey-mustard
1 tablespoon white wine vinegar
2 teaspoons olive oil
½ teaspoon soy sauce

1. In a large bowl, toss together the
melon balls, turkey, celery, scallions,
basil, and walnuts.

2. In a small bowl, whisk together the
honey-mustard, vinegar, oil, and soy
sauce. Toss the dressing with the melon
mixture just before serving. Serves 4.

*Per serving: Calories 211; Fiber 2g;
Protein 19g; Total Fat 8g; Saturated Fat 2g;
Cholesterol 36mg; Sodium 869mg*

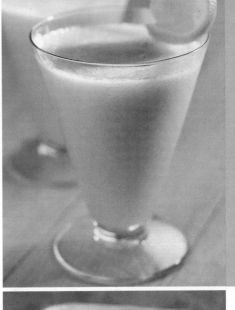

**Virgin Honeydew
Margarita** In blender,
combine 2 cups honey-
dew chunks, ½ cup
orange juice, 1 tbsp.
lime juice, 1 tbsp.
honey, and 4 ice
cubes. Purée. Pour into
2 tall glasses. Serves
2. *[Cal 121; Fat 0g;
Sod 19mg]*

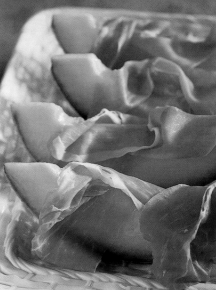

**Prosciutto & Melon
with Honey-Lemon
Dressing** Halve and
seed 1 cantaloupe
(2¾ pounds). Cut into
12 wedges. Drape
each wedge with a thin
slice of prosciutto
using about ¼ lb. total.
Whisk ⅓ cup honey
with ¼ cup lemon
juice. Serve wedges
with the lemon sauce.
Serves 4. *[Cal 208;
Fat 5g; Sod 543mg]*

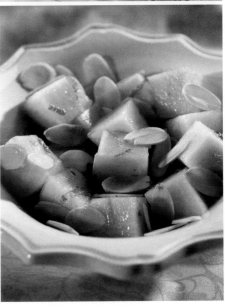

**Melon in Syrup with
Toasted Almonds** In
small saucepan, bring
⅓ cup water, 3 tbsp.
sugar, and 1 tsp.
grated lime zest to a
boil. Boil 3 minutes.
Cool. Add 1½ cups
honeydew cubes and
1½ cups cantaloupe
cubes. Serve sprinkled
with ½ cup toasted
sliced almonds. Serves
4. *[Cal 149; Fat 6g;
Sod 13mg]*

Oranges & Tangerines

Nutritional power
These popular snack fruits are outstanding sources of vitamin C; they also supply folate and fiber as well as flavonoids—cancer-fighting compounds.

Healthy Highlights

Tangerines
PER 1 MEDIUM

Calories	37
Fiber	1.9g
Protein	1g
Total Fat	0.2g
Saturated Fat	0g
Cholesterol	0mg
Sodium	1mg

NUTRIENTS

	% Daily Value
Vitamin C	43%
Vitamin A	16%

Did you know? . . .
Tangerines and oranges contain compounds called terpenes, which seem to limit the body's production of cholesterol. Terpenes also fight cancer by deactivating carcinogens.

Citrus fruits contain pectin, a type of dietary fiber that can lower blood cholesterol levels.

Shrimp & Tangerine Salad

PREP: 25 MINUTES / COOK: 5 MINUTES

This summer-bright salad is a treat in the winter—peak season for tangerines.

- ¾ teaspoon salt
- ½ teaspoon each dried oregano and black pepper
- 1 pound medium shrimp, peeled and deveined
- 6 tangerines or clementines
- 3 tablespoons light mayonnaise
- 2 tablespoons reduced-fat sour cream
- ⅛ teaspoon cayenne pepper
- ½ cup diced red bell pepper
- ½ cup diced green bell pepper
- ¼ cup finely chopped red onion
- 1 stalk celery, halved lengthwise and thinly sliced

1. In a large bowl, combine ¼ teaspoon of the salt, the oregano, and black pepper. Add the shrimp, tossing well to coat; set aside.

2. Separate 5 of the tangerines into sections. Cut each section into thirds and remove the pits. Juice the remaining tangerine and measure out ¼ cup. In a large bowl, whisk together the tangerine juice, mayonnaise, sour cream, cayenne, and remaining ½ teaspoon salt. Add the tangerine sections, bell peppers, onion, and celery.

3. Preheat the broiler. Broil the shrimp 6 inches from the heat for 2 minutes per side or until just cooked through. Cool to room temperature and add to the bowl, tossing to combine. Serve at room temperature or chilled. Serves 4.

Per serving: Calories 214; Fiber 3g; Protein 21g; Total Fat 7g; Saturated Fat 2g; Cholesterol 146mg; Sodium 674mg

Tangerine & Lamb Stir-Fry

PREP: 25 MINUTES / COOK: 10 MINUTES

Bite-size bits of tangerine bring a burst of flavor to this spicy stir-fry.

- 2 tablespoons cornstarch
- 2 tablespoons lower-sodium soy sauce
- 1 teaspoon ground coriander
- 1 teaspoon grated tangerine zest
- ½ teaspoon each sugar and salt
- ⅛ teaspoon cayenne pepper
- 1 pound well-trimmed boneless leg of lamb, cut into ½-inch-wide strips
- 2 teaspoons vegetable oil
- 1 red bell pepper, cut into ½-inch squares
- 3 cloves garlic, minced
- 4 scallions, thinly sliced

½ cup chicken broth
4 tangerines, peeled, separated into sections, halved, and pitted
¼ cup chopped cilantro

1. In a medium bowl, combine 5 teaspoons of the cornstarch, the soy sauce, coriander, tangerine zest, sugar, ¼ teaspoon of the salt, and the cayenne. Add the lamb, tossing well to coat.

2. In a large nonstick skillet, heat 1 teaspoon of the oil over moderately high heat. Add the lamb and stir-fry for 2 minutes or until lightly browned. With a slotted spoon, transfer the lamb to a plate. Reduce the heat to moderate, add the remaining 1 teaspoon oil, the bell pepper, garlic, scallions, and the remaining ¼ teaspoon salt, and stir-fry for 4 minutes or until the pepper is crisp-tender.

3. In a small bowl, whisk the broth into the remaining 1 teaspoon cornstarch. Add to the pan and bring to a boil. Return the lamb to the pan, add

Shrimp & Tangerine Salad *The creamy dressing is made with tangerine juice.*

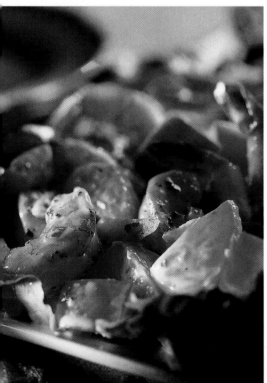

the tangerines, and cook for 1 minute or until the sauce is lightly thickened and the lamb is heated through. Stir in the cilantro. Serves 4.

Per serving: Calories 242; Fiber 3g; Protein 25g; Total Fat 8g; Saturated Fat 2g; Cholesterol 73mg; Sodium 796mg

Frozen Vanilla-Orange Mousse

PREP: 1 HOUR 20 MINUTES
COOK: 5 MINUTES / CHILL: 2 HOURS
This is reminiscent of that classic ice-pop duo: vanilla ice cream and orange sorbet.

1 cup evaporated milk
¼ cup malted milk powder
1 teaspoon grated orange zest
2 envelopes unflavored gelatin
2½ cups orange juice
½ cup sugar
1 teaspoon vanilla extract
⅛ teaspoon salt

1. In a large bowl, with an electric mixer, combine the evaporated milk, malted milk powder, and orange zest. Place in the freezer until ice crystals begin to form, about 1 hour.

2. In a glass measuring cup, sprinkle the gelatin over ½ cup of the orange juice and let stand for 5 minutes or until softened. Place the cup in a pan of simmering water and heat for 4 minutes or until the gelatin has dissolved. Cool to room temperature.

3. Beat the partially frozen evaporated-milk mixture until thick. Gradually beat in the sugar. Add the gelatin mixture. Beat in the remaining 2 cups orange juice, the vanilla, and salt. Spoon into 4 dessert bowls and chill for 2 hours or until set. Serves 4.

Per serving: Calories 326; Fiber 0g; Protein 10g; Total Fat 6g; Saturated Fat 4g; Cholesterol 21mg; Sodium 258mg

At the market
Oranges are widely available all year round; tangerines and their kin are most bountiful in the winter.

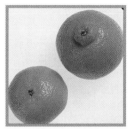

Two members of the tangerine family: the diminutive clementine (left) and the Minneola tangelo (a tangerine-grapefruit cross).

Look for Select firm, heavy oranges and tangerines. Choose thin-skinned oranges such as Valencias for juicing; use navel oranges for snacking and cooking (they're seedless and easy to peel).

Prep Remove all the white pith when peeling an orange. Tangerines are easy to peel but must be seeded: Snip the top of each segment and squeeze out the seeds.

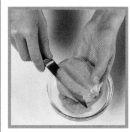

To section an orange, cut along both sides of each dividing membrane to release the segments.

Chicken Bigarade is a delectable, classic French dish that's made without butter or cream.

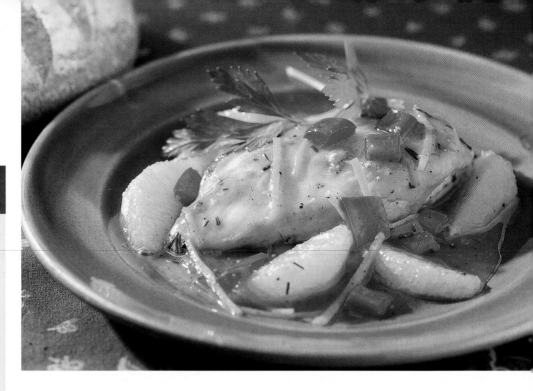

Healthy Highlights

Oranges*
PER 1 MEDIUM

Calories	64
Fiber	3.4g
Protein	1g
Total Fat	0.1g
Saturated Fat	0g
Cholesterol	0mg
Sodium	1mg

NUTRIENTS

	% Daily Value
Vitamin C	133%
Folate	12%

navel

Did you know? . . .
Oranges contain a phytochemical called limonene, which seems to have an anticarcinogenic effect in the body. Oranges also contain glucarase, another cancer-fighting compound, as well as plenty of vitamin C, an antioxidant.

If you usually drink a small glass of orange juice at breakfast, consider eating a whole orange instead: You'll get the same amount of vitamin C, but the whole fruit also provides fiber.

Winter Fruit Shortcakes

PREP: 25 MINUTES / COOK: 15 MINUTES

A creamy, fresh orange filling is sandwiched in a homemade buttermilk biscuit.

- **4** navel oranges
- **2** tablespoons packed light brown sugar
- **⅓** cup plain low-fat yogurt
- **¼** cup reduced-fat sour cream
- **½** teaspoon vanilla extract
- **1** cup flour
- **2** tablespoons granulated sugar
- **1** teaspoon baking powder
- **¼** teaspoon each baking soda and salt
- **2** tablespoons cold unsalted butter
- **1** tablespoon solid vegetable shortening, chilled
- **⅓** cup low-fat (1.5%) buttermilk
- **1** egg white

1. Preheat the oven to 425°F. With a small paring knife, peel the oranges. Working over a bowl to catch the juice, separate the orange sections from the membranes; reserve any juice that collects in the bowl.

2. Transfer the orange segments to a bowl with ¼ cup of the reserved orange juice. Add the brown sugar, yogurt, sour cream, and vanilla, tossing well to combine. Cover and refrigerate while you make the shortcakes.

3. In a medium bowl, combine the flour, 1 tablespoon plus 2 teaspoons of the granulated sugar, the baking powder, baking soda, and salt. With a pastry blender or two knives, cut in the butter and shortening until the mixture resembles coarse meal. Add the buttermilk and stir just until combined.

4. Transfer the mixture to a lightly floured surface and knead 5 or 6 times until the mixture forms a dough. Pat out to a ½-inch-thick round 5 inches in diameter. Cut the round into quarters. Place the wedges on an ungreased baking sheet. Brush with the egg white and sprinkle with the remaining 1 teaspoon sugar. Bake for 15 minutes or until golden brown and baked through.

5. Transfer the biscuits to a wire rack to cool completely. With a serrated knife, slice off the top one-third of the biscuits to create a bottom that is thicker than the top. Spoon the orange mixture over the bottom of each biscuit and add the biscuit top. Serves 4.

Per serving: Calories 368; Fiber 4g; Protein 9g; Total Fat 12g; Saturated Fat 6g; Cholesterol 23mg; Sodium 393mg

Chicken Bigarade

PREP: 15 MINUTES / COOK: 20 MINUTES

A classic bigarade is made with tart Seville oranges. We add vinegar to recreate that zing.

- 1 tablespoon olive oil
- 4 skinless, boneless chicken breast halves (4 ounces each)
- 2 tablespoons flour
- 1 red bell pepper, diced
- 2 tablespoons sugar
- ¼ cup red wine vinegar
- 1 tablespoon thinly slivered orange zest
- ½ cup orange juice
- ½ cup chicken broth
- ½ teaspoon salt
- ¼ teaspoon each rosemary and black pepper
- 1 teaspoon cornstarch blended with 1 tablespoon water
- 2 navel oranges

1. In a large skillet, heat 2 teaspoons of the oil over moderate heat. Dredge the chicken in the flour, shaking off the excess. Sauté the chicken for 2 minutes per side or until lightly golden. Transfer to a plate. Add the bell pepper and the remaining 1 teaspoon oil and sauté for 3 minutes or until crisp-tender. Add to the plate with the chicken.

2. Add the sugar to the pan and cook for 3 minutes or until caramelized. Add the vinegar and cook for 30 seconds. Add the orange zest, orange juice, broth, salt, rosemary, and black pepper, and bring to a boil.

3. Return the chicken and bell pepper to the pan, reduce to a simmer, cover, and cook for 7 minutes or until the chicken is just cooked through. Stir in the cornstarch mixture and boil for 1 minute, stirring, until lightly thickened.

4. Meanwhile, with a small paring knife, peel the oranges. Separate the orange sections from the membranes and stir the segments into the pan. Serve the chicken with the sauce and oranges. Serves 4.

Per serving: Calories 254; Fiber 2g; Protein 28g; Total Fat 5g; Saturated Fat 1g; Cholesterol 66mg; Sodium 496mg

Orange-Banana Breakfast Smoothie

In blender, combine ¾ cup orange juice, ½ cup sliced banana, 2 tsp. brown sugar, and ⅛ tsp. almond extract. Add 2 ice cubes and blend until thick and smooth. Garnish with a mint sprig. Serves 1. *[Cal 189; Fat 1g; Sod 6mg]*

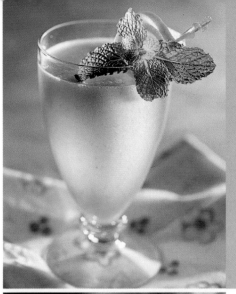

Modern Ambrosia

In large bowl, combine 3 tbsp. honey and 1 tbsp. lime juice. Add 6 peeled and segmented mandarins or clementines, 1 cup diced mango, ⅓ cup flaked coconut, and ¼ cup dried cranberries. Toss well. Serves 4. *[Cal 183; Fat 2g; Sod 19mg]*

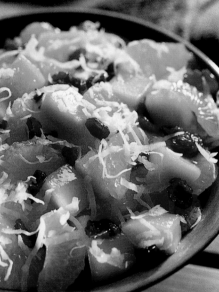

Caramelized Orange Compote

Place 4 peeled and segmented navel oranges in gratin dish or shallow broilerproof baking dish. Sprinkle with ¼ cup brown sugar, ¼ teaspoon cinnamon, and 1 tbsp. slivered orange zest. Broil 2 minutes or until sugar melts. Serves 4. *[Cal 118; Fat 0g; Sod 7mg]*

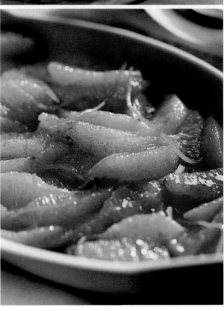

Papayas

Nutritional power

Take your vitamin C in the form of this luscious tropical fruit and you'll replenish potassium and folate, as well. There's a good amount of fiber, too.

Healthy Highlights

PER 1 CUP	
Calories	55
Fiber	2.5g
Protein	1g
Total Fat	0.2g
Saturated Fat	0.1g
Cholesterol	0mg
Sodium	4mg

NUTRIENTS	
	% Daily Value
Vitamin C	145%
Folate	13%
Potassium	12%

Did you know? . . .
Papayas are a wise choice for snacking: Ounce for ounce, papayas contains more than ten times as much vitamin C as apples, and more than twice as much potassium.

An enzyme in uncooked papaya keeps gelatin from setting, so you shouldn't use papaya in gelatin desserts.

Tropical Fruit Salad

PREP: 30 MINUTES

If necessary, you can substitute two nectarines or peaches for the mango—a little less tropical but still delicious.

- ⅓ cup papaya or apricot nectar
- 3 tablespoons lime juice
- 2 tablespoons honey
- ¼ cup chopped fresh mint
- 1 mango (1 pound), peeled and cut into 1-inch chunks
- 1 cup fresh or canned pineapple wedges
- 1 large banana, thickly sliced
- 2 kiwifruits, peeled and cut into ½-inch chunks
- 1 papaya (¾ pound), peeled and cut into ½-inch chunks

1. In a large bowl, whisk together the papaya nectar, lime juice, honey, and mint. Add the mango, pineapple, banana, and kiwi, tossing to combine. Refrigerate until serving time.

2. At serving time, add the papaya and toss again. Serve immediately. Serves 4.

Per serving: Calories 192; Fiber 4g; Protein 2g; Total Fat 1g; Saturated Fat 0g; Cholesterol 0mg; Sodium 9mg

Papaya-Raspberry Crisp

PREP: 10 MINUTES / COOK: 15 MINUTES

The crunchy topping for this crisp covers a tempting combination of fruit that's accented with lemon and, surprisingly, salt and pepper.

- 2 papayas (1½ pounds total), peeled and cut into 1-inch chunks
- 1 teaspoon grated lemon zest
- 2 tablespoons lemon juice
- ¼ teaspoon each salt and pepper
- ⅛ teaspoon ground allspice
- ¾ cup raspberries
- 2 tablespoons granulated sugar
- 2 tablespoons packed light brown sugar
- 1 tablespoon unsalted butter
- 3 tablespoons flour

1. Preheat the oven to 450°F. In an 8-inch round ceramic or glass baking dish, toss together the papayas, lemon zest, lemon juice, salt, pepper, and allspice. Scatter the raspberries on top.

2. In a small bowl, combine the granulated sugar, brown sugar, and butter with your fingers. Mix in the flour until the mixture is crumbly. Sprinkle the crumb mixture over the fruit. Bake for

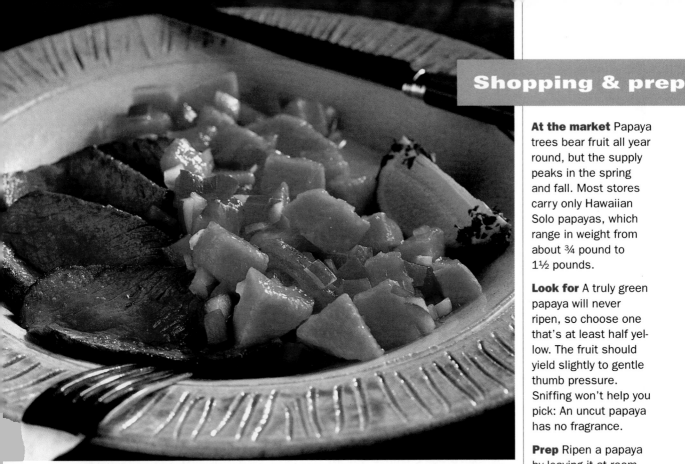

Broiled Steak with Fresh Papaya Chutney *A burst of tropical color and flavor.*

At the market Papaya trees bear fruit all year round, but the supply peaks in the spring and fall. Most stores carry only Hawaiian Solo papayas, which range in weight from about ¾ pound to 1½ pounds.

Look for A truly green papaya will never ripen, so choose one that's at least half yellow. The fruit should yield slightly to gentle thumb pressure. Sniffing won't help you pick: An uncut papaya has no fragrance.

Prep Ripen a papaya by leaving it at room temperature in a paper bag for a few days. When ripe, store it in the refrigerator and use as soon as possible. To serve, just halve the fruit lengthwise and spoon out the seeds, which are edible. Scoop out the flesh with a spoon or melon baller, or peel the papaya halves with a swivel-bladed vegetable peeler.

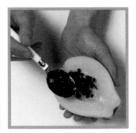

Scoop out papaya seeds with a spoon; you can use them as an edible garnish.

12 to 15 minutes or until the top is lightly browned and set and the fruit is heated through. Serves 4.

Per serving: Calories 180; Fiber 2g; Protein 2g; Total Fat 6g; Saturated Fat 4g; Cholesterol 16mg; Sodium 144mg

Broiled Steak with Fresh Papaya Chutney

PREP: 20 MINUTES / COOK: 10 MINUTES

This freshly made relish is refreshingly different from sticky-sweet bottled chutney. It supplies about 110mg of vitamin C, more than any commercial chutney.

- ¾ teaspoon salt
- ½ teaspoon sugar
- ½ teaspoon dried oregano
- ¼ teaspoon black pepper
- 4 well-trimmed sirloin steaks (6 ounces each)
- 2 papayas (1½ pounds total), peeled and cut into ½-inch chunks
- 1 red bell pepper, cut into ¼-inch dice
- 1 small red onion, cut into ¼-inch dice
- ¼ cup lime juice
- 2 tablespoons apricot jam

1. Preheat the broiler. In a small bowl, combine ½ teaspoon of the salt, the sugar, oregano, and black pepper. Rub the mixture into the steaks; set aside.

2. In a large bowl, combine the papayas, bell pepper, onion, lime juice, jam, and the remaining ¼ teaspoon salt. Cover and refrigerate the fresh chutney until serving time.

3. Place the steaks on the broiler rack and broil 6 inches from the heat for 3 minutes per side for medium-rare. Thinly slice each steak on the diagonal and serve with the chutney. Serves 4.

Per serving: Calories 340; Fiber 2g; Protein 40g; Total Fat 10g; Saturated Fat 4g; Cholesterol 114mg; Sodium 509mg

Peaches & Nectarines

Nutritional power
These closely related tree fruits are good sources of beta carotene, vitamin C, and potassium. They also supply some fiber.

Healthy Highlights

Peaches
PER 1 MEDIUM

Calories	42
Fiber	2.0g
Protein	1g
Total Fat	0.1g
Saturated Fat	0g
Cholesterol	0mg
Sodium	0mg

NUTRIENTS

	% Daily Value
Vitamin A	11%
Vitamin C	10%

Nectarines
PER 1 MEDIUM

Calories	67
Fiber	2.2g
Protein	1g
Total Fat	0.6g
Saturated Fat	0.1g
Cholesterol	0mg
Sodium	0mg

NUTRIENTS

	% Daily Value
Vitamin A	20%
Vitamin C	12%
Potassium	10%

Did you know? . . .
Cooking has very little effect on beta carotene.

Peach-Filled Dessert Crêpes

PREP: 15 MINUTES / COOK: 15 MINUTES

The crêpe batter can be made several hours ahead of time and refrigerated, covered.

- ¾ cup flour
- 1 teaspoon granulated sugar
- ¼ teaspoon salt
- 1 cup low-fat (1%) milk
- 1 egg
- 1 tablespoon unsalted butter, melted
- ⅓ cup peach or apricot nectar
- 2 tablespoons plus 2 teaspoons light brown sugar
- ¼ teaspoon ground ginger
- 1 pound peaches or nectarines, sliced ¼ inch thick
- 2 tablespoons reduced-fat sour cream

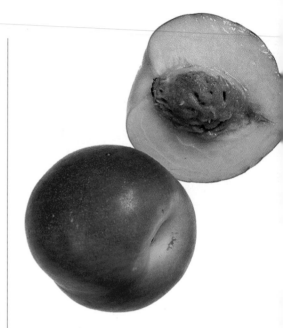

1. In a medium bowl, combine the flour, granulated sugar, and salt. Whisk in the milk, egg, and melted butter until well combined. Let the batter stand for at least 10 minutes.

2. Spray an 8-inch nonstick skillet with nonstick cooking spray and heat over moderate heat. Spoon the batter, a scant ¼ cup at a time, into the pan, swirling so that the batter covers the bottom. Cook for 30 seconds or until lightly browned on the bottom. Turn the crêpe over and cook for 10 seconds on the second side. Transfer the crêpe to a plate and cover with a sheet of wax paper. Continue cooking and stacking the crêpes until you have used all the batter (you should have 8 crêpes).

3. In a large skillet, bring the nectar, 2 tablespoons of the brown sugar, and the ginger to a boil over moderate heat. Add the peaches, reduce to a simmer, and cook for 4 minutes or until the peaches are tender. Reserving the juices in the skillet, remove the peaches with a slotted spoon.

4. In a small bowl, stir together the sour cream and the remaining 2 teaspoons brown sugar. Spoon one-eighth of the peaches (about ¼ cup) in a strip down the center of each crêpe. Fold the sides of the crêpes in over the peaches until they almost meet in the center, then roll up from the short end. Serve drizzled with the reserved pan juices and dolloped with the sweetened sour cream. Serves 4.

Per serving: Calories 255; Fiber 2g; Protein 7g; Total Fat 6g; Saturated Fat 3g; Cholesterol 66mg; Sodium 191mg

Peach Pandowdy

PREP: 25 MINUTES / COOK: 40 MINUTES

Pandowdy is a deep-dish fruit dessert with a sweet, biscuit-like topping. The topping can be simply spooned on (as shown here); or, for a less "dowdy" pandowdy, it can be piped over the fruit in a lattice pattern.

- 3 **pounds large peaches or nectarines, sliced**
- 2 **tablespoons lemon juice**
- ½ **cup finely chopped dried apricots**
- ⅔ **cup packed light brown sugar**
- 1½ **cups flour**
- ¾ **teaspoon cinnamon**
- ¼ **cup granulated sugar**
- 1 **teaspoon baking powder**
- ¼ **teaspoon salt**
- 1 **egg**
- 1 **tablespoon unsalted butter, melted**
- 1 **teaspoon vanilla extract**
- 2 **cups vanilla nonfat frozen yogurt**

1. Preheat the oven to 400°F. In a large bowl, combine the peaches, lemon juice, and apricots. Sprinkle with the brown sugar, ¼ cup of the flour, and the cinnamon, tossing well to combine. Transfer to a 7 x 11-inch baking pan.

2. In a medium bowl, whisk together the remaining 1¼ cups flour with the granulated sugar, baking powder, and salt. Make a well in the center and add the egg, butter, vanilla, and ⅓ cup of water. Whisk the liquid ingredients in the center until blended. Then quickly incorporate the dry ingredients just until blended. Spoon or pipe the topping over the fruit.

3. Bake for 35 to 40 minutes or until the topping is golden and the fruit is bubbly. Serve warm with a scoop of frozen yogurt. Serves 8.

Per serving: Calories 329; Fiber 3g; Protein 5g; Total Fat 2g; Saturated Fat 1g; Cholesterol 30mg; Sodium 169mg

Peach Pandowdy *Serve this old-fashioned dessert warm and "à la mode."*

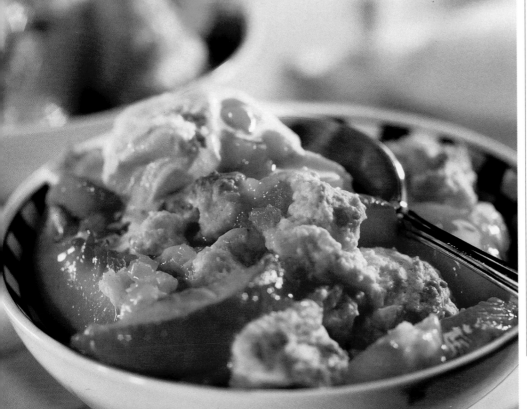

At the market
Domestically grown peaches are available from April through October; nectarines are on the market during the summer months. Imported peaches and nectarines are available at other times of year.

Look for Locally grown peaches and nectarines are tastiest; those grown for shipping are picked when still hard, and these fruits don't ripen further after picking (although they will become softer). Choose fruits with a yellow undertone (not greenish). They should yield slightly to thumb pressure along the "seam."

Prep If a recipe requires you to peel peaches, you'll need to blanch them in boiling water for about 2 minutes—not enough to cook them, but just enough to loosen the skin. Cool the fruit in a bowl of ice water, then peel them.

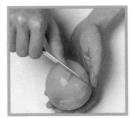

Peaches are easy to peel if you first blanch them briefly in boiling water.

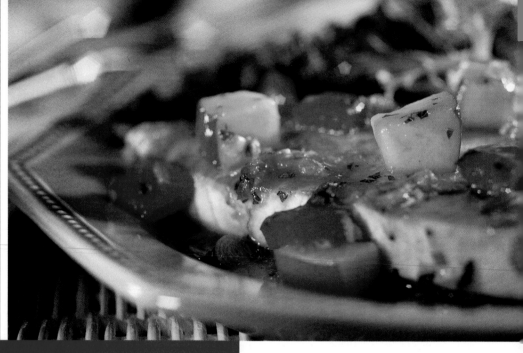

Swordfish with Fresh Nectarine Relish
The chunky fruit "salsa" is sweet, spicy, and touched with the freshness of mint.

Did you know? . . .
Ounce for ounce, a peach or nectarine contains more potassium than a navel orange.

Fully ripe peaches and nectarines supply more vitamin C than do unripe fruits.

Some frozen peaches have as much as 20 percent more vitamin C than fresh peaches. That's because ascorbic acid is added to maintain the fruit's color.

White-fleshed peaches are considered a delicacy, but nutritionally they're inferior to yellow peaches and nectarines, which are a good source of beta carotene.

Peaches and nectarines are not only sweeter, softer, and more fragrant when they're fully ripe; they also contain more vitamin C.

Refrigerator Peach Jam

PREP: 20 MINUTES / COOK: 20 MINUTES

A special type of fruit pectin for making low-calorie preserves lets you create a thick fruit jam with relatively little sugar. If you can't find this type of pectin, you can make tasty refrigerator "preserves" instead. Simply omit the pectin and cook the peaches until slightly thickened.

3	pounds peaches
2	tablespoons lemon juice
1	package (1¾ ounces) fruit pectin for light jam
¼	teaspoon allspice
1	teaspoon cinnamon
3½	cups sugar

1. Bring a large pot of water to a boil. Add the peaches in batches and cook for 2 minutes to blanch. Peel and pit the peaches, transfer them to a large saucepan, and mash them with a potato masher.

2. Add the lemon juice, pectin, allspice, and cinnamon, stirring until the pectin is dissolved. Bring to a full boil over high heat. Add the sugar all at once, stirring constantly. Bring to a full rolling boil and cook for 1 minute. Skim off the foam.

3. Ladle the jam into four 1-pint containers rinsed in boiling water; fill to within ½ inch of the top. Cover with tight lids and let stand at room temperature overnight; then store in the refrigerator for up to 3 weeks. Makes 7 cups.

Per tablespoon: Calories 32; Fiber 0g; Protein 0g; Total Fat 0g; Saturated Fat 0g; Cholesterol 0mg; Sodium 6mg

Peach-Cherry Oat Crumble

PREP: 15 MINUTES / COOK: 25 MINUTES

4	cups sliced peaches
2	cups cherries (8 ounces), pitted and halved
½	cup granulated sugar
1	tablespoon cornstarch
1	teaspoon vanilla extract
½	teaspoon grated lemon zest
⅓	cup old-fashioned rolled oats
3	tablespoons packed light brown sugar
3	tablespoons flour
1½	tablespoons unsalted butter, cut up

1. Preheat the oven to 375° F. Spray a 9-inch glass pie plate with nonstick cooking spray.

2. In a medium saucepan, combine the peaches, cherries, granulated sugar, and cornstarch, and bring to a boil over moderate heat. Remove from the heat and stir in the vanilla and lemon zest. Spoon into the pie plate.

3. In a medium bowl, combine the oats, brown sugar, and flour. With a pastry blender or 2 knives, cut in the butter until the mixture is crumbly. Scatter over the fruit, place the pie plate on a baking sheet, and bake for 20 minutes or until the filling is bubbly and the top is browned. Serve warm or at room temperature. Serves 4.

Per serving: Calories 343; Fiber 4g; Protein 4g; Total Fat 6g; Saturated Fat 3g; Cholesterol 12mg; Sodium 5mg

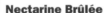

Swordfish with Fresh Nectarine Relish

PREP: 20 MINUTES / COOK: 10 MINUTES

- 2 **tablespoons honey**
- 2 **tablespoons chili sauce**
- 2 **tablespoons red wine vinegar**
- ¼ **teaspoon salt**
- 1 **pound nectarines or peaches, cut into ½-inch cubes**
- 1 **red bell pepper, cut into ½-inch squares**
- 2 **scallions, thinly sliced**
- ¼ **cup chopped fresh mint**
- 4 **swordfish steaks (6 ounces each)**
- ½ **teaspoon each ground coriander and cumin**

1. In a medium bowl, whisk together the honey, chili sauce, vinegar, and salt. Add the nectarines, bell pepper, scallions, and mint, tossing to mix. Refrigerate until serving time.

2. Preheat the broiler. Rub the swordfish with the coriander and cumin. Broil 6 inches from the heat for 3 minutes per side or until lightly browned and just cooked through. Serve topped with the relish. Serves 4.

Per serving: Calories 285; Fiber 2g; Protein 32g; Total Fat 7g; Saturated Fat 2g; Cholesterol 59mg; Sodium 388mg

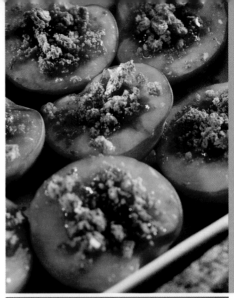

Amaretti-Stuffed Peaches Preheat oven to 350°F. Halve 4 peaches and place cut-sides up in 7 x 11-inch baking dish. Spoon 1 tsp. red currant jelly into each hollow. Spoon 1 crushed amaretti cookie into each hollow. Cover with foil and bake 25 minutes or until tender. Serves 4. *[Cal 97; Fat 1g; Sod 5mg]*

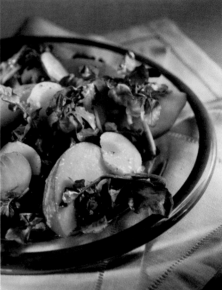

Savory Peach Salad with Watercress In large bowl, combine ¼ cup red wine vinegar, 1 tbsp. Dijon mustard, 1 tbsp. olive oil, ½ tsp. each salt and pepper. Add 2 bunches watercress, 4 peaches or nectarines cut into thick wedges, and ½ cup sliced water chestnuts. Toss well. Serves 4. *[Cal 118; Fat 4g; Sod 401mg]*

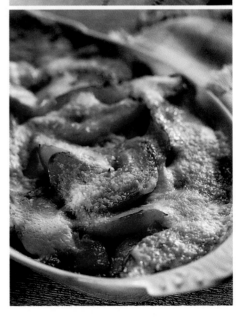

Nectarine Brûlée Preheat oven to 350°F. Cut 4 nectarines or peaches into thin wedges. Toss with 1 tbsp. lemon juice and 1 tbsp. sugar. Spoon into an 8-inch gratin dish (or other broiler-proof pan) and bake 10 minutes. Preheat broiler. Top fruit with ½ cup reduced-fat sour cream. Sprinkle with ⅓ cup brown sugar. Broil 5 minutes or until sugar is melted and bubbly. Serves 4. *[Cal 197; Fat 5g; Sod 24mg]*

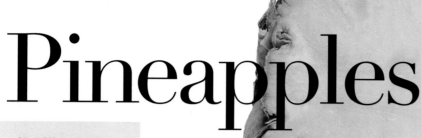

Pineapples

Nutritional power

Serve luscious pineapple in place of candy or cake and you reap the advantages of vitamin C and manganese, a mineral that helps build strong bones.

Healthy Highlights

PER 1 CUP FRESH

Calories	76
Fiber	1.9g
Protein	1g
Total Fat	0.7g
Saturated Fat	0g
Cholesterol	0mg
Sodium	2mg

NUTRIENTS

	% Daily Value
Manganese	128%
Vitamin C	40%

Did you know? . . .
When buying canned pineapple, opt for the juice-packed type; pineapple packed in heavy syrup has lots of added sugar and about 50 calories more per serving.

Fresh pineapple can be used as a meat tenderizer, as it contains an enzyme, bromelain, which breaks down protein. Bromelain is used to make commercial meat tenderizers.

Pineapple-Barbecued Shrimp

PREP: 30 MINUTES / MARINATE: 30 MINUTES / COOK: 5 MINUTES

A grill topper—a smooth, flat, perforated metal grilling "sheet"—is great for shrimp.

- 3 tablespoons honey
- 2 tablespoons lime juice
- ¾ teaspoon chili powder
- ½ teaspoon salt
- ¼ teaspoon crushed red pepper flakes
- 3 cups fresh pineapple chunks (¼ inch)
- ½ cup diced red bell pepper
- ½ cup diced cucumber (¼ inch)
- ¼ cup diced red onion
- ½ cup pineapple juice
- 2 teaspoons olive oil
- ½ teaspoon dried oregano
- 1 pound large shrimp, peeled and deveined

1. In a large bowl, whisk together the honey, lime juice, ¼ teaspoon each of the chili powder and salt, and the red pepper flakes. Add the pineapple, bell pepper, cucumber, and onion, tossing well to combine. Cover the salsa and refrigerate until serving time.

2. In a large bowl, whisk together the pineapple juice, oil, oregano, the remaining ½ teaspoon chili powder and ¼ teaspoon salt. Add the shrimp and toss well. Marinate for 30 minutes.

3. Preheat the broiler (or preheat the grill with a grill topper). Broil the shrimp 6 inches from the heat (or grill 8 inches from the heat) for 2 minutes per side or until just cooked through. Serve with the pineapple salsa. Serves 4.

Per serving: Calories 233; Fiber 2g; Protein 20g; Total Fat 3g; Saturated Fat 1g; Cholesterol 140mg; Sodium 364mg

Pineapple Brown Betty

PREP: 10 MINUTES

Amaretti are Italian almond cookies; light as air, they're made without shortening.

- 4 ounces amaretti cookies (20 medium)
- ¼ cup pecans
- ⅓ cup packed light brown sugar
- 1 tablespoon unsalted butter, cut up
- ½ teaspoon cinnamon
- 1 teaspoon vanilla extract
- 2 cans (20 ounces each) juice-packed pineapple chunks, drained

1. Preheat the oven to 350°F. In a food processor, combine the amaretti, pecans, brown sugar, butter, cinnamon, and vanilla, and pulse until the cookies are finely ground.

2. In an 8-inch square glass baking dish, toss the pineapple with the crumb mixture. Bake for 30 minutes or until the pineapple is piping hot and the crumbs are crusty. Serves 4.

Per serving: Calories 435; Fiber 3g; Protein 4g; Total Fat 11g; Saturated Fat 2g; Cholesterol 8mg; Sodium 24mg

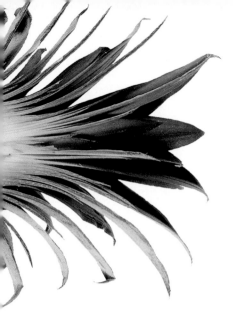

Pineapple Foster

PREP: 15 MINUTES / COOK: 10 MINUTES

Bananas Foster is a beloved New Orleans dessert, created in the 1950s at Brennan's Restaurant. This pineapple variation, in which the fruit is sautéed in butter and brown sugar and then flambéed, will bring raves.

- 4 teaspoons unsalted butter
- 3 tablespoons packed light brown sugar
- ¼ teaspoon ground nutmeg
- 6 slices (¾ inch thick) fresh pineapple, cored and cut into thirds
- 3 tablespoons dark rum
- 2 tablespoons Grand Marnier or other orange liqueur
- 1⅓ cups vanilla frozen yogurt

1. In a large skillet, melt the butter over moderate heat. When it begins to foam, add the brown sugar and nutmeg, and heat until the sugar has melted. Add the pineapple and cook, tossing often, for 4 minutes or until the pineapple is warmed through.

2. Remove the pan from the heat, sprinkle the rum and Grand Marnier over the pineapple, and ignite the alcohol with a long match. Return the pan to the heat and shake until the alcohol burns off.

3. Serve the pineapple slices and sauce with the frozen yogurt. Serves 4.

Per serving: Calories 240; Fiber 2g; Protein 3g; Total Fat 5g; Saturated Fat 3g; Cholesterol 14mg; Sodium 46mg

At the market Fresh pineapples are available all year round.

Look for Once picked, a pineapple won't get any sweeter. Fruit labeled "jet-shipped" is your best bet for peak ripeness. Choose a large, plump, heavy specimen with fresh green leaves; a ripe pineapple may have a sweet fragrance, but if it's chilled, that may not be detectable.

Prep To cut pineapple, first remove the crown (see below). For crosswise slices, first pare off the skin with a sharp knife, then slice the fruit (cut out the woody core after slicing). For chopped fruit, it's simpler to quarter the unpeeled fruit lengthwise and then cut the fruit off the skin before chopping.

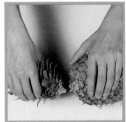

To remove the crown, grasp it in your hand and twist.

Basic cooking The bromelain in fresh pineapple will prevent gelatin from setting. So use only cooked (or canned) pineapple in gelatin desserts.

Pineapple Foster is a seductive pairing of warm sautéed fruit and frozen yogurt.

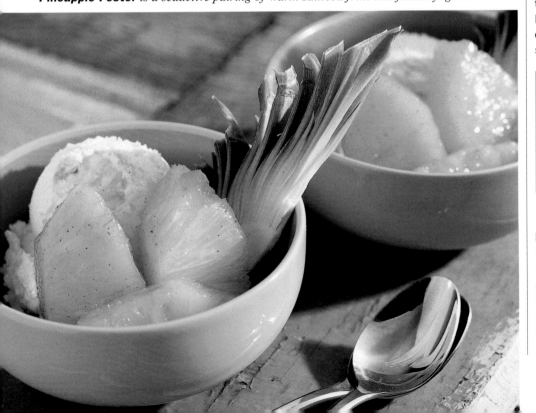

Plums

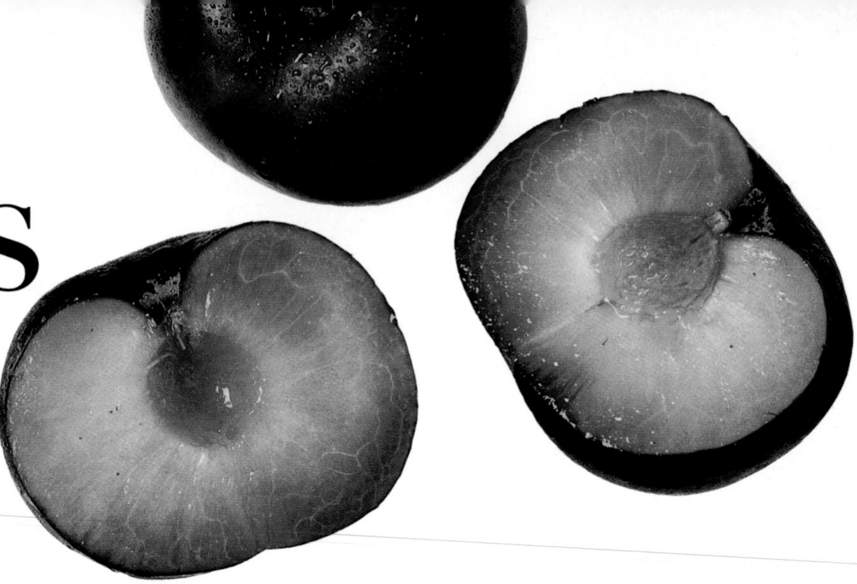

Along with vitamin C, beta carotene, potassium, and fiber, plums are a source of lutein, a lesser-known carotenoid that is lacking in many people's diets.

Healthy Highlights

PER 1 CUP

Calories	91
Fiber	2.5g
Protein	1g
Total Fat	1.0g
Saturated Fat	0.1g
Cholesterol	0mg
Sodium	0mg

NUTRIENTS

	% Daily Value
Vitamin C	27%
Vitamin A	11%
Potassium	10%

Did you know? . . .

Lutein, which is also found in leafy greens, parsley, and pumpkin, helps protect your retinas against the damaging effects of free radicals.

In the USDA's evaluation of total antioxidant capacity of fruits, plums won third place, behind blueberries and strawberries.

Plum Clafouti

PREP: 15 MINUTES / COOK: 45 MINUTES

Clafouti, a rustic recipe from the Limousin region of France, is a charmingly simple dessert best described as a moist oven-baked pancake. The fruit rises to the surface as the batter bakes.

1½	**pounds black or red plums, cut into ⅓-inch-thick wedges**
1	**tablespoon plus ½ cup granulated sugar**
2	**eggs**
2	**egg whites**
½	**cup flour**
1	**cup low-fat (1%) milk**
¼	**cup reduced-fat sour cream**
1	**teaspoon vanilla extract**
1	**teaspoon grated orange zest**
¼	**teaspoon salt**
1	**tablespoon confectioners sugar**

1. Preheat the oven to 400°F. In a medium bowl, toss the plums with 1 tablespoon of the granulated sugar; set the plums aside.

2. In another medium bowl, whisk together the whole eggs, egg whites, and the remaining ½ cup granulated sugar. Slowly beat in the flour, milk, sour cream, vanilla, orange zest, and salt. Arrange the plums in a 10-inch quiche pan or pie plate. Pour the egg mixture over. Bake 30 minutes or until the custard is just set. Dust with the confectioners sugar and serve warm. Serves 6.

Per serving: Calories 241; Fiber 3g; Protein 7g; Total Fat 4g; Saturated Fat 2g; Cholesterol 76mg; Sodium 155mg

Spiced Plum Tart

PREP: 30 MINUTES / CHILL: 1 HOUR
COOK: 40 MINUTES

The plums are sprinkled with a mixture of flour, brown sugar, ginger, and (surprisingly) black pepper. Used in many European gingerbreads and spice cookies, pepper has a bite that points up the ginger's flavor.

1	**cup plus 4 teaspoons flour**
1	**tablespoon granulated sugar**
¼	**teaspoon salt**
3	**tablespoons unsalted butter, cut up**
2	**tablespoons reduced-fat cream cheese (Neufchâtel)**
2	**tablespoons reduced-fat sour cream**
1	**egg white, lightly beaten**
1¼	**pounds purple plums, cut into ¼-inch-thick wedges**
⅓	**cup packed light brown sugar**
¼	**teaspoon ground ginger**
⅛	**teaspoon black pepper (optional)**

1. In a large bowl, combine 1 cup of the flour, the granulated sugar, and salt. With a pastry blender or 2 knives, cut in the butter and cream cheese until the mixture resembles coarse meal. In a small bowl, combine the sour cream and 2 tablespoons ice water. Stir the sour-cream mixture into the flour mixture until just combined. Flatten the dough into a disk, wrap in plastic wrap, and refrigerate for at least 1 hour.

2. Preheat the oven to 375°F. On a lightly floured surface, roll the dough out to a 13-inch round. Place on a baking sheet and roll the edges over once to form a neat edge and an 11-inch circle.

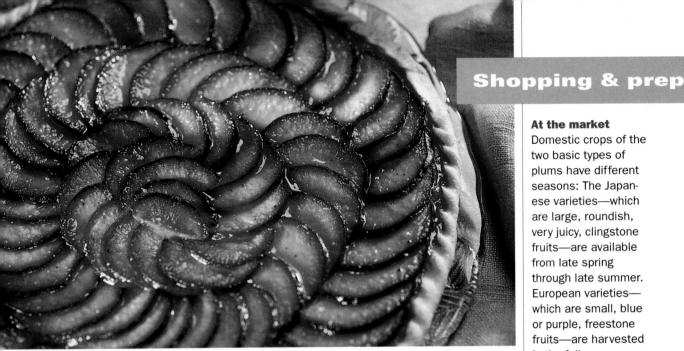

Spiced Plum Tart The secret of its tender low-fat crust is reduced-fat cream cheese.

3. Brush the dough with the egg white. Lay the plum wedges on top in overlapping concentric circles. In a small bowl, combine the brown sugar, ginger, pepper, and the remaining 4 teaspoons flour. Sprinkle evenly over the plums. Bake for 40 minutes or until the plums are tender and the crust is golden. Serves 6.

Per serving: Calories 276; Fiber 3g; Protein 5g; Total Fat 8g; Saturated Fat 5g; Cholesterol 20mg; Sodium 133mg

Stir-Fried Pork with Plums

PREP: 20 MINUTES / COOK: 15 MINUTES

Chinese plum sauce from a jar has little to offer nutritionally, but this stir-fry is made with fresh plums, which supply beta carotene, potassium, and vitamin C.

- **1 tablespoon vegetable oil**
- **1 pound well-trimmed pork tenderloin, cut into 1 x ½-inch strips**
- **1 tablespoon plus 1½ teaspoons cornstarch**
- **1 large carrot, thinly sliced on the diagonal**
- **3 scallions, thinly sliced**
- **2 cloves garlic, minced**
- **1 pound purple, red, or black plums, cut into ½-inch-thick wedges**
- **1 cup chicken broth**
- **2 tablespoons plum jam**
- **1 tablespoon rice or cider vinegar**
- **1 tablespoon lower-sodium soy sauce**
- **½ teaspoon ground ginger**

1. In a large nonstick skillet, heat the oil over moderately high heat. Toss the pork with 1 tablespoon of the cornstarch, rubbing it into the meat. Stir-fry the pork for 5 minutes or until lightly browned and just cooked through. With a slotted spoon, transfer the pork to a plate.

2. Reduce the heat to moderate. Add the carrot, scallions, and garlic to the pan and cook for 1 minute. Add the plums and cook for 4 minutes or until they begin to soften.

3. In a small bowl, whisk together the broth, jam, vinegar, soy sauce, ginger, and the remaining 1½ teaspoons cornstarch. Pour into the skillet and bring to a boil. Boil for 1 minute. Reduce to a simmer, return the pork to the pan, and cook for 2 minutes or until heated through. Serves 4.

Per serving: Calories 287; Fiber 4g; Protein 26g; Total Fat 8g; Saturated Fat 2g; Cholesterol 74mg; Sodium 485mg

At the market
Domestic crops of the two basic types of plums have different seasons: The Japanese varieties—which are large, roundish, very juicy, clingstone fruits—are available from late spring through late summer. European varieties—which are small, blue or purple, freestone fruits—are harvested in the fall.

Look for Red, yellow, green, purple, or "black" (really blue-black), plums offer many varieties to choose from. Pick firm (but not hard) plums that are full and plump, not shriveled or bruised. For recipes that require the plums to be pitted, freestone varieties, such as Italian prune-plums, are the best choice.

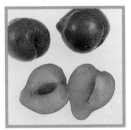

The Kelsey plum is a Japanese variety that turns a red-blushed gold as it ripens. It can be used interchangeably with other Japanese plums.

Prunes

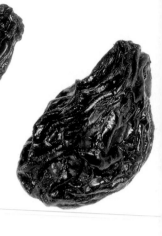
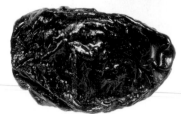
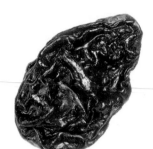

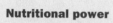

Nutritional power
These dried plums are a highly nutritious snack and a healthful cooking ingredient. They're rich in beta carotene, potassium, iron, and fiber.

Healthy Highlights

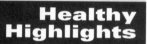

PER ¼ CUP	
Calories	102
Fiber	3.0g
Protein	1g
Total Fat	0.2g
Saturated Fat	0g
Cholesterol	0mg
Sodium	2mg

NUTRIENTS	
	% Daily Value
Vitamin A	17%
Potassium	11%

Did you know? . . .
Prune butter can replace up to half the shortening in many baking recipes —a substitution that greatly cuts fat and increases fiber and nutrient content. Baked goods with intense flavors, such as chocolate cookies or spice cake, are good candidates for this trick. To make 1 cup of prune butter, process 8 ounces of pitted prunes with 6 tablespoons of water in a food processor.

Pork & Prunes with Port

PREP: 15 MINUTES / COOK: 30 MINUTES

The heady flavor of port—a sweet, fortified red wine—adds a deep, rich "bass note" to the complex flavors of this dish. The pork and prunes are cooked in a sauce that also includes scallions, garlic, and mustard.

- 1 tablespoon olive oil
- 1 pound well-trimmed pork tenderloin, cut into 8 slices
- 2 tablespoons flour
- 1 yellow or red bell pepper, cut into ½-inch squares
- 2 scallions, thinly sliced
- 1 clove garlic, minced
- ½ cup dry red wine
- ½ cup ruby port
- ½ cup chicken broth
- 1½ cups pitted prunes (8 ounces)
- 2 teaspoons Dijon mustard
- ½ teaspoon each salt and black pepper

1. In a large nonstick skillet, heat the oil over moderate heat. Dredge the pork in the flour, shaking off the excess. Sauté for 2 minutes per side or until lightly browned. With a slotted spoon, transfer the pork to a plate.

2. Add the bell pepper, scallions, and garlic, and sauté for 4 minutes or until the pepper is crisp-tender. Add the wine and port, increase the heat to high, and cook for 3 minutes or until slightly reduced.

3. Add the broth, prunes, mustard, salt, and black pepper; reduce the heat to low and cook for 5 minutes.

4. Return the pork to the pan and cook for 7 to 10 minutes or until the pork is cooked through but still juicy and the prunes are tender. Serves 4.

Per serving: Calories 379; Fiber 5g; Protein 26g; Total Fat 8g; Saturated Fat 2g; Cholesterol 74mg; Sodium 546mg

Curry Cream-Stuffed Prunes

PREP: 25 MINUTES / COOK: 10 MINUTES

For this tempting hors d'oeuvre, look for the extra-large prunes that are often sold loose (in gourmet shops and health-food stores); the smaller packaged prunes can be tedious to stuff. If you don't have—or don't care for— crystallized ginger, substitute 2 tablespoons of chopped mango chutney.

- ¼ cup walnuts
- 3 ounces reduced-fat cream cheese (Neufchâtel)
- 1 tablespoon milk
- 2 tablespoons finely chopped crystallized ginger
- ½ teaspoon curry powder
- ¼ teaspoon black pepper
- 24 large pitted prunes

1. Preheat the oven to 350°F. In a small baking pan, toast the walnuts for 7 minutes or until fragrant and crisp.

When cool enough to handle, finely chop the walnuts.

2. In a medium bowl, stir the cream cheese and milk together until soft. Stir in the crystallized ginger, curry powder, pepper, and toasted walnuts.

3. With a paring knife, make a slit in each prune. Spoon the cream cheese mixture into the prunes. Serves 6.

Per serving: Calories 188; Fiber 4g; Protein 3g; Total Fat 6g; Saturated Fat 2g; Cholesterol 10mg; Sodium 68mg

Spiced Prunes

PREP: 15 MINUTES / COOK: 20 MINUTES

If you're looking for a change from apple- or cranberry sauce, cook up a pot of these fragrant, exotically spiced prunes. Try them with roast chicken, turkey, or pork.

- ⅔ **cup red wine vinegar**
- ⅓ **cup sugar**
- ½ **teaspoon each ground ginger, salt, and black pepper**
- ½ **teaspoon mustard seeds**
- ⅛ **teaspoon ground allspice**
- 1 **box (12 ounces) pitted prunes, halved**
- 1 **red bell pepper, cut into ½-inch squares**
- 1 **tomato, cut into ½-inch cubes**
- 1 **small red onion, cut into ½-inch cubes**
- 1 **teaspoon vanilla extract**

1. In a medium saucepan, combine the vinegar, sugar, ginger, salt, black pepper, mustard seeds, and allspice. Bring to a boil over moderate heat.

2. Stir in the prunes, bell pepper, tomato, and onion. Return to a boil, reduce to a simmer, cover, and cook for 10 minutes. Uncover and cook for 5 minutes or until the prunes are tender and the liquid is reduced to a thick syrup. Stir in the vanilla. Serve warm, at room temperature, or chilled. Makes 3½ cups.

Per ¼ cup: Calories 86; Fiber 2g; Protein 1g; Total Fat 0g; Saturated Fat 0g; Cholesterol 0mg; Sodium 86mg

At the market Dried prunes, whole or pitted, are sold in bags, boxes, and cans, and also in bulk. You can buy jars or cans of cooked prunes packed in light or heavy sugar syrup, as well as prune butter, which can replace fat in baking (see "Did you know?" on opposite page).

Look for When buying prunes in bulk, shop where the fruit is kept in closed containers, and check to be sure that the prunes are still plump and moist.

Prep To remove the pits, snip each prune with kitchen shears dipped in hot water (to keep the blades from sticking). Squeeze out the pits.

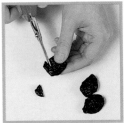

It's easier to snip prunes with scissors than to chop them with a knife. Dip the blades in hot water, or oil them lightly, to keep them from sticking.

Spiced Prunes *are a fine accompaniment for roast meat or poultry.*

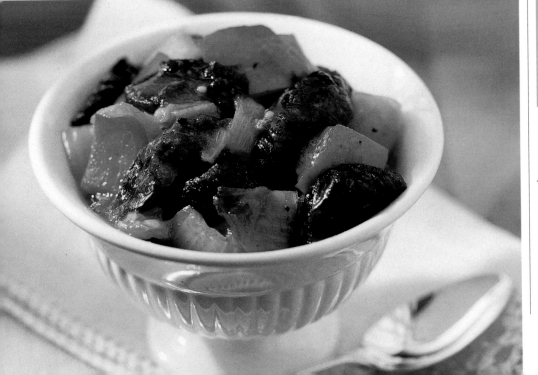

Blackberries & Raspberries

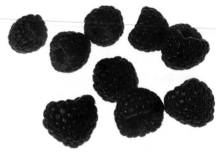

Nutritional power

These luscious berries are loaded with pectin, a type of fiber that can lower cholesterol; they also contain cancer-fighting ellagic acid and carotenoids.

Healthy Highlights

Blackberries
PER 1 CUP

Calories	75
Fiber	7.6g
Protein	1g
Total Fat	0.6g
Saturated Fat	0g
Cholesterol	0mg
Sodium	0mg

NUTRIENTS

	% Daily Value
Vitamin C	50%

Raspberries
PER 1 CUP

Calories	60
Fiber	8.4g
Protein	1g
Total Fat	0.7g
Saturated Fat	0g
Cholesterol	0mg
Sodium	0mg

NUTRIENTS

	% Daily Value
Vitamin C	52%

Did you know? . . .
One cup of raspberries or blackberries supplies roughly one-third of your daily fiber requirement.

Raspberry Coffeecake

PREP: 30 MINUTES / COOK: 40 MINUTES

Crunchy walnut streusel covers juicy berries that in turn top a light, lemony cake.

- ¼ cup packed light brown sugar
- 2 tablespoons chopped walnuts
- 1 teaspoon cinnamon
- 2 tablespoons plus 2 cups flour
- 2 tablespoons vegetable oil
- 2 tablespoons unsalted butter, melted
- 1 cup granulated sugar
- 1 tablespoon baking powder
- ¾ teaspoon salt
- 1 egg
- 1 cup low-fat (1.5%) buttermilk
- 1 teaspoon grated lemon zest
- 2 cups fresh or frozen unsweetened raspberries
- ¼ cup seedless raspberry jam

1. Preheat the oven to 400°F. Spray a 9-inch square baking pan with nonstick cooking spray.

2. In a small bowl, combine the brown sugar, walnuts, cinnamon, and 2 table-spoons of the flour. In another small bowl, blend the oil and butter. Add 1 tablespoon of the butter mixture to the walnut mixture and stir until crumbly.

3. In a large bowl, stir together the remaining 2 cups flour, the granulated sugar, baking powder, and salt until combined. Make a well in the center. Add the egg, buttermilk, lemon zest, and the remaining butter mixture. Blend the wet ingredients, then stir in the dry ingredients just until combined.

4. Scrape the batter into the prepared pan. Top with the raspberries and dab on the jam. Sprinkle with the walnut topping. Bake for 40 minutes or until a cake tester inserted in the center comes out clean. Serves 8.

Per serving: Calories 378; Fiber 3g; Protein 6g; Total Fat 9g; Saturated Fat 3g; Cholesterol 36mg; Sodium 421mg

No-Bake Raspberry Cheesecake

PREP: 30 MINUTES / COOK: 5 MINUTES
CHILL: 4 HOURS

- 1 cup evaporated skimmed milk
- 3 cups fresh or frozen unsweetened raspberries, thawed
- 1 cup sugar
- 2 teaspoons cornstarch mixed with 1 tablespoon water
- 2 packages unflavored gelatin
- 1 package (8 ounces) nonfat cream cheese
- 1 package (8 ounces) reduced-fat cream cheese (Neufchâtel)
- 2 cups low-fat (1%) cottage cheese
- ½ cup reduced-fat sour cream
- 2 teaspoons grated lemon zest
- 2 tablespoons lemon or lime juice

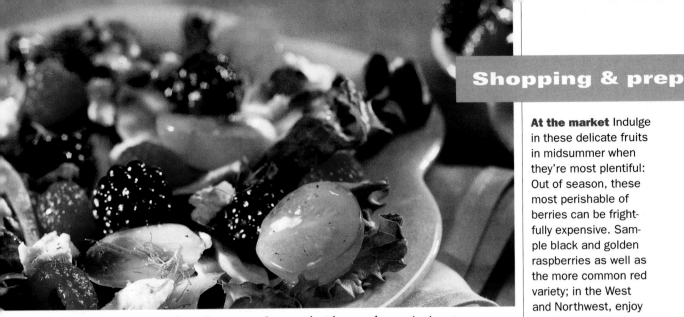

Savory Berry Salad *The fruit flavor is underscored with a raspberry vinaigrette.*

At the market Indulge in these delicate fruits in midsummer when they're most plentiful: Out of season, these most perishable of berries can be frightfully expensive. Sample black and golden raspberries as well as the more common red variety; in the West and Northwest, enjoy locally grown blackberry variants—loganberries, boysenberries, marionberries, and olallieberries. Unsweetened frozen berries can stand in for fresh in many recipes.

Look for Be sure that these fragile berries are in good condition, uncrushed and free of mold. If the bottom of the box is stained, some of the berries have gotten mashed.

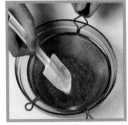

A seedless raspberry sauce is a delectable luxury. To eliminate the seeds, use a rubber spatula to press the berry purée through a sieve.

1. Pour the evaporated milk into a metal bowl; place in the freezer until ice crystals form. Spray a 9-inch springform with nonstick cooking spray.

2. Meanwhile, in a blender or food processor, purée 1 cup of the raspberries and strain through a sieve into a small saucepan. Add ¼ cup of the sugar and the cornstarch mixture. Bring to a simmer, stirring, and cook for 1 minute or until thickened. Set aside to cool slightly.

3. Place the gelatin in a small bowl and sprinkle on ⅓ cup of cold water to soften. Place the bowl over a pan of simmering water and stir to dissolve the gelatin. In a food processor, combine the cream cheeses, cottage cheese, sour cream, lemon zest, lemon juice, and the remaining ¾ cup sugar, and process until smooth. Add the dissolved gelatin and process until smooth. Scrape into a large bowl and refrigerate until the mixture begins to mound.

4. With an electric mixer, whip the partially frozen evaporated milk until soft peaks form. Fold half of the raspberry sauce into the cream-cheese mixture, then fold in the whipped milk. Fold in the remaining 2 cups raspberries. Scrape the mixture into the prepared springform pan. Dollop the remaining raspberry sauce on top and

swirl it with a knife. Chill for 3 to 4 hours or until set. Remove the sides of the springform and slice. Serves 8.

Per serving: Calories 307; Fiber 2g; Protein 19g; Total Fat 7g; Saturated Fat 5g; Cholesterol 25mg; Sodium 547mg

Savory Berry Salad
PREP: 15 MINUTES

- ¼ **cup raspberry vinegar or balsamic vinegar**
- 4 **teaspoons olive oil**
- 2 **teaspoons honey**
- 2 **teaspoons Dijon mustard**
- ¼ **teaspoon each salt and pepper**
- 8 **cups torn mixed salad greens**
- 1 **cup thinly sliced fennel or celery**
- 1 **cup raspberries**
- 1 **cup blackberries**
- 1 **cup yellow cherry tomatoes, halved**
- 2 **ounces mild goat cheese, crumbled**

1. In a small bowl, whisk together the vinegar, oil, honey, mustard, salt, and pepper.

2. Arrange the greens on 4 salad plates. Top with the fennel, raspberries, blackberries, tomatoes, and goat cheese. Drizzle with the dressing. Serves 4.

Per serving: Calories 170; Fiber 5g; Protein 5g; Total Fat 8g; Saturated Fat 3g; Cholesterol 7mg; Sodium 303mg

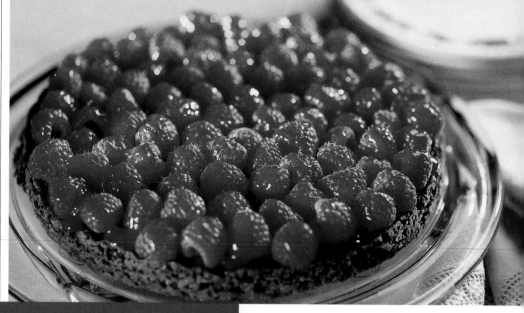

Raspberry-Topped Brownie Cake

Treat family or guests to this luscious combination of chocolate and berries.

Did you know? . . .
The high fiber content of raspberries and blackberries is due in large part to the fact that they are usually eaten seeds and all.

Raspberries and blackberries contain at least five cancer-fighting phytochemicals.

The Evergreen variety of blackberry, long popular in the Northwest, has the highest fiber content of all blackberry varieties.

Along with ellagic acid and beta carotene, blackberries and raspberries contain other cancer-fighting phytochemicals: monoterpenes, catechins, and phenolic acids. Monoterpenes also inhibit cholesterol production.

If you're seeking a potassium source, consider blackberries, which are superior to blueberries, cranberries, raspberries, and strawberries in potassium content. This vital mineral helps to regulate blood pressure.

Raspberry-Topped Brownie Cake

PREP: 15 MINUTES / COOK: 30 MINUTES

- 2 **tablespoons vegetable oil**
- 2 **tablespoons unsweetened cocoa powder**
- 1 **egg**
- ¾ **cup sugar**
- ½ **cup flour**
- ¼ **teaspoon baking soda**
- ¼ **teaspoon salt**
- ¼ **cup coarsely chopped pecans**
- 3 **cups raspberries**
- 1 **tablespoon cornstarch mixed with 2 tablespoons water**

1. Preheat the oven to 350°F. Spray an 8-inch round cake pan with nonstick cooking spray. In a large bowl, combine the oil, cocoa powder, egg, ¼ cup of water, ½ cup of the sugar, the flour, baking soda, and salt. Mix until well combined. Fold in the nuts. Pour the batter into the prepared pan and bake for 20 minutes or until a toothpick inserted in the center comes out clean. Cool in the pan on a rack.

2. Meanwhile, in a medium saucepan, combine 1½ cups of the raspberries and the remaining ¼ cup sugar, and cook, stirring, for 4 minutes or until the berries are juicy. Stir in the cornstarch mixture and cook, stirring, for 4 minutes or until thickened. Strain through a sieve to remove the seeds. Cool for 10 minutes, then spoon over the brownie base. Arrange the remaining 1½ cups berries on top. Serves 8.

Per serving: Calories 193; Fiber 3g; Protein 3g; Total Fat 7g; Saturated Fat 1g; Cholesterol 27mg; Sodium 115mg

Raspberry Swirl Sorbet

PREP: 25 MINUTES / FREEZE: 4 HOURS

- 2 **mangoes, peeled and pitted**
- 2 **tablespoons lime juice**
- ½ **cup sugar**
- ¼ **cup plus 2 tablespoons honey**
- 2 **cups fresh or frozen unsweetened raspberries**
- ⅓ **cup seedless raspberry jam**

1. In a food processor, purée the mangoes with ¾ cup of water, the lime juice, sugar, and ¼ cup of the honey. Place in a metal pan and freeze for 2 to 3 hours or until almost frozen.

2. Meanwhile, in the food processor, purée the raspberries, jam, and the remaining 2 tablespoons honey. Strain through a sieve to remove the seeds. Place in a metal pan and freeze for 2 to 3 hours or until almost frozen.

3. Cut the frozen mango purée into chunks and process in a food processor until smooth; transfer to a bowl. Repeat the process with the raspberry purée. Add the raspberry sorbet to the mango sorbet, swirl together, and return to the freezer to refreeze. Serves 6.

Per serving: Calories 238; Fiber 3g; Protein 1g; Total Fat 0g; Saturated Fat 0g; Cholesterol 0mg; Sodium 10mg

Summer Pudding

PREP: 25 MINUTES / CHILL: 8 HOURS

This classic British dessert is a sort of uncooked bread pudding. As the pudding stands, the berry juice saturates the bread.

- **2 cups blackberries**
- **2 cups raspberries**
- **1 cup blueberries**
- **½ cup seedless raspberry jam**
- **¼ cup honey**
- **¼ cup sugar**
- **1 tablespoon lemon juice**
- **10 slices firm-textured white sandwich bread, crusts removed**
- **⅓ cup heavy cream, whipped**

1. In a medium saucepan, combine the blackberries, raspberries, blueberries, jam, honey, and sugar. Bring to a simmer and cook for 2 minutes. Stir in the lemon juice and set aside to cool.

2. Line a 1-quart soufflé dish or mixing bowl with plastic wrap, leaving a 5-inch overhang. Slice the bread in half on the diagonal and line the bottom and sides of the dish (there will be bread left over for the top).

3. Spoon the berries and juices into the bowl. Cover with the remaining bread, trimming all sides. Cover with plastic wrap and fold the overhang over the top. Weight down with a skillet or heavy can. Refrigerate for at least 8 hours. Unmold onto a serving plate, remove the plastic, cut into wedges, and serve with the whipped cream. Serves 8.

Per serving: Calories 259; Fiber 4g; Protein 3g; Total Fat 5g; Saturated Fat 3g; Cholesterol 14mg; Sodium 166mg

Spicy Raspberry Vinegar In medium bowl, crush 2 cups raspberries with 2 tbsp. sugar. Transfer to large jar with 3 cups distilled white vinegar, 1 tsp. red pepper flakes, and let stand 24 hours. Drain. Makes 3 cups. *[1 tbsp. serving: Cal 5; Fat 0g; Sod 0mg]*

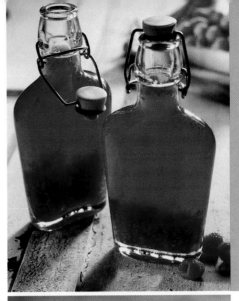

Blackberry Fool In food processor, purée 2 cups blackberries with ½ cup sugar. Stir in ½ cup reduced-fat sour cream. Whip 1 cup very well chilled evaporated whole milk until stiff peaks form. Fold in the blackberry mixture. Serves 4. *[Cal 269; Fat 9g; Sod 83mg]*

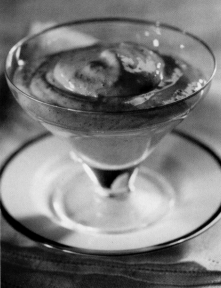

Raspberry Dessert Sauce Purée 12-oz. bag thawed frozen unsweetened raspberries with ¼ cup honey, 2 tbsp. orange juice, and 1 tsp. vanilla. Strain out seeds. Serves 4. *[Cal 118; Fat 1g; Sod 1mg]*

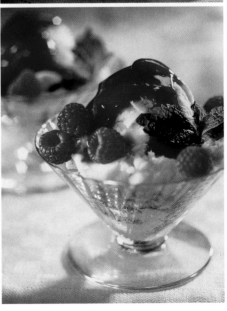

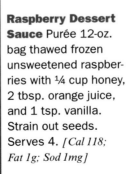

Strawberries

Nutritional power
Strawberries are a primary source of ellagic acid, a phytochemical that fights carcinogens. Strawberries are also an excellent source of vitamin C and fiber.

Healthy Highlights

PER 1 CUP SLICED	
Calories	50
Fiber	3.8g
Protein	1g
Total Fat	0.6g
Saturated Fat	0g
Cholesterol	0mg
Sodium	2mg

NUTRIENTS	
	% Daily Value
Vitamin C	157%
Manganese	24%

Did you know? . . .
In the USDA's assessment of the antioxidant power of various fruits, strawberries placed second, after blueberries.

One cup of strawberries supplies more vitamin C than a whole orange.

Strawberries contain respectable amounts of folate—a heart-healthy B vitamin—and potassium.

Strawberry-Ricotta Crêpes

PREP: 25 MINUTES / STAND: 30 MINUTES
COOK: 15 MINUTES

- ½ cup milk
- ⅓ cup flour
- 1 teaspoon plus ¼ cup granulated sugar
- 1 egg
- 1 egg white
- 2 teaspoons unsalted butter, melted
- ¼ teaspoon salt
- 1 cup part-skim ricotta cheese
- 1 teaspoon vanilla extract
- 3 cups strawberries, hulled and thinly sliced, plus 4 whole strawberries for garnish
- 1 tablespoon confectioners sugar

1. In a blender, combine the milk, flour, 1 teaspoon of the granulated sugar, the whole egg, egg white, melted butter, and salt. Process until smooth. Let stand for 30 minutes.

2. Spray an 8-inch nonstick skillet with nonstick cooking spray. Heat over moderate heat. Spoon the batter, a generous 2 tablespoons at a time, into the pan and swirl to coat the bottom. Cook for 15 seconds or until lightly browned on the bottom. Lift and turn the crêpe over and cook for 5 seconds or until cooked through. Slide the crêpe onto a plate, cover with wax paper, and continue making crêpes and stacking them with sheets of wax paper in between. You will need 8 crêpes (if you are adept at making crêpes, you may get more than 8).

3. In a large bowl, combine the ricotta, vanilla, and the remaining ¼ cup granulated sugar. Fold in the strawber-ries. Spoon the mixture onto the center of each crêpe, fold the ends over, and roll up. Place 2 crêpes on each of 4 dessert plates, sprinkle with the confectioners sugar, and garnish with a whole strawberry. Serves 4.

Per serving: Calories 286; Fiber 3g; Protein 12g; Total Fat 11g; Saturated Fat 5g; Cholesterol 82mg; Sodium 266mg

Strawberry Salad

PREP: 25 MINUTES / COOK: 10 MINUTES
If the idea of strawberries in a savory salad sounds odd to you, remember that tomatoes, like strawberries, are juicy red fruits!

- ¼ cup pecan halves
- 4 cups strawberries, hulled
- 2 tablespoons balsamic vinegar
- 2 teaspoons olive oil
- 1 teaspoon light brown sugar
- ¼ teaspoon each salt and pepper
- 6 cups Boston lettuce, torn into bite-size pieces
- 1 cucumber, peeled, halved lengthwise, seeded, and thinly sliced
- ¼ cup snipped fresh dill
- 4 ounces mild goat cheese, thinly sliced

1. Preheat the oven to 350°F. In a small baking pan, toast the pecans for 7 minutes or until crisp. When cool enough to handle, coarsely chop.

2. In a large salad bowl, mash ½ cup of the strawberries. Thickly slice the remaining strawberries; set aside.

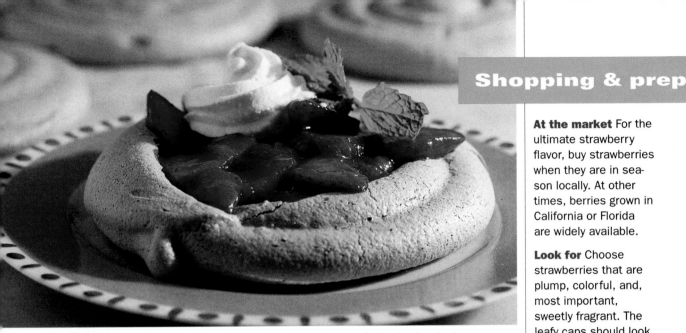

Strawberry Angel Tarts *A mint sprig is a fine finishing touch for this lovely dessert.*

At the market For the ultimate strawberry flavor, buy strawberries when they are in season locally. At other times, berries grown in California or Florida are widely available.

Look for Choose strawberries that are plump, colorful, and, most important, sweetly fragrant. The leafy caps should look fresh and green. Check the bottom of the box —stains there suggest that the berries at the bottom may be crushed or spoiled.

Prep Rinse berries in cold water, then hull them (see below). If you hull the berries *before* rinsing, they will absorb excess water.

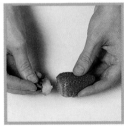

Hulling a strawberry involves more than removing the leafy caps; you also need to remove the white "core" attached to the cap. Use a small paring knife to dig it out.

3. Whisk the vinegar, oil, brown sugar, salt, and pepper into the mashed strawberries. Add the lettuce, cucumber, dill, and sliced strawberries, tossing to combine. Sprinkle the salad with the goat cheese and pecans. Serves 4.

Per serving: Calories 211; Fiber 6g; Protein 8g; Total Fat 14g; Saturated Fat 5g; Cholesterol 13mg; Sodium 258mg

Strawberry Angel Tarts

PREP: 30 MINUTES
COOK: 1 HOUR 5 MINUTES

These tarts are miniature versions of the meringue-based angel pie.

4	large egg whites
¼	teaspoon cream of tartar
1	cup sugar
3	tablespoons unsweetened cocoa powder, sifted
1	teaspoon vanilla extract
4	cups strawberries, hulled
3	tablespoons seedless raspberry jam
2	teaspoons cornstarch blended with 1 tablespoon water
¼	cup heavy cream, whipped

1. Preheat the oven to 300°F. Line a baking sheet with parchment paper. Draw four 4½-inch circles on the parchment; set aside. In a large bowl, with an electric mixer, beat the egg whites and cream of tartar until soft peaks form. Gradually add the sugar and beat until stiff peaks form. Fold in the cocoa and vanilla.

2. Spoon the mixture into a pastry bag without a tip or into a heavy-duty plastic bag with a small bit of one corner cut off. Pipe the mixture in a spiral on the 4 circles, making 4 flat disks. Bake the disks for 1 hour or until the meringue is set. Remove the tart shells and cool to room temperature.

3. Meanwhile, place 1 cup of the strawberries in a small saucepan and mash with a potato masher. Slice the remaining strawberries and set aside. Stir the jam into the mashed berries and bring to a boil over moderate heat. Stir in the cornstarch mixture and cook, stirring constantly, for 1 minute. Off the heat, stir in the sliced berries.

4. Just before serving, beat the cream until stiff peaks form. With the back of a spoon, break the center of the cooled meringue shells to create a depression. Spoon the strawberry mixture onto the shells. Top with the whipped cream. Serves 4.

Per serving: Calories 361; Fiber 5g; Protein 6g; Total Fat 7g; Saturated Fat 4g; Cholesterol 20mg; Sodium 70mg

A

Acorn squash, about, 120
   apricot-maple acorn squash, 121
Alfredo, fettuccine, with green
   noodles, 132
Allyl sulfides, 10, 86
Almonds, about, 194-196
   almond brittle, 194
   brown rice & nut pilaf, 171
   chicken salad with almond
     dressing, 197
   chocolate-almond bars, 197
   fig & almond cookies, 302
   granola macaroons, 164
   green beans amandine, 197
   melon in syrup with toasted
     almonds, 317
   pasta with almond-basil pesto, 196
   pumpkin-date muffins with
     almonds, 118
Alpha carotene, 46
Ambrosia, modern, 321
Amino acids, about, 10
Anthocyanosides, 296
Antioxidants, about, 10
Appetizers/first courses. *See also*
   Salsas; Soups
   artichokes with lemon-herb
     mayonnaise, 44
   avocado & ham antipasto with
     guacamole dressing, 292
   baked spinach-stuffed clams, 220
   California crab roll, 222
   caprese salad, 115
   curried lentil dip, 185
   curry cream-stuffed prunes, 332
   garlic-dill yogurt cheese, 129
   hummus, 180
   liptauer cheese, 132
   mockamole, 93
   mushroom roll-ups, 156
   prosciutto & melon with honey-
     lemon dressing, 317
   raspberry yogurt cheese, 129
   scallion pancakes, 84
   scallion-pepper yogurt cheese, 129
   shrimp cocktail, 231
   spiced walnuts, 197
   spicy cantaloupe antipasto, 316
   tomato bruschetta, 112
   vegetable antipasto, 67
   vegetable-stuffed mushrooms, 82
   white bean garlic dip, 78
Apples, about, 284-285; how to
     core, 35
   apple pie with Cheddar crust, 285
   apple-pear crisp, 287
   banana, apple & peanut salad, 198
   chicken Normandy, 286
   chunky apple & pear sauce, 287

parsnip-apple purée, 88
souffléed omelet with apple
   topping, 144
squash & apple soup, 284
sweet potato & apple bake, 108
warm winter salad, 58
Apricots, dried, about, 288-290
   apricot "poundcake," 289
   apricot danish, 290
   apricot-cornbread stuffing, 272
   apricot-pecan stuffing, 290
   Argentinian beef & fruit kebabs,
     241
   carrot-apricot muffins with pecans,
     65
   chocolate-dipped apricots, 291
   peach pandowdy, 325
   pork rolls stuffed with apricots,
     250
   sweet noodle kugel with apricots,
     135
   warm apricot compote, 291
Apricots, fresh, about, 288-290
   apricot bavarian, 288
   fresh apricots poached in syrup,
     291
   grilled chicken with fresh apricot
     sauce, 288
Artichokes, about, 44-45
   artichokes with lemon-herb
     mayonnaise, 44
   autumn artichoke stew, 44
   pasta shells & artichoke hearts in a
     creamy green sauce, 45
Arugula, about, 102-103
   arugula salad with spicy
     vinaigrette, 102
Ascorbic acid. *See Vitamin C*
Asparagus, about, 46-47; how to
     trim, 34, 47
   angel hair with asparagus & lemon
     cream sauce, 153
   asparagus & chicken stir-fry, 47
   asparagus & red pepper frittata,
     144
   bow-ties with smoked ham
     & asparagus, 253
   creamy asparagus & sweet potato
     bisque, 46
   linguine with roasted asparagus
     & pecans, 46
   stir-fried steak with vegetables, 243
Avocado, about, 292-293
   avocado "sushi" salad, 292
   avocado & ham antipasto with
     guacamole dressing, 292
   California crab roll, 222
   Maryland crab cakes with tomato-
     avocado relish, 223
   mixed greens with creamy avocado
     dressing, 293

romaine salad with avocado
   & oranges, 101

B

Baked beans, molasses, 179
Bananas, about, 294-295
   banana bran muffins, 157
   banana pudding pie, 295
   banana raita, 294
   banana, apple & peanut salad, 198
   banana-chocolate shake, 192
   banana-pecan bread, 294
   orange-banana breakfast
     smoothie, 321
   tropical smoothie, 131
Barley, about, 158-159
   broccoli & barley soup, 54
   old-fashioned mushroom-barley
     soup, 158
   spiced barley & corn, 159
   summery barley-vegetable salad,
     158
Beans, dried or canned, about,
     176-180. *See also Black beans;*
     Chick-peas; Kidney beans; Pinto
     beans
Beans, fresh. *See Snap beans*
Beef, about, 234-243; how to broil
     and carve flank steak, 41;
     how to cut flank steak for
     stir-fries, 41
   Argentinian beef & fruit kebabs,
     241
   barbecued beef sandwich, 241
   beef & tomato pasta sauce, 237
   beef moussaka, 235
   beef Stroganoff, 239
   broiled flank steak with
     chimichurri sauce, 242
   broiled steak with fresh papaya
     chutney, 323
   chunky beef chili, 237
   chunky beet, potato & beef soup,
     48
   deviled hamburger, 241
   double-pepper steak, 238
   fajitas with spicy tomato relish,
     240
   grilled herb-rubbed steak, 239
   Italian beef & broccoli sauté, 56
   Italian beef rolls, 237
   Louisiana beef stew, 234
   pepper steak, 52
   pot roast with carrots & sweet
     potatoes, 234
   quick beef Burgundy, 238
   shepherd's pie, 236
   spaghetti Bolognese, 151
   steak & pasta salad, 242
   steak & potato salad, 240

D

PHOTO CREDITS

Cover photographs by Angelo Caggiano
(pasta recipe), David Murray, Vernon
Morgan, Jules Selmes. All interior recipe
photography by Mark Ferri, with the
following exceptions: Beatriz daCosta:
Pages 83-85, 87 (top & center), 89, 93-97,
99 (top), 141, 149-153, 289, 291 (top &
center), 313. Lisa Koenig: Pages 184-187,
189, 205-230, 231 (top), 252-255, 259-267,
285-287, 293-297, 301, 313, 319, 321, 325-
327, 331, 335-337. Steven Mark
Needham: Pages 67 (center), 71, 73-79.
All how-to and ingredient identification
photographs by Lisa Koenig.

METRIC CONVERSIONS

LENGTH

When you know:	If you multiply by:	You can find:
INCHES	25	MILLIMETERS
INCHES	2.5	CENTIMETERS
FEET	30	CENTIMETERS
YARDS	0.9	METERS
MILES	1.6	KILOMETERS
MILLIMETERS	0.04	INCHES
CENTIMETERS	0.4	INCHES
METERS	3.3	FEET
METERS	1.1	YARDS
KILOMETERS	0.6	MILES

VOLUME

When you know:	If you multiply by:	You can find:
TEASPOONS	4.9	MILLILITERS
TABLESPOONS	14.8	MILLILITERS
FLUID OUNCES	29.6	MILLILITERS
CUPS	0.24	LITERS
PINTS	0.47	LITERS
QUARTS	0.95	LITERS
GALLONS	3.79	LITERS
MILLILITERS	0.03	FLUID OUNCES
LITERS	4.22	CUPS
LITERS	2.11	PINTS
LITERS	1.06	QUARTS
LITERS	0.26	GALLONS

WEIGHT

When you know:	If you multiply by:	You can find:
OUNCES	28.4	GRAMS
POUNDS	0.45	KILOGRAMS
GRAMS	0.035	OUNCES
KILOGRAMS	2.2	POUNDS

TEMPERATURE

When you know:	If you multiply by:	You can find:
DEGREES FAHRENHEIT	0.56 (AFTER SUBTRACTING 32)	DEGREES CELSIUS
DEGREES CELSIUS	1.8 (THEN ADD 32)	DEGREES FAHRENHEIT